T0337846

Domestic Animal Behavior for
Veterinarians and Animal Scientists

Domestic Animal Behavior for Veterinarians and Animal Scientists

Seventh Edition

Katherine A. Houpt

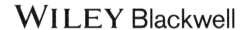

Limit of Liability/Disclaimer of Warranty
While the publisher and author have used their best efforts in preparing this book, they make no representations or warranties with respect to the accuracy or completeness of the contents of this book and specifically disclaim any implied warranties of merchantability or fitness for a particular purpose. No warranty may be created or extended by sales representatives or written sales materials. The advice and strategies contained herein may not be suitable for your situation. You should consult with a professional where appropriate. Neither the publisher nor author shall be liable for any loss of profit or any other commercial damages, including but not limited to special, incidental, consequential, or other damages. Further, readers should be aware that websites listed in this work may have changed or disappeared between when this work was written and when it is read. Neither the publisher nor authors shall be liable for any loss of profit or any other commercial damages, including but not limited to special, incidental, consequential, or other damages.

For general information on our other products and services or for technical support, please contact our Customer Care Department within the United States at (800) 762-2974, outside the United States at (317) 572-3993 or fax (317) 572-4002.

Wiley also publishes its books in a variety of electronic formats. Some content that appears in print may not be available in electronic formats. For more information about Wiley products, visit our web site at www.wiley.com.

Library of Congress Cataloging-in-Publication Data

Names: Houpt, Katherine A., author.
Title: Domestic animal behavior for veterinarians and animal scientists /
   Katherine A. Houpt.
Description: Seventh edition. | Hoboken, New Jersey : Wiley-Blackwell,
   [2024] | Includes bibliographical references and index.
Identifiers: LCCN 2023055133 (print) | LCCN 2023055134 (ebook) | ISBN
   9781119861102 (hardback) | ISBN 9781119861126 (adobe pdf) | ISBN
   9781119861119 (epub)
Subjects: MESH: Animals, Domestic | Behavior, Animal
Classification: LCC SF756.7 (print) | LCC SF756.7 (ebook) | NLM SF 756.7
   | DDC 636.089–dc23/eng/20240126
LC record available at https://lccn.loc.gov/2023055133
LC ebook record available at https://lccn.loc.gov/2023055134

Cover Design: Wiley
Cover Image: © Charles Houpt

Set in 9.5/12.5pt STIXTwoText by Straive, Pondicherry, India

SKY10075283_051624

To all the furry and feathered creatures who have enriched my life.

Contents

Acknowledgment

To Charles Edward Houpt for his help with every aspect of my life and especially with the chickens

About the Companion Website

This book is accompanied by a companion website:

www.wiley.com/go/houpt/7e

Scan this QR code to visit the companion website:

There you will find valuable material designed to enhance your learning, including:

- Videos
- Question and Answers
- Multiple choice questions

1

Communication

Introduction

Communicating with animals, in particular learning to understand the messages the animal is sending, is the most important part of diagnosis. Communication is a vital part of animal husbandry and the art of veterinary medicine and a very useful adjunct to the science of veterinary medicine. Before ordering a complete blood count and liver function tests, the astute clinician already will know that a dog is suffering from abdominal pain because it assumes an abnormal posture with rump high and head low, or that a horse that paces in its stall and kicks at its belly is suffering from colic.

Another important aspect of communication between veterinarian and patient or between handler and stock is assessment of an animal's emotional state or temperament. Adequate restraint or, preferably, a quiet, tractable patient is necessary for thorough examination and diagnosis. Most practitioners learn eventually to recognize animals that will be aggressive or fearful and, therefore, require tranquilization, muzzling, or more stringent methods. It would be helpful for agriculture and veterinary students to learn in advance how to recognize animals' moods. Learning by experience to recognize behavior problems may occur at the expense of a badly bitten hand or kicked leg. For their own safety, as well as for accuracy of diagnosis, clinicians should learn to listen to and watch for the messages their patients are transmitting both to them and to each other. Farmers can prevent injury to themselves and to their stock if they can interpret the animals' messages.

Animals communicate not only by auditory signals, as humans do, but also by visual and olfactory signals. Many olfactory messages cannot be detected by humans, although male odors, such as those contained in the urine of tomcats and the very flesh of boars and billy goats, are quite discernible to humans. Goats and cattle can distinguish conspecifics by means of urine. Male urine is more easily distinguished than is female urine.[138] We are all aware of vocal communication by animals, but many of these calls remain to be decoded. It is the visual signals made by ear, tail, mouth, and general posture that are of most benefit in gauging the temperament and the health of the patient.

Perception

Vision

Acuity

Communication in animals depends on their ability to perceive messages. The sensory abilities of domestic animals, with the exception of dogs and cats, have not been studied systematically. The perception of animals is almost always compared with that of humans. Dogs and cats have a higher critical flicker fusion (point at which a flickering light appears to be fused, or a steady light) than humans, which means that dogs and cats can see television, but in some cases the image may appear jerky to them.[438] Cats respond to television, especially rapidly moving animations (mice, birds, or inanimate objects such as balls), and will spend 6% of their time watching the screen.[634] Cats can discriminate illumination at one-fifth the threshold of humans, but their resolving power is only one-tenth that of humans.[658] Cross-eyed Siamese cats do not have stereoscopic vision; other cats do.[1750] Environmental conditions affect visual acuity. Free-ranging cats have been shown to be hypermetropic, whereas caged cats are myopic.[225] The visual acuity of cattle, measured by using a closed or partially opened circle at various distances from the cow, is inferior to that of humans.[639] Bulls have fairly poor vision; they are able to discriminate a 36 cm solid black disk from a similar disk with a white center, if the center is 1 cm or larger and the bull is within 1.5 m.[1916] This indicates a visual acuity of only 23°, similar to the horse (23°) or the dog (10°).[1588] Cattle have horizontally oriented pupils and, as a result, are better at discriminating vertical than horizontal details.[2946] The visual acuity of sheep is between 11.7 and 14.0 cycles/degree. Chickens can perceive 7 cycles/degree.[2812]

In some studies, pigs have been found to have poorer visual acuity than cattle – a hundredth or a thousandth of a human's. In the Snellen system, humans have 20/20 acuity, whereas horses have 20/30, dogs have 20/85, and cattle and pigs 20/200 acuity.[2521] This means that what a person could see from 200 feet a bull would have to be within 20 feet to see. Cattle can discriminate objects at 2 lux of illumination. Cattle are also poorer in brightness discrimination compared to humans. They have a brightness discrimination threshold of 66 lux in bright light and 4.8 lux in dim light, whereas humans have discrimination thresholds of 105 and 4.2 lux.[1810] Horses can see in dimmer conditions than humans; they can make visual discrimination at a level of light equivalent to the illumination in a dense forest on a moonless night.[899] They can discriminate a difference of 14% in circle size, which is worse performance than humans. They use length rather than area to discriminate size. They pay more attention to local components than to global shapes, in contrast to humans.[2273]

Within-Species Recognition

Sheep can recognize faces of other sheep and differentiate them on the basis of photographs. They can remember at least 25 different sheep faces for more than a year. Goats can discriminate familiar from strange goats, even if their horns are not visible.[1189]

Cattle can discriminate a photo of a cow from that of other ruminant species.[460] They can recognize familiar cattle and learn to recognize unfamiliar ones, but have more difficulty learning to differentiate cattle of different coat patterns, especially all white cattle.[461] When presented with photographs of cow heads, they are more likely to explore and lick the images of familiar cattle than unfamiliar ones, and they never lick a photograph of a pony. Heifers rewarded for choosing images of unfamiliar conspecifics pointed their ears backward more frequently (indicating confrontation with unfamiliar stimuli).[461] In contrast, pigs do not appear able to discriminate between photographs of other pigs.[819]

Horses were more likely to approach photographs of horses displaying facial expressions associated with positive attention and relaxation, and to avoid stimuli displaying an expression associated with aggression. When presented with photographs of conspecifics, both horses and sheep identified emotional signals based on visual cues of changes in facial expressions.[2984,2852]

Chickens recognize breed differences, in that a rooster will attack members of a breed if another chicken of that breed was subordinate to him and avoid a chicken of a breed that was dominant to him.

We do not use one sense alone to identify individuals, and neither do animals. We recognize people by their voice and their appearance. Horses are also able to match the neigh of another horse with its picture.[1865,1866] Dogs can be taught to differentiate dogs of various breeds from other animals.[114]

Cross-Species Recognition

An important question is, "Can an animal tell the difference between different people?" The answer is definitely yes.[2851,2864,3097] Areas that respond to human or dog faces, in particular the temporal cortex in the brain, have been located in dogs, pigs, and sheep.[488,1196] Dogs and cats appear to interpret each other's signals correctly even when the behaviors have opposite meanings in the two species, for example, tail wagging, which signals annoyance in cats and pleasure in dogs.[688]

Pigs can tell people apart, even if olfactory cues are masked, on the basis of visual cues such as height and facial appearance. They can even distinguish humans apart in dim (20 lux) light.[1242] They can recognize familiar people and base their behavior on how that human treated them. Piglets will approach a stationary human even if that human has scared them, but will try to escape if that person or an unfamiliar person approaches them.

Cattle recognize people by their faces or the color of their coveralls, and use height to discriminate between people.[1646,2012] Sheep are able to recognize human faces, but a photograph of a familiar stock person is not as effective as the stock person himself in calming an isolated lamb.[2225]

Dogs associate their owner's voice with their face, and when a strange voice is played while the owner's picture is displayed the dogs gaze longer, indicating that there is a mismatch.

A dog can match a female voice by looking at a woman, but only if the dog lives with more than one person of each sex.[1904] They cannot distinguish the smiling face from a blank face of a stranger of the opposite sex from the owner.[1662] Dogs looked longer at faces when the voice being played at the same time matched the emotion of the face (i.e., angry voice – angry face).[2645] Pupil sizes of dogs were significantly larger when viewing angry faces than happy faces.[2989] D'Aniello et al.[3102] reported that dogs are able to recognize human emotions from body odor because they displayed behaviors indicating stress only when being presented with human odor of fear.

When dogs were trained to lie still in an magnetic resonance imaging (MRI) device and were exposed to various stimuli, the reaction to the majority of happy stimuli led to increased activation of the caudate nucleus associated with reward processing and angry stimuli led to activations in limbic regions.[3075] Oxytocin seems to be involved in attachment of dogs to people.[2889] After receiving oxytocin, dogs fixated less often on the eye regions of angry faces and revisited (glanced back at) more often the eye regions of smiling (happy) faces. Viewing the caregiver activated brain regions associated with emotion and attachment processing in humans. In contrast, the stranger elicited activation mainly in brain regions related to visual and motor processing, and the familiar person relatively weak activations overall.

Whether the pictures were of dogs or humans dogs will look at their owners more often if they are retreating from a stranger. They will look sooner at a stranger, but are slower to approach.[599] Dogs will gaze at photographs of humans and dogs interacting. They gaze longer at humans than at dogs, whereas people gaze more at dogs than at people. Both species gaze more at images in which the two subjects (human or dog) interact. Dogs will whine or whimper more often if their owners gaze at them, but are no more likely to approach or paw at them.[1730] They will approach their owner or even strangers when they cry.[494] When approached by a stranger in a threatening manner, dogs will avoid or threaten, but not if the stranger approaches in a playful manner. The owner is approached in a playful manner even when threatening.[876]

Canine domestication took place tens of thousands of years ago, and over the course of those centuries the two species have evolved a close relationship. Oxytocin is a neurohormone involved in mother and offspring bonding as well as the physiological effects of milk letdown and uterine contraction. When a dog gazes into the eyes of its owner, the human releases oxytocin and is more affiliative to the dog that in turn releases oxytocin. Both dog and owner release oxytocin in a positive feedback loop.[1663] Oxytocin does not always increase affiliative behavior. When owners approached their own dogs in a threatening manner, the dogs reacted more aggressively after oxytocin treatment.[1000]

Whether dogs yawn empathetically when humans yawn is controversial. If someone yawns for five minutes with auditory as well as visual stimuli, dogs will also yawn, but if a person yawns without sound for three minutes the dogs do not yawn.[1156,1729,2817]

Dogs are more attracted to dog-directed speech (essentially, high-pitched baby talk) than to adult-directed speech.[2660,3005]

Cats show more positive behaviors (e.g., ears forward and relaxed body posture) when their owner exhibits a positive (smiling) rather than negative (angry) facial expression, but showed no significant difference when voices exhibited the same emotions.[784] Cats recognize their owner's voice in that they discriminate between strangers' voices and the owner's.[2015]

Horses can learn to recognize human faces and are able to discriminate members of a pair of identical twins. They can transfer recognition from a two-dimensional photograph to a real person.[1041] They can match the appearance and smell of a familiar person with his or her voice.[1299] Horses can match adults' and

children's faces and voices cross-modally.[2809] Horses' heart rates increase when listening to children's voices.[2809] Horses react differently to human faces when they have previously been shown an angry face of that individual. The horse is more likely to gaze at the photo with the left eye (right brain).[2939] See Chapter 9 for more discussion of laterality.

Using "baby talk" or "pet-directed" speech, which is higher pitched and more variable in pitch than adult-directed speech, is more likely to result in a horse's attempt to mutually groom the speaker who is scratching them.[2850] During a pointing task in which the experimenter pointed at the location of a reward with their finger, horses who had been spoken to with pet-directed speech found the reward more often.[2843]

All people do not look the same to sheep, cattle, dogs, horses, or pigs, and probably this is true of most domestic animals. Therefore, the animals can remember who has treated them well or painfully.[1647]

Emotional Perception

In pigs, lower frequency vocalizations are produced more in positive situations; however, within grunts, higher frequencies reflect positive situations. In horses, more snorts and shorter, lower frequency whinnies could be linked to positive situations. In cows, closed-mouth vocalizations (lower in frequency) might be more common in positive emotions. Food calls and fast clucks may be linked to positive emotions in chickens. In goats, the fundamental frequency shows less fluctuations during positive compared to negative situations.[3081]

Animals seem to be able to discriminate emotions of conspecifics and humans.[2700] Dogs looked longer at faces when the voice being played at the same time matched the emotion of the face (i.e., angry voice and angry face, whether the pictures were of dogs or humans).[2645] Cats also have this ability.[2940,3901]

When goats were shown photographs of goats displaying negative emotion (ice had been applied to their udder) they spent more time with their ears forward indicating interests than they did when they saw goats with a positive emotion (being groomed by a human). This may indicate that the observers were more concerned about possible danger than about pleasant things.[2659] Pigs appear to be empathetic in that they exhibited more negative behavior (standing alert with ears back) when accompanying a pig that had been isolated.[2948] Cows can discriminate human emotion based on chemosignals.[2721]

Horses can recognize human emotions on the basis of olfaction as well as vision.[2692] They can also differentiate the sweat of frightened people (who watched a horror movie) from that of the same people after watching a cartoon. The horses raised their head more after sniffing the sweat of frightened people. It is interesting that people can differentiate sweat of a calm versus a stressed horse.

Horses can also recognize intentionality. When presented with a person who gave them food, one who could have given food but did not or tried to give food, but dropped it, the horse looked mostly at the willing person who dropped the food.[3010]

Color Vision

A question often put to a behaviorist is whether animals have color vision. All species of domestic animals have been shown to possess color vision in that they will make discriminations based on color, but color probably is not as relevant to these animals as it is to birds, fish, and primates. For example, teaching cats to discriminate between colors is very difficult, although they learn other visual discriminations with ease and have two types of cones that absorb green and blue. Nevertheless, cats,[1936,2074] dogs,[1682] horses,[866] cattle,[496,822] pigs,[1237,1681] goats,[352] and sheep[1645] can all make discriminations based on color alone. Color vision in domestic animals is not identical to that in humans. In the most carefully conducted studies, dogs appear to see the world not in shades of gray but rather in shades

of violet, blue, and yellow. Their vision is similar to that of color-blind or dichromat humans, who see the green traffic light as pale yellow, the yellow as yellow, and the red as dark yellow. Chickens unlike mammalian domestic animals can see ultraviolet, which probably aids in identification of flowers and other food stuffs.[2938]

Ruminants can discriminate medium and long wavelengths (yellow, orange, and red) better than they can short wavelengths (violet, blue, and green). Cattle can discriminate red from blue and green but have difficulty discriminating green from blue. Animals can not only perceive colors but also be influenced behaviorally by color. For example, calves are more active in red light and less startled by loud noises in green light.[1813] Bulls, indeed, can perceive the matador's red cape.[1938] Horses can discriminate red from blue, but some horses have difficulty distinguishing green or blue green (wavelength 480 nm) from gray.[391,1438,1818,2144] Color may be a more important feature of the equine environment than previously thought because horses do not habituate to objects of different colors and shapes, but do habituate if all the objects are the same color. Apparently, one blue blob is similar enough to another blob that the horse realizes it is not a threat.[423] Some colors – blue, black, white, and yellow – cause more reaction when the horse encounters them on the ground than others – brown, green, red, and gray.[887]

Monocular and Binocular Vision

Eye placement in the skull also affects vision. Horses have eyes set quite laterally and can, therefore, see to the side and far to the rear. They cannot see well right in front of their heads. Lateral vision is necessarily monocular, and horses see binocularly only in the 70° directly in front of the head. They can see objects at 132° to the side.[900] Contrary to many popular and scientific sources, horses do not have a ramped or slanted retina; the retina is similar to that of other animals.[2134] Figure 1.1 illustrates the field of vision of the horse. The

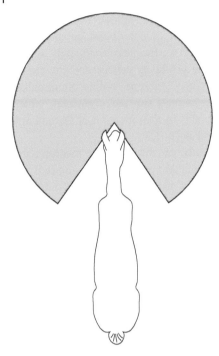

Figure 1.1   Field of vision of the horse.
Source: Courtesy of Charles E. Houpt.

binocular overlap (areas where the horse is viewing objects with both eyes simultaneously) is down the nose and not straight ahead. Chickens also have laterally placed eyes and may be able to see 180° to the side.

The most interesting thing about chicken vision is that they cannot move their eyes so must move their heads to view their environment. The result is the typical jerky movement of a chicken.[2909]

Horses can see clearly with their heads lowered, contrary to popular belief.[176] They do so by adjusting their eyeball to a horizontal position. When the horse lowers its head, the binocular field is directed toward the ground for grazing and the monocular fields are in position to scan the lateral horizon. When the head is raised with the nose pointing forward, the horse uses the binocular field (both eyes) to scan the horizon, and the monocular (single eye) lateral vision becomes limited.[915]

Cattle are capable of depth perception and have a fear of heights that can be demonstrated when they are first exposed to a milking pit.[96]

Audition

Acuity

In hearing, as in vision, cats and dogs appear to perceive more than humans. Humans can hear 8.5 octaves; cats can hear 10. Cats have 40,000 cochlear fibers and humans have 30,000, although the range of hearing in cats is only 1.5 octaves greater than that of humans because higher frequency detection requires a disproportionate increase in cochlear nerve fibers; the number of fibers needed per octave is not constant but, rather, rises with the rise in frequency.[1965] Cats, despite their mobile pinnae, can discriminate between sounds 5° apart, whereas humans can discriminate sounds 0.5° apart. The pinnae significantly lower the auditory threshold in the cat. The absolute upper limit of hearing in cats is 60–65 kHz (kilohertz = kilocycles per second) and 45 kHz in dogs.[965] Dogs and cats can discriminate one-eighth to one-tenth tones.[658,1678] Sheep also appear to perceive higher frequencies than do humans.[53] The auditory acuity of dogs has been used in silent dog whistles and ultrasonic (but not to the dog) distracting devices.[379] Dogs and adult cats are not known to produce ultrasonic calls, but rodents do make ultrasonic noises[47] that the carnivores use to locate them. Chickens can hear from 200 to 8,000 Hz.[2909]

The dog brain has the capacity to detect speech naturalness and distinguish between languages. Longer headed dogs' greater auditory sensitivity to speech naturalness, indicates breed differences in processing human auditory cues.

Practical Application

The importance of hearing to cattle is indicated by the fact that they will avoid the side of a maze where milking facility noises are played.[97] Dogs are quieter when classical music is played but more reactive when heavy metal is played.[2417]

Acuity

Olfaction is to animals what writing is to humans – a message that can be transmitted in the absence of the sender. The sender must be present for auditory or visual signals to be sent, but an odor persists for minutes (or days) after the sender has gone. Olfactory acuity is probably the most important sense of domestic animal species because individual odor recognition and pheromonal release are important parts of their communication. There are breed differences in the number of olfactory receptors: Bloodhounds have 300 million receptors, and Dachshunds 125 million. Dogs can detect aliphatic acids at one-hundredth the concentration detectable by humans;[1638] the lowest concentration of amyl acetate that dogs can detect is two parts per thousand.[2375] They can distinguish between the odors of identical twins[1166] and detect the odors of fingerprints six weeks after the fingerprints were placed on glass.[1226]

In the dogs highly soluble odorants are deposited anteriorly in the sensory region, particularly along the dorsal meatus, while less soluble odorants are deposited more uniformly.[2684] The olfactory epithelium in cats is concentrated on the medial aspect of the olfactory recess, with less olfactory epithelium being distributed peripherally; hence, there is less surface area to detect moderately soluble and insoluble odorants.

Dogs frequently are trained to sniff out drugs and natural gas leaks, and Bloodhounds have been used for centuries to track people; apparently, no modern invention is as reliable as the canine olfactory mucosa. However, when thermally stressed or physically tired, dogs' rate of detecting explosives falls from 91 to 81%.[804] They also have difficulty detecting an explosive in a mixture of odors following training on the pure explosive.[2583]

Boredom, fatigue, lack of appropriate stimuli, no bond with the handler, or handler insensitivity to the signals sent by the dog, in addition to other factors such as health status or age affect ability to identify odorants. There are dietary components which can negatively/decreasing (coconut oil) or positively/increasing olfactory acuity (corn oil, eicosapentaenoic acid (EPA), diphenylamine (DHA), DPA (docosahexaenoic acid), animal-based proteins). Dogs can also be trained to identify areas contaminated with dangerous substances.

In the case of hyposmia in dogs caused by endocrinological disorders such as hyperadrenocorticism, hypothyroidism, or diabetes, a neural mechanism is probably involved. Oral administration of the antibiotic metronidazole degraded the ability of working dogs to detect the odors of explosives. Similarly, the use of steroids (dexamethasone or hydrocortisone) caused a significant elevation in the olfactory detection threshold of dogs, without any observable structural alteration of the olfactory tissue using light microscopy.[659,2831]

Dogs can be trained to match a human scent from one part of the body, for example, the hands, with another part such as the elbows, but it appears to be a difficult concept for them to grasp. This is probably because they can easily discriminate odors from different body parts.[335,2089] The same dog can learn to detect at least 10 different odors.[2458] Dogs can be trained to detect cadavers and live scent. Dogs trained to do both are less accurate – more distracted by cadaver odor when commanded to find a live human scent.[1401] Dogs appear to be able to detect cancer in the exhaled breath of lung and breast cancer patients, but are poor in detection of cancer in urine samples from breast or prostatic cancer patients.[1636]

Pheromones, chemicals secreted by one animal that affect the behavior of another animal of the same species, have been identified in the intermammary area of lactating sows, bitches, mares, and doe goats as well as the cheek glands of cats,[1753] and these may be of value in reducing aggression and fear and encouraging feeding. The use of synthetic versions of these pheromones and that of the feline cheek glands is discussed under the appropriate species.

The vomeronasal organ lies between the hard palate and the nasal cavity in all species except humans. It is a paired tubular organ into which nonvolatile material can be aspirated. Receptor neurons in the lining of the organ detect pheromones and send information more directly to the hypothalamus than neurons in the main olfactory system. In ruminants and horses, flehmen or lip curl accomplishes this by closing the nostril while the animal breathes deeply. Cats gape and dogs tongue, using their tongue to move material into the opening of the incisive ducts that open into the vomeronasal organ. Each neuron expresses only one pheromonal receptor gene. In mice, the vomeronasal organ allows recognition of sex. Individuals are recognized by combinatorial activation of neurons.[958] Domestic animals are not as dependent as rodents on the vomeronasal organ for reproduction, but it still plays a role as will be discussed for each species.

Horses

Vocalizations

Neigh

The neigh (or whinny) is a greeting or separation call that appears to be important in maintaining herd cohesion. It is most often heard when adult horses or a mare and foal are separated.[2484] Stallion neighs contain lower frequencies than those of mares or geldings. Horses appear able to discriminate between familiar and unfamiliar horses on the basis of their neighs alone.[1339]

A separated mare and foal will neigh repeatedly. These neighs appear to be nonspecific distress calls, which the mare, but not the foal, may recognize individually.[2483] The neighs of a mare separated from her foal can be distinguished from those anticipating feeding by analysis of their spectral frequencies.[1837]

Nicker

The nicker, a low-volume call, is a care-giving (epimeletic) or care-soliciting (et-epimeletic) call. It is given by a mare to her foal upon reunion and probably is recognized specifically by each.[2300] A horse may also nicker to its caretaker and a stallion to a mare in estrus.

Snorts, Squeals, and Roars

Nickers or neighs usually elicit a reply; other equine vocalizations, such as snorts, squeals, and roars, do not. The roar is a high-amplitude vocalization of a stallion and is usually directed to a mare. A sharp snort is an alarm call. More prolonged snorting or sneezing snorts appear to be a frustration call given when horses are restrained from galloping or forced to work. Snorts and nickers are sounds from the nostrils. The mouth is closed. Other calls are given with the mouth open.

When two strange horses meet, or when horses have been separated for some time, they greet each other by putting their muzzles together nostril to nostril (Figure 1.2). The nostrils are flared, but if any vocal signals are given, they are inaudible to humans. Usually one, the other, or occasionally both of the horses will squeal and strike or jump back, although neither has been bitten or threatened. The squeal is, therefore, a defensive greeting. It is heard frequently when horses are forming a dominance hierarchy and many bites are being exchanged. Mares that are not in estrus squeal and strike when a stallion approaches too closely. A squeal may also be a response to the sudden onset of pain.

Visual Signals

Expression

The horse's ears are probably the best indicator of its emotions. The alert horse looks directly at the object of interest and holds its ears forward. Ears pointed back indicate aggression, and the flatter the ears are against the head, the more aggressive the horse.[2291] The submissive horse holds its ears to the side (Figure 1.3).

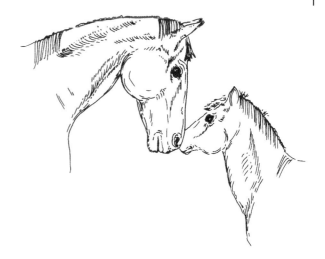

Figure 1.2   Greeting. Nostril-to-nostril investigation, in this case by a horse and pony.

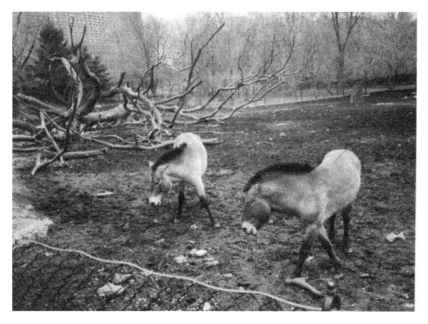

Figure 1.3   The aggressive and submissive postures of horses. The ears of the aggressive horse on the right are back, while those of the submissive horse on the left are pointed sideways.

Other facial expressions of the horse are subtler; nevertheless, they can be used profitably to understand a horse's mood. Facial expression (ears forward and relaxed lips) linked to oxytocin release indicate positive emotion.[2844] A submissive horse turns its ears outward. Young horses (less than three years old) have a more dramatic display, snapping, also called "champing" or "tooth-clapping," in which the lips are retracted, exposing the teeth that are sometimes clicked together (Figure 6.10). This expression is shown by a yearling colt to an approaching stallion or toward an adult that is threatening him. The sexually receptive mare shows a unique expression, the mating face, in which her ears are swiveled back and her lips hang loose (Figure 1.4). She may also exhibit

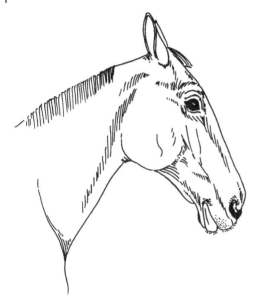

Figure 1.4 The mating expression of the mare. *Source:* Houpt [1042].

snapping. The flehmen response, or curled upper lip, of the courting stallion is discussed further in this chapter. A horse that sees but cannot reach food, or is anticipating food, makes chewing movements and sticks out its tongue (Figure 1.5). This may be a submissive signal, indicating that the horse is ambivalent and reluctant but motivated to approach.

As a horse become less satisfied (a neighbor horse is fed, but he is not) the shape of the eye of the unfed horse changes to more round, and the number of wrinkles in the eyelid increases due to contraction of the inner eyebrow raise.[2790]

More difficult to identify is the horse in pain. It is important for veterinarians and horse owners to recognize when the horse is in pain: the pain grimace in horses is characterized by ears laid stiffly back, orbital tightening, tension above the eye area, prominent strained jaw muscles, strained mouth and nostrils, pronounced chin, and flattening of the profile (Figure 1.6).[499] It may be possible to use machine recognition for this purpose because otherwise humans need extensive training.[3050] Before a horse is in such pain with colic that it kicks at its belly, it will repeatedly swivel its ears back as if attending to its abdomen. In addition to the facial expressions shown in Figure 1.6, there are changes in posture, limb position, and vocalizations that indicate pain in horse as illustrated in Torcivia and McDonnell.[3098]

The various facial and postural expressions of horses have been illustrated by McDonnell.[1505] A very detailed description of equine facial expression has been made.[2393] Horses tend to position their ears in the same direction in

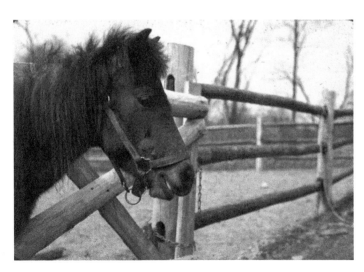

Figure 1.5 The food-anticipating expression of the horse.

Stiffly backwards ears		

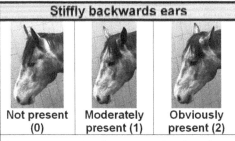

Not present (0)	Moderately present (1)	Obviously present (2)

The ears are held stiffly and turned backwards. As a result, the space between the ears may appear wider relative to baseline.

Orbital tightening		

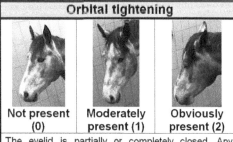

Not present (0)	Moderately present (1)	Obviously present (2)

The eyelid is partially or completely closed. Any eyelid closure that reduces the eye size by more than half should be coded as "obviously present" or "2".

Tension above the eye area		

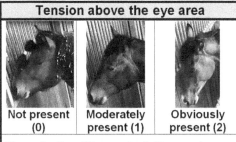

Not present (0)	Moderately present (1)	Obviously present (2)

The contraction of the muscles in the area above the eye causes the increased visibility of the underlying bone surfaces. If temporal crest bone is clearly visible should be coded as "obviously present" or "2".

Prominent strained chewing muscles		

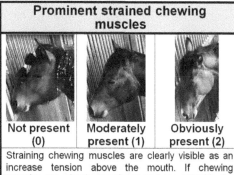
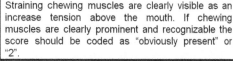

Not present (0)	Moderately present (1)	Obviously present (2)

Straining chewing muscles are clearly visible as an increase tension above the mouth. If chewing muscles are clearly prominent and recognizable the score should be coded as "obviously present" or "2".

Mouth strained and pronounced chin		

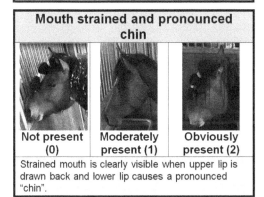

Not present (0)	Moderately present (1)	Obviously present (2)

Strained mouth is clearly visible when upper lip is drawn back and lower lip causes a pronounced "chin".

Strained nostrils and flattening of the profile		

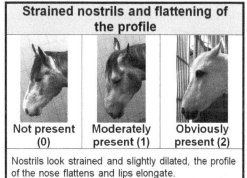

Not present (0)	Moderately present (1)	Obviously present (2)

Nostrils look strained and slightly dilated, the profile of the nose flattens and lips elongate.

Figure 1.6 The horse grimace scale. *Source:* Dalla Costa et. al. 2014 / PLOS / CC BY 4.0.

which they are looking. Thus, when the horse's ears are pointed straight ahead, it is looking straight ahead. This can be a clue that the horse is about to shy at an object. Usually, the rider can identify the frightening object by looking where the horse's ears are pointing. The horse can then be coaxed to investigate and conquer its fear of the object. When the horse turns its ears to the side and back, it is looking to the side. There are signs of conflict in horses, in this case conflict between what the rider wants and what the horse wants. Jumping horses will pull the reins from the rider's hands, and dressage horses lash their tails.

Horses are aware of other horses' facial expressions, so they will approach a feed bucket toward which a photographic image of a horse is looking or pointing its ears toward the bucket.[2392]

Posture

The posture and bodily actions of the horse are also useful in interpreting its moods. The relaxed horse stands quietly, whereas its nervous counterpart prances and chafes at the least restraint. The aggressive horse, when threatening to kick, lashes its tail and may even lift one of its hind legs. The frightened horse tucks its tail tightly against its rump and stands with its feet close together. Muscle guarding is seen, especially if the animal anticipates pain. A few mares will urinate and lash their tails, splattering urine, as they are being chased, and it should not be confused with the frequent urination with deviated tail seen in estrous mares. The stallion moving his mares assumes a unique posture, called "herding," "driving," or "snaking," with head down, nearly touching the ground, and ears flattened (Figure 1.7).

Horses paw the ground not in aggression but rather in frustration when they are eager to gallop or, more commonly, when they want to graze and are restrained by rope or reins. Pawing to eat may be a behavior derived from pawing through snow for grass and might be considered a form of displacement behavior. Tail lashing and pawing can be signs of discomfort.[1183]

When being groomed gently a horse exhibits "pleasure expression" with eyes half-closed, lip(s) extended forward and twitching, or immobile.[2842]

Tactile Sense

Horses can detect a fly on their skin and respond by either moving their skin or swishing their tails. Riders make use of the horse's ability to perceive a slight pressure on his flank in order to signal dressage movements. Very light pressure on the skin is used to calm a horse.[2238] Another use of the horse's tactile sense (or, more likely, pain receptors) is the twitch. When the horse's upper lip is twisted with a chain or rope, endorphins are released and analgesia is produced.[1296]

Olfactory Signals

Scent Marking

Olfactory communication plays an important part in the sexual behavior of horses. Stallions curl their upper lip in the flehmen or "horse laugh" position when they smell the urine of a mare (Figure 1.8). Estrous urine alone does not stimulate more episodes of flehmen by stallions than does non-estrous urine, but the frequency of flehmen by a stallion toward a particular mare in his herd increases as she approaches estrus, perhaps because the mare urinates more frequently.[1461,2167] After the stallion investigates urine by putting his lips in it, his lips are raised in the flehmen

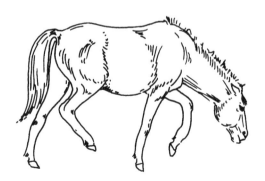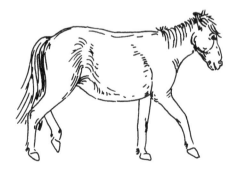

Figure 1.7   Driving posture of the horse. The stallion, left, drives a mare. This behavior is also called "snaking," "herding," or "driving" (rounding).

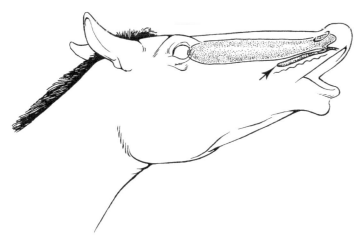

Figure 1.8   The flehmen response, or lip curl. The location of the vomeronasal organ is indicated by the arrow.

position, the nostril opening is partially blocked, and the horse, by breathing deeply, aspirates the urine into the vomeronasal organ. Although stallions flehmen most frequently, geldings and mares also exhibit the behavior in response to olfactory or gustatory stimuli. Cough medicine or a new bit often causes the horse laugh, or flehmen – but it is obviously not a sign of amusement. Stallions usually urinate on the urine (scent mark) as they are exhibiting flehmen.

Horses can distinguish the skin odors of one horse from another.[1798] Although they can distinguish their own feces from that of other horses, they do not distinguish those of familiar from unfamiliar horses. They sniff most at feces from horses that are aggressive to them.[1272] Mares can discriminate the urine of different individuals.[1041]

Wild stallions use manure piles, or stud piles, along well-used pathways, possibly to scent mark.[677] These piles may separate bands of horses both spatially and temporally. Even in a pasture, stallions and some geldings select one place to defecate and then back into the pile to eliminate, so the pile does not grow much wider. On the other hand, mares and most geldings face outward, gradually increasing the diameter of the pile. Because horses do not eat grass contaminated with feces, a pasture containing mares and geldings rapidly becomes "horsed

out" or inedible.[1721] Despite the discrimination of older horses against feces, foals show coprophagia, as discussed in more detail in Chapter 6, "Development of Behavior." Horses respond to predator odor by increased sniffing, but only seem frightened (refuse to eat and increase heart rate) when the odor is combined with the sound of a plastic bag being dragged over the ground.[418] Horses have individual sensitivities. Some are more reactive to odors, others to tactile or auditory stimuli, but there is no general sensory sensitivity. A horse that responds strongly to a sound is not necessarily going to respond strongly to a spicy taste.[1308]

Artificial Pheromones

The equine appeasing pheromone, from the intramammary sulcus of the lactating mare, can reduce the signs of fear and the elevation of heart rate in response to a novel stimulus – a bridge.[664]

Donkeys

The visual signals of donkeys are similar to those of horses, but their long ears make it easier to determine aggression in this species than in horses. Donkey vocalizations consist of the bray, grunt, growl, and whuffle.[2711] The signs of pain in donkeys are shown in Figure 1.9.

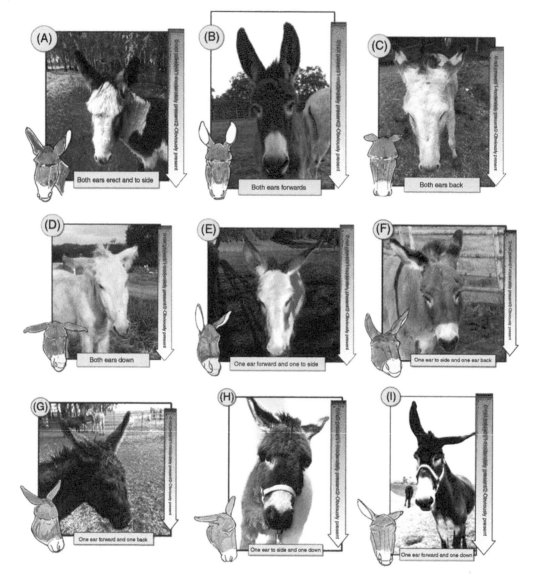

Figure 1.9 An ethogram describing ear position related to grimace scale (0: not present, 1: moderately present, and 2: obviously present). Ear positions that maybe associated with pain or discomfort include both ears back (C), down (D), one ear forward and one to the side (E), one ear to the side and one back (F), one ear to the side and one down (H), and one forward and one down (I) along with other facial action units associated with pain. Ear positions that are less likely to be associated with pain would include both ears are erect to side (A), both ears are forward (B), one ear forward and one to the side (E), and possibly one ear forward and one ear back (G).

Dogs

Vocalizations

The common vocal communications of dogs are the bark, whine, howl, and growl.

Bark

Barking is a territorial call of dogs. It is used to defend a territory and to demarcate its boundaries. Stray dogs, whose resting places may be quite temporary, rarely bark.[213] As a stray dog passes the yards of owned dogs, however, it precipitates territorial barking. Barks recorded in aggressive situations were characterized by lower fundamental frequency and reduced harmonic content with a shorter inter-bark interval. Affiliative vocalizations had a higher fundamental frequency and included more harmonics.[2934] The observant owner can recognize various types of barks. The bark to be let in the house differs from that directed at human intruders, which may differ from that directed at canine intruders.[10] People obtain dogs because they bark and can serve to warn their owners of the approach of intruders. Unfortunately, dogs are much more likely to bark in response to another dog's bark than to the sound of a human intruder.[11,12] The barking trait can become a problem in a highly urbanized environment. Two thousand two hundred complaints about barking are filed in Los Angeles per year.[2082] For this reason, a dog's barking can be a problem for the owner. A more acute problem is the barking of kenneled or caged dogs in a veterinary clinic. The noise level generated by barking can exceed the 90-decibel limit of the Occupational Safety and Health Act (OSHA).[15] Animal hospitals must, therefore, be constructed with very good sound insulation.

Whine and Howl

Whining is an et-epimeletic or care-soliciting call of the dog. It is first used by puppies to communicate with the mother, who provides warmth and nourishment. Mature dogs whine when they want relief from pain or are in even a mildly frustrating situation, such as when they want to escape outdoors or reach a rabbit for which they are digging.

Howling is a canine call that has not been deciphered well. It occurs more frequently in some breeds of dogs, such as Huskies, Malamutes, and to a lesser extent hounds, often in response to auditory stimuli or when isolated.

Growl

Growling is an aggressive or distance increasing call in dogs, but there are distinctions between play growls and growls directed at a threatening stranger. Play growls have a higher fundamental frequency and a pulsing rhythm.[665]

Acoustic signals are more important than visual signals, and dogs react by either retreating, approaching, or not responding to the sound. Dogs that retreat have higher levels of salivary cortisol.[2487] Dogs look at a picture of a normal-sized dog when they hear an aggressive growl, but at the picture of a larger than normal dog if they are hearing a play growl.[158]

Visual Signals

A dog's emotional state can be determined by observation of its ears, mouth, facial expression, tail, hair on its shoulders and rump, and overall body position and posture (Figure 1.10). The calm dog stands with ears and tail hanging down. When it becomes alert, its tail and ears are pointed upward. The dog may point with one front leg; this can be a sign of anxiety. As the dog becomes more aggressive, the hair on the shoulders (hackles) and the rump rises and the lips are drawn back. The ears remain forward, and the tail may be slowly wagged. With increasing aggression, the lips are retracted and the teeth exposed in a snarl. The dog stands straight. As the dog becomes frightened, the ears go back until they are flattened against the head and the tail descends until it is between the legs. Dogs are more apt to exhibit displacement or appeasement behaviors after a familiar person (rather than an unfamiliar one) pets their head or holds their paw. Because dogs communicate more openly with familiar than unfamiliar people, the unfamiliar person may be unaware of the dog's distress and therefore more likely to be bitten.[1282]

Dogs shed tears when reuniting with their owner after a five-hour separation which is the first example of weeping in an animal.[2895]

Posture

The posture of the fear-biting dog, the one most likely to injure a veterinarian, is that of a frightened dog with tail and ears down and the

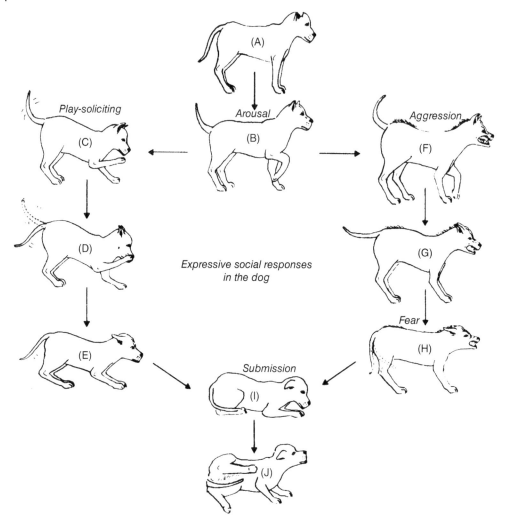

Figure 1.10 Body postures of the dog. (A, B) Neutral to alert attentive positions; (C) play bow; (D, E) active and passive submissive greetings – note tail wag and shift in ear position and in distribution of weight on fore and hind limbs; (F–H) gradual shift from aggressive display to ambivalent fear-defensive aggressive posture; (I) passive submission; and (J) rolling over and presentation of inguinal-genital region.[724]

body leaning away from the source of fear. It will have raised hackles and lips retracted in a snarl, which may expose the molars as well as the canines. Care must be taken when approaching a dog to notice any lifting of the lip, because this may be the only prediction of defensive aggression or fear biting. The fear biter will escape if possible; but if it is approached within its critical distance, which may be a yard (approximately a meter or less) from it, it will attack.

More common, fortunately, is a dog in which fear is not mixed with aggression. The fearful dog crouches with its tail between its legs and its ears flattened down. If the dog is abjectly submissive, it will lie on its side and lift its hind leg, displaying the inguinal area. It may also make licking intention movements, that is, sticking its tongue out but not contacting anything. Finally, it may urinate. This behavior probably represents a reversion to puppy habits in which the puppy lies down on its side, presents the inguinal area to the mother (who is, of course, dominant over the puppy), and allows her to lick and clean it.

General posture is also a good indication of the dog's mood. A lowered body posture with depressed tail is associated with fear and fear-based aggression, and a tall (especially rigid) posture with stiff, raised tail is associated with offensive aggression.[948] See Chapter 9, in which the laterality of tail wagging is discussed.

During a submissive approach, dogs curve their bodies, wiggling toward the superior, whereas a dominant dog stands straight and walks stiffly with tail and ears erect. This stiffening of posture can be used to predict when an initially friendly greeting is about to become an attack. There is considerable debate about whether dogs display guilt when they have transgressed. There is neither a difference in the behavior of guilty versus innocent dogs nor in the owner's estimation of the dog's guilt.[963,1742]

Dogs greet their owners as they did their mothers: by licking their faces. As puppies, dogs lick their mothers' faces to beg for regurgitated feed. Although wild canids frequently regurgitate food for their pups, not all domestic dogs do so; nevertheless, the begging behavior is shown by domestic puppies. The behavior persists in the adult dog that either licks the owner or, if prevented by discipline or its small stature, makes licking intention movements. Licking their own lips, yawning, and even falling asleep sitting up are all signs of ambivalence in dogs. A few dogs will "grin" as a submissive greeting. They show their teeth with flattened ears.

Dogs have a play signal; it is necessary to signal that the action that follows is play because, otherwise, the recipient of the playful act will consider it genuine aggression or sexual activity and respond in kind. A bowing with the forequarters lowered and the hindquarters elevated and topped by a rapidly wagging tail is the signal for canine play.[223] Often, one paw is waved or rubbed at the dog's own muzzle. Interspecific communication is important,

too.[3094] People use various motions and vocalizations to signal that they want to play with a dog. The most successful are lunging or bowing toward the dog while whispering or speaking in a high-pitched voice.[1960]

Figure 1.11 indicates the facial expressions of a dog.

Olfactory Signals

The legendary olfactory acuity of dogs has already been mentioned. Because dogs can smell so well, it is not surprising that dogs use odors as a means of communication.

There are applied uses of canine olfactory abilities too. Although olfactory repellents are seldom effective in dogs, odors can have a positive effect. Lavender oil reduces canine vocalization and locomotion during car travel.[2416] A chemical has been synthesized from the epithelial cells of the bitch's mammary sulcus and is available commercially as Adaptil®. It has been used for a variety of behavior problems, but the studies of its efficacy were not well controlled.[736]

Urine
Male dogs and the occasional female dog raise a hind limb to urinate. The importance of olfactory communication to dogs is exemplified by the diligence with which male dogs scent mark vertical objects by urinating. Dogs are believed to be capable of identifying species, sex, and even individuals from the odor of the urine. Dogs scent mark much more frequently in areas where other dogs have marked. The record may be 80 markings by one dog in 40 hours.[2162] Even though male dogs rarely empty their bladders completely, such efforts exhausted this dog's supply; the last urinations were dry. Older dogs urine marked more than adult dogs that urine marked more than juvenile dogs. The height of a urine mark may have significance because small adult male dogs may place urine marks higher, relative to their own body size, than larger adult male dogs.[3066] Castration reduces the raised limb (scent marking) position.[3085]

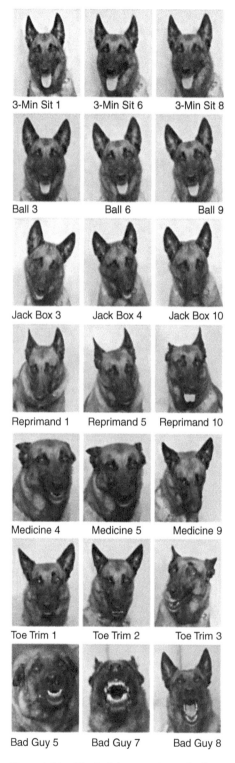

3-Min Sit 1   3-Min Sit 6   3-Min Sit 8

Ball 3   Ball 6   Ball 9

Jack Box 3   Jack Box 4   Jack Box 10

Reprimand 1   Reprimand 5   Reprimand 10

Medicine 4   Medicine 5   Medicine 9

Toe Trim 1   Toe Trim 2   Toe Trim 3

Bad Guy 5   Bad Guy 7   Bad Guy 8

Figure 1.11   The facial expressions of a dog. *Source:* Bloom and Friedman (2013).[2661]

The most powerful means of olfactory communication in the canine species is the urine of an estrous bitch. Male dogs are more strongly attracted to the urine of an estrous bitch than to vaginal or anal sac secretions.[568] Dogs "tongue," that is, flick their tongues against the palate just behind their incisor teeth, introducing estrous urine into the vomeronasal organ. This is the canine equivalent of flehmen.

There is a marked preference by an estrous bitch for male urine as compared with either estrous or non-estrous urine.[588] The urine contains pheromones. In estrous urine, these compounds are probably estrogen metabolites. The urine of a bitch in heat can attract males from great distances. The attractant effect of the bitch's pheromone is usually considered a nuisance, but it has practical applications. For instance, the pheromone could be used to attract stray dogs that could then be easily captured. One might expect that male dogs would inevitably be attracted to the urine of a receptive female, but a dog without mating experience does not investigate estrous urine in preference to anestrous urine, whereas sexually experienced dogs do.[195]

Elimination Postures

Although standing and lifting the hind leg are typical innate male behaviors mediated by testosterone, males urinate in other positions 3% of the time.[236] Bitches assume not only the squatting position (68% of the occasions that they urinate), but also lift their hind legs (2%) and use various combinations of the two postures.

Urine marking is the most common form of scent marking in dogs, but vertical objects may also be marked with feces; this behavior is termed "middening." Again, males are more likely than females to mark with feces.[2162] Castration reduces scent marking in male dogs.[923] Dogs that cannot smell (anosmic) and that, therefore, cannot identify other dogs' urine mark less frequently and, in contrast to intact dogs, do not urinate on the urine of other dogs. When dogs scratch after eliminating, they are not making rudimentary burying movements but are spreading the scent and possibly adding the odor of secretions from interdigital sebaceous glands. Intact male dogs mark more during the breeding season; lactating bitches mark around their nest area.[1756]

Anal and Aural Secretions

Urine is not the only olfactory means by which dogs communicate. The anal gland secretions normally are eliminated with the feces and, no doubt, give them a unique odor.[568] Dogs, on meeting, usually sniff under each other's tails. This behavior is probably one of identifying the individual by its smell. A very frightened dog can express its anal sacs forcefully; the resulting odor is pungent enough to be smelled by humans and may function as a fear pheromone.[561] The secretions of the ears are also believed to function in individual identification,[730] and investigation of one another's ears is a common greeting behavior of dogs.

Submissive Urination

Submissive urination is a frequent behavioral problem. It occurs more often in young dogs and small dogs. Punishing the dog for urinating in fear or excitement aggravates the problem. The dog is already afraid, and punishment only confirms and reinforces that fear. The wisest course is to avoid overexciting the dog. Submissive urination often declines as the dog matures.

Cats

Vocalizations and Audition

Many more feline vocalizations exist than those described in Table 1.1; some of these vocalizations may not be recognized by every owner.[317] The wild ancestor of cats, *Felis silvestris lybica*, is less vocal and meows in fewer contexts; its call is longer and lower in frequency and deemed less pleasant by humans.[1688] Apparently, we have selected cats to communicate with us in "pleasant" voices. Humans can distinguish positive and negative affect in feline vocalizations.[1689] Purring can be a pleasure vocalization or, when a higher frequency is incorporated, a food-soliciting call.[1497] Agonistic calls are longer in duration and lower in frequency than affiliative calls. Other positive vocalization are the trill and the squeak.[2737] Feline vocalizations can be recognized automatically.[2912]

Cats orient to the sound of their own names from other words and discriminate their own names from the names of other cats in the household.[3103] Cats can discriminate speech specifically addressed to them from speech addressed to adult humans, when sentences are uttered by their owners.[2710] Females and kittens have higher fundamental frequencies characteristics and solid-colored coated cats presented higher fundamental frequency than other coat colors.[3104] Because cats can hear ultrasound, it has been used to deter cats from entering an area, and, although the technique is only moderately effective, the efficacy increases with time.[1684]

Visual Signals

Posture

The postures and facial expressions of the cat are shown in Figure 1.12A and 1.12B. A cat carries its tail high when greeting, investigating, or frustrated. The tail is depressed and the tip wags during stalking. When walking or trotting, the tail is held out at a 40° angle to the back, but as the cat's pace increases, the tail is held lower.[1213] A relaxed cat, as does a relaxed dog, usually stands with tail hanging, but the cat's ears are usually forward. When the cat's attention is attracted, the tail is raised and both ears are pointed forward and held erect. The aggressive cat walks on tiptoe with head down. Because the cat's hind legs are longer than its front legs, it appears to be slanting downward from rump to head. Its tail is held down but arched away from the hocks; it is partially piloerected. Its ears are held erect and swiveled, so

Table 1.1   The vocalizations of cats.

Murmur	A soft, rhythmically pulsed vocalization given on exhalation. Murmurs are the request, or greeting call, which can vary from a coax to a command; and the acknowledgment, or confirmation call, which is a short, single murmur with a rapidly falling intonation.
Chirp	A vocalization given by a queen to her own kittens when approaching the nest or nursing.
Purr	A soft, buzzing vocalization that is easy to recognize. It occurs only in social situations and may indicate submission or a kitten-like state. Remmers and Gautier[1596] have shown that purring is associated with rapid contraction of the muscles of the larynx. The laryngeal muscles are driven by a central pattern generator with a cycle of contraction every 30–40 ms.[640]
Growl	A harsh, low-pitched vocalization,[309] usually of long duration and given in agonistic encounters.
Squeak	A high-pitched, raspy cry given in play, in anticipation of feeding, and by the female after copulation.
Shriek	A loud, harsh, high-pitched vocalization given in intensely aggressive situations or during painful procedures.
Hiss	An agonistic vocalization produced while the mouth is open and teeth are exposed. This vocalization is probably defensive and can be used to gauge whether a cat is defensively or offensively aggressing.
Spit	A short, explosive sound given before or after a hiss in agonistic situations. Saliva is expelled.
Chatter	A teeth-chattering sound made by some cats while hunting or, more commonly, when restrained from hunting by confinement.
Estrus call	A call of variable pitch, lasting a half-second to one second. The mouth is opened and then gradually closed. It is given repeatedly by queens in estrus, which is termed "calling" because the vocalization is so characteristic.
Howl and yowl of an aggressive cat	These are loud, harsh calls.
Mowl, or caterwaul, of the male cat	A variable-pitch call, usually given in a sexual context.
Mew	A high-pitched, medium-amplitude vocalization. Phonetically it sounds like a long "e." It occurs in mother–kitten interactions and in the same situations as the squeak.
Moan	This is a call of low frequency and long duration. The sound is "o" or "u." It is given before regurgitating a hair ball or in epimeletic situations, such as begging to be released to hunt.
Meow	This characteristic feline call, "ee-ah-oo," is given in a variety of greeting or epimeletic situations just as the mew and squeak are. Anyone who has tried to restrict a cat's food will not be surprised to know that cats can be trained to meow twice a minute for two hours when the reward is food.[647]

the openings point to the rear. Its whiskers are rotated forward, and its claws are protruded. Subordinate cats crouch in the presence of a dominant cat.

The frightened cat crouches with ears flattened to its head, and it salivates and spits.

The pupils of the aggressive cat are constricted; as the animal becomes more defensive, the pupils dilate. The light-colored iris of the cat's eye makes an especially prominent signal of the cat's mood; it is probably an important intraspecific signal and should be used also to

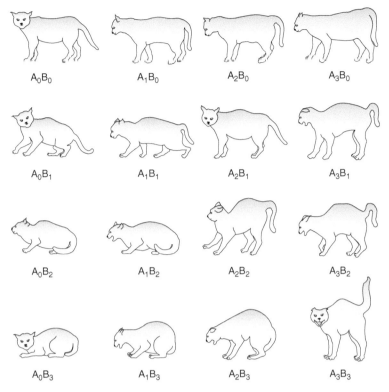

Figure 1.12A Body postures of the cat. Aggressiveness is increasing from A_0 to A_3, fearfulness from B_0 to B_3. A_3B_0 is the most aggressive cat, A_0B_3 the most fearful, and A_3B_3 the defensively aggressive cat[1360] from Overall[1745] with permission Elsevier.

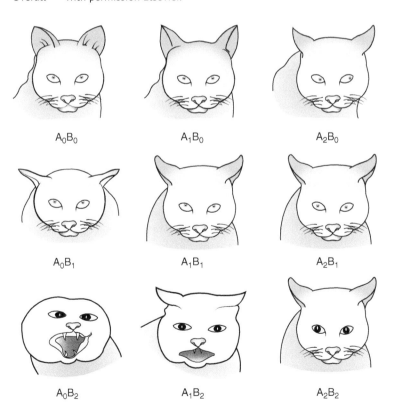

Figure 1.12B Facial expressions of the cat. A_2B_0 is offensively aggressive; A_0B_2 is defensively aggressive from Overall [1745] with permission Elsevier.

(A)   (B)

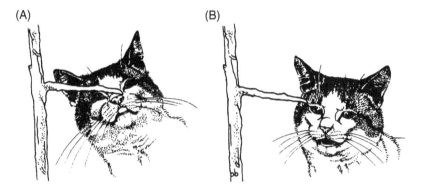

Figure 1.13 The gape expression of a cat. (A) The cat touches the investigated object with its nose and may lick its nose; then (B) it opens its mouth while gazing in a preoccupied fashion. *Source:* Courtesy of Priscilla Barrett, Cambridge, UK.

advantage by the veterinarian. The eyes of an excited cat appear red because the retinal vessels can be seen through the dilated pupils. Contrary to popular belief, the "Halloween cat" is not the most aggressive one; this cat, with arched back, erect tail, and ears flattened, which is piloerected and hissing, corresponds to the fear-biting dog. The cat is fearful but will become aggressive if its critical distance is invaded. One clue to the cat's emotions is that the hind feet appear to be advancing while the front feet retreat; the paws are gathered close together under the cat. A grimace scale has been developed for cats (Figure 1.13).[2730]

In general, tail up is directed to higher ranking cats and may precede rubbing.[368] There are many tail positions and actions: (a) tail extended straight, but end curled over; (b) tail extended, and the tip moves forward or backward, or to one side; (c) tail held upright, and entire tail "vibrates" from the base to the tip; (d) when the cat is lying down or sitting, tail moves from side to side; (e) rhythmic movement of tail backward and forward; (f) tail erect and points straight up, skyward; and (g) in any position, the tail becomes tightly wrapped around the body or the handler. Positions (b) through (d) are negative reactions.[635]

Cats roll on their backs, but sex differences appear in this behavior. Most female rolling occurs during estrus and is directed toward males, whereas most rolling exhibited by

young males is toward adult males and is presumably a sign of submission.[679]

The gape is a response to a strange smell. This expression is most commonly seen when the cat smells a strange cat's urine, and it is the feline equivalent of the flehmen response of the ungulates. The mouth is opened, and the tongue is flicked behind the upper incisors where an opening in the hard palate communicates with the vomeronasal organ (Figure 1.13). At the same time, an autonomic response to the odor occurs whereby the urine brought to the hard palate is aspirated into the vomeronasal organ during parasympathetic stimulation. Fluid is flushed from the vomeronasal organ during sympathetic stimulation.[616]

Olfactory Signals

The olfactory epithelium in cats is concentrated on the medial aspect of the olfactory recess, with less olfactory epithelium being distributed peripherally; hence, there is less surface area to detect moderately soluble and insoluble odorants.[2684]

Scent Marking

Male cats scent mark – that is, spray urine – more than females, but both sexes do it. They spray trees along their most frequently traveled path. Spraying is also done by cats that are subjects of aggression.[1671] Free-ranging tomcats spray a dozen times per hour.[2298] Queens spray once an hour and are more likely to spray when they are in heat. Cats probably also use scent marking to arrange their activity temporally with other cats. Much of the signal value of urine is lost within 24 hours, as evidenced by a comparison of interest in fresh and older urine marks by male cats.[520] Cats can apparently distinguish the urine of familiar cats from that of strange cats.[1669] The smell of male cat urine is quite detectable by humans and usually objectionable to them. The smell of tomcat urine is probably caused by the sulfur-containing amino acid, felinine, which is present in highest quantity in tomcat urine and may be an important olfactory component in territorial spraying.[994] Cats are less stressed when their owner is present, but olfactory cues of the owner are not sufficient.[3051]

Anal Secretions

Cats are well known for their fastidious covering of their feces, but in some situations, such as outside their core living area, cats may leave their feces uncovered. This may be a form of middening, marking with feces. Cats probably use fecal and anal sac odor for communication; two strange cats spend considerable time circling one another, attempting to sniff in the perianal area. If the cats are not too antagonistic, they will eventually permit each other to sniff.

Rubbing

Cheek rubbing (bunting) behavior may also be a form of olfactory communication in that glandular secretion from the cat's face is deposited on the object bunted. Cats bunt the objects to which they respond with a gape. Urine up to three days old can elicit these responses.[2348]

Cats also rub each other. In general, the subordinate cat rubs the dominant one. This behavior serves to exchange odors among all the cats in a group, that is, they all smell the same. Cats scratch vertical surfaces or, less often, horizontal surfaces for 10 seconds three times a day which can be a problem if furniture is scratched.[3101]

Communication with Humans

Cats seem to have a come-hither communication – a slow blink which indicates communicate a positive emotion. Slow blink sequences typically involve a series of half-blinks followed by either a prolonged eye narrow or an eye closure. If the owner mimics that expression the cat is more likely to approach.[3071]

It can be difficult to recognize pain in cats but lowering the ears, tightening the muzzle, tightening the orbital muscles, pushing the whiskers forward, and lowering the head appear to be signs.[2759] The facial expression of a cat in pain is seen in Figure 1.14.

Pigs

Vocalizations

Vocal signals are probably the most important means of communication in pigs. Twenty calls have been identified, and half a dozen are easily recognizable to humans.[881] Porcine vocalizations can be classified according to the emotional valence positive calls, whether they are low frequency (LF) or high frequency (HF), are shorter and contain less amplitude modulations than negative calls.[2674]

Grunt, Bark, and Squeal

The common grunt is 0.25–0.4 seconds long and is given in response to familiar sounds or while a pig is rooting. The staccato grunt or short grunt is, as the name implies, shorter (0.1–0.2 seconds); it is given by an excited or investigating pig and may precede a squeal. A crescendo of staccato grunts is given, for example, by a threatening sow and may precede an attack on anyone who disturbs her litter. In a milder form, it can be a greeting. The bark is given by a startled pig. Pigs respond to an adult sow's bark by freezing or fleeing, but not to juvenile pig barks.[407] The long grunt (0.4–1.2 seconds) may be a contact call and is associated with pleasurable stimuli, especially tactile ones.[1456] The squeal is a more intense vocalization indicating arousal, and a pig that is hurt will scream.

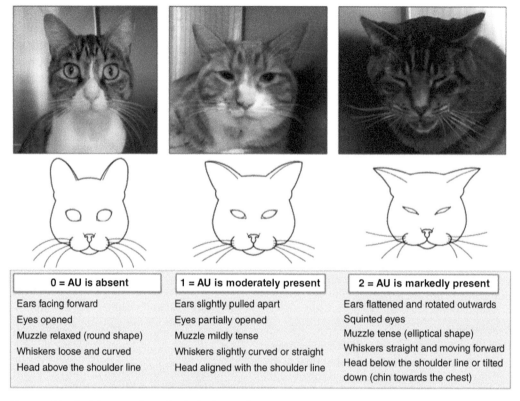

0 = AU is absent	1 = AU is moderately present	2 = AU is markedly present
Ears facing forward	Ears slightly pulled apart	Ears flattened and rotated outwards
Eyes opened	Eyes partially opened	Squinted eyes
Muzzle relaxed (round shape)	Muzzle mildly tense	Muzzle tense (elliptical shape)
Whiskers loose and curved	Whiskers slightly curved or straight	Whiskers straight and moving forward
Head above the shoulder line	Head aligned with the shoulder line	Head below the shoulder line or tilted down (chin towards the chest)

Figure 1.14 Facial expressions of pain in the cat. Evangelista et al., 2020 / PeerJ / CC BY 4.0.

The various grunts and combinations do not appear to have specific meanings, but the intensity of the vocalization varies with the intensity of the situation. A common sequence is to proceed from common grunts to staccato grunts to repeated grunts without interruption to grunt squeals to screams as the animal is approached, chased, picked up, and injected. Staccato greeting grunts are given by pigs that are reunited after a separation, and a series of 20 grunts with no pause may be given by the hungry pig. Nursing calls are described in Chapter 5, "Maternal Behavior." Changes in the frequency and length of calls can indicate need. When separated from the sow, hungrier piglets call more frequently and at a higher frequency than do satiated ones.[2396] Sows can discriminate the calls of their own piglets from those of others. When reunited with the sow, piglets emit a contact call.[2396]

Isolation in a strange place causes pigs to vocalize. Short grunts are followed by screams. At the same time, the rate of defecation increases.[745] They do not react behaviorally or physiologically to recordings of distress calls of unfamiliar pigs.[597] When anticipating an aversive event (e.g., climbing a ramp), pigs will emit a high-pitched vocalization.[1108] Mature pigs often react to restraint by tantrum behavior accompanied by very loud calls, but with no increase in heart rate.[1458] When disciplining a subordinate pig, a dominant pig will give a sharp bark as it feints with its snout. The pig in chronic pain grinds its teeth.

Posture

Possibly because the vocabulary of swine is so large, visual signals do not appear to be as important. One can learn something about pig thermoregulatory problems, if not about their moods, by observing their posture. Newborn pigs are relatively deficient in fur or fatty insulation, and their surface-to-volume ratio is large; therefore, maintaining body temperature is difficult. Pigs have compensated for their poor physiological abilities with several behavioral strategies to reduce heat loss. A warm piglet lies sprawled out, but a cold one crouches with its legs folded against the body. The surface area is thus reduced, and contact with a cold floor is minimized.

The facial expression of a pig in pain is seen in Figure 1.15.

Tail Position

The tail, particularly in piglets, is a good index of general well-being in most breeds. Although Vietnamese mini-pigs do not curl their tails, a tightly curled tail indicates a healthy pig in most breeds, and a straight one indicates some sort of distress. The pig's tail is elevated and curled when greeting, when competing for food or chasing other pigs, and during courting, mounting, and intromission. The tail straightens when the pig is asleep or dozing, but curls again when the pig rouses unless the animal is isolated, ill, or frightened. The tail will twitch when the skin is being irritated. Amputation of pigs' tails removes a valuable, if crude, diagnostic aid.

Group Behavior

Group behavior is important among pigs. Pigs, especially newborn ones, huddle when they are cold. They thereby convert several small bodies into one large one, both decreasing their surface area and using one another for insulation. Pigs can select an optimal temperature when a gradient is present, both in the laboratory and on the farm. Therefore, heat lamps are provided, and newborn pigs, except those brain damaged by anoxia at birth, stay under the lamp at a comfortable 29°C (85 °F). Adult pigs still huddle when they are cold, but their thermoregulatory problem is more apt to

be one of hyperthermia. Pigs do not sweat, and although they pant, it is not sufficient for cooling. Again, behavioral thermoregulation takes over and pigs wallow in mud, which is more effective than plain water for evaporative heat loss.[1640]

Olfactory Signals

Boars may use behavioral signs more than pheromones to determine the sexual receptivity of the sow. Boars are the only male ungulates that do not exhibit flehmen. Instead, they gape as a cat does when they encounter sow urine. Females can identify intact males, probably by the strong boar odor produced by the androgen metabolites present in both the saliva and preputial secretions of boars.[2123] Sex differences exist in the ability to detect androstenone.[566] Boars may habituate to this odor because it is present in their saliva. Females can detect the pheromone at one-fifth the concentration that intact boars do.[566]

Olfactory stimuli serve to identify pigs individually, for pigs can distinguish conspecifics by means of odor, including urine odor.[1563,1547] When visual, auditory, and olfactory stimuli were available separately and together, olfaction appeared to be the most important sense in individual recognition.[1539] Pigs investigate any newcomer or any pig that has been temporarily removed by nosing it. The ventral body surface is a preferred site for sniffing. The ability of pigs to form a dominance hierarchy while blindfolded indicates that olfactory and auditory, rather than visual, signals are important to pigs.[656]

Cattle

Visual Signals

Cattle posture indicates alertness, aggression, and submission (see Chapter 2). A subtle sign, the showing of the whites of the eyes (>15% of the eye), can be elicited even by mild frustration such as visible but unreachable food or by

Ear Position

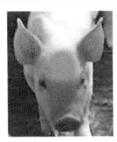 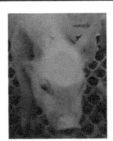 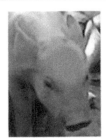

Absent (0) Moderately present (1) Obviously present (2)

When the animal is in pain, the ears are drawn back from forward (baseline) position

Cheek Tightening/Nose Bulge

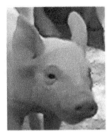 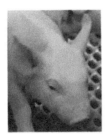 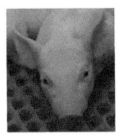

Absent (0) Moderately present (1) Obviously present (2)

When the animal is in pain, a bulge of skin is apparent on the snout in response to cheek tightening

Orbital Tightening

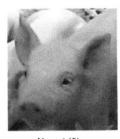 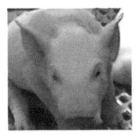

Absent (0) Present (1)

When the animal is in pain, the orbital area is narrowed as the eyelids
are squeezed together (scored on a two-point scale)

Figure 1.15 Facial expressions of pain in the pig. *Source:* Cieri *et al.* (2014).[2697]

social frustration such as removal of the cow's calf or anticipation of food.[2020–2022] Treatment with diazepam several hours before the frustrating experience decreases the percentage of visible eye white.[2023] Pain in cattle is characterized by ears that are tense and backward or held low, and eyes that may have a tense stare or a withdrawn appearance. Tension of the muscles above the eyes may be seen as "furrow lines." The muscles on the side of the

EP1 EP2

EP3 EP4

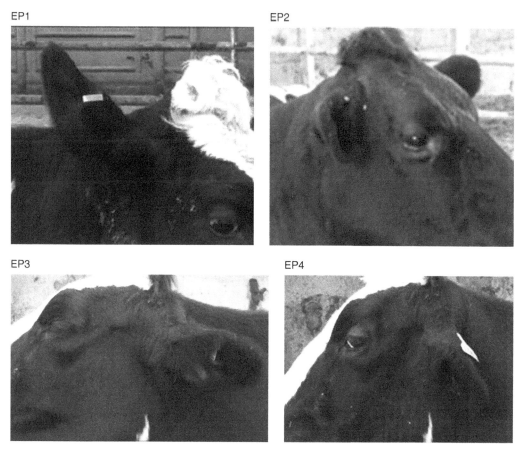

Figure 1.16   The ear postures of the cow are: Ear posture one (EP1) was characterized by the ear being held upright, above the focal cow's head and neck, and the ear pinna faced either forward or was rotated to the side. In ear posture two (EP2), the ear pinna was directed forward, in front of the cow, and the ear was held horizontally. Ear posture three (EP3) was when the ear was held backward on the cows head, but was not passively drooping or upright. In ear posture four (EP4), the ear was hung down loosely, naturally falling perpendicular to the head, with the ear pinna facing downward. *Source:* Proctor and Carder (2014)[3092]/ Reproduced with permission of Elsevier.

head may be tense, the nostrils may be dilated, and there is increased tonus of the lips (Figures 1.16 and 1.17).[826]

The typical aggressive and submissive postures of cattle are described in Chapter 2, "Aggression and Social Structure."

Vocalizations

The moo is low pitched.[1211] The other common vocalization – the call, hoot, or roar – is higher pitched and consists of repeated brief calls, usually by a distressed cow. A threatening bull gives a roar of high amplitude. A very hungry calf will give a high-intensity "menh" call. During copulation, grunting sounds are heard. Some humans can recognize cows by voice, so it would not be surprising if cattle were able to recognize one another. Cattle appear to respond to a vocalization with a vocalization of similar intensity. An excited call is answered by excited calls. Calves have a special moo, almost a baa, or play call.[347]

Vocal communication in a prey species such as cattle may be most important in transmitting information about general safety or danger. It may have been more important for cattle

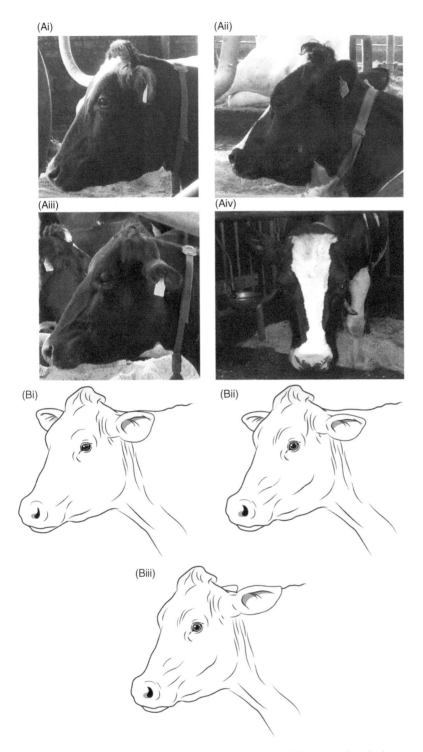

Figure 1.17 (A) Photos of a cow relaxing, not in pain (i) and three cows in pain: lameness (ii), compromised vascular system, udder sore, few and week peristaltic movements (iii) and post-surgical pain after rumen fistulation (iv). The features of the pain face of the cow comprise changes in 4 areas: (1) Ears: ears are tense and backwards (ii) or low/lambs ears (iii). (2) Eyes: eyes have a tense stare (ii + iv) or a withdrawn appearance (iii). Tension of the muscles above the eyes may be seen as 'furrow lines' (iii + iv). (3) Facial muscles: tension of the facial muscles on the side of the head (ii + iii). (4) Muzzle: strained nostrils, the nostrils may be dilated and there may be 'lines' above the nostrils. There is increased tonus of the lips (ii + iii + iv). (B) Illustrations of the Cow Pain Face. The scientific illustrations aim at accentuating the important changes in the facial expression without disturbances of the specific cow's individual expression. (i) Relaxed cow. (ii) Cow in pain with low ears/ lambs ears. (iii) Cow in pain with ears tense and backwards.[826]

(and horses) to be alert and ready to flee than to communicate more precise information in their calls.

Sheep

Visual Signals

The ears of sheep can be pointed forward, backward, or horizontal (hanging passively and loosely). The horizontal posture corresponds to a neutral state. Sheep point their ears backward when they face unfamiliar and unpleasant uncontrollable situations, hence likely to elicit fear; they point their ears up when facing similar negative but controllable situations. The ears are in asymmetric posture in very sudden situations likely to elicit surprise.[278] The auricle can point backward or downward. Frequent ear-posture changes are associated with situations inducing negative states, and a high proportion of passive ear postures or axial ears (perpendicular to the head–rump axis) are associated with situations likely to induce positive emotional states. Tail wagging in sheep is indicative of a positive emotion.[3004] A raised tail is seen when sheep are isolated – a very stressful situation for the species.[1914] The eye's aperture is wider in a fearful sheep.[1915]

Submissive postures are the lowered neck and the headshake given mostly by small sheep in the presence of larger ones. Sheep have a visual signal for defensive aggression: they stamp. Threats in sheep are the foreleg kick, often repeated several times and sometimes actually contacting the opponent. The horn threat is movement of the head sharply downward. The twist and low stretch involves stretching the neck and twisting the head with accompanying tongue flicks. Some rams threaten by standing stiffly with their heads up, which causes their necks to bulge. Rams rub their horns on one another's face, probably spreading pre-orbital secretions. The other visual signals used in courting behavior are discussed in Chapter 4. Sheep rarely will huddle facing one another; head-to-head orientation is aggressive behavior in this species. The facial expression of sheep in pain is seen in Figure 1.18. Orbital tightening, depressed ears, and flehmen are the signs of pain.

Adult sheep continue to use vocalizations as contact calls. Sheep also are able to distinguish conspecifics by means of olfaction.[147]

Communication with Human

The facial expression of sheep in pain is seen in Figure 1.18.

Sheep are aware of human visual activity. They look at a staring human more than a non-staring human, and they are more active and urinate more often.[207]

Vocalizations

Vocal communication in sheep consists of bleating in distress or to initiate contact. Ewes rumble to their newborn lambs (see Chapter 5), and rams make a similar call while courting. The snort is an aggressive communication in sheep.

Goats

Visual Signals

When goats are aroused, their ears point forward more and to the side less, and they emit higher frequency calls. Their ears are oriented backward less often and their tails are up in positive (food-anticipating) situations compared to when they are isolated.[331]

Vocalizations

Goats stamp and produce a high-pitched sneeze when threatened. Kids have a distress call and an isolation bleat. The unique behaviors of caprine courtship are discussed in

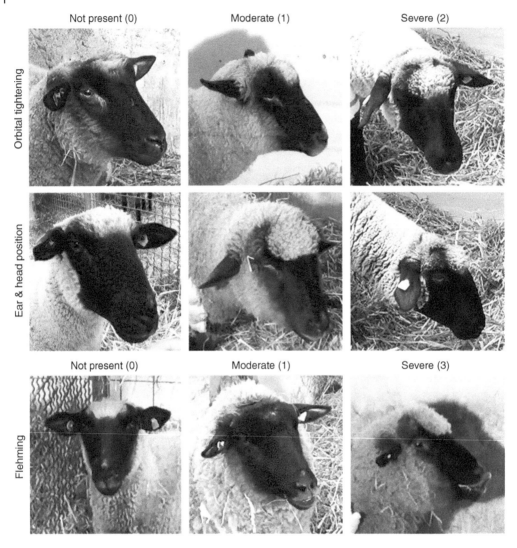

	Not present (0)	Moderate (1)	Severe (2)
Orbital tightening			
Ear & head position			

	Not present (0)	Moderate (1)	Severe (3)
Flehming			

Figure 1.18   Facial expressions of sheep in pain.

Chapter 4, and the ontogeny of goat "language" is discussed in Chapter 6.

Olfactory Signals

Olfactory communication is very important for sexual activity in ruminants. The flehmen response is shown by all male ruminants in response to female urine. Goats have pedal glands on only two feet and a tail gland. Aspiration of nonvolatile material into the vomeronasal organ has been demonstrated in goats.[1295]

Chickens

Chick vocalizations are the twitter, peep, trill, and shriek. The twitter is a pleasure call. The trill is a response to a startling situation. The peep is a distress call and the shriek is a response to pain. Hens emit a gackle call before laying.[3055] Hens communicate with their chicks even before hatching and they learn her voice. After hatching the chicks respond to her food call as well as her broody call and roosting call.

Roosters crow and is one reason they are often legislated against in urban areas. The purpose of crowing is to announce the bird's social status; crows contain information on the bird's size and hormonal status. Roosters do serve as a defense against predators for the hens and emit very different vocalizations when an aerial threat (a hawk) is present than when a ground threat (a fox) is present.[2909]

Head shaking and scratching might be a good indicator of bird frustration or a response to disturbing stimuli. Raised hackles indicate aggression and a low crouch is submissive.

When anticipating positive events chickens exhibit comfort behaviors such as preening and wing flapping, but when anticipating negative events, they showed more locomotion and head movements.[3045]

Tonic immobility. Although facial expressions and physiological reactions such as heart rate or corticosteroid levels are used to measure fear, there is a unique method that can be used in chickens, termed "tonic immobility." It is also seen in other species, for example, playing possum in opossums. To test tonic immobility duration, the chicken is held gently on its side, with light pressure applied to the body and neck region for 30 minutes. The time from the end of the restraint to the bird moving is a measure of how fearful the bird was at the time of testing.

2

Aggression and Social Structure

Sociability

The sociability index (SI) is equivalent to the relative proportion of time that an individual spends as the nearest neighbor of other animals in the group, and it is scaled to have an expectation of 1.0 under the null hypothesis of random mixing. A highly sociable individual will therefore have a value >1.0, while low sociability is defined by a value <1.0. Sociability is reflected in the speed with which a cow will rejoin its herd, for example. Those who are slower to approach have fewer nearest neighbors and are more apt to be at the periphery of the group.[816] This can be applied to interspecific relationships as well. Dogs that are friendlier to humans (i.e., more social) will continue to gaze at people even when the behavior is unrewarded.[1125]

Introduction

Aggression is not a unitary phenomenon, but serves a variety of functions in an animal's life. In some cases, aggression is used to obtain food; in others, it may facilitate access to a sexual partner or establish an animal's place in a social hierarchy. In some situations, aggression is highly desirable, as when fighting takes place to establish a dominance hierarchy. The importance of such fighting is that after the dominance hierarchy is formed, it provides the animals in the group a means by which additional serious combat may be minimized. For the animal practitioner, the problem is not to eliminate all aggression but to determine the type of aggression with which he or she is dealing; only then can the problem of control be dealt with effectively. For example, castration may stop a tomcat from fighting with neighborhood cats, but it may have little influence on his hunting behavior.

Categories of Aggression

Social or Dominance-Related Aggression

Social aggression occurs when animals live in groups. It serves to establish the dominance hierarchy, that is, who will be dominant over whom. When adult animals that have never been penned together previously are brought together for the first time, intense aggressive encounters may occur for several days until each animal has established its position in what generally turns out to be a hierarchy of dominant-submissive relationships. This type of social grouping contains an alpha animal, who is seldom challenged by subordinates; a beta, or second-ranked, animal, who is challenged only by the alpha animal; and so on. Within this organization, the type of aggressive encounter changes after the rank of each animal has been determined. No longer is an attack and subsequent fight needed for an alpha animal to establish its rights over a beta animal. Now, a direct stare, or the threat of a charge, usually serves to deter the beta animal from further confrontation. This assertion of dominance in the absence of physical combat is called "ritualized aggression." Although perception of an extensive hierarchy is questionable in domestic species, the relationship between any two animals certainly is recognized. The scarce resource over which social dominance is expressed can be food, a comfortable place to rest, a mate, or any action by one animal that is perceived as a threat or challenge by the other. One of the best examples is of two horses sharing one bucket of food, with one horse displacing the other at the bucket and obtaining the scarce resource. Another example is of two dogs who usually coexist peacefully, but who fight when the owner tosses a ball.

This type of aggression was first described in chickens and is, therefore, called a "pecking order."[2969] One chicken, the alpha bird, can peck all the other chickens in her group and none can peck her. The next chicken, the beta chicken, will not peck the alpha chicken, but can peck everyone else. Finally, there is the omega or bottom chicken who everyone else can peck, but who pecks no one. Chickens recognize breed differences, in that a rooster will attack members of a breed if another chicken of that breed was subordinate to him and avoid a chicken of a breed that was dominant to him.

Territorial Aggression

Territorial aggression keeps others out of a particular geographical area. This is the type of aggression a domestic dog displays when it becomes a snarling menace to the delivery person. In essence, the dog is defending a territory that it considers its own, and strangers – whether canine or human – simply are not welcome.

Pain-Induced Aggression

Pain-induced aggression develops directly out of induced pain or fear of pain. The function, of course, is to reduce the pain by eliminating the source. When an animal breaks a leg, it does not discriminate between the pain that comes from the break and the unavoidable pain induced by the veterinarian who tries to set the broken leg. A defense reaction of many species, including dogs and cats, is to attack the cause of pain.

The veterinarian must expect to encounter pain-induced aggression frequently, for any animal will attempt to retaliate if it is suffering acute pain. The fact that pain increases aggression should help to explain why corporal punishment of an aggressive dog may exacerbate, rather than attenuate, its undesirable behavior.[3117]

Fear-Induced Aggression

Fear-induced aggression can be related to pain, but in some cases, it is motivated by neophobia (fear of the unknown) or fear of a particular person or animal for no apparent cause. This type of aggression is usually accompanied by more physiological and visceral signs than those seen in pain-induced aggression, for example, crouching, spitting, and dilated pupils in a fearful cat or retreating with tail down and ears back in a dog.

Maternal Aggression

Maternal aggression is directly related to the protection of young. Although the male is generally considered the more aggressive of the two sexes, maternal aggression can equal the ferocity of any male attack.

Predatory Aggression

Predatory aggression is usually directed toward another species, and its purpose is to obtain food. Cats that are fully satiated will often hunt and not eat the catch, indicating that predatory aggression is not entirely governed by hunger. During predatory aggression, the predator adopts an inconspicuous posture and usually does not vocalize.

The Biological Basis of Aggression

With this classification scheme in mind, now we can analyze aggression species by species. In the remainder of this chapter, the major forms of aggression in domesticated species are discussed. Some species, such as the canids, show a much wider spectrum of aggression than others, or perhaps we observe a wider spectrum because of our close association with the species. We omit pain-induced aggression because it occurs in all species.

Genetic Factors: Breed Differences

These are discussed in Chapter 9.

Environmental Control of Aggression

Various environmental factors can increase aggression. Hunger and crowding are the primary ones. Almost every study has found that decreasing enclosure size increases the rate of aggression. This is true of dairy cattle,[1572] beef cattle,[2239] and pigs.[1140] Most aggressive interactions occur at the time of feeding. Unpredictability of feeding time also increases the rate of aggression.[386]

Hormonal Control of Aggression

In many species, the male is more aggressive than the female, at both the interspecies and intraspecies levels. Some notable exceptions exist, however, such as the female with young. At other times, female aggression is generally limited to discouraging male suitors when the female is not sexually receptive and to maintaining the female's place in a female hierarchy if she lives in a group, such as a dairy herd. Female dogs do show territorial defense, but usually not with the gusto that males do.

Testicular Hormones
Testicular hormones appear to play two distinct roles in the control of aggression. During very early development, the presence of testicular hormones establishes a heightened potential for aggression. This is one of the organizational effects of androgens on the brain. In the absence of testicular hormones, this aggression fails to develop. Hence, in the male, the presence of androgens during sexual differentiation enhances the potential for aggression, whereas the female escapes this influence.

Cats show sex differences in aggressiveness that are dependent on the neonatal hormonal environment. An organizational effect of testosterone can occur in female puppies of a predominantly male litter; these females are more apt to be aggressive after spaying.[293,1115] Female puppies treated with testosterone in utero and after birth were, as adult dogs, more successful in competing for a bone than were normal females, but they still were less successful than males.[199] Testosterone administration increased dominance rank in cows[301,302] and aggression in sheep.[1771] Castration has been practiced for centuries to improve tractability as well as to prevent breeding. Bulls, for example, are more aggressive than steers; the difference increases with age. Bulls also mount one another, which may be an expression of dominance rather than homosexuality.[1232]

In addition to their developmental effects, androgens have well-known activational effects upon aggression. Exposure to androgens during adulthood increases the probability that the male will show various forms of aggression (territorial, sexual, social, or dominance); androgens, however, have little to do with predatory aggression.

Chicken

The wild ancestor of the domestic chicken, the jungle fowl lives in a small group usually composed of several hens and a rooster. Commercially they are kept in huge groups, but it seems that the chickens prefer to be within 75 cm (30 in.) of one another.[2737] High-producing layer hens are less social than low-producing hens, but not more fearful.[2725] They may be conserving energy for egg production.

There are separate male and female hierarchies. In contrast to mammals, there are physical markers of dominance in chickens, a large comb. When hens are placed together for the first time, they set up a dominance hierarchy – a pecking order. Dominant hens defeat subordinates by pecking at them, jumping on them, or clawing them. Subordinates show submission by crouching or trying to get away.[2791]

Cocks will fight one another and this is the basis of the "sport" of cock fighting. The roosters leap in the air like hens do, but have been selected for clawing and pecking at their rival until one of the animals is dead. Even "backyard" roosters are aggressive and show this aggression toward humans. This is a common reason their owners seek a veterinary behaviorist.

If chickens observe an encounter between a strange and a familiar bird they will alter their behavior according to the outcome of that encounter. If the stranger wins the observer chicken may avoid a fight, but if the stranger loses, the chicken may attack. Chickens are more likely to imitate a dominant chicken than a subordinate one. Chicken do not appear to have preferred associates. When flock sizes are large the rate of aggression is low.

Cattle

Free-Ranging Cattle

In contrast to most other domestic species, cattle are not often found in the feral state. Their large size and nutritional requirements may account for this. One group of cattle has remained relatively unmanaged on an estate in England for more than 500 years. These animals, the Chillingham or White Park cattle, form cow and calf herds, but the bulls live separately, either alone or in groups of two or three. They join the cow herds during the breeding season.[1321] Their home ranges are stable, but different areas may be used in different seasons. More aggression occurs among the cows than among the bulls or between cows and bulls when they are artificially fed.[889] The bulls maintain a hierarchy through displays with little overt aggression, but bulls from different home ranges rarely breed the same group of cows.

Confined Cattle

Social Behavior

Although cattle cannot choose their social group, they do form bonds with the cattle with which they associate. If released in a communal pasture, they remain close to and groom with cows from their own farm.[2220] They can learn to distinguish between cattle[883] and are less stressed in a frightening situation when familiar cattle are present, even if each cow has been placed in an individual stall. When a familiar or an unfamiliar steer is penned next to him, a steer is more likely to stay closer to the unfamiliar animal and is less likely to move away from him to obtain a food reward. Despite this, when penned together, a steer will stay farther from an unfamiliar steer than a familiar one and spend less time resting.[1777] Cows associated more with conspecifics of similar lactation number. There was also positive assortment by breed and milk production.[311]

Social Aggression

The dominance hierarchy in cattle is known as the "bunt order" in polled cattle and the "hook order" in horned cattle. Dominance can be determined by observing the stances of the two cows involved. The dominant cow, when threatening the submissive one, will stand with her feet drawn well under and with her head down, but perpendicular to the ground. The ears will be turned back with the inner surface pointing down and back. The submissive cow also stands with lowered head, but her head is parallel to the ground and her ears are turned so that the inner surface points to the side. In the absence of horns, cattle use their heads as battering rams, pummeling each other's heads and shoulders until one can reach the more vulnerable flanks or simply inflict overpowering punishment on the other. They can push with their bodies, block another cow's access, or simply threaten with a swing of the head. The recipient can ignore, withdraw, avoid, or retaliate.[815] Equally matched cows may fight for long periods, interrupting active aggression to rest in clinches; one cow will put its muzzle between the hindquarters and the udder of the other, effectively immobilizing her (see Figure 2.1).

Aggressive bulls turn perpendicular to the opponent and display their full height and length. Some may paw and drop to their knees to horn the ground. Aggression is expressed, in

the absence of horns, by bunting or striking the opponent with the head.

Determinants of Dominance

The determinants of dominance in cattle appear to be height, weight, age, sex, presence or absence of horns, and territoriality, with horns, age, and weight being most important. The cow with horns dominates a polled animal. In general, the heavier animal is dominant over the lighter one, but in one study, height was found to be negatively correlated with dominance.[444,300,301] In an established herd, the older cows tend to be dominant, probably because initially the older cows are larger than the younger ones; after the hierarchy is formed, it remains stable.[203,2043] The dominant cows are closer to the front of the herd during both

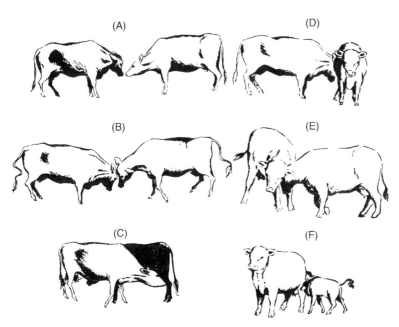

Figure 2.1 Patterns of agonistic interactions in cattle. (A) Cows meeting after an active approach. The one on the left is threatening, whereas the one on the right has assumed a submissive posture. Note the head and leg positions of each cow. (B) Physical combat: a fight. The cows bunt or push against each other head to head, each striving for a flank position. (C) The clinch. One contestant of an evenly matched pair slips alongside the other; the head of the former is pushed between the legs and udder of the latter. In unusually prolonged contests, the cows rest briefly in the clinch between bouts of bunting. (D) Flank attack. The animal that gains a flank position is at a decided advantage over the other. The flanked animal either submits and flees or strives to regain the head-to-head position. (E) The butt. A dominant animal directs an attack against the neck, shoulders, flank, or rump of a subordinate, which in turn submits and avoids the aggressor. (F) Play fighting. The calf butts the mother. *Source:* Hafez (1975).[879]

traveling and foraging. Foraging and short-distance traveling movements of cows are not led by any particular individual, but rather are influenced by a graded type of leadership; that is, the more dominant a cow is, the stronger the influence she may have on the movements of the herd. Cows associate more with conspecifics of similar lactation number in and sort themselves by breed, gregariousness, and milk production.[2667] In single-breed groups of cattle, age had the largest influence on social dominance rank. The longer cattle had been in a group (i.e., longevity) may impact social dominance rank more than age or breed following changes in group.[2803] Dominant dairy cattle on pasture spend more time in the shade than subordinate ones.[2716,2747]

If strange cattle are added to the herd, they tend to be subordinate even if they are older and heavier. The reason is, presumably, that the cattle on their own territory have an advantage over those just introduced.[2043] Bulls were dominant over cows in a study of Holstein cattle.[2147]

The same cow does not "win" every interaction. To be dominant, a cow must win most of the interactions with the other cow.[2449] Dominance hierarchies can be observed simply by noting all agonistic interactions between cattle. However, this can be a slow process. Only 0.1 agonistic encounters per hour were noted in free-ranging Highland cattle, whereas they found that ponies engaged in agonistic behavior 1.9 times per hour.[434] Provision of food to hungry cattle almost always provokes aggressive behavior and can be a technique for determining food-related dominance quickly. Cattle of the same rank feed within 2 m (6.6 ft.) of one another at a trough, but the greater the difference in their rank, the farther apart they will be. Presumably, the lower ranked cow is the one responsible for the separation.[1453] The cow that delivers the most blows and spends the most time controlling the food is dominant. Physical contact is necessary for dominance to be determined, but vision is not. When two cows are in separate pens with the bucket anchored between the pens, both attempt to eat from it; neither retreats. If the cows are in the same pen, one defers to the other, with or without a struggle. The same process occurs even if the cows are blindfolded.[300] A unique way to determine dominance is to put the animals facing one another in a passage that is too narrow for them to turn around. The animal that is forced to back out of the passage is the submissive one.[2196]

Dominance hierarchies are similar, whether determined by aggressive interactions in many situations or just in feeding situations. Free-stall housing contains many areas where cattle compete: narrow passageways, drinkers, feeders, and cubicles. Most aggressive interactions among dairy cows occur at the feeder, but most grooming occurs in the lying area or the alley.[2747] Entry into the milking parlor is not directly related to rank, although middle-ranking cattle tend to come first, with dominant cows in the middle and low-ranking cattle last.[780,1221] In most cases, no correlation exists between milk production and dominance, but in at least one study, high-ranking cattle tended to be good producers.[319,547] Herds in which the average behavior in the milking parlor is better (i.e., less restless and aggressive) have higher milk production than herds with poor behavior.[1877]

The trend to automated milking results in interesting effects on cow behavior. Dominant cows spend more time chewing when entrance to feeding stations in an automated milking system is limited, although intake is similar in high- and low-ranking animals.[1554] High-ranking cows spend less time in the waiting area before automatic milking than low-ranking ones.[1553] Large herds have many triangular relationships because the number of cows is so much larger than a natural herd of cattle, which consists of a dozen cows.[899,1809] Furthermore, hierarchies fluctuate because dairy herds have so many changes in composition because of culling of poor producers, addition of replacement heifers, and movement of dry and calving cows to separate facilities.

Cattle apparently remember one another, so when a cow leaves her herd and then returns within a few weeks, she will assume the same rank.[445] Sick cows and heavily pregnant ones will withdraw from the herd and, therefore, show a change in status – a fact that the stockperson and veterinarian should note.[219]

When cattle are driven, the least dominant animals are first and the dominant animals are in the middle of the herd,[221] although when grazing freely, the dominant animals are the farthest from an observer.[219] When feed is available from a stall in which only one animal can eat at a time, animals that are dominant in other situations do not supplant subordinate animals.[2195] Perhaps having protection on three sides allows the subordinates to maintain their position.

Problems can arise when crush gates are used to speed entry into milking parlors; subordinate cows that would enter last are pushed into dominant cows. Aggressive interactions may result. Nonpregnant cows precede pregnant ones in the crush order.[560] Most cattle that refuse to enter a crush do so consistently. More bulls than steers were very agitated, and more steers (40%) than bulls (25%) were calm.[849]

The individual distance of grazing cattle is about 20 m (66 ft.), and intrusion into this area may be met with threats or bunts.[434] Cattle high in the hierarchy have an inter-animal distance smaller than that of cattle that are low in the hierarchy; that is, they are not reluctant to approach another animal. Bulls tend to have greater inter-animal distance than steers.[1013] Inter-animal preferences may also be related to dominance because animals found close to one another in a field are also close in rank.[2214] The dominant cow is not the first into the milking parlor but is the first to a feeding area. Having arrived at a feeding area, the dominant cow spends more time eating and less time moving from place to place than does a low-ranking cow.[21] This is true both in the feedlot and on pasture. There are several interactions of reproductive status and dominance. Dominance increases with estrus and decreases with

pregnancy.[220,1986] These physiological changes may be the reason that 25% of cows change rank in the course of a year in a stable herd.[1809] Prolactin levels are negatively correlated with dominance.[74]

Stage of lactation and adaptation to a challenging environment can have a destabilizing effect on dominance hierarchies. For example, when pastured in the Alps, Holsteins were subordinate to the native Swiss breeds, although one would have expected the larger Holsteins to be dominant.[1713]

When formed, dominance hierarchies reduce overt aggression; only the lowest ranking animals may suffer deprivation of food when supplies are scarce or feeding space is limited. The importance of this can be seen when cows choose to eat a non-preferred food alone than a preferred food next to a dominant cow.[1937]

Most aggression is seen during the initial stages of formation of a hierarchy. Stock managers should mix unfamiliar animals with care and avoid putting hungry animals together. When a previously unacquainted group of cattle is created, the hierarchy takes 24 to 28 hours to form. Four to 40 days can elapse before nonphysical interactions (i.e., threats) replace physical ones.[1248] In addition to physical injury, cattle may also suffer from lack of rest because of the general turmoil. The normal pattern of standing and lying as a group does not emerge for at least 48 hours after the group is formed. The stress resulting from lack of rest as well as decreased rumination is added to the stress of transportation that usually precedes the formation of a new group.[2444] These considerations may explain why cattle are more susceptible to such diseases as the shipping fever complex when new groups are formed. Regrouping heifers up to 16 times does not decrease their aggressiveness or hasten the time to form new hierarchies.[1905]

Bulls are sometimes kept in groups with resulting problems.[503,1220] Bulls mount other males, and these animals retaliate by butting.[1606] Mounting in this case is probably motivated by dominance, not sex. Keeping bulls together can result not only in injury to the animals but also damage to the substrate, because the bulls paw and horn the ground.[1124] Aggression can be reduced if the bulls are kept in the group with which they were raised; not only are they less aggressive, but also they are less fearful at slaughter.[1639] Bulls who were hand reared individually were more aggressive toward other bulls than were group-reared bulls.[1850]

Maternal Aggression

Cows will attempt to protect their young, and caution always is warranted when a mother is with her offspring. Angus cows may be especially protective.

Grooming

Mutual grooming (licking) occurs, but this occupies only a few minutes per day. Cattle groom their age mates, their kin, and the cows closest to them. One cow solicits grooming, either by approaching submissively with head lowered and chin stretched forward or by approaching more vehemently (head only slightly lowered, chin not stretched forward), which may be accompanied by slight head butts or horning.[1297] Most licking is of the head and neck.[2034,2035] The recipient of grooming is calmed in that her heart rate decreases. If she is lying, her heart rate may increase; the licker's heart rate also may increase.[1297]

In a free-housing situation, most grooming takes place at feeding time. If feeding space per cow is reduced from 0.6 m/cow to 0.3 m/cow, grooming decreases and agonistic encounters increase.[2317] Older and larger cattle receive and give more grooming than younger cattle do. Milk production and milking order (order of entrance into the milking parlor) are also correlated with the amount of grooming received.[2486]

Environmental enrichment is often decreed to improve the welfare of confined animals. "Toys" do not seem to be used by many animals over the age of two months, but devices that, when manipulated, provide food or devices on which a cow can rub or scratch and groom itself are used.[2463]

Sheep

Free-Ranging Sheep

Feral sheep in a natural setting form separate ewe and ram flocks. The ewe flocks also include lambs and immature rams. A flock seldom has more than 20 adult ewes. Ram flocks are much smaller (about six animals) and less stable. This type of social organization is seen in Soay sheep, which are a primitive form of domestic sheep, and among mountain sheep.[807,863] Domestic as well as wild sheep "camp" in one particular area at night. These areas are theorized to be useful because information can be exchanged between animals, even though energy must be expended in traveling from food sources to the night camp.

In a large pasture, sheep divide into flocks with individual, but overlapping, territories. Newly introduced sheep, even offspring separated since weaning, are not allowed to join the original flocks but are relegated to less productive parts of the pasture, which may explain their tendency to wander. Lambs may follow their mothers for up to two years after weaning, varying with the population.[1316,1986,2060]

Flocking

The formation of large commercial herds of hundreds of sheep is usually accompanied by a cacophony of baaing as the small flocks are lost within the large one and the individual sheep give separation calls. The formation of smaller or larger groups of sheep in farm situations is somewhat unnatural. Three sheep do not readily form a flock, and they tend to disperse; therefore, three sheep are often used in sheepdog trials as a test of the dog's ability to control the sheep. Sheep tend to select sheep of the same breed as flock mates when randomly mixed.[91,2470] Familiarity is very important to sheep. They quickly form associations that are slow to break down.[2471]

The nearest-neighbor distance on pasture is approximately 5 m.[2118] Sheep are closest while resting and farthest apart when their activity is not synchronized, that is, when some sheep are resting and others active.[1575]

The leader sheep tend to be on the edge of the flock and move their heads more. The flock is less dispersed and more vigilant before moving. The first followers are preferential partners of the first mover.[1890]

Dominance

Within an established, related flock of sheep, the oldest ewe is dominant over other ewes and is usually the leader in movements. Dominance is not related to body weight in commercial flocks of sheep of similar age. Very little overt aggression is seen among sheep, but dominance can be determined by limiting feeding space. Dominant sheep push out subordinates.[92,2164] One can observe the dominance hierarchy by entering a pen of sheep. The farthest sheep will be the most dominant.[573] The subordinate sheep will lie down less than dominant ones when the lying area is restricted. Displacements increase from seven to almost 30 instances per day.[273] Aggressive sheep shoulder push; then, after the dominant animal has established itself, it displays behaviors toward the subordinant that appear identical to those used in courtship, that is, nudging, with head low and nose up, while striking with the front limb.

Age and weight, but not sex, are also important in determining dominance.[2060] Appearance must be important because shearing may reduce the rank of a dominant ewe. The importance of flock living to sheep is demonstrated by the fact that (1) they are less fearful of an orange umbrella in a flock than alone, and (2) the larger the flock, the less frightened they are, based on escape attempts.[838]

Sexual Aggression

Sexual aggression in sheep can actually interfere with breeding. Among rams, the dominant ram will usually breed more ewes than his subordinates unless he is so aggressive that his battles distract him from the ewes.[2113] Two rams may breed fewer ewes than one alone if they are often engaged in the butting contests typical of ram aggression. If three rams are present in a flock, two may fight while the third one, which may be less aggressive but evolutionarily more competent, impregnates the ewes.

Feral goat herds can range in size from one to 100 goats, but the mean size is four,[2090] and the optimal size is 12; above that size, the group is more apt to fission.[2169] Goats form sexually segregated flocks, except in mild climates where breeding takes place throughout the year. As with sheep, goats tend to spend each night in a particular area, a night camp. Home ranges of male goats are larger than those of females and vary with the season. The total range is 10–40 ha (25–99 acres).[1715]

Because goats, as an introduced species, are a threat to native wildlife, goats may be captured and removed. Use of a "Judas" goat that will lead the captors to the feral goats or attract the males when she is in heat is a technique that takes advantage of caprine social structure.[376]

Does live in small, stable groups (heft groups), each group composed of three to four animals and occupying its own range. Goats continue growing with age. Horn size as well as body size increase; therefore, older goats are dominant over younger ones and males, who are larger, are dominant over females. This applies until the goats are five or six years old. Thereafter, the bucks decline in dominance; despite larger horn size, they may not be as strong and have a high mortality rate. Females decline more slowly. Does dominate kids except for their own, who are as likely as their dam to win a contest. Goats compete for food, and the rate of aggression increases as food availability and day length decrease in the fall. Most contests are resolved without overt aggression. The initiator approaches, and the subordinate leaves the feeding spot and moves 3 m away.[2101] Most aggressive interactions occur when the goats are eating heather or other small shrubs rather than grass, which is distributed more continuously.

Confined Goats

Aggression is expressed as:

1) Frontal clashing: A position where the actor is rearing onto the hind legs with the head and torso twisted, followed by descending forcefully onto the front legs and delivering a powerful strike forward and downward, reaching the head of the receiver.
2) Butting: Contact (sudden and forceful movement) with the head toward another goat.
3) Pushing: Pressing the head to any part of another goat, slowly.
4) Threatening: Pawing, rushing toward, or directing the forehead toward the opponent without physical contact, biting, or attempting to bite another goat.

These behaviors are more common when density is higher, whereas the socially positive behaviors of grooming and nosing do not change.[2337]

Individual distances are shorter during resting than feeding in heterogeneous age groups, but not in homogeneous age groups. There were no differences in individual distance (2–3 m) during resting between the different age groups. Overall, young goats appear to be more tolerant to having other individuals of similar age in close proximity, and they keep the longest distance to adult goats.[274]

Dominance

In goats, as with horned sheep, the presence of horns is an important determinant of dominance. Because horns confer dominance, most agonistic interactions are brief feints or rushes in which the dominant animal lowers its head and

points its horns at the subordinate. Horns, size, and age determine dominance.[174,274,1976,1977,2061] When the animals are of equal or undetermined rank, long fights occur in which horns and heads are clashed together repeatedly. The goats that act as leaders have been born in the area and have more kin in the flock than do non-leaders. Introducing a new goat to a group is harder on the introduced animal than the original members of the group. Introduced goats, for example, were on the receiving end of a relatively high number of agonistic behaviors from resident goats on day 0, emerged as losers in most of these confrontations, spent most of their time during the introduction period withdrawn, and considerably increased the length of time they spent lying whilst substantially decreasing the amount of time spent feeding and ruminating.[2928] A novel food will increase the level of aggression within a goat herd.[644,2213] Restricting feeding space increases aggression, but the effect depends on the type of forage; there is more aggression over hay than over silage.[1161] Goats do bite, especially polled goats who are three years old or older.[2268]

Grooming

A goat grooms itself by scratching its head and neck with a hind hoof and by oral grooming of the rest of the body surface. The oral grooming consists of an upward scraping motion of the lower canine and incisor teeth, a behavior that is suppressed by testosterone. Intact male goats groom orally less than wethers or does.[1619] More self-grooming occurs following aggressive interactions, possibly indicating anxiety. Affiliative contact, through muzzle-to-muzzle contact or allogrooming by the aggressor, appears to reduce the post-conflict anxiety.[2945]

Horses

Free-Ranging Horses

Horses live in small groups called "bands," which are composed of a stallion, several mares, and their offspring. A number of bands living in the same area are referred to as a "herd." In a free-ranging horse band, each stallion is associated with 2–28 mares (mean: 4–12). Band size is optimal at five to seven mares. An older or larger mare is apt to be the highest ranking female, and she leads the herd in flight and in daily journeys to rest or to a new grazing area. The stallion drives the herd from behind, going to the front only to confront another stallion. Nevertheless, the stallion is usually, but not always, dominant over his harem.[238,1049,2419]

Mares apparently choose the stallion and the band that they ultimately join. Fillies usually leave their natal band at puberty, possibly to avoid an incestuous breeding with their sire.[1195] The mares may switch bands several times, but by five years they are usually in their permanent band; they remain in the same general area, often joining a band that shares the same home range.[1396] They may join another band or a bachelor band. The small percentage that does remain in its natal band has very low foaling rates, indicating that inbreeding depression of reproduction does occur.[1195]

There are many ways that a young stallion may acquire a band: (a) joining unguarded females, (b) defeating a harem stallion, (c) raiding a harem and taking some of the mares, (d) becoming a satellite or secondary stallion, and (e) remaining in the natal band and inheriting it.[1190,1208] The dominant stallion within the bachelor band is the one most likely to become the harem stallion. The stallion has more chances of siring a foal as a secondary stallion than as a bachelor.[106,673] Some bands have more than one stallion. There is usually a harem stallion, a "lieutenant" stallion who helps with harem defense against other stallion and tag stallions who follow the band, but are peripheral members.[3076]

The feral ponies on Assateague Island, off the coast of Maryland, are known as "Chincoteague ponies." About 20% of mares change bands. Mares may leave bands for reasons having to do with the stallions. They are less likely to leave larger bands with older

stallions who have had a harem for several years.[2008] Mares who change bands have a lower foaling rate than those who remain. Although this could be due to many factors, the fact that contracepted mares (to control horse populations, the zona pellucida vaccine is used on many island populations), like naturally foal-less mares, change bands more often than fertile mares indicates that reproduction may play a role.[1711] Culling of feral horses is another method of controlling the population size. When only young horses were removed, band size was reduced and stallions spent less time herding their mares, but more time harem tending (defense of a band female or recruitment of a new female into the band).[1900]

If a mare enters a new band, the resident mares are aggressive toward her, but the stallion will protect her. The larger the herd, the higher the aggression rate per mare. Dominant mares interrupt nursing bouts of subordinates. The highest rate of aggression occurs at water holes.[2010] Dominance is important not only for immediate access to scarce resources but also for the reproductive success of one's offspring. Stallions born to dominant mares sire more foals.[672] The dominance hierarchies remain stable in undisturbed feral herds, and age appears to be the most important determinant of dominance.[1192] Movements of the herd can be initiated by any member of the herd. Dominant animals are more likely to be followed.[1274]

Stallions defend their mares, not a fixed territory. Two herd stallions, upon meeting, usually prance toward each other. When they are close enough to do so, they investigate each other with their nostrils. They then defecate and sniff at the manure. The most dominant animals within bachelor herds defecate last.[677] These displays between stallions can lead to a fight, but aggression is much more likely to result in the absence of the displays when a bachelor stallion tries to abduct a mare. Within bachelor herds of Przewalski horses, a dominant animal may intervene when another horse is threatened.[1276]

Stallions may evaluate their rivals on the basis of vocalizations. Subordinate stallions have shorter squeals that also begin at a lower frequency than those of dominant stallions.[1990] Rival stallions may be more likely to challenge a subordinate after having heard him squeal.

Large bands may have more than one stallion.[239,1590] The dominant stallion in the herd does most of the breeding; the subordinate stallion engages in most of the fighting with any other stallions that approach the band. The subordinate stallion sires 25% of the foals.[673] Bands of horses compete for fresh water; the band drinking usually will not be ousted by an intruding band.[739] The order of drinking is stallion, mares, and then juveniles. Only juveniles will be displaced by an intruder. Large, multi-male bands tend to supplant smaller bands at water sources.[1591] Multi-male bands have an advantage in that fewer mares leave these bands during the winter, when food is scarce.[1397] Some disadvantages of being in a multi-male band exist: the mares are in poorer body condition and carry a heavier parasite load; they have traveled more and rested less. The foaling rate is lower and foal mortality higher in multi-stallion bands.[1397] The stallions in a multi-male band are aggressive to the mares. When their subordinate stallions are removed, the dominant stallions seem to be able to defend their mares, so the advantages of having a subordinate stallion are not clear.[1398]

Bands of horse are not stationary; they move from one grazing area to another or to water. Within a band, movements are more likely to be initiated by bold horse and preferred partners follow each other.[673] Before departure individual horses become more active, oriented, and cohesive and begin departure. Individuals start to move toward the future goal area by positioning themselves along the front to back axis. Presumably the horses share the motivation to drink or find shade so move in the same direction.[2673] Horses are more likely to follow a horse with higher social status even when the leader makes the wrong choice.[3017]

In interspecies relationships, feral horses dominate cattle[2300] but domestic horses are afraid of them and they approach them less closely than they would a moving box of the same size.[3035] Infanticide is reported in the domestic horse, but has also been observed in free-ranging Przewalski horses living in zoos,[310] in semi-natural reserves,[674] and reintroduced into the wild in China and Mongolia.[411] The stallion kills a newborn foal, usually a colt and usually not his own offspring.

Domestic Horses

What is a band? Judging by the decrease in walking and increase in grazing compared with those of smaller groups, three horses are a band.[1289] Although the strict order by sex and age just described may be observed in wild horses, quite a different picture emerges when herds of domestic horses are studied. Dominance hierarchies tend to be linear unless the group is large, in which case triangular and more complex relationships appear. Weight and age are important determinants of dominance in some groups, but not in others.[434,865,1057,1613] Przewalski horses have linear dominance hierarchies even on <30-ha (74-acre) pastures. The position of the stallion in the hierarchy is variable.[88, 1049] Yearling fillies are more aggressive than yearling colts in a feeding situation.[1637] When yearling Icelandic fillies and geldings maintained in separate herds were compared, both formed linear hierarchies, but the fillies showed more submission and less escalation or ignoring of aggression from another horse.[2391] High-ranking Icelandic horses had more access to hay and used the bodies of the other horses as windbreaks. As a result, the higher ranking horses improved in condition over the Icelandic winter, whereas the lower ranking horses lost condition.[1109] The presence of adults reduces aggression in subadult horses.[304]

Horses that are stabled singly are more aggressive than those kept in groups.[419] Spacing feed buckets widely apart is the easiest way to prevent aggression between horses by reducing competition over resources; the resource is usually food. Wire partitions along a feed trough allow a subordinate horse to eat in the presence of a dominant one.[1026] Feed containers must be 10 m apart, and the ratio of feed containers to horses should be 1.5, that is, four horses should have six containers.[1423]

There is less total aggression if a new horse is introduced to two resident horses rather than introducing each horse separately.[934] Bites by young, but not adult, horses can be reduced by meetings in adjacent stalls before the horses are released together, and threat behavior predicts contact aggression when the horses are together.[902] Following a conflict, the two horses are more likely to show nonaggressive interactions to one another, or reconciliation behavior.[461,1238] When horse groups, even of familiar horses, are manipulated there are changes in behavior. Low-ranking horses perform fewer aggressive behaviors.[2971] The remaining horses are more vocal, have higher heart rates, and are more active (irrespective of the rank of the horse removed).[2995]

Mothers are not necessarily dominant over their daughters. The daughters of dominant mares tend to be dominant within their own groups.[1053] Little change occurs in the rank of mares when they foal.[646]

Within a herd, the mares appear to have preferred associates – "friends," anthropomorphically – with whom they mutually groom, especially when their winter coats are shedding. Preferred associates synchronize their behavior more than non-preferred associates in the same herd.[946] Mares appear to be more socially dependent than geldings.[2763] Preferred associates share resources without competing. When the relationships of the mares are known, the preferred associates often are mother and daughter or siblings, and are usually animals close in social rank.[434,2300] Horses will use brushes to self-groom and while self-grooming exhibit the pleasure face and are likely to initiate mutual grooming with another horse.[2842] When a member of a pair of preferred associates is allogrooming with another horse, the other partner may intervene, either stopping the bout or replacing the non-partner. The more subordinate animal of a pair is more likely to intervene. Subadult mares intervene in play bouts by males.[2333] Foals of high-ranking mares receive fewer aggression from other horses than those of low-ranking mares.[971]

Mares are more likely to choose another horse rather than food in a two-choice test, probably because, mares live in herds their entire lives, but males leave bachelor herds to establish their own harems.[2765] Our modern manner of keeping horses in box stalls separated by bars prevents formation of relationships between adjacent horses despite olfactory and visual contact.[419] Apparently, horses must have direct contact to form a dominance relationship. Proximity does not cause horses to become preferred associates. In summary, the determinants of dominance in horses appear to be more closely related to the animal's temperament and the position of its mother in the band than to physical characteristics.

Although most equine sports involve solitary horses, they may be driven in pairs (or teams of larger numbers). Aggression between the two horses may occur, especially when first harnessed together. The aggression was less if the stallion had tactile contact with another horse while in his stall.[2760]

Types of Aggression

Fighting can include a variety of responses in horses – running, chasing or fleeing, circling, neck wrestling, biting, and kicking – but most aggressions consisted of displacements or threats rather than kicks or bites.[1235] Horses neck wrestle and nip at one another in play, but biting or biting attempts with ears flattened to the head and lips retracted are signs of serious aggression (Figure 2.2). Kicking is considered to be the horse's most aggressive act, and, although some have hypothesized that kicks are defensive – that is, directed up the dominance hierarchy – kicking more likely occurs

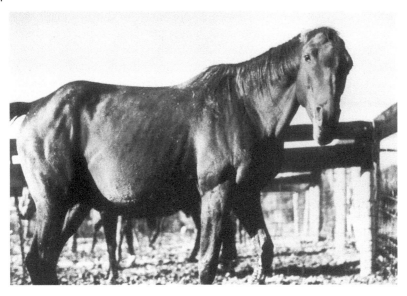

Figure 2.2   An aggressive expression in a horse. A threat to bite.

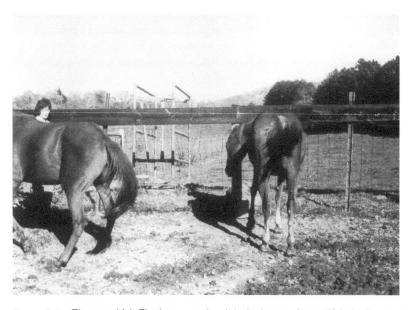

Figure 2.3   Threat to kick. The horse on the right is threatening to kick the horse on the left. Note the lashing tail of the threatening horse and the tucked tail of the threatened horse.

when either the challenge or the danger is from the rear (Figure 2.3).[2419]

Aggression between stallions can take many forms. Prefight behavior includes the arched neck threat, fecal pile display, head bowing, striking, threatening to bite, squealing, snorting, prancing in parallel, and pushing.[1504] The levade (rearing with deeply flexed hind limbs) is part of untrained stallions' interactions. This is probably the reason that Lipizzaner stallions, rather than mares, are used by the Spanish Riding School. Stallions may rear and box with their forelegs. A horse may avoid the lunge of another horse by swinging its head in

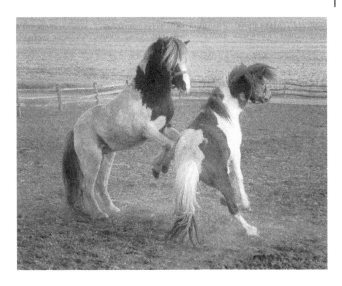

Figure 2.4 Balking behavior by stallion on the right. *Source:* Courtesy of Dr. Sue McDonnell, University of Pennsylvania.

a dorsolateral direction away from an apparent threat while the hind legs remain stationary, a posture termed the "balk" (Figure 2.4).[1505] A less intense version of this is seen when two horses share feed over which they might have been expected to fight. The horses turn away from each other. Avoiding eye contact as well as physical contact may be the goal of this behavior. Elements of sexual behavior such as resting the chin on the opponent's rump, rump presentation, and mounting also occur. These behaviors are seen in bachelor herds of stallions and may be play or determination of the hierarchy. The activities practiced in the bachelor herd are used to defeat a band stallion when a former bachelor acquires mares.

Horses can be severely injured in the process of forming a hierarchy, especially if they are so confined that the loser cannot escape. Horses that have been stalled separately for a few months may show much more aggression than when they have been together on a daily basis. Because neither age, weight, nor sex appears to be an important determinant of dominance, one should hesitate to predict a hierarchy in horses. It is safest to leave horses in the same group. Exercise on a treadmill does not change aggression level.[1337] A good management practice, therefore, is to introduce (or reintroduce) horses to one another across a fence. The

horses can investigate and threaten each other but will be able to escape easily without being kicked, although the danger of injuring their limbs on the fence while striking or kicking is always present.

Grooming

Horses mutually groom one another. Licking of the foal is seen only in the short period after the foal's birth, but horses will stand shoulder to shoulder and nibble at each other's withers and back. Horses tend to groom animals close to their own rank in the dominance hierarchy, which are also the horses nearest to them.[434] This behavior is more pronounced in the spring, when the heavy winter coats are being shed. Horses that have been kept in individual stalls groom more when placed in a social situation, indicating a build-up of motivation for grooming.[419,1062] Horse owners assume the role of grooming partner when they curry their horses. Grooming in the withers area reduces the horse's heart rate.[675]

Summer weather brings horses irritating companions: flies, many of which are biting species. To escape flies, horses spend many of the daylight hours in the shade,[2300] in grassless areas, or, if available, in the snow or surf.[1194] Some horses have a particularly effective way to deal with flies. They stand side-by-side, nose to tail, and keep the flies off one another's faces with their tails. Not all horses form pairs, despite the obvious advantages, but most will stand closer to one another during times of high fly density.[595]

Causes of Equine Aggression

Aggression is an all-too-common behavior problem of horses. Aggression can be directed at people or other horses. Aggression toward people is seen most often in the stall, a small, easily defended space. Its appearance in the stall is probably a form of resource guarding and is influenced by the caretaker.[941]

Pain is a common, and often overlooked, cause of aggression in horses. Misbehavior toward the farrier often resolves when the lameness is cured.[1452] The more vertebral abnormalities found in a horse's spine, the more aggressive it was.[775]

Few horses are aggressive to people as they approach, but if the person carries a saddle or halter, a greater percentage are aggressive. The same horses that threaten humans who signal work are the ones that will not cross a novel surface.[777]

Donkeys

Although feral donkeys do not form herds, domestic donkeys form pair bonds and will choose to be with that donkey in preference to a strange or a familiar donkey.[2897]

Pigs

Free-Ranging Pigs

Numerous populations of feral swine exist. They form groups of approximately eight, consisting most commonly of three sows and their offspring. The males are solitary for much of the year but may form all-male groups in the late winter.[851] The males travel farther than the females. Young pigs do not leave the sow until

they weigh 27–32 kg (60–70 lb.). The pigs have overlapping home ranges of 121–809 ha (300–2000 acres).[1286] When domesticated pigs are released, they too form groups, but the size varies with their activities: approximately five pigs when grazing and 13 when resting.[1947]

Confined Pigs

Social Aggression

Teat Order Pigs have the most intriguing of hierarchies because the ranks are formed soon after birth, not by uncoordinated pushing for a nipple as exhibited by puppies, but by vicious blows with the appropriately named "needle teeth" possessed by piglets at birth. To reduce the injury and infection from snout lacerations during the neonatal period, most swine producers clip the teeth to the gumline.[747] The resource over which the piglets are fighting is the preferred pair of teats, usually the most anterior pair that produces the most milk and has the lowest incidence of mastitis. In addition, pigs sucking at these teats are much less likely to be kicked by the sow's hind legs. The hierarchy is formed within the first two days after birth; the heaviest and first-born pigs are usually dominant.[1485] Because the anterior teats produce the most milk, the pigs that suckle these teats grow fastest and remain dominant;[613,1486,1487] after its formation, the teat order of hierarchy remains stable, especially the top and bottom ranks.[655] By the sixth day after birth, the same teat is suckled by the same pig 90% of the time.[983]

Hierarchy Formation

When unfamiliar weanlings or older pigs are mixed, a hierarchy must be formed.[1487,1903] If the group consists of six pigs, the hierarchy is linear, but only quasi-linear in a group of 12. It is unclear whether this phenomenon, which appears to be true across species, is due to inability to recognize relationships with a large number of animals.[682] When mixed with 28 other pigs right after weaning, the pigs engaged in 40 fights during the first two days, but six weeks later only six fights.[2200] Plasma triiodothyronine levels were higher in the most aggressive pigs than in the least aggressive pigs.[2978]

The larger the group, the less aggression, and pigs from large groups are less aggressive when transferred to a smaller group.[2018] A meta-analysis of 45 studies of aggression in pigs indicated that, in the absence of bedding, aggression increased with group size. Provision of environmental enrichment objects, especially hanging deformable objects, decreased aggression.[115]

When young pigs (seven to eight weeks old) are introduced, they spend a minute or two nosing one another, sniffing the face and anogenital regions – these investigations are longer between unfamiliar pigs – and then begin to butt the head and body and bite, especially the head and ears.[2153] Up to 80 bites may be inflicted before one turns away and retreats; the winner will continue biting.[1143] Even week-old pigs will fight with strange piglets, although the fights are short. In older pigs, the process of hierarchy formation takes several days.[1546] Although most aggression is seen in the first 24 hours after mixing strange pigs, the food intake and weight gain of pigs are inhibited for more than 24 hours after mixing, and increased fighting continues for as long as six weeks.[624]

Mixing litters before weaning may be advantageous.[1828] "Socializing" piglets by letting two litters mingle from 10 to 30 days of age led to differences in their behavior when they were mixed with strange pigs at 51 days. The socialized piglets initiated aggression sooner, but formed hierarchies sooner (within 10 days) than unsocialized piglets.[527] There is more mounting between pigs in the mixed groups as compared to littermate groups.[2685] The more pigs are regrouped, the quicker they form hierarchies and the less serious the injuries, even when the pigs are always complete strangers to one another.[2331] Other consequences of regrouping occur as well: pigs that have been regrouped are less likely to approach people than are pigs that have remained in a stable group; and, apparently, regrouping makes the pigs more fearful.[956]

Affiliation (social preference) in pigs may be a result of choice of activity; pigs chose their lying partners influenced by sex and dominance rather than choice of individual, that is, both pigs chose to lie down at the same time, influenced by sex and dominance. Young pigs spend most of their lying time in contact with other pigs, but interact socially with different pigs than the one next to whom they lie.[2686]

Even simple physical factors such as a draft can cause pigs to be more aggressive.[2042] Pen size and shape can also affect aggression when strange pigs are mixed. Less aggression arises in a rectangular pen.[169] At weaning the most aggressive pigs had lower triiodothyronine than the least aggressive pigs.[2978]

When strange pigs are mixed, size disparity reduces the initial fighting; not surprisingly, however, the smaller pigs do not gain as well or remain as healthy as they do in groups of similar-sized pigs.[1615] When pigs of disparate size must be mixed, however, smaller pigs fare better if the larger pigs are added to the pen so that the small pigs have the advantage of an established territory. The younger pigs are when mixed – between 5 and 26 days – the shorter the time spent fighting.

When two pigs are introduced, the most aggressive pig bites first but may not win.[371] Weight predicts success in encounters among newly mixed pigs, but aggressiveness predicts bullying behavior (one-sided aggression) and persistence of aggression.[526] Even at four weeks of age, intact piglets are more aggressive when mixed than castrated pigs.[1642] Females fight longer than castrated males.[2189] Boars are presumably dominant over sows, but when barrows (castrated males) and sows are penned together, the males might not be dominant. Pigs from male-biased litters (>60% males) are more aggressive than those from female-biased liters.[2977] More aggressive pigs express more negative emotionality at the start of an agonistic encounter.[2918]

When pigs are removed for 25 days or sows for six weeks from a group that has been together for months, they assume their original rank, but the 12-week-old pigs that were dominant in a group formed for only five days may not be dominant when reintroduced to that group three weeks later.[81,655,1743] Small pigs and newcomers to an established group are usually subordinate.[744] Littermates show less aggression to one another than to unfamiliar pigs except over food, when similar levels of aggression are seen.[1874] The reduced aggression among littermates relates to familiarity, not kin recognition, as indicated by the fact that littermates cross-fostered onto another sow are treated like strangers.[2190] After separation, the dominant pig lies down and lets its belly be nosed by the other pigs. This behavior, the function of which remains unknown, is seen most often when the dominant pig has returned to its group after a separation.[744] Immunocastration with a GNRF (gonadotropin-releasing factor) vaccine reduces both aggression and sexual behaviors in male pigs as well as boar taint in their meat.[326]

Sows The hierarchy of pregnant sows (240 kg) is more stable than that of younger feeder pigs (40 kg).[1766] Dominant sows give birth to more male piglets than do subordinate ones.[1551,1561] The biological significance of this is that the offspring of the dominant animal is more likely to grow large and strong and to be dominant itself. The male offspring of a dominant sow has a better chance to dominate other boars, to gain access to estrous sows, and, therefore, to sire many piglets. If the sow is not dominant, a greater risk exists that her sons will not sire any piglets. A safer way to ensure that her genes are passed on is to produce daughters, all of whom will have at least some offspring. Dominant sows give birth to piglets that are more active, more vocal, and faster to touch a novel object (a large red container) than piglets of low-ranking sows.[1560] The best predictor of the dominance rank of a sow is the rank of her mother.[579] Pregnant sows form dominance hierarchies based on parity; the greater the number of litters the sows has had the lower her rank.[2847,2940] Low-ranking sows will lose weight unless feed is provided ad libitum.[342] A subordinate sow in a group may produce small litters or low-birth-weight piglets,[1560] not because she lacks the genetic potential but because she cannot obtain adequate nourishment. Sows were exposed twice a week for three weeks to different dominant sows, and, although their salivary cortisol rose immediately after the first five defeats, by the sixth confrontation cortisol did not rise. The subordinate sow avoided the dominant pig or remained passive rather than fighting back by the third confrontation.[2327] Age affects dominance among sows; older sows are dominant, feed more often, and gain more weight.[1250] The immune status of subordinate pigs is inferior to that of dominant pigs,[2292] but both dominant and subordinate pigs may be immunosuppressed in a hot environment.[1633]

As in other species, after the hierarchy is formed, fighting is replaced by threats; these consist of a sharp, loud grunt and a feint with the snout by the dominant pig. Aggressive behaviors include thrusting the head upward or sideways against the head or body of the opponent. These activities may be accompanied by biting. Levering, in which the snout is put under the body of the opponent, usually from behind, also occurs. The submissive gesture in pigs consists of twisting the head away from the opponent.[1139] The subordinate pig quickly gives ground (see Figure 2.5). Leadership on a novel pasture is not correlated with dominance.[1545]

Not surprisingly, the sows that received the most aggressive acts showed the least estrous behavior. They did not mount or nose other sows as much as did high-ranking sows.[1783] The level of aggressiveness is not correlated with age or weight.[1641] Pigs in their home pen have some advantage over intruders.[2228] The greater the number of unfamiliar, as opposed to familiar, pigs, the more fighting will occur.[82]

Confinement in gestation crates is controversial and has been banned in Europe. The alternative is housing sows in groups, which may lead to aggression when the sows are mixed after insemination. Forming stable groups that live together until farrowing would result in the

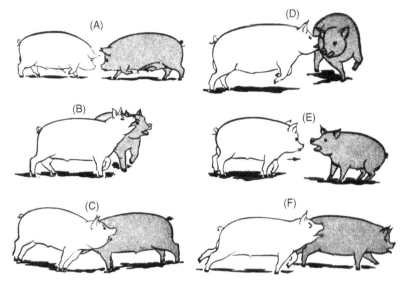

Figure 2.5   Agonistic behavior in boars. (A) Pawing the ground during initial encounter. (B) Strutting. (C) Shoulder-to-shoulder contact and slashing. (D) Perpendicular biting attack. (E) Submission of pig on the right. (F) Pursuit of the loser. *Source:* Hafez and Signoret.[881]

least aggression. When new sows are added to a group, there is four times more aggression directed at the new sows, and increased aggression persists for three weeks.[1264,2187]

Aggression can be a problem in pregnant sows, but management practices can reduce the fighting. If sows are returned to the group a week after they left to be bred, there is much less aggression than if they were gone for four weeks.[2165] Newly added sows rest apart from the original residents in a less desirable area of the pen, the dunging area. Only after three weeks does integration of the new and resident sows occur.[1614]

Vision is not necessary for dominance hierarchy formation in pigs, as indicated by the fact that pigs that have been temporarily blinded with opaque contact lenses form a hierarchy, although overt aggression is reduced.[656] The lack of vision has advantages for a producer, resulting as it does in less aggression if strange pigs are mixed at night.[170] Producers routinely keep pigs in dim light to reduce aggression. Anosmic pigs are not as aggressive as normal pigs, perhaps because they have difficulty discriminating among pigs.[1544]

Most aggressive behavior appears in relation to food. If trough space is limited, the subordinate pigs are forced to eat at night, and they gain less weight.[1902] Average production may be acceptable, but the dominant pigs will gain too much weight, and the subordinate ones too little.[809] Pigs may show aggression over entrance to an electronic feeder and form a queue in order of dominance.

The importance of confinement as a factor in dominance is that less aggression and milder consequences occur for subordinate pigs when they are housed outside.[1468] Crowding increases aggression in most species, and pigs show more aggression when the stocking rate is increased.[350]

Boars   A classic example of porcine sexual aggression is the confrontation of two boars. Pigs tend to use loud vocal communications in general, but two boars threatening one another are eerily quiet. They strut shoulder to shoulder, champing their jaws, from which fall clumps of thick, white saliva containing an androstenol pheromone (refer to Figure 2.5). When they face each other, they often paw the ground, a sign of aggression in many artiodactyls. The animals meet in frontal assault. They slash at each other's shoulders with their well-developed tusks, inflicting severe lacerations. The stronger pig will achieve a flank attack and, consequently, victory. The winner of a conflict usually chases the loser. Aggression between sows and barrows is similar to that of boars, except that champing and strutting are restricted to intact males.

Preventing Aggression among Newly Mixed Pigs

Strange pigs typically are mixed in two types of circumstances: when pigs are grouped by sex or size after weaning or after sale to a feeder pig operation; and when sows are grouped for breeding and gestation.

Many methods are available for minimizing aggression among newly mixed pigs: tranquilization, provision of shelters, addition of tryptophan to diet, and boar pheromone. The aggression can be reduced by tranquilizers such as azaperone 2.2 mg/kg[2215] or amperozide 1 mg/kg,[254] but these are not readily available. Head hides, small recesses in the pen into which a pig could put its head, reduce aggression.[1524] The reason that hiding the head reduces aggression is not clear. Perhaps the sight of the head stimulates aggression in the more aggressive pig. A simpler explanation is that the pig's head is protected. Furthermore, his weapons are the teeth and snout, and if they are in the hides they are not being used on other pigs. Provision of toys can reduce aggression.[255]

Simple masking odors have no effect on aggression.[168] Spraying or dabbing the boar pheromone 5a-androstenol on the pigs reduces aggression among young pigs, but not older ones.[1520–1522] Perhaps the explanation is that young pigs are always submissive to adult boars, whereas an older pig may challenge an adult male or a pig that smells like one. A more practical method of reducing aggression is to add the amino acid tryptophan and reduce the amount of other neutral amino acids because

these compete with tryptophan for the carrier across the blood–brain barrier. Tryptophan will be converted into serotonin in the brain. When fed a 0.35% tryptophan diet, aggression is reduced, especially in three-month-old pigs.[2610] When pigs are exposed to a dominant pig, those fed tryptophan have lower levels of cortisol before and two hours after the confrontation, although their behavior during the conflict is not affected.[1253] Little information exists about reducing aggression when sows are mixed, although more should be learned before gestation crates are no longer used. The presence of a boar does not reduce aggression among sows and actually increased their salivary cortisol level.[2076] Providing partitions longer than the body length of the sows and between which individual sows can eat reduces aggression. Feeding a diet diluted with water also helps.[54]

Tail Biting

Another type of aggression that is seen mostly in penned pigs housed on artificial floors is tail biting.[653] Crowding encourages the outbreak of tail biting,[655] but the main cause appears to be lack of opportunity for oral stimulation in a species that normally spends seven hours a day rooting on pasture.[881] This is substantiated by the finding that tail-biting pigs spend more time in contact with a novel object than victim or noninvolved pigs.[2253] Electronic feeder information can be used to predict tail biting because low feeding frequencies predict future tail biting in a pen as early as nine weeks before the first tail injuries. Moreover, increased feeding frequencies occur in victims before the tail biting ensues, after which they eat much less frequently.[2379] Other predictions of tail biting are the presence of one tail-bitten victim, often a small pig, and pigs with tails tucked under as if to protect them.[2174,2521] Quite possibly, bored pigs begin to nibble on each other's tails for lack of anything else to do. After a tail has been bitten severely enough to bleed and the bleeding has been aggravated as the victim swishes its injured tail, the pigs become much more aggressive and bite in earnest.[2329] The blood itself appears to be the stimulus for play to become true aggression.[750] Some pigs are killed outright, but more often losses occur as the result of infection of the wounded tails. If only one or two pigs are responsible for most of the biting, they should be removed. Often, simply giving the pigs corn on the cob to chew will stop an outbreak of tail biting that has not progressed to the cannibalistic stage. Tail biting can be reduced by providing a rooting source such as soil that is also a source of iron;[69] this soil is helpful because iron deficiency can be a cause of tail biting.[751] The incidence of tail biting increases when pigs are housed without bedding on slatted floors and are fed automatically. Feeding by hand and providing straw bedding and manipulatable objects decrease the incidence.[313] Docking of the pigs' tails at birth is performed on many hog farms. This approach eliminates the target but not the vice, and ear biting may arise instead.[1791]

Grooming

Subordinate pigs groom dominant ones. The dominant pig lies on its side, while the subordinates nibble at its belly. The pig has areas that it cannot reach with its own snout or hind feet (Figure 2.6). These areas, the flanks and back, are groomed by other pigs. Singly penned pigs scratch themselves on inanimate objects instead. If scratching seems particularly prolonged or intense, skin parasites may be present.

Pigs frequently nose one another (18 times per hour), but this behavior is unrelated to dominance. It may be an affiliative behavior or simply a means of acquiring olfactory information.[372]

Dogs

Social Behavior

Males are dominant to females in each age group. Most aggression occurs over food or

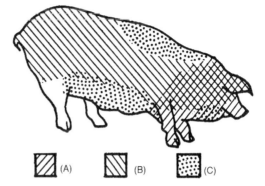

Figure 2.6 Grooming behavior of the pig. (A) The area scratched by the hind legs. (B) The area rubbed on vertical objects. (C) The area licked and nosed by other pigs. *Source:* Hafez and Signoret (1969).[881]

estrous females. Subadults are often the recipient of aggression, but juveniles rarely are.[367] The best postural correlates of dominance are high posture of the dominant and low posture, especially low tail wag, of the subordinate. In some cases, muzzle biting is a dominant gesture, whereas licking the mouth and passing under the other dog's head are signs of subordination.[2325] Inadequate socialization, inactivity, and urban living environment are associated with social fearfulness in pet dogs.[2940]

Urban dogs either are solitary or form small groups, most often of two or three, although larger groups may attend an estrous bitch.[213,243,507,508,730,1338] Social affiliation involves tail wagging, playing, allogrooming, and resting in physical contact with another dog, and is bidirectional. Social prestige is measured by the amount of submissive behavior – muzzle licking – the dog receives.

If suburban feral dogs are fed, the packs are larger – up to 12 dogs.[284] There is an interesting dynamic within these large packs; the larger the pack, the less likely an individual dog is to confront a rival pack. Dogs that are more social within the pack are more likely to confront another pack. Rural dogs form packs that often contain two to five dogs.[2069]

Regardless of the size of a canine group, social relationships are formed. The importance of a companion of the same species is illustrated by a study of dogs afraid of thunder. Their corticosteroid levels rose over 200%, but they rose less if there was another dog in the household.[577] Dogs are more likely to approach a novel object (bike, teddy bear, pail, or ball) if a pack mate, especially a related dog, is present. Higher ranking dogs investigate a novel object longer.[1621] Dogs do seem to form dominance hierarchies.[284] Resource-holding potential relies on the animal valuing the item more than it fears the other dog. For that reason, a dog might guard a bone, but not a bowl of dry dog food, from another dog or from its owners. Dominance is a function of the relation between two individuals, and in some pairs of dogs, dominance is very apparent. A dominant dog typically assumes a T-position in relation to the submissive dog's shoulder. The submissive dog turns its head away, avoiding the eye contact that might elicit an attack. The submissive animal often remains stationary because running usually elicits an attack or chase.[724] Dogs seem to be able to identify their own breed and will choose their own littermates in a two-choice test.[997] Adult males choose the scent of a nonrelated dog; presumably, this serves to prevent inbreeding.[894] There is not only preference for their own breed but also aversion to others. For instance, the attack of fox terriers will be more aggressive toward a dog of another breed. When greeting another dog sniffing is directed to the head twice as often as to the rear. Pet dogs are more likely to sniff if their owners are communicating and male dogs sniff more than females. Dogs sniffed the head as the first area on the recipient's body twice as often as the rear and ten times more often than the abdomen.[2794]

The Ainsworth separation test was originally devised to test babies' reactions to separation from their mothers, but now has been used to test attachment of dogs, horses, and cats to their owners. The test involves the owner and animal sitting in a room with a stranger. After a few minutes the owner leaves and the animal's behavior is recorded – does he wait at the door for the owner's return, does he interact with the stranger, does he play with the toys provided. The animal's reaction when the owner returns is also recorded. Will he now play with the toys or approach the stranger? An animal who is attached to the owner will not only greet the owner, but also be willing to interact with the stranger once the owner, the "secure base" is present.[3007] Dogs, but not cats, are more secure when their owner is present.[2935]

Maternal Aggression

See Chapter 5, "Maternal Behavior," for a description of pseudopregnancy in bitches that may be accompanied by aggression. There are non-maternal forms of female aggression. Spayed females tend to be more aggressive than intact ones, possibly because the source of progesterone has been removed, especially if females were outnumbered by males in their litters.[1724] Lactating bitches may aggressively protect their puppies. Pronounced aggression by a lactating bitch with a large litter may be a sign of lactation tetany.

Predatory Aggression

Guard Dogs for Predator Control

In the western United States, coyotes are the major predator of sheep; in the eastern United States, dogs are the primary predator. In both areas, guard dogs, not herding dogs, have been moderately successful. The breeds used are the Anatolian Shepherd, Maremma, Shar Planinetz, Spitz, Komondor, and Great Pyrenees. Great Pyrenees are best when small predators such as coyotes are involved, but the larger, more aggressive Shar Planinetz may be necessary when wolves or bears are the predators. From 60 to 70% of sheep producers who use these dogs believed that they were economically beneficial. The major problem is that 25% of the guard dogs injure or kill the sheep themselves, but most dogs can be trained not to chase the sheep.[456,852] Bonding sheep or goats to cattle may be a better means of reducing losses from predation.[58,60,1084] The bonding will succeed more often if only one heifer is added to a flock of sheep.[58] If two or more heifers are present, they may not stay with the sheep. Llamas and donkeys have also been used as sheep-guarding animals. Dogs can be used to guard cattle, but care must be given to introduce them only after they have been bonded to a calf at 6–10 weeks, and later are introduced to adult cattle at three to six months.[2349]

Cats

Free-Ranging Cats

It has been hypothesized that cats have formed social groups only since they were domesticated and that the behaviors used in social encounters are derived from kitten-to-mother behavior.[314] Feline social organization is very variable. Group size varies from fewer than 10 on most farms to more than 30 in some urban areas where an abundant food source is located in a confined area.[2298]

In a rural setting, cats have territories as large as 200 ha per female cat and 600 ha per male cat,[1432,2298,2483] or 1 cat/km^2, whereas in an urban setting the density can be 1000 cats/km^2 (or ~2,000 cats/mi.^{2}).[514,1669] Cats were considered to be a nonsocial species because they do not live in groups as adults if they are living on natural prey,[2298] but cats have been able to modify their social organization and live in groups, even multi-male groups. Cats can adapt to a concentrated food source such as that found in dumps, fishing villages, and farms by living in groups, but these groups are of matrilineal female kin. Females rarely transfer from group to group, although males can. In general, the dominant tom's territory encompasses the females' (Figure 2.7). Although he will not hunt on the females' territories, he will repel any marauding male, and the females will repel any female intruder. The larger the male's home range, the more female territories he encompasses and the greater his reproductive success. The males may make excursions outside their home range to mate with additional females.[2036] When free-ranging urban cats were studied, intact females were bolder (would approach a rat in a cage or jump into a box for food) than neutered females, and a positive correlation was found between cortisol levels and food dominance scores.[316]

Crowell-Davis and her colleagues have studied several groups of free-living cats and found many signs of affiliative behavior, especially cheek and tail rubbing of other group members.[175,474,486]

Confined Cats

Social Aggression

When two cats approach each other aggressively, they walk on tiptoe, slowly lashing their tails about the hocks and turning their heads from side to side while making direct eye contact. This threat may intimidate a subordinate cat so that it slinks off; evenly matched rivals will continue to approach one another (Figure 2.2). They will walk slightly past one another before one cat will spring, trying for a grip on the nape of the opponent's neck. The attacked cat throws itself on its back, thus protecting the nape. The two adversaries will both lie on the ground belly to belly while they claw, vocalize, and bite at each other. After a few moments, one cat, usually the original attacker, will jump free. The other cat may adopt a defensive posture, attack, or run away. The victor usually pursues the vanquished.[1361] Cats that are aggressive toward other cats are not necessarily aggressive toward people, and vice versa.[2298] Poor socialization to humans and a history of being a rescue cat were associated with higher fearfulness.[2887]

Cats that are compatible will rub one another and sleep together and groom one another. Cats may also rub on their owners after a separation.[3051] When placed together in a home, laboratory, or farm, cats will form dominance

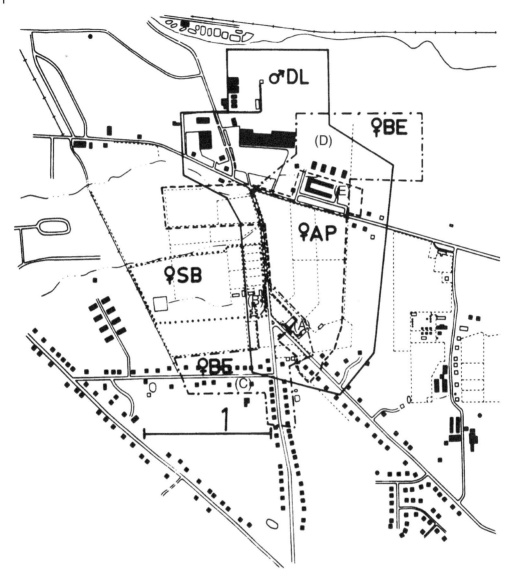

Figure 2.7   Ranges used concurrently by three adult female (AP, BE, and SB) and one adult male (DL) cats in 1979. AP and BE shared three of four barns at the home farm (A) and most of the yards and pastures immediately surrounding the barns. SB was the only female at her farm (B). BE used the southern section of her range (C) through most of 1978 and 1979, and started using the northern area (D) in the late summer of 1979 in a series of foraging excursions with that year's litter. One female kitten remained and eventually reproduced in this section of the range, whereas BE and a male kitten disappeared from this area in late 1979. The two sections of BE's range were connected only by the road between SB's and AP's ranges; BE hunted frequently along the road shoulders, and SB and AP foraged only in the adjoining pastures. AP and BE shared the area around an apartment complex (E), but never were noted to contact one another there. DL's range included large areas of each female's range, and on most evenings DL visited each barn complex at least once. The enclosed line at the lower end of the map represents 500 m. Immediately above it, the north–south axis is indicated. Dark quadrangles represent homes, apartments, and stores; open quadrangles, barns and other outbuildings. Narrow dotted lines indicate fence lines. *Source:* Wolski (1982).[2483]

hierarchies,[172,439,1314] but marked aggression may persist in this originally solitary species. When feral cats, who voluntarily determine the group composition, are studied, a hierarchy emerges that varies with body size in females and age in males.[2500] More closely related cats are less aggressive.[317] The rank of cats for food may differ from their rank in social space in intact female laboratory cats,[600] but it is the same in a large group of neutered cats of both sexes confined in one household and yard.[1241] Larger, older cats and male cats tend to be dominant over smaller, younger female cats. Cats may divide up a house: one's territory may be the first floor, and the other's the second floor. Roommates may find that the two cats belonging to one person will gang up on the single cat belonging to the other. Urination in the house, especially on beds or rugs, often occurs when strange cats are introduced. Cats in multi-cat household may or may not be stressed, but are less aggressive to people.[2742,2729] The method of forming multi-cat households – littermate kittens versus unacquainted adults – probably accounts for the different outcomes. Cats in groups are most apt to aggress just before feeding.[2718] Cats with high cortisol and testosterone concentrations established less contact with others, and individuals with high oxytocin concentrations did not exhibit affiliative behaviors as much as expected. Additionally, the higher the frequency of contact among the individuals, the greater the similarity in gut microbiome.[2834] See Chapter 9.

Territorial Behavior

Males maintain nonoverlapping territories in the nonbreeding season, but overlap considerably in the breeding season. Therefore, in both free-ranging and pet cats, intraspecies aggression among intact male cats is a very common problem. Many tomcats are presented repeatedly for treatment of bite wounds and abscesses resulting from fighting behavior. Castration is approximately 90% effective in eliminating roaming and fighting in adult male cats,

although the disappearance of one behavior may not be associated with a decline in the other.[930]

In highly concentrated populations in which cats compete for food, males are dominant over females. The larger, older males are dominant over younger, smaller ones in competition for food or for females.[2500]

Cats can form harmonious social groups, but adding a new cat leads to fighting in 50% of households, and there is a greater risk of fighting if the cats are allowed access to the outdoors. Ten percent of the cats are still aggressive a year after introduction.[1350]

Predatory Behavior

The tall posture of the cat engaged in territorial or sexual aggression is to be contrasted with the stalking posture of predatory aggression. The predatory cat carries its body as closely as possible to the ground. It moves toward its quarry slowly, taking advantage of any natural cover. The closer the cat gets to its prey, the more slowly it advances. Almost inevitably, the cat will pause before leaping to attack. Only the tip of the tail will move as the cat lies in wait. There are usually two or three bounds from hiding to the prey. When attacking a large animal, cats try to make a nape bite to sever the spinal cord.[1361]

Predatory aggression is innate but has some learned aspects. Kittens raised with a mother who killed rats in their presence killed at their first opportunity; kittens raised alone seldom did, whereas those raised in a cage with a rat never did.[1247] Apparently, kittens learn to direct various innate predatory motor patterns to the prey (see Chapter 6) their mother brings to them. She does not simply let them eat the prey; she lets the prey go and catches it again. If the kittens attempt to catch or eat the mouse, the mother will compete with them for it. In this manner, the kittens are stimulated by the hunting game and, apparently, learn by observation. The types of prey brought to the kittens may influence the range of prey hunted by the kittens as adults. Although the mother can influence kittens' predatory skills by bringing prey and interacting with it, adult cats without such learning experience also become competent predators, so a kitten that is not a good hunter can acquire the skills as an adult.[2298]

Most cats will kill rats if fasted for two or more days, but they still prefer to eat commercial cat food rather than their prey.[5] Success of predatory attempts can be lowered by fitting the cat with a belled collar, a collar that emits beeps every seven seconds, a colorful ruff, or a bib.[888,1684] The number of prey animals taken by owned cats is controversial because they are a threat to birds and endangered species. Only 20% bring prey back to their homes; they either consume or simply leave it. The use of video cameras worn by the cat made possible true estimates of the rate of predation. House cats catch prey every other day.[2589] The species of prey will vary with the environment, from amphibians in the southeastern United States to rodents in rural England and ground-foraging birds in many areas. Feral cats kill three times more than owned cats, resulting in the death of over one billion birds and seven billion mammals in the United States each year.[1414]

One feline characteristic that is distasteful to some people is that cats sometimes play with their prey before and after it is dead. They will catch a mouse, let it go, and catch it again. After it is dead, they will throw it up with their paws and leap upon it. The function of this behavior is obscure, although it may be appetitive or, perhaps, displacement behavior, but it does indicate that the difference between predatory play and true predation is small. Truly hungry cats rarely play with prey; they eat it as soon as it is dead and they have recuperated from the predatory effort.

Grooming

Feline grooming is an important part of daily activities. Cats sometimes lick one another; this is most likely to occur when a mother continues to groom her adult offspring, but long-term associates also allogroom, and licking is part of courtship behavior. The more closely related and

the longer cats have co-habituated, the more likely they are to groom one another.[493] One of the simplest types of grooming is licking the nose and lips. These are two distinct motions that rarely overlap. Licking the nose occurs after gaping, for example, and the tongue goes dorsally on the midline and then is pulled immediately vertically and into the mouth. A common licking problem is an exaggeration of this behavior in which the nose is chronically irritated by the abrasive tongue. Licking the lips involves movement of the tongue along the edge of the upper lips to the corners of the mouth; this behavior is seen after eating or drinking.

Feline face washing always occurs in an invariant pattern. The cat is in a sitting position and applies saliva to the medial aspect of the front leg, which is held horizontally. The paw is rubbed from back to front over the nose with a circular upward motion. This motion is repeated a few times; each time, the paw reaches out a little farther until it reaches behind the ear (only after three rubs) and then travels downward over the ear, forehead, and eye. Other areas of the body are cleaned, but not in the invariant order in which the face is washed. The tongue is drawn over the coat in long strokes, mostly in the direction of the hair. If deprived of grooming by an Elizabethan collar, for example, cats will groom more when again free to do so, indicating the importance of the behavior. Grooming functions in external parasite control; we know this because when they are prevented from grooming, cats have more fleas.[619]

During normal grooming, the saliva applied is licked up again, but in a hot environment the saliva is allowed to remain to aid in thermoregulation. The neck, chest, shoulders, and front paws receive the most grooming. The stomach, rear legs, back, croup, tail, and anal areas receive less attention. All the former regions are licked as the cat sits. The cat lies to lick the sides, stomach, rear legs, tail, and front paws (Figure 2.8).[1361] A cat may sit like a bear on its haunches to lick the penis; this can be a sign of urethral obstruction. Grooming can also be a post-conflict

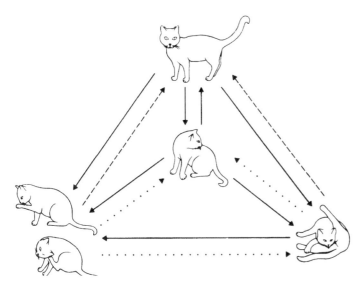

Figure 2.8 Grooming postures of the cat. (Top) Non-grooming. (Center) Flank grooming. (Clockwise) Grooming of hindquarters; scratching ears; the first step of face grooming, licking the front leg. Solid arrows indicate grooming sequences of normal cats. Dotted and dashed arrows indicate sequences in cats with tectal lesions. *Source:* Swenson and Randall (1977).[2212]

(cat–cat or cat–human) stress response.[2323] It is easy to understand how psychogenic overgrooming can result when a cat is stressed.

Clinical Problems of Canine and Feline Aggression

Inactivity and urban living environment are associated with social fearfulness in pet dogs.[2040] Poor socialization to humans and a history of being a rescue cat were associated with higher fearfulness.[2887] Female cats and cats whose owners said "No" or picked them up when they misbehaved were more likely to be aggressive. [2914]

Beaver,[208] Borchelt and Voith,[290] Hart et al.,[932] Hunthausen,[1092] Landsberg et al.,[1037] Overall,[1745] Stelow[3105] Deneneberg,[3084] and Horwitz and Nelson[863] have addressed the problem of aggression in dogs and cats as well as other less common behavior problems.

3

Biological Rhythms and Sleep and Stereotypic Behavior

Introduction

Animals do appear to have a sense of time, which can explain the phenomenon of the dog that wakes up and stands at the door shortly before the owner appears at the end of the working day. Pigs remember when they have been confined for a longer or shorter period in identical cages and will choose the place where confinement was shorter.[2161]

One should be aware of the activity and sleep patterns of animals so that abnormality can be detected. A horse that is lying down at night is probably sleeping; an adult horse that lies down during the day (especially a cold, cloudy day) is abnormal and should be observed carefully because this is an unusual time for a horse to be recumbent. Time budgets can be used to examine welfare.[2654]

The patterns of behavior, especially those of activity and sleep, reflect internal rhythms. There are several types of rhythms of differing duration. The circadian rhythms, occurring in approximately 24-hour periods, are the best known and best studied. The activity cycles of most animals are circadian in that the periods of activity and inactivity add up to approximately 24 hours. Other types of rhythms are high-frequency, ultradian, infradian, and annual cycles. Biological clocks are found in single cells. The various clocks appear to be linked in a hierarchal organization that allows temporal coordination. The master clock appears to be located in the suprachiasmatic nucleus.[1683]

High-Frequency Rhythms

High-frequency rhythms, for example heart and respiration rates, occur in periods of less than 30 minutes. Heart rate varies inversely with body weight, so the heart rate of a cat (110–130 beats per minute) is considerably higher than that of a horse (28–40 beats per minute). Respiratory rate does not vary linearly with body size, so the cow breathes 10–30 times per minute, and the pig 8–18 times per minute. Respiratory cycles have an effect on cardiac rate, which increases during inspiration. This effect, called "sinus arrhythmia," is more marked in dogs than in other domestic species. The endogenous nature of biological rhythms can be best appreciated by a consideration of the contraction rate of the embryonic heart, especially that of the chick embryo, which does not have even the maternal heart rate to influence it.

Ultradian Rhythms

Ultradian rhythms are more frequent than 24 hours; one example is the fluctuations of growth hormone output from the pituitary,

Domestic Animal Behavior for Veterinarians and Animal Scientists, Seventh Edition. Katherine A. Houpt.
© 2024 John Wiley & Sons, Inc. Published 2024 by John Wiley & Sons, Inc.
Companion website: www.wiley.com/go/houpt/7e

which in cattle occur in 3.5-hour cycles.[268] Body temperature also varies in ultradian cycles of approximately one hour in cats.[952] The physiological bases for, or influences upon, these short cycles are unknown but are believed to result from oscillations of cells in central pattern generators. A most interesting ultradian behavior rhythm is that of feeding. When food is available ad libitum, nearly all species eat 9–12 meals a day. This pattern is seen in dogs and cats,[1172,1643] sheep,[406] horses,[1315] pigs,[246] and cattle.[1878]

Circadian Rhythms

A circadian rhythm is self-sustaining, is maintained under conditions of constant light or dark, and has a cycle of approximately 24 hours.

Zeitgebers

Circadian rhythms are endogenous, that is, they persist under conditions of constant light or constant dark; but they usually are influenced by, and entrained to, external factors, which set the biological clock. Some of these factors are temperature, barometric pressure, various drugs, hormones, and light. Of these factors, the most important is light. These factors are called *zeitgebers* (German for "time givers") because they set the rhythms just as one might set a clock.

Light

Circadian rhythms are entrained to light; that is, although under conditions of constant illumination a rhythm may have a period of approximately 24 hours, under naturally occurring light, the rhythm will be that of the light–dark cycle. The light must be present during a specific portion of the endogenous rhythm. Hamsters, for example, entrain to a 12-hour-light/12-hour-dark day and to a 6-hour-light/12-hour-dark day, but not to a six-hour-light/30-hour-dark day.[631]

Considerable practical advantage has been taken of the entraining function of light to bring mares into estrus early or, conversely, to avoid injuries during hierarchy formation by keeping pigs in the dark. Even the simple act of putting a cover over a parrot's cage makes use of the effect of light on avian activity. The photoreceptors responsible for entraining circadian rhythms are not the same as those for vision, and some may even be extraocular.[376] Not all types of light are equally effective in entraining circadian rhythms. Green light is most effective and red light is least effective; therefore, red light may be used when visibility is desirable but interference with an animal's circadian rhythms and dark activities is not.[1535] When *zeitgebers* are removed, the resulting desynchronization of internal rhythms may have deleterious results; for example, thermoregulation may be impaired.[767] When one travels, *zeitgebers* are removed or are not present at the proper period of time in the endogenous rhythm, causing jet lag because rhythms are not synchronized.

Barometric Pressure

The influence of other factors on circadian rhythms has not been as well studied, but barometric pressure has been shown to influence activity patterns. Mice show higher activity levels when barometric pressure is increasing.[2163] Although the phenomenon has never been quantified, farm animals, such as horses and dogs, show high levels of activity before storms, and tail-biting episodes often occur in swine just before storms.

Drugs

Drugs can affect rhythms. Examples are caffeine and theophylline[623] and lithium.[536,1153,1516] The action of lithium on the circadian rhythms of humans and animals may be the basis for its amelioration of depression and aggression. The two compounds that may be useful for treatment of jet lag and sleep disturbances are melatonin (see the "Pineal Gland" section) and benzodiazepines.[2077,2296]

More important from a clinical standpoint is that a given drug may have a greater effect and/or have lower toxicity at one time of day than at another. Hypoglycemic agents, if administered while liver glycogen and plasma glucose are low, are more apt to precipitate hypoglycemic convulsions than if administered at another point in the cycle.[1154]

Pineal Gland

The pineal gland is probably an important intermediary in the synchronization of circadian rhythms because it demonstrates marked rhythms of output of several hormones and neurotransmitters.[788] Melatonin is produced by the pineal gland and is present in higher quantities in plasma and cerebrospinal fluid at night (Figure 3.1).[964] Melatonin has an antigonadotropic effect in long-day breeders and a pro-gonadotropic effect in short-day breeders. It may be the means by which the hypothalamus is informed of day length, the link between circadian rhythms and annual sexual cycles, for melatonin would increase as dark-period length increases, and the increased melatonin levels would depress gonadal activity. The practical application of this role of melatonin is that short-day breeders such as sheep may be brought into estrus earlier by oral administration of melatonin in the afternoon for several months.[80] Efficacy of melatonin for treatment of behavior problems remains to be investigated.

The peak level of the neurotransmitter serotonin is 180° out of phase with melatonin. Serotonin is a precursor of melatonin. The activities of the enzymes catalyzing the reaction (serotonin to melatonin) are influenced by light.[1517] Day length will influence the relative amounts of serotonin and melatonin present in the pineal gland, thereby influencing the organism's sleep–wakefulness cycle and reproductive condition. Aggressive behavior also may be influenced. Most owners are bitten by their dogs at night, when serotonin levels are low. Drugs that increase serotonin activity decrease aggression.[1745]

Examples of Circadian Rhythms

In addition to gross activity, a number of cellular and endocrinological parameters vary in a circadian rhythm. Many hormones have been demonstrated to have circadian rhythms. Corticosteroids, including both cortisol and corticosterone, increase during the day in pigs and horses, with peak levels in late morning (Figure 3.2).[298,2432] The peak of cortisol precedes that of activity by about five hours in horses.[813] Optimal athletic performance may be achieved when exercise times and competition times coincide because exercise influences circadian gene expression.[2896]

Both salivary and serum cortisol peak in the morning, but the amplitude of the salivary circadian variation is much smaller.[275] Horses that do not show circadian patterns of cortisol secretion are at risk of colic.[1325] Both pigs and horses are diurnal (day-active) animals and show diurnal peaks in adrenocortical activity and adrenal responsiveness to adrenocorticotropic hormone (ACTH) during the day, whereas cats show increased adrenal activity at night.[2059] In stallions and boars, testosterone levels are highest during the day.[628,1229] Some hormones, such as vasopressin in the cat, show circadian rhythms in the cerebrospinal fluid but not in the blood.[1928]

There are age-related effects on the expression of circadian rhythms. For example, although there are circadian rhythms that occur in cortisol concentration in adult dogs, rhythms are not observed in either puppies or old dogs (>12 years of age).[1761] These age-dependent changes may be related to some of the problems of restlessness seen in older dogs (see Chapter 7, "Learning").

Not all hormones are secreted in greatest quantity during the day in diurnal animals; growth hormone, for example, decreases in output during the day in pigs.[2277] Circadian rhythms of heart rate, body temperature, white blood cell number, metabolic rate, liver glycogen and glucose, and glucose absorption from the gut have also been identified.[107,647]

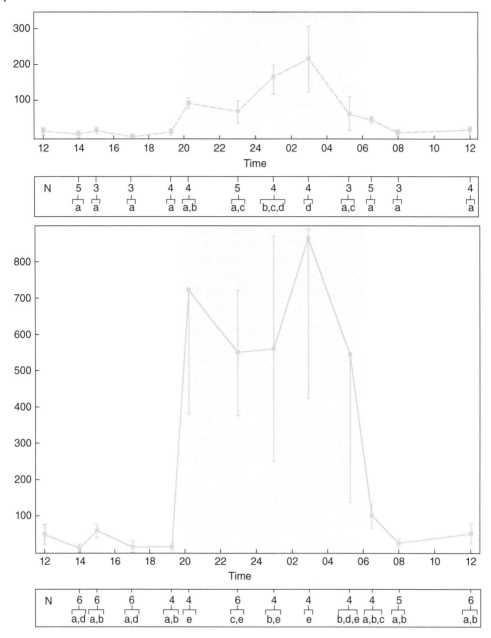

Figure 3.1 Nyctohemeral cycle of melatonin concentration in calf plasma (upper) and cerebrospinal fluid (lower) at selected times of the day. The lights were on from 0600 to 2000 hours. Data points are means ±1 standard error of samples from number (N) of calves. Letters indicate that when two means do not have any letter in common, they are significantly different. *Source:* Hedlund *et al.* (1977).[964] Reproduced with permission of The American Association for the Advancement of Science.

Dogs show circadian rhythms of body temperature that have a period of 23.7 hours.[1174] There is a circadian rhythm of body temperature in calves, peaking in the afternoon and reaching a nadir in early morning.[1431] Not all hormones exhibit a circadian rhythm. Insulin-like growth factor, unlike cortisol, has no circadian rhythm in horses.[1699] Lactate

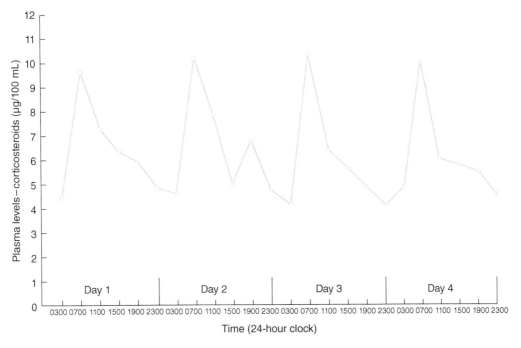

Figure 3.2 Circadian rhythms of corticosteroid secretion in pigs. The graph is based on the mean results from six pigs. The peak of corticosteroid output occurs in late morning. *Source:* Baldwin and Stephens (1973).[143] Reproduced with permission of Elsevier.

and urea show diurnal changes, but in opposite directions so that the postprandial efficiency of protein metabolism is greater, whereas efficient carbohydrate metabolism is decreased after an evening meal in comparison to a morning meal.[1253]

Feeding

Feeding not only is rhythmic but also can entrain other rhythms. When an animal has meals imposed on it instead of freely feeding (the situation for most domestic animals), the animal anticipates the meal with an increase in activity. In order for this rhythm to be entrained, the meal must contain calories.[1604] Daily variations occur in activity and core body temperature of sheep, but these are entrained by feeding.[1814] And a period of activity occurs approximately 24 hours after a meal (when one meal a day is fed).[1605,2346] Rhythms of intestinal enzymes are also secondary to feeding.[698] Although animals usually drink prandially, that is, at the time they eat, evidence exists that drinking bouts may have a different rhythm than feeding. Goats drink mostly just before dawn and just after dark.[1981]

Other Rhythms

Infradian rhythms have cycle periods less frequent than 24 hours. Circatrigintan rhythms are rhythms of approximately 30 days. The sexual cycles of polyestrous domestic animals show periods of approximately three weeks. The sow and cow come into heat every 21 days. Examples of species that are seasonally polyestrous include the mare, which comes into heat every 17–24 days in the spring, and the ewe, which comes into heat every 16–17 days in the fall.[669] These cycles may represent rhythms of hypothalamic, pituitary, or ovarian activity.

Annual Rhythms

Annual or seasonal cycles are somewhat better understood. Horses and sheep are seasonal breeders. Horses are anestrous in the fall and winter, and begin to show estrus as day length increases in late winter. Sheep show an opposite response in that they begin to be sexually active when days shorten in the fall. The evolutionary advantages to both species are obvious. The offspring of horses and sheep are born in the spring, when food is abundant. Dogs now show sexual cycles of approximately six months' duration, but there is reason to believe that they, too, were once annual breeders. Basenjis, for example, still show an annual fall breeding season.[2066] Domestication, abundant food, and selective breeding also may have caused cattle and swine to become polyestrous throughout the year rather than during one season.

Not all annual cycles are reproductive. Cats show annual cycles of corticosteroids, thyroxine, and epinephrine levels. Peak levels of these three hormones occur during the winter.[2013] More familiar are the cyclic changes in hair coat. Hair-follicle activity in cats is highest in late summer and lowest in late winter, and as a result, fur is 0.5 mm (0.2 in.) longer in winter than in summer.[2013]

Adult ewes show a seasonal variation in heart rate, with a minimum in winter. In wethers, serum concentrations of prolactin, insulin, insulin-like growth factor, and thyroxine were all higher in the spring and summer than in the fall or winter; meal sizes were also larger when the days were longer.[1931]

Horses show seasonal rhythms in carbohydrate metabolism, but these may be related to training.[823] In a seminatural environment, horses also show a decrease in intake from 10 kg/day in late summer to 7 kg/day in late winter when the losses of body heat while foraging are greater than the gain from nutrient-poor winter forage.[1284]

Sleep Functions and Types

Sleep occupies one-quarter (for ruminants) to one-half (for dogs) of the lifetime of animals, but the function of sleep remains unknown. One possible function is replenishing of neurotransmitters. A device to conserve energy, a means of remaining inconspicuous, a period for consolidation of memory, or simply a way to fill up time not needed for foraging are other hypothetical functions of sleep.[2515]

Sleep can be classified into two types: the "sleep of the mind," slow-wave sleep (SWS), or quiet sleep; and the "sleep of the body," paradoxically active, or rapid eye movement (REM) sleep. The two types can best be differentiated from wakefulness and from one another by means of electroencephalography.

The electroencephalogram (EEG) of the alert animal is characterized by low-voltage, fast waves that are not synchronized. SWS is characterized by synchronous waves of high-voltage, slow activity. During paradoxical sleep, the EEG shows low-voltage, fast activity similar to that seen in the wakeful state (Figure 3.3), but very little muscular activity occurs; therefore, this type of sleep is called the "sleep of the body." Although overall muscle tone is very low during paradoxical sleep, the muscles of the eyes frequently contract, hence the term "rapid eye movement." The low-voltage, fast activity of REM sleep does not result in many body movements because the medulla has an inhibitory area that, in effect, paralyzes the muscles of the body.[1629] Humans awakened from REM sleep report that they have been dreaming; the twitching of the face and legs (which are not completely inhibited) and whining during canine sleep indicate that dogs may also be dreaming. We can only speculate as to the presence or content of animal dreams. Total deprivation of either type of sleep is fatal. Deprivation of REM sleep results in behavioral abnormalities in all species

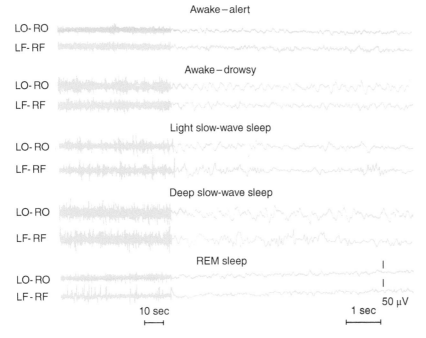

Awake – alert

LO- RO

LF- RF

Awake – drowsy

LO- RO

LF- RF

Light slow-wave sleep

LO- RO

LF- RF

Deep slow-wave sleep

LO- RO

LF- RF

REM sleep

LO- RO

LF- RF

10 sec   1 sec   50 µV

Figure 3.3   The stages of vigilance and sleep in the cat. Polygraphic record at the speed of 30 mm per second showing the stages identified. LO-RO: electroencephalographic record from the left and right occipital area; LF-RF: electroencephalographic record from the left and right frontal area. *Source:* Ursin (1968).[2308] Reproduced with permission.

tested, and rebound or extra REM sleep occurs during recovery from deprivation.[1992,1993,2309]

Patterns of Sleep and Activity in Domestic Animals

Sleep varies considerably among species.[378] The activity patterns of the various species described here are reported under specific environmental conditions. The behavior patterns may be different under different environmental conditions, and, therefore, the numbers given should not be considered applicable to every animal under every condition. One hypothesis is that sleep time is inversely related to the danger of predation for a given species.[48] See Figure 3.4 for activity patterns of three species in the same pasture.

Dogs

Sleeping dogs often lie in a characteristic posture with their hind legs tucked up and their heads turned caudolaterally. Their eyes may be open or closed. REM sleep may be accompanied by leg movements, vocalizations, and either polypnea or apnea. A dog awakened abruptly from REM sleep may bite, so it is best to let dreaming dogs, or at least sleeping dogs, lie, or to awaken them gently. Dogs show short periods of activity interspersed with periods of rest when free ranging,[213] when tethered outdoors,[2505] and when caged.[951] Dogs are likely to sleep less during their first two days in the shelter.[3019] Shelter dogs slept for 660 minutes over the 24-hour period (72% of the nighttime and 3% of the daytime).[3088] Kenneled dogs spend less time lying or sitting inactive in a noisy environment, while increasing the time

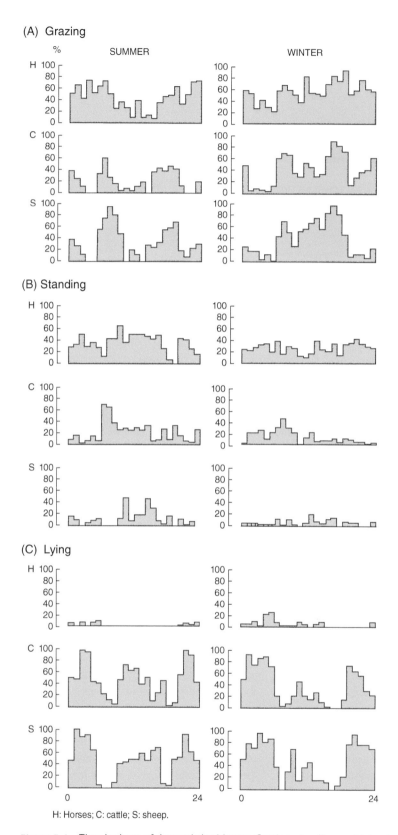

(A) Grazing

(B) Standing

(C) Lying

H: Horses; C: cattle; S: sheep.

Figure 3.4   Time budgets of domestic herbivores. Grazing, standing, and lying behavior of cattle, sheep, and horses living on the same pasture during two seasons. *Source:* Arnold *et al.* (1981).[95] Reproduced with permission of Elsevier.

they spend standing and in locomotion. Dogs sleep less as environmental temperature rises.[2973]

Pet dogs appear to sleep at night, but their behavior may be entrained to that of their owner (see Figure 3.5). Active (REM) sleep occupies only 6% of their time.[10,11] Dogs sleep in cycles of 16 minutes asleep and 5 minutes awake. House dogs and caged dogs sleep more than free-ranging dogs, but even the latter sleep 60% of the night.[12] Dogs that were more attached to their owners showed longer non-REM sleep (NREM) sleep duration during a visit to a laboratory with their owners.[2690] Dogs show more REM sleep and less drowsiness after a negative interaction (separation from owner and a threatening stranger) than a positive interaction (playing and petting).[2829]

Dogs show a "first night effect" in that they napped less during the first two days they were taken to a laboratory, especially if they had fewer experiences of sleeping away from home.[2947] Meal patterns affect sleep in that napping bouts decreased and napping duration increased in dogs fed twice daily rather than once daily. Twice-daily feeding was also associated with earlier sleep onset time at night and onset of morning activity, as well as shortened sleep interval. Older dogs sleep more during the day and arise later in the morning.[2515]

Although sleeping dogs are relatively easily roused, owners who wish their dogs to guard property must be aware that dogs will sleep where they are most comfortable, that is, on soft surfaces and not necessarily at the property line.[12] In the case of caged dogs, 30-minute to two-hour periods of activity alternate with longer quiescent periods. Dogs in groups in kennels spend 7–24% of their time in active behavior (walking or trotting), 5–10% socializing with other dogs, and the majority of the time inactive (sitting, standing, or resting), with 20% of inactive time in light slow-wave sleep (LSWS), 25% in deep slow-wave sleep (DSWS), and 10–12% in REM sleep.[1009,1016,1075] Dogs position themselves so that they can see other dogs, but neither their activity level nor

their barking rate changes when other dogs are visible.[2417] Free-ranging feral urban dogs are most active in early morning and in the evening. Foraging for food, usually garbage; socializing with other dogs; and traveling from alley to street to park are their major activities and are usually interspersed with periods of rest.[213] Similar periods of activity occur just after sunrise and an hour or two before sunset in sled dogs tethered to their doghouses by 240 cm (8 ft.) leads. Under these conditions, dogs spend more than 80% of their time, night and day, lying down and sit only 2% of the time, mostly while observing another dog or a person.[2505]

Dogs exhibit similar behavior patterns whether in runs or on a tether; they are mostly lying down.[2505] Dogs with access to an outdoor run are more active and are outside for over 2 h/day in 100 trips/day.[2157] Dogs housed in group pens spend 40% of their time inactive, 12% moving around, and 5% in maintenance behaviors such as eating and eliminating.[1706]

A pet dog's activity is controlled by its owner. Dogs are walked or let out early in the morning when their owners arise and in early evening when their owners return from work.[243] A peak can also occur at noon in communities where people apparently return home for lunch.[1338] Dogs left at home during the day spend most of their time lying down, with smaller percentages of time spent orienting to their environment, whining, or playing. Dogs sleep more as they age.[3038] In mild climates, people often confine their dogs in their backyards rather than in the house. These dogs spend most of their time inactive, but do walk, run, chew, and explore. They spend a lot of time visiting the door into the house. Problems in these dogs such as barking and chewing were more likely to occur in untrained dogs.[1243]

The behavior of dogs in shelters is important because of concerns about long-term welfare of dogs that are not adopted in a no-kill (euthanasia only for medical problems or aggression) shelter. Time spent sleeping can be used as an indicator of welfare.[3030] Interaction with a human for 15 minutes a week results in dogs

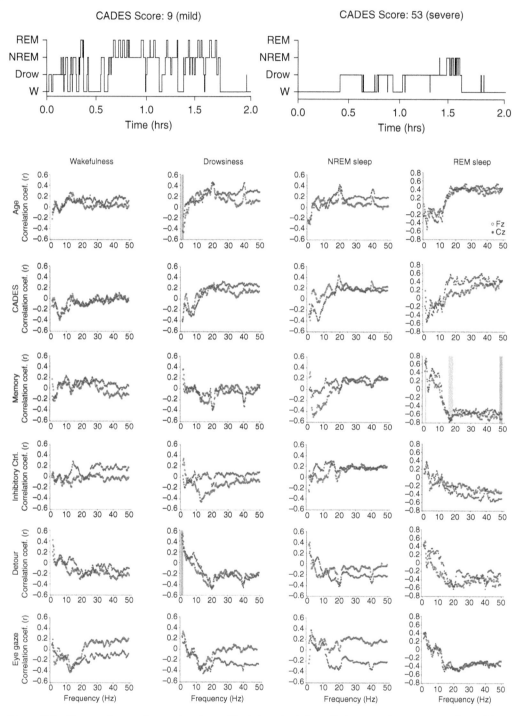

Figure 3.5 Sleep patterns of normal and cognitively impaired dogs. Cades score is a measure of cognitive impairment. Red lines indicate dogs with cognitive dysfunction.

that spend more time visible to the public and that wag their tails more often, which should increase adoptability.[1706]

Cats

General Activity

In the laboratory, cats, like dogs, show short bursts of activity (one to two hours of activity distributed throughout the day) and are 1.4 times more active during the day than at night.[2186] During the day, group-housed laboratory cats spend 36% of their time in maintenance behaviors such as resting, sitting, ingesting, or eliminating and another 30% in comfort behaviors such as grooming and stretching. A quarter of their time is spent in motion.[1832] Caged cats in shelters spend 70% of their time in alert (easily disturbed) rest, 11% asleep, 14% sitting, and 6% active.[1278] Catnip and the odor of prey animals have soporific effects on cats, decreasing their activity and increasing their sleeping time.[633] When caged cats are presented with television for 3 h/day, they spent only 6% of their time looking at it, but if the program showed moving objects, animate or inanimate, the cats slept less.[634] Disruption of schedule can result in sickness behavior in cats, so consistency in the environment of caged cats is very important.[2628] Farm cats spend 40% of their time asleep, most of it at night. The rest of the farm cat's time is divided into 22% resting, 14% hunting (although this will vary from cat to cat), 15% grooming, 3% traveling, and 2% feeding.[1764] Feral cats living on a barrier island were inactive 90% of their time, roaming 9% of the time and 0.9% hunting, but they were provided with food, which may account for the low percentage of hunting.[2787] Cats can wear cameras to allow their activity and location to be identified.[2803] Global positioning system (GPS) tracking has allowed us to determine just how active and far cats range. Danish cats roamed over 1–113 ha (2.5–225 acres).[2786] Unowned cats shift home range seasonally probably reflecting prey availability, but owned cats do not.[2691]

Indoor cats show circadian changes in activity and feeding which change seasonally; they are most active during the spring and fall. They are most active at night. Cats are minimally active and least likely to be eating at midnight and midday.[2926] When cats kept indoors for 23 h/day were compared to cats with free access to the outside during the day and forced to remain outside at night, the outside cats were much more active, especially at night, indicating the indoor cats were adjusting their rhythms to that of humans.[1817] Cats are more likely to interact with food enrichment objects in the morning than in the afternoon, so owners should adjust their behaviors accordingly.[504] Compared with the younger age groups cats in the prime age group (3–7 years) showed a significant reduction in physical activity, which then remained constant in the mature 7–11 years and senior (11–15 years) age groups.[2983] See Figure 3.6.

Sleep

Caged cats spend 10 h/day sleeping. SWS occupies 39% of the day, and REM sleep 8%. During REM sleep, the nictitating membrane covers the eye. SWS of cats, like that of dogs, can be subdivided into LSWS and DSWS, based on electroencephalographic characteristics and ease of arousal.[2308] The usual sequence of sleep stages in the cat is from wakefulness to LSWS

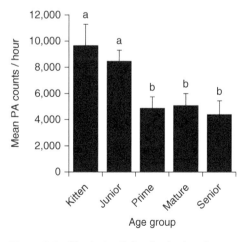

Figure 3.6   Physical activity of cats at various ages.

to DSWS to REM to either LSWS again or to wakefulness. The two major sleep epochs occur at night. Drowsiness varies with feeding schedule. Cats fed three times a day drowse more than those fed once a day, and fasted cats drowse even less.[1995] Older cats (>10 years of age) show less REM sleep, more SWS, as well as briefer episodes of wakefulness than do younger cats.[305]

Elimination

Because house soiling is such a common behavior problem of cats, it is important to know how often they eliminate and the behaviors that surround the act of elimination. Cats eliminate three to five times a day. They spend 12 seconds digging before elimination; sniff the litter for 18 seconds afterward, especially if it is within their core area (where they spend 75% of their time); and cover for 12 seconds.[2204] House-soiling cats dig less before eliminating, implicating litter qualities such as odor or texture as factors discouraging cats from using the litter. Cats avoid fecally contaminated litter.[2822]

Pigs

Pigs, despite thousands of years of domestication, still forage optimally, that is, they obey the marginal value theorem and spend longer in each food patch when the cost of moving from patch to patch is higher.[871] Pigs are active from 0500 to 2100 in the summer and somewhat fewer hours in the winter. Twenty percent of their time is spent rooting, even in the presence of *ad libitum* food.[3107] Under most modern conditions, pigs usually are kept in confinement so that the seven hours of rooting (e.g., food searching) noted on pasture[2491] fall to two hours per day of eating in a pen. If all oral, nasal, and facial activities are summed, sows housed outdoors spend 46 minutes of the two-hour post-feeding period engaging in these behaviors in comparison to the 26 minutes spent in those ways by crated sows.[498] Sows living outdoors with access to shelters spend 25% of their time foraging and half their

time outside, but newly farrowed sows spend 85% of their time in the shelters.[353]

Pigs in a seminatural environment spend 24% of their time rooting.[2993] The hungrier pigs are, the more time they spend rooting and the less time lying down. When kept in pens and supplied with peat in which to root, pigs still spend 10% of their time rooting, indicating that the behavior persists even when no food reward occurs.[2198] Hunger, too, may predispose to tail biting by increasing rooting time.[519] Increased time spent rooting results in decreased time spent manipulating pen-mates, a behavior that leads to tail biting. The motivation for rooting can be hunger or curiosity (approaching novel stimuli) about the environment, which is the reciprocal of boredom (avoiding familiar stimuli). The ideal rooting material can be manipulated and destroyed, like straw or peat.[2198] Frustration (e.g., from the presence of inaccessible food) leads to changes in behavior. Oral activity is increased, and the pigs are more likely to sit or lie on their sternums and less likely to lie on their sides, which is the more relaxed position.[1357]

Pigs in sounders of 12 travel 600 m/day, although those kept in groups of six traveled less and activity decreased as the pigs grew.[323] Pigs spend more time resting than do any other domestic animals.[939] They are recumbent 19 h/day. They drowse 5 h/day. SWS occupies 6 h/day. REM occupies 1.75 hours in 33 periods. Pigs are characterized by extreme muscle relaxation during sleep (see Figure 3.7). Evaluating muscle tonus in a 400-pound sow is difficult, but when a sleeping piglet is picked up, it is as relaxed as a rag doll. Only 1–3 h/day are spent in other activities, such as drinking, walking, playing, or fighting.[741] Domestic pigs are diurnal; therefore, most activity takes place during the day.[1630] As do most diurnal species, pigs have higher melatonin levels during the scotopic, or dark, phase of the day; however, particularly bright light is necessary for entrainment.[859] Although motor activity and food intake increase during the day in pigs, these rhythms disappear in constant light,

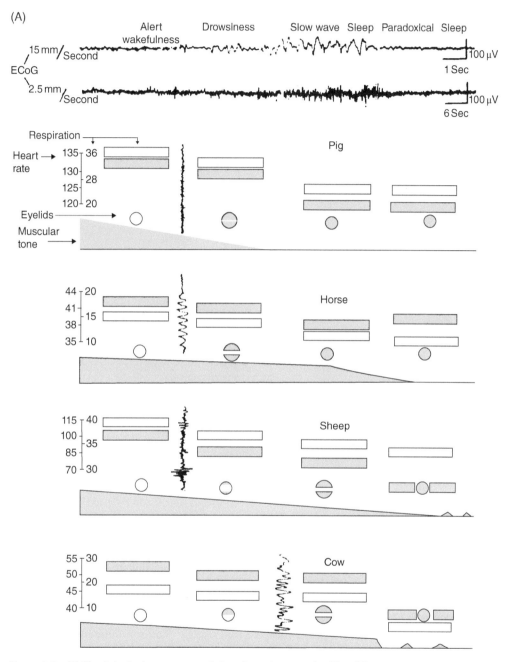

Figure 3.7 (A) Physiological parameters of sleep in various species. The different electrocorticogram (EcoG) patterns for each species are shown at a speed of 15 mm per second: theta rhythm (horse), delta rhythm (ruminating cow), spincles (sheep), and alpha rhythm (pig). (B) Mean comparative data of sleep and wakefulness states and of postures during nighttime. The inner circle shows the relative duration of the EcoG pattern (rapid eye movement [REM] in dark green), and the outer circle shows the relative duration of the postures. *Source:* Ruckebusch (1972).[1992] Reproduced with permission of Elsevier.

(B)

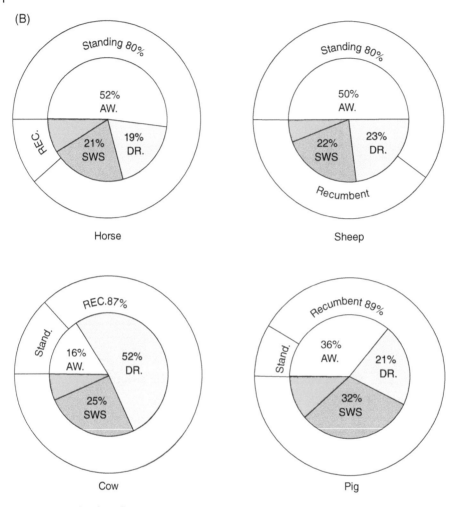

Figure 3.7 (Continued)

indicating that they are not circadian. Rhythms of body temperature depend on feeding and do not occur in pigs fed ad libitum.[1112] Pigs can entrain to nine hours of light and nine hours of dark, as well as to 12:12 cycles.[1113] There are changes in feeding behavior with changing intensity of light. Pigs use different feeding strategies during different times of the day: from 0700 to 1400 h, pigs behave as "nibblers and slow eaters"; from 1400 to 2000 h, pigs show a "meal eater and fast eater" strategy; and, from 2000 to 0700 h, animals followed a "meal eater and slow eater" strategy.[683]

Feral pigs and wild boars are more nocturnal in habit during the summer months, probably to avoid predation. Even wild pigs are not very active. Trapping and re-trapping indicated that sows were usually found within 0.3 km (0.19 mi.) of the point at which they were originally trapped; boars were within 2.0 km (1.24 mi.).[1469] The sex difference may be in range rather than in activity.

Circadian rhythms are disrupted by changes in physical, social, or reproductive conditions. For example, putting a pig into a group after it had been housed individually, or tethering a pig, will disrupt circadian rhythms of cortisol for one to four days, as will surgery or estrus.[214]

Pigs defecate four to seven times a day; the number decreases with body size and age.

They urinate three to five times a day. Elimination mainly occurs during daytime following the activity and drinking pattern.[2647] When kept in partly slatted pens, pigs will lie on the slats when the temperature is warm and increase the number of defecations on the solid part, probably because there is little space on the slatted portion.[1100]

Horses

Equine activity varies with the season; during the summer, locomotor activity, resting heart rate, and total water turnover are greater than in winter.[334] Horses are most active at the vernal equinox and least active during the winter solstice. They are most active at the middle of the photoperiod.[2536] Horses are able to drowse and even to engage in SWS while standing by means of the unique stay apparatus of the equine limbs, but they lie down[885] when engaging in REM sleep. The horse in REM sleep lies either in lateral recumbency or in sternal recumbency with its muzzle touching the ground so that its head is supported during the atonia accompanying that phase. See Figure 3.8 for lying and rising postures. A healthy horse seldom remains lying when it is approached, probably because a standing horse is better able to flee or to defend itself.

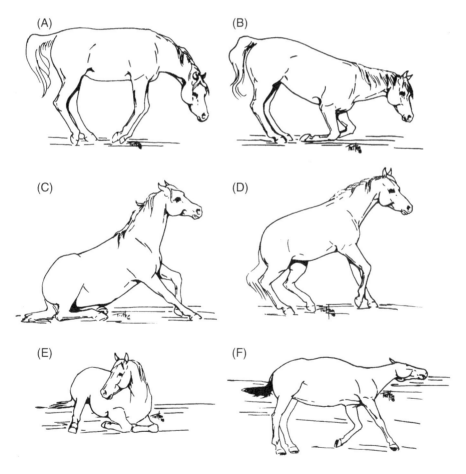

Figure 3.8   The postures of the horse when lying down and getting up. (A, B) Lying down; (C, D) getting up; (E) sternal recumbency: the horse not lying symmetrically but with the lateral surface of one foreleg on the ground; (F) lateral recumbency: the upper foreleg anterior to the lower one. The horse exhibits REM sleep in (F) or in (E) with the muzzle touching the ground.

A dominant stallion lies down first, that is, before subordinate horses lie down.[1994]

A review of 12 papers revealed that horses spend 10–64% of their time eating, 8–66% resting, 3–27% lying, and 0.02–19% in locomotion.[2654] During the day, the horse is awake 88% of the time, and during most of this time the animal is alert. Nighttime grazing also increases when days shorten. Both changes serve to keep grazing time, and therefore food intake, constant.[594] Even at night, the horse is awake 71% of the time, but it drowses for 19% of the night.[1994] Stabled horses are recumbent 2 h/day in four to five periods. Ponies are recumbent 5 h/day, and donkeys even more.[1403] SWS occupies 2 h/day, and REM sleep occurs in nine five-minute periods. Horses, in contrast to ruminants, show tachycardia, leg movements, and an increase in respiratory rate during REM sleep.[1994]

Management practices can affect equine sleep patterns. Sleep time has implications for equine welfare.[2767] Forced activity influences sleeping time in horses. Racehorses subject to training on continual days have lower physical activity in the nighttime than those that train on intermittent day.[2959] They lie down more when stalled alone than when in a group.[3040] Playing classical music to horses for several hours a day increased the time they spent eating and decreased the time they spent standing alert, indicating relaxation.[2805]

Previously stabled horses sleep less on pasture; they do not lie down during the first night, and total sleep time remains low for a month. Horses prefer bedding to no bedding.[1089] Bedding affects how long horses lie; they lie longest on coconut husks, rarely on sawdust or coconut fiber, and for an intermediate time on straw.[1654] They also are in lateral recumbency and REM sleep for a longer time on straw than shavings.[823,2423] Care must be taken not to deprive horses of sleep inadvertently. This is most apt to occur when horses are transported long distances or when they must be tied in straight stalls. If horses are tied short in a straight stall so that they cannot lie down, they may not have REM sleep. The horses compensate by sleeping while free during the day. Diet also affects length of sleep in horses as it does in ruminants. An increase in lying occurs when the protein content of grasses increases in the spring; a similar trend, an increase in lying, occurs when oats are substituted for hay. Fasting has the same effects.[500,501]

Horses turned out for two hours a day as a group lie down more than those restricted to a box stall.[2421] Ponies on pasture lie 7% of the night, 2% in lateral recumbency. Lying in lateral recumbency occurs almost always in the hours just after midnight. In stalls, the same ponies lie 12% of the time, probably in response to the drier stall environment. Horses can be seen lying in lateral recumbency during the day, usually after bad weather has kept them from lying down. Horses fitted with a urine collection harness lie down for only 0.5% of the time, in contrast to control mares who lie down 3% of the time.[1160] Horses feed, lie, stand, and travel, but the main activity is feeding, either grazing or eating hay when that is available as a free choice. Grazing time varies from 50 to 80% of the 24 hours, taking place both day and night. The time of day when grazing takes place varies with the presence of biting insects.[595,1194] Horses graze 15 minutes less for every extra hour of sunlight per day in the spring. Lactating mares graze more than barren or pregnant mares, reflecting the greater energy demands of milk production. Table 3.1 lists the percentage of time spent grazing by different populations of free-ranging or pastured horses and ponies. There are breed differences in activity patterns. Thoroughbreds move, eat, and drink more often than Haflingers.[3040]

The circadian rhythms of most of our domestic animals are influenced by the provision of meals. This is especially true of herbivores, such as horses and ruminants, who normally would have access to grass at all times and whose hour-to-hour behavior would not depend on access to food. The large amount of time occupied by oral behavior indicates the reasons for the appearance of oral stereotypies,

Table 3.1 Percentage of time grazing by various populations of free-ranging feral horses.

					Time of day (h)									
0600	0800	1000	1200	1400	1600	1800	2000	2200	2400	0200	0400	Season	Population	References
98	95	33	85	70	80	80	81	–	–	–	–	Winter	W. Alberta	2619
100	65	45	90	70	80	92	80	–	–	–	–	Summer	W. Alberta	2619
80	77	83	83	75	72	75	–	–	–	–	–	Summer	Assateague Is. MD–VA	1190
–	–	–	–	–	–	–	63	53	53	40	70	Summer	Assateague Is. MD–VA	2576
					55–64[a]							Winter	Camargue, France	593
					51–60[a]							Summer	Camargue, France	593
					25–50[a]							Summer	Grand Canyon, CO	238
80	80	75	85	80	85	70	75	70	–	–	–	Winter	Shackleford Is., SC	2618
70	70	60	55	50	60	65	65	60	–	–	–	Summer	Shackleford Is., SC	2618

[a] Average percentage of time spent grazing over total time period.

such as wood chewing, in stalled horses on low-roughage diets.

Insects also affect equine time budgets and locations. Horses swish their tails 29 times an hour, skin twitch 11 times an hour, and shake their heads three times an hour. When flies are prevalent, tail swishing increases to once a second (360/h) and skin twitching to 13 times a minute.[3108] These behaviors are reduced on cool, windy, rainy days.[2564] Biting insects drive the horses to refuge in snow, water, barren areas, or indoor shelter when available.[595,1194] Rolling and self-grooming maintain the horse's coat. Horses roll daily, mostly in the morning for about 30 seconds, and prefer soil to straw or sand as a substrate.[2597]

The amount of traveling a horse does depends on two things: the availability of nutrients and the horse's social status. Young bachelor stallions travel more than harem stallions or mares, but otherwise, the distance that must be traveled to procure water or enough forage determines the amount of movement.[239] Isolated horses walk considerably more than those in sight of other horses. This type of walking, like that of the bachelor stallion, is presumably a search for companions. Camargue horses grazing on a large pasture walk 7–10% of the day, as do horses in a grassless corral.[593,1051] Rapid traveling, that is, trotting and cantering, occupies a very small fraction (less than 1%) of the time budgets of adult horses studied in a variety of environments.

Pasture or paddock design influences activity. Horses in rectangular paddocks make many more abrupt turns than those in square ones. The abrupt turns and stops can lead to leg injury.[1288] Horses do not spend as much time traveling at night as they do during the day. Ponies on lush pasture walk 3% of the night, whereas stalled horses and ponies walk less than 1% of the night. If hay is provided ad libitum, the time that fresh hay is added does not affect the activity period, which is diurnal.[1816] Horses are more active if the resources are distributed through the paddock and available only at prescribed times.[1968]

Rolling is a form of self-grooming by horses. Horses roll frequently following intense exercise when they have sweated. They paw and sniff at the substrate before rolling and may rub their neck. They may roll completely over, from right to left side, for example.[2858]

Standing is the behavior that occurs when horses are not engaged in acquiring food, socializing, or sleeping deeply. Standing increases when feeding decreases (see Table 3.2 for time budgets of horses and ponies on a variety of diets, and Table 3.3 for time budgets of tethered horses) and when horses are satiated. Foraging in the bedding of the stall is a sign of hunger.[1696] Standing is also influenced by weather conditions in pastured horses. Horses stand rather than lie when it rains, and stand 20 minutes more per day for every Celsius degree drop in environmental temperature.[594] They stand in the shade during times of peak summer solar radiation and spend more time moving and eating in the shade.[1022] Shelter should be provided for horses because when the weather is windy and either rainy or snowy, horses will seek shelter, although overall use is low.[978]

Many riding horses are stalled most of the day and turned out in paddocks of varying sizes. The larger the paddock, the more active the horse, but 45 minutes of exercise on an automatic walker decreased activity in all paddock sizes.[1163] When turned out with another horse in a 35 × 10 m paddock, horses travel 2 km in two hours; less if they have just been ridden.[2421]

Horses turned out for only 2 h/week trot, canter, and buck, but graze less than those turned out 12 h/week. Similarly, horses confined for two weeks are more active when released than those turned out daily.[2571]

The activity of mares is higher in the three days prepartum than postpartum. Most interesting is that the acrophase (highest point) of locomotor activity of mares is opposite to that of their foals, who are more active when the mare is inactive.[814]

The time budget of a young horse depends on the housing. When first placed in individual

Table 3.2 Time budgets of stabled horses and ponies

Time/equid	Environment	Diet	Percentage of time					
			Feeding	Standing	Moving	Drinking	Lying	References
Day/horse	Metabolism cage	Limited hay	50	45	0	1	4	2636
		Concentrates	32	62	0	1	5	2210
Day/pony	Box stall	Ad libitum hay	76	19	3	2	1	2209
Day/horse	Corral	Limited hay and grain	53	27	6	–	0	1051
Night/pony	Box stall	Limited hay and grain	15	17	1	–	13	1089
Night/horse	Box stall	Limited hay and grain	27	67	0.3	–	6	2093
24 h/pony	Pen	Ad libitum grain	17	–	–	2	–	1315
24 h/pony	Pen	Ad libitum pellets	31	–	–	–	–	2616
Day/pony	Pasture		53	34	0.6		2	947

Table 3.3 Time budget of tethered horses.

Feeding	Standing	Stand resting	Lying	Drinking	References
50–58	19–22	20–24	1	2	2553
48	8	39	0	1	1062
32	25		6.7		2599
36	58	19	6	1	2607

stalls, two-year-old horses eat less, are more often vigilant, but sleep more than pair-housed horses. Although this difference in feeding and sleep disappears after two weeks in individual stalls, the individually housed horses continue to nibble walls and buckets, neigh, snort, and paw more than group-housed horses.[2363]

Time budgets of Przewalski horses have been recorded in various zoos, semi-reserves, and the wild in Mongolia. The biggest difference is in walking, which increased when the horses were released into the wild and persisted for at least three years. The increased locomotion is most marked in the stallions,[308,310] although this was not observed

with all Przewalski.[2990] The reason for this increase in walking may be increased vigilance. Seasonal differences appear, with horses grazing more at night in midsummer. Activity is lowest in the winter and highest in the late summer (see Table 3.4).[237] In fact, during the Austrian winter, heart rate and body temperature of Przewalski horses dropped, increasing again in May.[98]

Stereotypic Behavior Problems in the Stable
Predisposing Factors
The prevalence of stereotypic behaviors varies from 5 to 16% in the United Kingdom and appears to be higher in Canada.[1419] Among

Table 3.4   Time budget of Przewalski horses.

Graze	Stand	Rest	Move	Environment	References
55	8	20	17	Free in tundra	308
46		35	11	Free in Gobi Desert	2991
54	12	24	8	Enclosure	308
51	20	13	13	Pasture	2539
48[a]	24	7	15	Yard	237
68[a]	18	0	12	Small pen	2540
44[a]	45	0	8.5	Large pen	2540

[a] Feeding.

Thoroughbreds, most stereotypic behavior was seen in mares and two-year-olds. A horse with one stereotypy is more likely to exhibit another.[1596] Lack of a variety of roughage, non-straw (shavings or paper) bedding, three meals per day, and few horses in the immediate environment are all risk factors.[1531,1532] The use of the horse was also important. Dressage and three-day-event horses and racing Thoroughbreds had a greater prevalence than did endurance horses and racing Standardbreds.[1531,1910]

Equine stable problems, the so-called vices, can be divided into oral and locomotor behaviors. These problems may be classified as stereotypies because they are repetitive, serve no known function, and occupy a large part (>10%) of the animal's time.[2967] Prevalence of stereotypies varies with the use to which a horse is put. Dressage horses have more stereotypic behavior than eventing and riding-school horses.[943] Cribbing, licking or biting walls and feeders, lip- or tooth-rubbing tongue play, and wood chewing are the common oral stereotypies, whereas stall walking, pawing, and weaving are the common locomotor behaviors. Although confinement is common to all these problems, cribbing and wood chewing appear to be influenced by diet. More than half of two-year-old Warmbloods placed in individual stalls for the first time begin to stall walk, weave, or crib.[2363]

Cribbing Cribbing is an oral behavior in which the horse grasps a horizontal surface (such as the rim of a bucket or the rail of a fence) with its incisors, flexes its neck, and aspirates air into its pharynx. Some horses aspirate air without grasping an object. This is called "aerophagia" or "windsucking"; the latter term can also be used to refer to pneumovaginitis. It was thought that the horse swallows the air, but this does not usually occur unless the horse is swallowing food between cribbing bouts.[1529]

Cribbing occurs in association with food, in particular eating grain or other highly palatable food.[824,1287] See Figure 3.9 for an illustration. The relation of cribbing to eating is similar to that of nonnutritive suckling in calves that occurs after drinking milk. Cribbing rate is highest during the eight hours following feeding.[432]

From 2.5% to 5% of Thoroughbreds and 0 to 6% of other breeds crib.[20,1048,2340] Cribbing occurs less frequently in endurance horses (3%) than in those used for dressage or eventing (8%), who are confined in their stall for much longer periods.[1531] When horses used for dressage were compared to those used for eventing, voltage, or lessons, the dressage horses were more likely to have multiple stereotypic behaviors, especially cribbing.[2567] Cribbers are less anxious than non-cribbers but equally trainable.[1666]

It is a clinical impression that cribbing occurs more frequently in confined horses, but once established, it may persist even when the

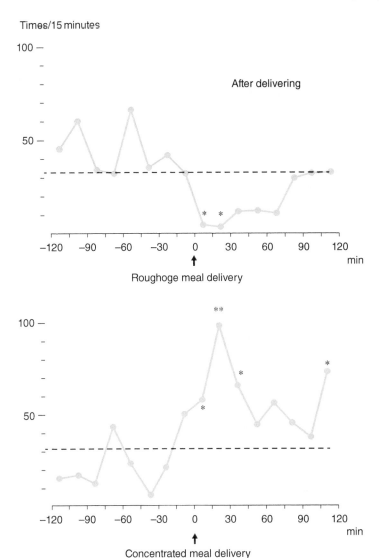

Figure 3.9 Mean frequency of cribbing before and after delivery of roughage meal (upper graph) and concentrated meal (lower graph). Dotted line indicates the mean level. *$P < 0.05$; **$P < 0.011287$.
Source: Kusunose (1992).[1287] Reproduced with permission of *Jpn J Equine Sci.*

horse is on pasture. It may be the cause, rather than the result, of gastrointestinal problems. Aspirating air or inflating the pharynx may be a pleasurable sensation to an animal. Although the opiate blockers such as naloxone will inhibit cribbing, opiates fall or do not change in the blood when horses crib.[558,1787] In fact, horses that crib have lower or similar blood levels of opiates than those of non-cribbing horses, but the blood levels may not reflect brain levels.[824,1787] There is a higher tactile sensitivity in crib-biters, in that they react (twitch the skin) more than non-cribbers to touch using Von Frey hairs (filaments consisting of a hard plastic body connected to a nylon thread, and calibrated to exert a specific magnitude of force on the skin, ranging from 0.008 to 300 g) although their responses to novel or frightening situations was similar to non-cribbers.[2753,3052]

Horses are more, not less, sensitive to pain when they crib.[1599] Cribbers seem to have less vagal tone – that is, their resting heartbeat is higher than that of non-cribbers. Cribbers do show an increased cortisol response to exogenous ACTH administration.[759] The anti-inflammatory cytokines interleukin-4 (IL4) and IL10 are higher and the pro-inflammatory cytokine TNF (tumor necrosis factor) is lower in cribbing horses.[18] When horses are deprived of the opportunity to crib, gastrointestinal motility slows.[1533] In addition, horses prevented from cribbing show more stress-related behavior than those who are free to crib.[1665] Cribbers have a higher level of ghrelin, a feeding-stimulating hormone, than non-cribbers and their gastrin levels in response to concentrates are higher, but they have no more gastric ulcers.[980,2440]

The simplest method used to prevent cribbing is to place a strap around the throat just behind the poll so that pressure is exerted when the horse arches its neck and even more pressure is exerted when the animal attempts to swallow. The horse is, in effect, punished for cribbing. If a plain strap does not suffice, a spiked strap or metal collar, or one that is held in place with a head stall, can be used. A common observation of a horse wearing a cribbing strap is that it continues to grasp horizontal objects with its teeth but does not swallow as much air. Many stables are designed or modified so that few horizontal surfaces are available, but water and feed containers usually provide the horse some opportunity to crib. Shock has also been used to punish horses that crib.[135] Muzzles may also be used. These are wire baskets that permit the horse to eat and drink but not grasp a horizontal surface. Some horses learn to grasp a stick, pull it into the muzzle vertically, and crib on that. The muzzles seem more frustrating for the horse than the straps, and the horse will try to pull them off. When horses are prevented from cribbing by a cribbing collar, they may show a post-deprivation rebound; that is, they crib more than they did before the collar was applied, but this is not observed in horses that have been cribbing for some time.[1533,2524]

There have been a variety of surgical treatments for cribbing. These treatments include buccostomy; cutting the ventral branch of the spinal accessory nerve (ninth cranial); myotomy of the ventral neck muscles; or a combination of partial myectomy of the omohyoideus, sternohyoideus, and sternothyrohyoideus and neurectomy of the ventral branch of the spinal accessory nerve.[693,716,855,895,1178,1747,2053,2297] The success rates of these treatments vary from 0 to 70%, and they are no longer recommended. More recently, extensive laser surgery of the ventral neck has been found to be 90% effective, but horses that have cribbed for a long time are less likely to stop cribbing.[529] Cribbing "braces" – rings placed over the horse's incisors so they cannot make contact with a surface – are initially effective, but can cause infections and frequently fall out or move out of place.[2524]

Beginning at 20 weeks of age, 10% of foals crib. Foals begin to crib when they are weaned into stalls and fed concentrate diet; those weaned on pasture do not begin to crib.[2391] One hypothetical result of cribbing is an increase in gastric acidity due to the oral stimulation (cephalic phase of digestion) of gastric acid output. Ulcers are more numerous and more severe in foals that crib.[1692] Dietary reduction of the cribbing rate may be possible by feeding antacid.[1596,1692] Another – not necessarily contradictory – reason is that some component of concentrate diet stimulates cribbing. When the cribbing rate was measured for 30 minutes before and after various feeds were given, it rose from 2/5 minutes to 27/5 minutes when the horse was eating sweetened grain or pellets, but rose to only 8/5 minutes when alfalfa pellets were fed.[758] Although it could be any of the grains – corn, oats, and soybean – the most likely culprit is molasses. Oats are least likely to stimulate cribbing, even when constituting 50% of the diet.[2635] Although toys may not help with oral problems, provision of a simple foraging device that delivers food as the horse rolls it might help.[1450,2475,2635]

Increasing the frequency of meals appears to reduce cribbing but increase locomotor stereotypies.[451]

Is it necessary to prevent cribbing? There are health risks to the horse, the most important of which are colic (in particular, epiploic foramen entrapment), temporohyoid osteoarthropathy, and excessive wear of the incisor teeth.[75,76,857] The rate of epiploic foramen entrapment is higher, possibly because air-filled viscera migrate around the abdominal cavity, especially when the horse exerts negative pressure while aspirating air. Abdominal pressure increases when a horse cribs.[2643]

Damage can be done to fences or to buckets because the horse exerts great pressure (~50 lb.) when flexing its neck. Cribbing is also considered to be contagious, and it has been shown that being stalled next to a cribbing horse increases the risk of cribbing; the same study showed that being stabled next to an aggressive horse increases the risk of cribbing much more.[1664] When owners of cribbing horses were surveyed, only 1% of horses exposed to a cribber began to crib.[20] Young horses may be more likely to learn the habit from an adult than are other adults.

Wood Chewing Both cribbing and wood-chewing (lignophagia) horses grasp horizontal surfaces with their teeth, but the wood-chewing horse actually ingests the wood, whereas the only damage the cribbing horse does is to mark the wood with its incisors. In contrast to cribbing, wood chewing appears to have a definite cause: a lack of roughage in the diet. Wood chewing is more common in dressage and eventing horses than in endurance horses which spend more time outside their stalls.[1531] Several investigators have noted that high-concentrate diets or pelleted diets increase the incidence of wood chewing. Feral horses as well as well-fed pastured ponies have been observed to ingest trees and shrubs, so it would seem that there is some need or appetite for wood even when grasses are freely available. Farm managers are well aware that trees,

especially young trees, must be protected from horses on pasture. Three-quarters of horses on Australian pastures ingested bark or wood.[2322] Horses cannot digest wood; nevertheless, there may be some role for indigestible roughage in equine digestion. Wood chewing increases in cold, wet weather.[1121]

Eliminating edges, covering edges with metal or wire, and painting the surface with taste repellents are the traditional methods for preventing horses from wood chewing, but providing more roughage is a better practice both behaviorally and nutritionally. If roughage is provided, the horse's motivation to wood chew is reduced rather than thwarted. An increase in exercise also reduces the rate of wood chewing.[1279]

Locomotion Problems

Stall Walking and Weaving This behavior may often occur as part of a herd-rejoining behavior, in which case more visual contact with other horses or a stall companion will help. In other cases, it is claustrophobia, in that the confinement itself, with or without other horses, is a problem. Finally, stall walking may occur as a stereotypy – a repetitive, functionless behavior. This form of stall walking is usually slower than the others, but is more difficult to interrupt. Horses that constantly circle their stalls may lose condition or fail to obtain it because they expend more energy walking than they ingest. Their performance is usually affected as well. Restraining the horse by tying it often converts a stall-walking horse into a weaver. Weaving is a behavior in which the horse stands in one spot but shifts its weight and its head from side to side, and it may involve lifting each hoof in turn and walking in place. The cause of the behavior appears to be confinement. The treatment is to maintain the animal on pasture with a run-out shed for shelter. Other treatments are stall toys and more work. The size of the stall does not seem to influence the stall-walking behavior; a horse given access to an entire barn still circled in one corner. Stress appears to aggravate the problem; horses circle more frequently the evening before a hunt or show. A small dose of tryptophan did not have any calming effect.[125]

Weaving may be similar in etiology to stall walking. It is a stereotypy that appears in many zoo animals as well. Confinement and frustration are causes, and horses in pain may also weave. There is some evidence that stall walking and weaving may be inherited and possibly related to endogenous opiate production.[559,2340] The form of self-stimulation probably offers the horse some comfort, as rocking does to humans. Horses may "nod" by raising and lowering their heads, especially when food is anticipated. Tail rubbing is also probably a form of comforting self-stimulation, but medical causes must be eliminated.

Weavers have higher levels of blood serotonin than non-weavers, whereas ACTH, thyroid-stimulating hormone, and melatonin are lower in weavers.[250] There are differences in the cytokine levels for normal and stereotypic horses: IL4 and IL10 levels were higher in cribbers, and TNF was lower in both weavers and cribbers.[18] Cortisol levels do not differ between stereotypic and non-stereotypic horses, indicating there is no difference in stress levels.[774] Stereotypic horses yawn more often than those that show neither motor nor oral stereotypies.[772]

Increasing the frequency of meals increases weaving and nodding. Anticipating food when other horses are fed has the same effect.[452]

Providing a horse with more opportunity to look out of its stall, or providing a mirror, can decrease weaving.[450,1483] It is interesting that a view of another horse reduces weaving, but horses that face one another in a stable are more likely to weave than those who do not face another horse.[1695] The stall door may be the critical factor as an obstacle between one horse and its companion. Weaving occurs before feeding and is negatively correlated with the amount of hay fed.[1695]

Pawing　Pawing is a response to frustration, a displacement activity that originated from the activity of uncovering food buried under snow.[1720] Horses have been noted to paw in a variety of situations: when restrained from moving, when eating grain, when expecting feed, at a recumbent foal that does not stand, and in order to reach another horse. The most extreme forms of pawing occur in horses that have barrier frustration, that is, they are seeking to escape from their stalls. A typical case is that of a Standardbred that had spent most of its life on pasture with a run-out shed for shelter. When confined in a box stall for training, it dug a hole measuring 1.5 m (4 ft.) in depth in his stall. Some horses habituate to stall confinement eventually; others may do extensive damage to themselves and the stalls as they try to escape by jumping over the walls. Pawing is a less dangerous activity, but it damages dirt or clay floors.

Pawing is exhibited by Standardbreds, but in many cases, the horses stand in the hole they created, taking pressure off their hindlimbs. In this case, the behavior has a function: comfort or pain relief.[2543] The second cause of pawing is an attempt to reach another horse. Horses are herd animals, and stallions, in particular, try to reach one another to play if they are young or to fight if they are mature. If dirt floors are replaced with concrete, the horses will stop pawing, but their motivation has not changed. The stallions may rear up to reach one another over stall walls that do not reach the ceiling or lean out the front of the stalls to make contact if that is possible. A concrete floor can be hazardous when slippery and is more stressful to the horses' limbs and feet because it is a rigid surface.

Pawing in anticipation of food is similar to kicking in anticipation of food and is discussed in the next subsection, "Stall Kicking." Pawing at recumbent foals may serve to stimulate the foal but can injure a foal, especially if the foal is unable to rise and the pawing continues for some time. The reason why horses paw when eating grain is unknown. One hypothesis is that they may be responding to the highly palatable food that can be prehended quickly, which are too unnatural, and therefore frustrating, qualities.

Stall Kicking Aggressive kicking is discussed in Chapter 2. Only kicking directed against stall walls is considered here. Most horses kick stall walls with their hooves; a few knock their hocks against the wall. Both activities produce unwanted concussion on the horses' bones and joints. Kicking can damage the walls as well. A small hole made by kicking is often enlarged by wood chewing. Stall kicking may also be a form of self-stimulation. The horse kicks to hear the sound its hoof makes as it strikes the wood. Sometimes, stabling a horse on a wooden floor that makes a similar sound (hoof on wood) as the horse walks on it will eliminate the kicking.

The most common form of pawing and kicking is that which the owner has operantly conditioned. The horse will tend to paw or kick at feeding time because it is frustrated to see or smell food (or the giver of food) but not be able to eat. This is reflected physiologically in the increase in heart rate observed in horses that see feed. The horse is, of course, fed, so the animal's behavior has been positively reinforced. It has learned that kicking or pawing is followed by food. The horse paws, and food appears. It will begin to paw or kick earlier and earlier. In effect, it is increasing the fixed ratio of number of responses (paws or kicks) for every reward. The longer the horse kicks before feeding, the longer it will take to extinguish the behavior. In order to extinguish the behavior, the owner should feed the horse only when it does not kick. The process will go much more quickly if many small meals a day are given. The horse must at first refrain from kicking for only two seconds before it is given a half cup of feed. Gradually, the criterion is raised so that there must be no kicking for 5 and then 10 and then 30 seconds before food will be given. Only when the horse refrains from kicking for a short time for several feedings or trials should a longer time be demanded. The training will go faster if the horse is taught a counter-command such as "Stand" for a food reward at the same time.

Recently, a depressive state has been described in horses. These animals stand with their head lowered, are not as responsive to their environment, and fail to habituate at the same rate as normal horses.[773,1944]

Head shaking is rarely a behavior problem.[1441] A lesion anywhere in the head or neck, especially in the nasal cavity, can cause head shaking. Some horses react to bright light with a reflexive sneeze. Goggles, essentially sunglasses, can help. Others are allergic and will head shake seasonally.[1441] These horses can be helped by a net over their noses.[1594] There have been many suggested drug treatments. Cyproheptadine and carbamazepine appear to be most helpful. One case was resolved by infrared diode laser deflation and coagulation of corpora nigra cysts.[240]

Narcolepsy

Narcolepsy is characterized by attacks of inappropriate sleep.[719] A familial syndrome occurs in Miniature horses, Fell ponies and Suffolk Punch horses and it can be triggered in foals by holding them and in adults by tightening the girth.[1420] Narcolepsy occurs in horses as well, but it must be distinguished from the much more common problem in which a horse goes into normal SWS and collapses when he goes into REM sleep without having lain down.[3064] This is most apt to occur when the horse is reluctant to lie down, because the substrate is too hard, he is uncomfortable socially, or the horse will be in pain if he flexes his limbs.

Cattle

Cattle are essentially diurnal. Their major activities are grazing, ruminating, and resting. Feral urban cattle (street cattle) exhibit peaks of foraging at noon, of activity at 1600, standing at 1900, and lying at midnight.[2964] Cattle lie down to sleep, to ruminate, or to drowse. Lying occupies nearly half the cow's day; when deprived of the opportunity to lie down, it will compensate by lying for longer periods when it is free to do so. This compensatory behavior indicates that rest is necessary. In fact, when both rest and food deprived, cattle lie down rather than eat when given the opportunity to do either.[1570] When limited in the time they can spend feeding, lying, or in social interactions, cows prioritize lying, but may compensate for the decreased time spent feeding by eating more quickly so that caloric intake is not reduced in proportion to the decrease in time spent feeding.[1648] Many cattle are kept indoors now, and the amount of space can be limited. As space increases from 2.5 to 4 m^2/animal, the time spent lying stretched out increases and the number of times an animal steps on another decreases.[875]

Lying occupies 13 hours of a dairy cow's day in a loose-housing environment, but this time will be reduced if the housing contains fewer cubicles than cows.[2450] Lying time is affected by the environment. Loose-housed cattle spend less time lying than cattle in tie stalls, although their feeding times are similar.[1269] Stall design has a large influence on the ease with which the cow lies. If the number of free stalls is diminished, the cattle lie less and stand idle in the alley more, but still spend 5 h/day eating.[1011] Apparently, feeding is a protected behavior. Dairy cows housed indoors have the shortest total lying time, 10.2 h/day, whereas beef cows at pasture lie 11.6 hours and indoor-housed beef cows lie 10.5 hours. The probability of cows standing up increases with lying time, but the probability of cows lying down does not increase with standing.[2267] Feed type also influences lying time; cows fed a ration with shorter particle size had a longer daily lying time and tended to have more lying bouts than cows fed a ration with longer particle size.[2782]

Milking frequency also affects resting patterns. Cattle milked three times a day have longer periods of lying and stand more easily than those milked twice a day, presumably because their udders are less engorged.[1739] Tethering reduces lying time and increases the time taken to lie down in comparison to box-stalled or pastured cows.[1136] If dairy cows are confined in a small area, they lie less if the substrate is concrete or mud, and more if bedding is present. They compensate for the loss of recumbent time by lying when they next have access to pasture.

Feeding a barren diet (restricted solid food provision or lack of straw to calves) resulted in more time spent inactive lying or standing inactive, but did not change their reactivity to novel objects.[3025] Space allowance or area affects activity patterns in calves. They eat and walk more in a larger pen, but ruminate and stand less.[2232]

Grazing

Most grazing takes place during the day.[110] Cattle on pasture spend anywhere from five to eight hours grazing. Grazing time is inversely proportional to the quality of the pasture. Cattle on moderately good pasture spend five hours actually gathering food with their prehensile tongues and two hours walking.[1155] As herbage is sparser, more walking between mouthfuls is necessary.

Grazing usually occurs in bouts and is engaged in by the entire herd; social facilitation is strong in cattle. Two major grazing bouts take place each day, one just after sunrise and the other during late afternoon until sunset.[1080] Midmorning and midafternoon are resting and idling times.[2376] Light may not affect grazing patterns immediately; a total solar eclipse shortened grazing times but did not affect rumination time.[2011]

By an hour after sunset, most cattle are lying down, although they will usually arise to graze during the night.[799] Night grazing may increase during warm weather and may also increase as day length shortens. Both changes in behavior serve to keep grazing time, and therefore food intake, constant.[2072] Cattle drink two to four times a day during the summer on the range but only once a day or even every other day during the winter.[459] Grazing is covered in more detail in Chapter 8, "Ingestive Behavior: Food and Water Intake."

Distance Traveled

The distance traveled by cattle or sheep can be measured by a rangemeter, a device that is similar to an odometer.[57,469] The distance covered by a grazing cow varies from 0.3 to 20 km/day (0.19–5.6 mi.), depending on the size of the pasture or range and the abundance of forage. The longest distances are traveled by cattle foraging in a desert.[1001] Beef cattle on range in Montana walk 3 km/day (1.9 mi.), while spending 11–12 hours grazing per day at a bite rate of 50–60 per minute.[771] In rugged terrain, cattle create paths that involve the least effort – the shortest distance and the least hilly.[787] Dairy cows with free access to a pasture, a yard, and a barn traveled 3 h/day in summer but less than 1 h/day in winter.[1269] Cattle walk 20 times faster when walking to a goal, for example to be milked (60 m/min), than when grazing (3 m/min).[530]

Housing and Management Conditions

Cattle live not only on the range but also in varying degrees of confinement. Dairy cattle are milked at least twice a day, and their grazing habits are organized around the milking schedule. The most intense grazing activity follows each milking. Two bouts occur after the afternoon milking, and one before the morning milking. A brief bout of rumination follows each grazing bout. A total of 5.5 hours during daylight are spent grazing, with an equal time being spent ruminating. In contrast, cattle in a loose-housing situation spend only half as much time eating and ruminating as do cattle on pasture. They spend six to seven hours loafing, that is, standing while neither grazing nor ruminating, and they spend 12 hours resting. Time spent walking decreases with the size of the idling area available to the cattle.

Walking speed varies with the flooring type. Cattle move slower on slatted concrete floors than on solid concrete or rubber floors and move quickest with the longest stride on sand.[2237] When deprived of activity for as little as one day, cows will walk more when given the opportunity.[2346]

Cattle on feedlots are in a highly unnatural environment, as reflected in their activity patterns. Grazing bouts are replaced by 9–14 feeding periods, 70–80% of which occur during daylight hours. If hay and/or silage is fed, a total of 5 h/day are spent eating, but the time decreases as the percentage of concentrates in the diet increases or if the roughage is ground.[1878] When given a choice between pasture and feedlot, the cattle eat in the feedlot, but spend most of their time on pasture: 75% during the day and 90% at night.[1327]

Weather affects the time budget in that lying time decreases in cold, wet weather.[697,836] This is particularly true for thin cows, that are not as insulated by fat stores. Cows lie in different positions depending on the weather. They will fold their forelimbs under the body if the ground is cold or muddy, and spend less time with their head touching the ground or their flank – the typical position for REM sleep.[2294] In hot climates, moving into the shade is another activity that appears to be a response to light rather than to temperature per se. Cattle should, of course, have access to shade, and shading behavior should be considered when management plans are made.

Elimination

Cattle defecate 7–15 times a day and urinate 5–13 times, producing 10 kg of feces and 10 kg of urine.[1737] The frequency of both excretory activities decreases in hot weather.[457] Cattle usually stand to defecate and actively move away from their feces. They defecate while walking only when the whole herd is moving.[2433] Rumination time also decreases under these conditions. When the environment is conducive – the cows are not confined – they will usually move away from their feces after deposition.[2434]

See Table 3.5 for activity patterns of cattle in different environments.

Sleep

The presence or absence of true sleep in ruminants has been controversial,[136,227,1567] but the extensive studies of Ruckebusch[1993,1997]

Table 3.5 Activity patterns of cattle in different environments.

Grazing (h)	Number of grazing bouts	Ruminating (h)	Lying (h)	Walking (h)	Standing (h)	Idling (h)	Type of cattle	References
Cattle on pasture								
5.5–7.5	6 (2 at night)	–	13	–	4	–	Dairy cows	110
5.5–10	–	–	–	–	–	–	Beef steers (Hereford)	2530
6.5	–	5.5	9.25	–	–	8.25	Dairy cows (Shorthorn)	2544
8	5–7 (1 at night)	5.5	9.25	–	–	3.50	Dairy cows (Shorthorn)	457
7–9	2	–	–	–	–	–	Beef cattle	2546*
7.25–7.5	4–5	4	–	–	–	2	Dairy calves	503
6	3	–	8.25	–	–	9	Beef cows (Charolais)	799
10–12	6 (1 at night)	8	–	–	–	4	Dairy cows	897
9	4 (1 at night)	8.5	9	–	15	6	Dairy cows (Holstein)	2566
7–8	–	4.5	5	0.25	3.25	–	Zebu cattle	912
9 (8–11)	2	–	–	–	–	–	Steers	2569
9–10	4	8	2	2–3	2	–	Beef cows (Hereford, Santa Gertrudis)	998
11.50	–	8.50	–	–	4	–	Dairy cows	2570
8	5	8	–	–	–	9	Beef steers (Hereford)	1080
7–8	–	7	12	–	–	–	Beef cattle (Hereford)	1155
11.50	5	7	–	1.25	–	5	Beef and dairy heifers	2570
7	2	7	–	–	–	–	Zebu and grade steers	2579
–	4	–	–	–	–	–	Dairy cows (Brown Swiss)	2569
6–8	4–8	–	–	–	–	7–12	Steers	2587
10–10.5	–	–	9–11	–	2–3.5	–	Beef cattle (Hereford)	2604
9.5–12	3	–	10–14	–	1.25–4	–	Nonlactating cattle	2606

8–9.5	4	–	–	–	–	–	Dairy cows	2072
10	2	–	–	1.5	–	–	Beef cattle	2624
–	3	–	–	–	–	–	Beef cattle	2376
7 (5.5–8)	5	6.25 (4.5–9.5)	–	–	–	–	Dairy cows (Ayrshire)	2633
9	6	7	5	1[a]	6	–	Beef steers (Hereford)	2638
				Cattle in confinement				
3–5	–	–	–	11	–	–	Dairy cows[b] (Holstein)	2557
4–5	–	–	–	8–11	–	–	Dairy cows[c] (Brown Swiss)	2584
3.5–5.25	9–12	–	–	–	–	–	Steers[d]	1878
3.5	4	7.5	9.5	6.5	14	1.25	Beef cows[d] (Hereford)	2040
3–4	–	–	–	12.25	–	6–7	Dairy cows[c] (Holstein)	2621
5	10	–	10.5	–	8.5	–	Dairy cows[d] (Ayrshire)	2631
6.25	18	–	–	–	–	–	Dairy cows[e] (Guernsey)	2402

[a] Daylight observation only.
[b] Free stall.
[c] Loose housing.
[d] Feedlot.
[e] Cowshed.

indicate that cattle show both REM sleep and SWS. REM sleep occurs in 11 periods, so the total of 45 minutes of REM sleep and 3.5 hours of SWS are divided into many short naps. When cattle are in REM sleep, they usually are lying down with their heads resting on the ground and turned back into the flank. Although behavioral observations overestimate non-REM sleep, they do accurately measure REM sleep.[2243] Cattle sniff the ground before lying down, and, on arising, lick and scratch themselves. Cows in slings are sleep deprived, as are cows that have not yet adjusted to stanchioning or newly mixed groups of cattle. The stress of sleep deprivation should be considered by clinicians and stock managers. When kept in a corral at night, cattle, or Zebu cattle at least, tend to sleep in areas that remain constant for each individual from night to night. The resting places do not appear to depend on dominance.[1919] Most characteristic of ruminants are the extensive periods of drowsiness usually associated with rumination. Cattle are in a drowsy state 7.5 h/day, divided into 25 periods that precede and follow sleep. Rumination and sleep are inversely related, so sleep time decreases with rumen development (see Chapter 6, "Development of Behavior") and decreases as the percentage of roughage in the diet increases.[136]

Environmental Influences
Social changes can disrupt activity rhythms in ruminants as well as in pigs. For example, calves in a stable group show definite diurnal activity patterns; those in continually changing groups do not.[1248] Calves are affected by the lighting regime. They prefer a lighted area and spend more time lying there.[2406]

In summary, the normal bovine day depends on the diet and on the housing conditions and, in general, consists of alternating periods of eating and ruminating interspersed with resting or loafing and short periods of sleep (refer to Figure 3.4). Activity patterns in cattle have been studied by other investigators in addition to those listed in Table 3.5.[709,897,912,1907,2096]

Sheep

Grazing and Traveling
Sheep flock activity, whether based on speed, distance traveled, or azimuth, fit a circadian rhythmicity. In the summer, particularly July and August, sheep exhibited a significant advance in the acrophase (the time at which the peak of a rhythm occurs), which might have been caused by day length and temperature.[2932] Until recently, sheep were seldom kept in confinement, so studies of their activities have dealt with range or pasture conditions (Table 3.6). Sheep on the range spend 50% of the daylight hours grazing,[459] of which seven hours are spent grazing and two hours traveling.[564] On the range, sheep travel 6–14 km/day (4–9 mi.), but they travel only 0.8 km/day (0.5 mi.) on pasture.[470] Two factors determine how the range is used: familiarity with the area and social integration into the flock. Newly introduced animals may wander 14 km (9 mi.), for example, when introduced to a new flock in an unfamiliar environment.[2390] In pasture, sheep spend 9–10 hours grazing in four periods, and they spend an equal amount of time ruminating in 15 bouts. Sheep allowed to graze only during daylight hours also spent nine hours grazing, similar to the time spent by sheep allowed 24 hours to graze.[241] As has already been noted in the case of cattle, more time is spent grazing on a poor pasture (up to 12 h/day), and twice as much distance is traveled as on a good pasture. See Table 3.7 for sheep activity patterns.

Sheep in particular are synchronized in their behavior in that all or most of the sheep will be doing the same thing at the same time. Sheep may all begin to graze simultaneously, but much greater variation occurs at the end of a grazing bout. The satiety factors (discussed in Chapter 8) are more important in ending a meal, whereas the behavior of the other sheep is more important in starting it.[1958] Even on pasture, the type of feed can affect behavior patterns. For example, sheep grazing clover spend less time grazing and ruminating than

Table 3.6   Mean values of comparative data of sleep–wakefulness states and attitudes in four species of farm animals (three subjects of each species).

| Species and time period | Duration and percentage | | | | | |
| | Wakefulness | | Sleep | | Attitude | |
	AW	DR	SWS	PS	Standing	Recumbent
Horse						
24-h period	19 h 13 min	1 h 55 min	2 h 05 min	47 min	22 h 01 min	1 h 59 min
	80.8%	8.0%	8.7%	3.3%	91.8%	8.2%
Nighttime (10 h)	5 h 14 min	1 h 54 min	2 h 05 min	47 min	8 h 01 min	1 h 59 min
	52.4%	19.0%	20.8%	7.8%	80.1%	19.9%
Cow						
24-h period	12 h 33 min	7 h 29 min	3 h 13 min	45 min	9 h 50 min	14 h 10 min
	52.3%	31.2%	13.3%	3.1%	40.9%	59.1%
Nighttime (12 h)	1 h 55 min	6 h 14 min	3 h 06 min	45 min	1 h 30 min	10 h 30 min
	16.0%	51.9%	25.8%	6.3%	12.5%	87.5%
Sheep						
24-h period	15 h 57 min	4 h 12 min	3 h 17 min	34 min	16 h 50 min	7 h 10 min
	66.5%	17.5%	13.6%	2.4%	70.1%	29.9%
Nighttime (12 h)	5 h 59 min	2 h 45 min	2 h 43 min	34 min	7 h 10 min	4 h 50 min
	49.8%	22.9%	22.5%	4.8%	59.7%	40.3%
Pig						
24-h period	11 h 07 min	5 h 04 min	6 h 04 min	1 h 45 min	5 h 10 min	18 h 50 min
	46.3%	21.1%	25.3%	7.3%	21.5%	78.5%
Nighttime (12 h)	4 h 23 min	2 h 30 min	3 h 52 min	1 h 15 min	1 h 20 min	10 h 40 min
	36.5%	20.8%	32.9%	10.5%	11.1%	88.9%

Source: Adapted from Rubin *et al.* (1980).[1991]

Table 3.7   Activity patterns of sheep.

Grazing (h)	Number of grazing bouts	Ruminating (h)	Standing (h)	Lying (h)	Walking (h)	References
7	–	5.5[a]	–	–	2	564[b]
9–12	5	9–10.5	2.5	3.5	0.5	638
9	2	–	3.5	11.25	0.25	1080
4–5.5	2	–	–	–	–	2627

[a] Includes idling and resting.
[b] Observed for 14.5 h/day (daylight).

do those grazing grass.[1790] Behavior is influenced by environmental temperature, and behavioral thermoregulation is, in turn, influenced by the animal's insulation. This is particularly true in sheep who are sheared of their fleece rather than shedding gradually. This is reflected in their choice of substrate. Unshorn sheep in pens prefer expanded metal flooring, whereas newly shorn ones prefer solid floors.[906] Unsheared sheep spend 65% of their time lying, falling to 40% after shearing in winter and only returning to pre-shearing levels after several weeks.[662] Activity is almost exclusively during the light period in both grazing and confined sheep; those fed limited amounts are most active while feed is available.[1815] Pregnant sheep kept indoors lie down for 13 h/day in 27 bouts of about half an hour, whereas those managed outdoor spent 12 h/day lying down in 19 bouts of 36 minutes; older ewes lay down more than younger ewes.[3033]

Sleep

Sheep are awake for 16 h/day. They drowse 4.5 h/day, far less than cattle. SWS occupies 3.5 h/day, and REM sleep occurs in seven periods for a total of 43 minutes.[1992] Sleep increases in sheep fed a low-roughage diet.[1620] While sleeping, they expend 10% less energy than while waking,[2286] so sleep deprivation would be expected to increase energy expenditure. They will stand up 8–11 times during the night, usually to urinate or defecate.[638] Activity patterns in confined sheep have also been studied.[2383] In many colder climates, sheep must be confined during the winter. Because sheep choose to sleep against a natural or an artificial wall, it would seem logical that adding walls would increase resting time and encourage sheep to lie down in bedded areas rather than on slatted floors, but a cross-shaped configuration increased aggression and cubicles increased time spent lying on the slats.[1162]

The EEG, muscle relaxation, and other physiological parameters that accompany the various states of vigilance in farm animals are shown in Figure 3.7A. The percentage of the night spent in sleep, wakefulness, and various sleep states and postures are shown in Figure 3.7B. Comparative data for sleep and wakefulness in farm animals are given in Table 3.6.

Goats

Adults goats spend 41–47% of the time foraging and kids spend 59–65%, depending on the stocking rate.[1869] Goats graze less and travel more when it is raining or when flies are abundant. These changes are more pronounced in shorn goats.[333] When food and water are available ad libitum, goats eat mostly at the beginning of the light phase and at the beginning of the dark phase.[1981]

Feral goats on the Island of Rum spend their nights in caves. During the summer, there are two or three peaks in feeding interrupted by resting, but the percentage of time they spend feeding increases in the winter and their resting time decreases (see Figure 3.10). Yearlings spend more time feeding than adults or kids.[2101]

For comparison of sleep duration in domestic mammals see Table 3.8.

Table 3.8 Comparative sleep duration.

Species	Slow-wave sleep (h)	REM sleep (h)
Horse	2.98	0.7
Cow	3.2	0.8
Sheep	3.3	0.6
Goat	4.7	0.7
Pig	6.4	1.9
Dog	7.1	1.6
Cat	10	3.2

Source: Adapted from Greening and McBride (2022).[2768]

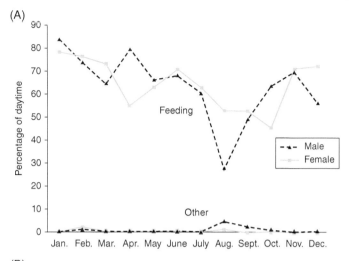

Figure 3.10 Comparison of monthly variation in patterns of activity budgets of male and female adult goats on Rum in (A) 1981 and (B) 2000. Only the proportions of daytime spent feeding and in other activities are shown. *Source:* Shi *et al.* (2003).[2102] Reproduced with permission of NRC Research Press.

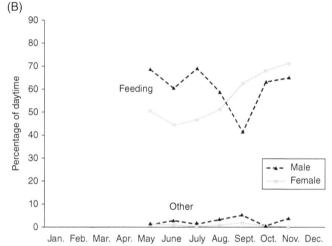

Chickens

Chickens rest several times during the day and at night. They prefer to perch rather than remain at floor level – probably predator avoidance behavior.

During sleep, domestic chicks (*Gallus gallus*) show brief and transient periods during which one eye is open while the other remains shut. Electrophysiological recordings showed that the hemisphere contralateral to the open eye exhibited an EEG with fast waves typical of wakefulness, whereas the hemisphere contralateral to the closed eye exhibited an EEG typical of SWS.[2906]

If chickens are exposed to constant light, they lose their circadian rhythms. Dustbathing is a self-grooming behavior in which the chicken lies down on a substrate of fine particles (sand or peat) shaking its wings and rubbing its head, activities which will remove old lipids and ectoparasites from its plumage.[2849] Other chickens may peck at the lice and other ectoparasites of the dust bathing chicken. When the chicken arises, it shakes itself. There does not appear to be a circadian rhythm to dust bathing, but it occurs daily or twice daily if a preferred substrate is present, but rearing environment can influence the behavior.[2648]

4

Sexual Behavior

Introduction

Sexual behavior is important in all species of animals. The importance lies not only in maintaining adequate levels of libido in breeding animals but also in controlling the various aspects of sexual behavior that persist in neutered animals.

Mating systems have evolved within the framework of the morphological and physiological parameters of the individual species under continual ecological pressures. Although we have drastically reduced the nutritional, climatic, and health stresses to which domestic animals are exposed and have selected heavily for "good breeders," we still find remnants of this long-term evolutionary selection hindering our goal of high reproduction rates. Thus, we may continue to see problems that hinder breeding and production schedules, such as seasonal breeding in housed stock subjected to artificial control of photoperiodicity; poor libido in some of our artificial insemination (AI) programs, despite the absence of organic disease; and mate selection preferences that do not coincide with our ideas of desirable matings. Figure 4.1 illustrates the factors that affect sexual behavior, using the stallion as an example.

Physiological Bases of Sexual Behavior

Adult male and female sexual behavior depends on a variety of factors – physiological, environmental, and psychological – for its expression. These factors are (a) the genetic sex of the animal, (b) perinatal organizational action of hormones, (c) past social and sexual experience, (d) adult activational action of hormone and anatomical status, (e) the attractiveness of the potential mate, and (f) the external environment.

Genetically Determined Sex

The sex of the animal is determined at the moment of conception, and the chromosomal sex will determine whether the indifferent fetal gonad develops into an ovary or a testis. Nevertheless, the potential for masculine and feminine behavior remains in both sexes. Studies on laboratory animals have revealed that the brain, and therefore behavior, is usually female unless the fetus is exposed to androgens during development. Similarly, without androgenic stimulation, the external genitalia will be female.

Organizational: Perinatal Hormonal Influences

The role of sex hormones during ontogeny has been studied in dogs. Male puppies have been castrated at birth, and their behavior compared with that of intact dogs and dogs castrated as adults. Anatomically, these neonatally castrated dogs were altered in that their penes were very small. Despite this anatomical change, they still urinated in the masculine

Domestic Animal Behavior for Veterinarians and Animal Scientists, Seventh Edition. Katherine A. Houpt.
© 2024 John Wiley & Sons, Inc. Published 2024 by John Wiley & Sons, Inc.
Companion website: www.wiley.com/go/houpt/7e

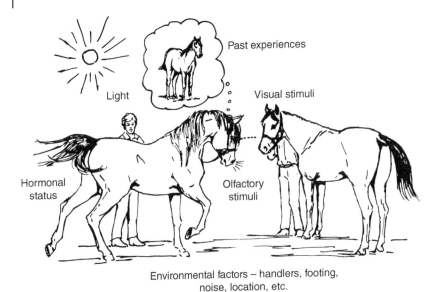

Light
Past experiences
Visual stimuli
Hormonal status
Olfactory stimuli

Environmental factors – handlers, footing, noise, location, etc.

Figure 4.1 Factors that affect sexual behavior.

posture and were no different in their response to exogenous testosterone from dogs castrated as adults.[191] They were attracted to estrous females and mounted them; however, their underdeveloped external genitalia prohibited normal intromission. Both sexes have the genetic potential for male or female behavior, but neonatal androgens "defeminize" males, that is, make them less likely to show female sexual behavior. Therefore, when treated with estrogen as adults, the neonatally castrated males show receptive behavior to other males.

Female puppies treated with androgens in utero and neonatally were markedly altered anatomically. They had no external vagina and did have small phalluses. They urinated in the masculine posture half the time. As adults, they were ovariectomized and treated with either female (estrogen and progesterone) or male (testosterone) hormones. The estrogen treatments revealed that the dogs had been defeminized; they would not stand or show any other signs of sexual receptivity. They were not even attracted to the male, as is a normal intact estrous female or an ovariectomized, estrogen-treated female. When treated with testosterone, the experimental dogs were

obviously masculinized because they were attracted to, and would mount, other female dogs that were in heat. These studies indicate the powerful effects of perinatal androgens on the anatomy and behavior of animals of either genetic sex.[194,196,199]

Sheep and cattle are also defeminized by their neonatal androgens. The freemartin cow (born twin to a bull) is an example of a naturally occurring manipulation of the perinatal hormonal environment; as is described later in this chapter, these females exhibit masculinized behavior, although their external genitalia are not masculinized. Pigs appear to be unique in that they are defeminized, not during the prenatal or neonatal period, but at puberty.[14]

Activational: Adult Hormonal Status

The most important feature of the hormonal basis of sexual behavior is that hormones have a permissive role; that is, an animal requires a certain level of hormones for normal sexual behavior, but a higher level of hormones will not increase libido or receptivity. Hormonal treatment will not cure a deficiency of sexual behavior unless a deficiency of that hormone exists.

The complex relationships of the central nervous system, gonadal hormones, and behavior are discussed in more detail in this chapter; in general, however, ovarian hormones result in an attraction to males and receptivity to male mounting. In some species (cats and pigs), the complete pattern of estrous behavior can be elicited by estrogen alone. In others (dogs and sheep),[192,244,2122] progesterone must also be administered. In ungulates, the behavioral action of estrogen is facilitated by a rapid preovulatory fall in progesterone, whereas in dogs a rise in progesterone is important. Progesterone is administered before estrogen in the ewe and after estrogen in the bitch to induce estrous behavior.

Ovariectomy and Castration

Ovariectomy (spaying) usually abolishes estrous behavior in females. Castration (orchiectomy) generally abolishes sexual behavior in males, but many exceptions exist. The more experienced the male, the longer sexual behavior, both arousal and copulation, will persist after castration. Pre-pubertal castration is, therefore, more effective than post-pubertal castration in eliminating sexual behavior. Species differences appear in the effectiveness of pre-pubertal castration. Cats are affected more than dogs.[921,1323,1972] Neutering affects other behaviors too. Spayed bitches are more aggressive than un-spayed ones.[2826] When owners rate their own dogs, gonadectomy had no affect on aggression to familiar people or dogs and severe aggression to strangers was somewhat more common in gonadectomized dogs.[2734]

Anatomical Factors

Anatomical factors are important because a small penis precludes successful intromission. Intact afferent pathways from the penis are also necessary; experimental or traumatic neural damage to the penis results in misorientation in tomcats[102] and failure to ejaculate in bulls.[216] Similarly, desensitization of the vagina inhibits ovulation in the cat, an induced ovulator.[546]

The species differences in the structure of the penis are also important. For anatomical reasons, castration reduces the copulatory ability of male cats and horses more than it does that of male ruminants and dogs. The muscular penis of the horse is more dependent on erection for successful intromission than is the fibroelastic penis of the ruminant. Similarly, the penile spines of the tomcat, which atrophy in the castrated male, are important for successful intromission and ejaculation as well as for induction of ovulation.

Social and Sexual Experience

It is much more common to observe animals that have been influenced by lack of adequate sexual experience than animals influenced by abnormal hormone levels. Male sexual behavior is affected by social influences. Having absolutely no social interactions – that is, being raised in isolation from weaning to adulthood – suppresses sexual behavior. The type of social interaction is important, but there are species differences. Whereas rams raised in all-male groups from weaning to one year are less sexually active than those raised (or even given brief exposure) with ewes, bulls, goats, and boars are independent of female exposure for normal behavior. Total lack of experience, homosexual experience only, too much sexual experience, or sexual experiences that are too unpleasant can all lead to sexual abnormalities.

Lack of Socialization

The concept of critical or sensitive periods of development is discussed in Chapter 6, "Development of Behavior"; it should be emphasized here, however, that the most obvious effect of lack of socialization to conspecifics is on sexual behavior. Dogs raised without physical contact with other dogs from the age of three weeks showed normal libido toward estrous bitches but were very poor at orientation; they would mount improperly and seldom achieved intromission. This is probably an effect of lack of mounting experience because mounting forms a large part of male puppy play.[188] Similarly, boars raised in isolation from the time they were three weeks old showed very little sexual behavior.[988]

Within all-male groups, individuals may direct their sexual attentions to other males or be subordinate to other males. The dominant males may continue to mount males even in the presence of an estrous female; the subordinate animals often have little or no mounting experience. Some of these inappropriate responses will cease over time, but breeding efficiency is affected (at least temporarily).

Negative Sexual Experience

Unpleasant experiences during mating will have a deleterious effect on future sexual behavior, especially if the animal is young and has not had many (pleasant) experiences. The negative associations can be the result of overt aggression on the part of the sexual partner, rough handling by a stockperson, or an injury sustained during mating.

Effect on Female Sexual Behavior

The effects of experience on sexual behavior have not been as thoroughly studied in females as in males. There may be less effect, in part because the female plays a less active role in mating in most management situations. Sows raised in isolation showed normal sexual behavior and were attracted to males when in heat.[2121] More research should be done on the effects of experience and age at weaning on female sexual behavior. Cats, in particular, may not be adequately socialized under normal rearing techniques and may reject toms, at least initially.

Attractiveness of Potential Mate

The element of attractiveness, or lack of it, of the sexual partner is not often considered, but higher mammals are influenced by this factor as well as by their hormonal levels. The attractivity of an estrous bitch's urine depends on her hormone state. If the donor of the urine is treated with estrogen, her urine becomes more attractive to males; if treated with testosterone, her urine is less attractive. Marking behavior of males is apparently an attempt to mask the attractiveness of bitch urine.[589,590]

Females may show individual preferences for one male over another. All females do not prefer the same male, indicating that the differences in attractiveness of males are based on the female's innate preferences and on past experience, rather than on some physiological characteristic of the male, such as pheromone release.

Male preferences can be based on physiological factors. For example, rams prefer ewes they have not bred before, as discussed later in this chapter. The action of ovarian hormones not only renders the female receptive but also increases her attractiveness, presumably by pheromonal release. Care must be taken when comparing the results of experiments on animals artificially brought into estrus with those involving females in natural estrus, because the latter may be more attractive than the former.

Males also show individual mate preferences that are apparently psychological or idiosyncratic. An evolutionary basis may exist for some of these preferences. Males may prefer females that are similar, but not too similar, to themselves so that inbreeding will not occur and yet the same gene pool will be propagated.[196] Evidence for such behavior influencing sexual behavior of sheep,[955,1335] cats,[1364] and horses[1195] has been found.

External Environment

The external environment is very important for optimal sexual behavior. Extremely inclement weather obviously will inhibit sexual behavior, but subtler environmental factors, such as too many human spectators or a slippery floor, may also inhibit it. Not all additions to the environment are detrimental. In some cases, the presence of another male may stimulate sexual behavior. This has been well documented in cattle and goats.[266,1863] Males generally are more influenced by the environment than are females, so the female is usually brought to the male. Nevertheless, environmental factors in female sexual behavior deserve study. Time of day, for example, is important in cows, which show more signs of estrus at night

The Central Nervous System and the Control of Sexual Behavior

Females
Hypothalamic Factors

In the female, gonadotropin-releasing hormone (GnRH) in the hypothalamus stimulates the release of follicle-stimulating hormone (FSH) and luteinizing hormone (LH) from the anterior pituitary. FSH induces follicular development, and FSH and LH together stimulate estrogen and progesterone production by the ovary. For most of the estrous cycle, estrogen and progesterone maintain low levels of LH and FSH through a negative feedback action on the hypothalamic–pituitary axis.

Near proestrus, however, the situation is reversed; rising estrogen levels have a positive feedback on LH secretion, resulting in the LH surge that causes ovulation. This preovulatory rise in estrogen is responsible for the hormonally based components of estrous behavior. The brain shows a refractory period during which biochemical changes presumably take place that will result in estrous behavior.[1574]

Cyclical Ovulation

In spontaneous ovulators (bitch, ewe, mare, and sow), the LH surge and, consequently, ovulation take place cyclically; but in induced ovulators, such as cats, external stimuli from the vagina by either natural coitus or artificial manipulation are necessary to trigger the LH surge. The relationship between hormone levels and sexual behavior in the bitch is shown in Figure 4.2. The female's active solicitation of the male is called "proceptive behavior."

The seasonal nature of reproductive behavior is also due to central neural variation in responsiveness to gonadal hormones. The same ewes had to be injected with a larger amount of estrogen to induce estrous behavior in the spring than was needed in the fall.

Olfactory Influences and Pheromones

Odors can have important effects on reproduction. This has been demonstrated in a variety of rodents, mice in particular.[338] In domestic animals, odor is probably not as important; nevertheless, the age at first puberty is lower in gilts exposed to a strange boar (continuous cohabitation with a boar will not produce the effect). Olfactory bulbectomy eliminates the effect, indicating that the odor is the important stimulus.[1230] Ewes show a similar response, called the "ram effect," but odor may not be essential. Post-pubertal cows show another response to odor; they will come into estrus sooner if exposed to the odor of estrous cow urine or mucus.[1118] The best studied farm animal pheromone is the boar odor, which stimulates the estrous sow to assume the immobile, rigid posture that permits the boar to mount her and that can be used for estrus detection.

Males
Hypothalamic Factors

The hypothalamic–pituitary axis is also involved in male sexual behavior. FSH is released in response to hypothalamic releasing factor. In the male, FSH stimulates spermatogenesis, and LH testosterone release. Testosterone, in turn, acts upon the anterior hypothalamus–preoptic area in conjunction with appropriate stimuli from an estrous female to produce male sexual behavior. Inhibin, a testicular factor produced in the spermatic tubules, acts as a negative feedback on the hypothalamus.[2088]

Considerable evidence is accumulating that it is not testosterone itself, but rather a metabolite of testosterone, estradiol, that acts on the central nervous system to produce male sexual behavior. In general, estrogen and testosterone

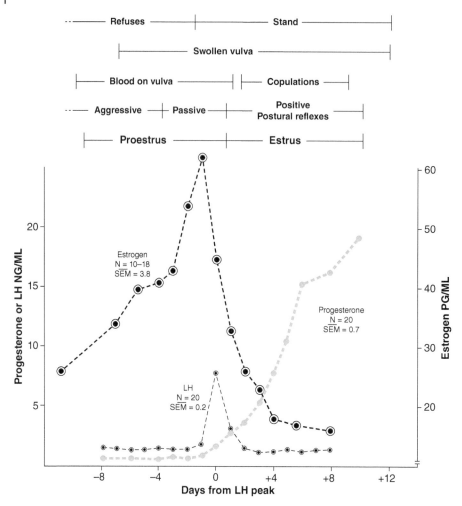

Figure 4.2 Relationship of estrogen, progesterone, and LH levels to behavior in the bitch. Times of onset of behavior and physical signs represent means of a range of times.[377] *Source:* Concannon *et al.* (1975).[447] Reproduced with permission of The Society for the Study of Reproduction.

have similar actions in stimulating male sexual behavior in castrated animals, but an androgen that cannot be metabolized to estradiol, dihydrotestosterone, does not.[401,431] When freemartins are treated with estrogens and androgens, both hormones increase aggressiveness, mounting, and sniffing of the vulva of other cows, but only testosterone stimulates the flehmen response.[853] Testosterone itself, rather than a metabolite, may be responsible for this response (see Figure 4.3). Dihydrotestosterone does stimulate enlargement of the penis and of the sex

glands, so when it is administered in combination with estradiol to castrated pigs, the full sequence of male sexual behavior, including intromission, occurs.[1772]

Stimulation of the brain by testosterone or its metabolites may facilitate the appearance of male sexual behavior; it is the appearance of a female, however, that triggers the behavior. The stallion, for example, will exhibit the flehmen response and begin the courtship rituals of nibbling the crest and rump of the mare. At the same time, stimulation of the parasympathetic nervous system results in

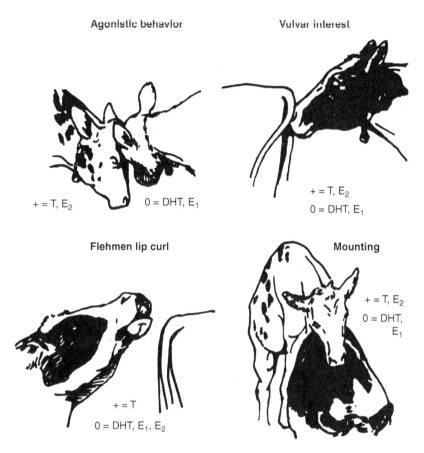

Figure 4.3 Effects of testosterone (T), estradiol (E$_2$), estrone (E$_1$), and dihydrotestosterone (DHT) on agonistic behavior, vulvar interest, the flehmen response, and mounting.[713] *Source:* Greene *et al.* (1978).[853] Reproduced with permission of Elsevier.

secretion of the accessory sex glands. The combination of penile stimulation after intromission and sympathetic stimulation leads to ejaculation.

Olfaction

Olfaction is, no doubt, important for identification of the estrous female; but elimination of the sense of smell by olfactory bulbectomy does not impair sexual performance of cats or rams, indicating that olfactory stimulation is not essential and that the male can identify the receptive female by visual or auditory means. The lack of resistance to his mounting attempts may be the most important information to the male.[101,926,1387]

Summary

In summary, hormones are important for normal sexual behavior, but the central nervous system can be relatively independent of them. This is indicated by the persistence of copulatory behavior in castrated male cats,[1972] dogs,[189] and rams[433] that had considerable precastration experience. Even pre-pubertal castration may not eliminate sexual behavior; one-third of pre-pubertally castrated bulls mounted cows.[707] A similar percentage of prepubertally castrated geldings showed sexual behavior.[1394] Apparently, after the brain is organized by androgens, external stimuli may be sufficient to trigger male sexual behavior.

Cattle

The Cow

The cow is a nonseasonal, continuously cycling breeder, but shows peak fertility from May to July and a nadir from December to February. Puberty occurs anywhere from 4 to 24 months of age, usually at 6–18 months. The estrous cycle is 18–24 days long (mean, 21 days), although it is somewhat shorter in heifers and in the *Bos taurus* (Zebu) breeds.

Onset of Estrus

Onset of estrus occurs more often in the evening and ceases in the morning. Actual sexual receptivity lasts 13–14 hours. The estrous cow shows a general increase in motor activity and a decrease in food intake (Figure 4.4).[1093] The more active a cow is, the higher her fertility.[2503] Investigative behavior such as flehmen, sniffing, rubbing, and licking increase, as does pre-mounting behavior such as standing behind the cow and resting the chin on the back of another, usually another estrous cow. She will bellow a great deal, switch her tail and raise or deviate it to one side, and urinate frequently. If a bull is available, she will approach it.[1330] When the cow stands to be mounted, estrogen levels are at a peak.[645,828] The cow that mounts is usually pre-ovulatory. The mounting cows are also usually dominant over the mounted cows. This represents an interaction between hormonally mediated behavior and social influences. Cows mount cows both before and after the period in which bulls would mount (Figure 4.5).[1222]

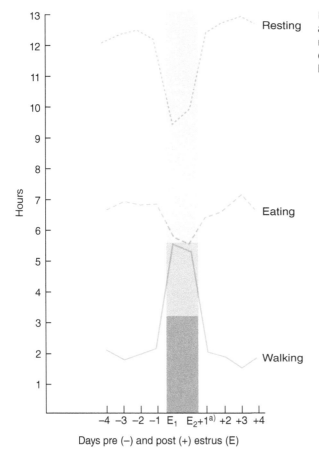

Figure 4.4 Average composition of daily activities of cattle during estrous and non-estrous stages of the reproductive cycle.[911] *Source:* Hurnik *et al.* (1975).[1093] Reproduced with permission of Elsevier.

Hours

Resting

Eating

Walking

Days pre (−) and post (+) estrus (E)

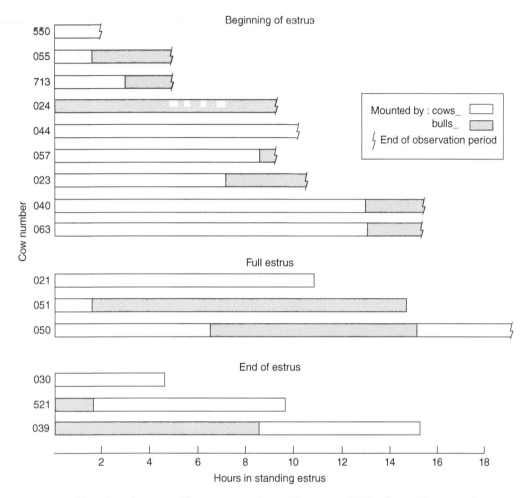

Figure 4.5 Mounting of cows at different stages of estrus by cows and bulls. *Source:* Kilgour *et al.* (1977).[1222] Reproduced with permission of New Zealand Veterinary Association.

Because visual cues are received over greater distances than olfactory cues, homosexual mounting may attract bulls who live apart from the cows (see Chapter 2, "Aggression and Social Structure"). Furthermore, bulls choose cows who are mounting and being mounted in preference to those who are not.[806] Homosexual mounting in cows may have been selected for in dairy cattle because as long ago as medieval times, bulls were not routinely kept with cows, so only those cows that the owner noticed to be mounting were taken to a bull and bred.[134] Beef cows mount much less frequently than dairy cows, confirming this hypothesis.

The male effect, discussed in more detail in this chapter, is weaker in cattle than in sheep and goats. The presence of a bull hastens the onset of estrous cycles in post-partum beef cows but not in high-producing dairy cows.[2111] This is unfortunate because delay in return to estrous cyclicity means a delay in becoming pregnant, which in turn means a financial loss to the dairy farmer. Mounting behavior by cows may not occur if a bull is present.[2046]

Aggressive behavior also increases markedly during estrus.[1093] The intensity of estrus can be measured using frequency of sniffing the vulva of other cows, chin resting, and mounting of head or rear. The intensity of sexual behavior is not related to the dominance hierarchy.[1736] Severely lame cows display less intense estrus as well as lower progesterone levels, but the incidence of behavioral estrus is unaffected.[2377] Once a cow has been mated she will no longer be receptive, but after an hour's rest she allows further copulation.[131]

Detection of Estrus

Detection of estrus becomes more and more critical in the dairy industry as AI becomes more widespread (more than 90% of Holstein calves are conceived via AI). The physical signs of estrus, such as a copious vaginal secretion and vulvar relaxation, may be weak or absent. Estrous behavior may be less noticeable in housed cattle than in yarded or pastured ones.[1811] Footing can also affect a cow's willingness to mount.[2313] Traditionally, the bull is the best detector of estrus in the cow, with humans doing a poor to fair second. An estimated 19% of heats may be missed because behavioral signs are absent (silent heats) even though ovulation occurs, and an additional 15% are labeled as estrous periods even though ovulation does not occur (false heats). Some silent heats may have been behaviorally evident but were not observed by the herders. Pregnant cows (3–15%), depending on the criteria used to label a cow as estrous, may also show signs of estrus.[549,741]

Mounting behavior is used by the farmer to aid in heat detection, but it may not occur around the milking time or when the cows are usually observed. A commercial estrus detection device, which consists of a plastic vial containing a red dye, is glued to the dorsal tail base of a cow suspected to be in estrus. As she is mounted by other cows in the herd, the dye is gradually expressed into a viewing chamber; a full chamber supposedly is correlated with a sufficient number of mountings to indicate a full estrus.[2460] Several cows may be in heat simultaneously and one may not be mounted, so even the mechanical heat detector can give misleading false negatives.[1659] Pedometers are used to determine estrus because the cow is more active then (see Figure 4.4), but the pedometers must be read several times a day to be accurate. Observations of chin resting and mounting are still the best indicators and correlate with estrogen levels.[1424]

A vasectomized bull or teaser bull with a surgically deviated penis may also be used to detect heat. The danger of keeping an unpredictably aggressive bull in close contact with people, however, has discouraged this practice. A freemartin heifer may be used satisfactorily. Fetal exposure to the androgens produced by the male fetus masculinizes the nervous system of freemartins; they are infertile and thus of little value as dairy animals. Freemartins are even more likely than the other cows in the herd to mount an estrous cow, and treatment with injectable androgens may heighten this behavior even further. Dogs have been trained to detect estrous cows, an interesting innovation presumably based on canine olfactory acuity.[1210] The dogs were 80–90% correct in detecting estrous cows.

Clinical Problems of Cows

Silent heats, a phenomenon to which heifers are especially subject, have already been discussed.

Nymphomania is more common in high-production dairy cows than in beef breeds. The cow shows intense estrous behavior either persistently or at frequent, irregular intervals. Herd milk production drops noticeably because these cows are often the best producers in the herd. Most commonly, the affected cow is four to six years old and has calved two to three times. Unlike a cow in normal estrus, however, the nymphomaniac does not stand for other cows. She actively seeks out other cows and mounts them. She paws and bellows like a bull and with time also becomes more male-like in voice and body conformation. Nymphomania is usually associated with follicular cysts, and treatment is sometimes successful using a source of LH, such as pituitary extract or chorionic gonadotropin.[1942]

The Bull

In contrast to rams, bulls' sexual performance is not improved by raising them with females or exposing them to females at the time of puberty.[296,1850] Rearing bulls in individual pens does suppress sexual performance.[1862] Residual seasonality occurs in bulls as in cows. LH treatment results in higher testosterone levels if administered during the summer rather than during shorter days.[1151] Bovine male courtship behavior is becoming an unobserved rarity in modern dairy farming with the advent and spread of AI. Bulls are now selected for (among other things) their willingness and ability to mount dummy cows, other bulls, or steers and to ejaculate into an artificial vagina. One might wonder how this willingness to leave behavioral interactions with the opposite sex up to random genetic drift eventually will affect the species. The courtship sequence is actually a series of reciprocal interactions between male and female. The female behavior has already been described.

Courtship Behavior

Starting late in the cow's proestrus, the bull will begin to graze beside the cow, guarding her from any other cattle. His attempts to mount will be repulsed by the cow. During proestrus, most females are attractive to the male and attracted to him but not yet receptive. The bull may attempt to herd the cow away from the rest of the herd.

Periodically, the bull will smell and lick the cow's vulva, often followed by the flehmen response (Figure 4.6). Some, but not all, dairy bulls flehmen to estrous urine, and they do so more often than to mucus or to non-estrous urine.[1063] Flehmen is followed by an increase in LH.[1421]

As estrus approaches, guarding becomes more marked as both other bulls and non-estrous cows are kept away. When the cow is in full estrus, the bull will have a partial erection while guarding her, and accessory gland fluid or precoital discharge will drip from the penis.[1205] The bull frequently nudges the female's flanks and either maintains head-to-head contact or, because of mutual genital sniffing and licking, stands in a reverse parallel (bigeminal) position with the cow. This position is common to the courtship sequence of all ungulates. The bull may rest his head across the cow's back while they stand in a T-position.[741] He makes several mounting attempts with a partial erection before the cow will stand for him. When she is ready, the cow remains immobile and the bull mounts immediately. He fixes his forelegs just cranial to the pelvis of the female as he straddles her. Ejaculation occurs within seconds of intromission and is noted by a marked, generalized muscular contraction (Figure 4.7). The bull's rear legs may be brought off the ground during this spasm. Dismounting and retraction of the penis follow rapidly. When bulls are used for hand breeding or for AI, lack of the stimulatory effects of the prolonged courtship may result in poor semen quality or poor reproductive behavior.

Sensory Stimuli

Experimental manipulations have shown that a variety of sensory stimuli are needed to elicit male sexual behavior. Tape recordings of cows will sexually stimulate a bull, but these sounds are probably of a non-specific arousal nature.[525] Bulls used for AI apparently become classically conditioned (see Chapter 7, "Learning") to the sounds in the collection arena, and these may help stimulate these animals. The stimulation of sexual behavior caused by a new female is called the "Coolidge effect." The Coolidge effect occurs in bulls so that the mounts with intromission and decreased mounting intervals occur when a novel female is provided hourly. There is also more flehmen. Alternating two females has an intermediate effect.[131]

Olfactory cues seem to be used by the bull during early estrus to monitor the stage of the reproductive cycle of the cow; however, no studies have been able to show sexual

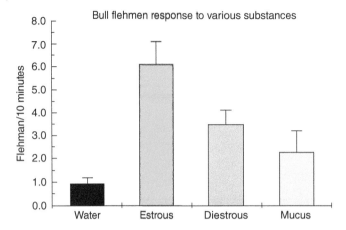

Figure 4.6 The mean (±SEM) response of bulls to estrous and non-estrous urine, mucus, and water. *Source:* Houpt *et al.* (1989).[1063] Reproduced with permission of Elsevier.

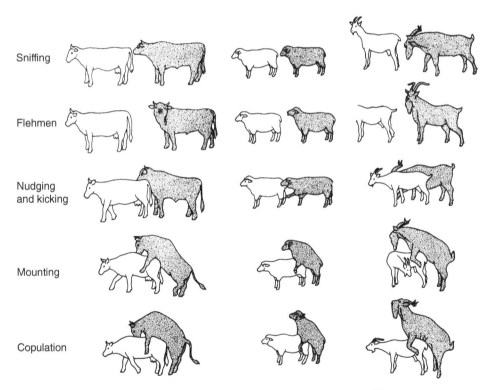

Figure 4.7 Sexual patterns in cattle, sheep, and goats. *Source:* Hafez (1974).[878] Reproduced with permission of John Wiley & Sons.

excitation caused by olfactory stimuli alone. Although volatile compounds have been isolated from estrous urine, these compounds do not elicit interest from bulls. Urine from a bull used as a teaser did elicit flehmen and other signs of interest, but none of these olfactory stimuli affected sexual performance of dairy bulls in an AI center.[1849]

Visual deprivation seems to hinder sexual response generally, but most markedly when the blinded individual is presented with a female in a novel situation.[884] The inverted U-shape seems to be the visual stimulus most likely to stimulate sexual behavior, whether this be in the form of a standing cow, a dummy, or an unfortunate person bending over. Without special conditioning, a wild bovid will mount only an estrous conspecific female. One of the aims of domestication has been to obtain "easy" breeders, that is, bulls that respond to a less specific series of stimuli than those offered by a female and that do so with little sexual foreplay.

Sexual responsiveness is influenced by the range of stimuli to which the male is exposed during ontogeny. Free-ranging or wild bovids gradually restrict their sexual behavior to interactions with females. Bulls not exposed to females do not establish this more narrowed range of sexual stimuli, hence the ability of some rather bizarre stimuli to instigate mounting and ejaculation. Dairy bulls are also rarely raised with females and so can be stimulated by other bulls.

Malnutrition rarely affects sexual performance, as evidenced by the continued reproductive success of starving cattle in parts of Asia and Africa. Underfed bulls actually are quicker to copulate than well-fed bulls.[2449]

Experiential Factors
Individual bulls show marked differences in their levels of sexual behavior as measured by such parameters as mounts or ejaculation, the number of ejaculations per unit time, the latency to ejaculation, the number of ejaculations required for satiation, and the length of time to recover from post-satiation refractoriness. It seems unwise, therefore, to continue breeding a male that shows limited interest in mounting females, because doing so will only perpetuate the defect. Early experience and management, in addition to genetic factors, are important determinants of sexual behavior. For instance, Zebu bulls raised in small groups had a faster reaction time (time to the first mount) than did those raised on the range in large herds.[1433]

Blockey[265–267] has developed a procedure for testing serving capacity (libido and copulation competence) in potential beef cattle sires whereby several bulls are tested for 20 minutes with heifers restrained in stanchions. The relative performance in this short test is well correlated with sexual performance in a 19-day pasture breeding test. Because dominance hierarchies are not strong in bulls under two years of age, they do not fight in the group-breeding situation, but they can interfere with one another.[791]

Hereford bulls will consistently mount females by nine months of age, but are a year or older before they ejaculate. Therefore, Hereford bulls should not be given serving-capacity tests before they are 18 months old, when their ejaculation frequency peaks.[1851] The sex ratio in serving-capacity tests should be 1:1, and breeds that differ in aggression (Hereford and Angus) should not be tested together.[1852]

Problems can arise with short-term tests of libido. A high environmental temperature can reduce libido, and the effect may not be the same in all the bulls, so one who normally has high libido may be more affected than one with low libido.[416] Other problems are that bulls are more responsive to pre-ovulatory than to post-ovulatory cows,[791] so cows should be at that stage.

Clinical Problems of Bulls
Masturbation
Although commonly noted among bulls, masturbation causes no known reproductive problem. In general, masturbation is frowned upon on an anthropomorphic basis. Sperm quality or counts do not seem correlated with the frequency of this "vice." The bull performs pelvic thrusts, with his back arched, with a partially erect penis. Thus, the penis moves in and out of the preputial sheath until ejaculation occurs. All bulls masturbate, especially at times of inactivity.[1045] As shown throughout this chapter,

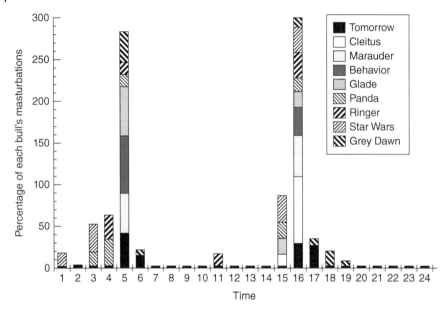

Figure 4.8   The occurrence of masturbation by time of day. The masturbations observed are plotted by the hour of the day in which they occurred as the percentage of each bull's masturbations. Some bulls were observed longer than others, so it was necessary to use percentages rather than absolute numbers of masturbations. *Source:* Houpt and Wollney (1989).[1045]

all domestic animals have been observed to masturbate, so it would be difficult to label this an abnormal behavior. See Figure 4.8 for patterns of masturbation in dairy bulls.

Impotence

Loss of libido must be approached as a clinical problem with a rather large differential diagnosis in mind. The problem may be secondary to almost any other organic disease. Bulls used for AI seem especially susceptible to musculoskeletal diseases, rendering them lame and unable or unwilling to mount. Obesity may be considered a pathological condition, and it caused many problems in the early development of the AI program. Obese bulls were difficult or impossible to arouse. Now the diets of bulls are more closely controlled; however, obesity should still be considered in assessing a case of loss of libido. Balanoposthitis or injury to the penis are specific conditions of the genital urinary tract that might be confused with a libido problem.[1942] Testicular atrophy

involving both the Leydig cells and the seminiferous tubules may occur and be recognized by the reduced size and soft consistency of the testis. This is one case in which androgen administration might be expected to lead to a return of normal sexual behavior. A sperm count is recommended, however, because a hypospermatic animal will still be an unsuitable breeder.

Management practices may influence male libido. A large bull may be unwilling to mount a teaser steer or a cow in an icy corral or on wet concrete floors. One or two slips may be sufficient to condition him to ignore the stimulus of the teaser. Distractions of other animals or human observers should be kept to a minimum; such distractions may present more of a problem for some bulls than others. By 2.5 years of age, most bulls are dominant over cows; before this age, a dominant cow may prevent a young bull from mounting. Restraint of the cow may be of value. Young bulls also lack experience, and their tentative approach while courting may stimulate aggression in a cow. If AI is not possible, and a proposed breeding is between animals far enough apart that one must be transported to the other, bringing the cow to the bull is advisable. Males seem more sensitive to environmental factors; a new or different surrounding may trigger a reluctance to mount. Fortunately, trucking a cow is usually easier than trucking a large, aggressive bull.

For reasons that must be classified as psychological, a bull trained to mount another male and ejaculate into an artificial vagina eventually may lose interest and refuse to mount, especially if he has been used too frequently. This inhibition may be overcome by changing the sexual stimulus to a new steer or bull (the Coolidge effect). A new teaser, preferably a cow or even better an estrous cow, or a moderate change in the environment or location of the mating arena, may be sufficient to stimulate sexual behavior, but because of the risk of disease, cows are not allowed at AI centers. Other bulls are found to be more attractive teasers than steers. Although psychological in its origin, the Coolidge effect has a physiological limit. The maximum number of ejaculations will be the same as that obtained by electroejaculation.

Restraining the bull from the teaser or allowing him to watch another bull being collected also may arouse a previously disinterested male.[266,1205,1440] A caution regarding the latter technique must be made: a submissive or young bull being allowed to observe an animal dominant to him may be further conditioned against servicing through intimidation. In most ungulate species, copulations are restricted to the dominant males. The lack of sexual activity in the remainder of the male population has been termed "psychological castration," although the effect is usually and quickly reversed if the dominant individual is removed.

The Buller Steer

Although most problems of sexual behavior in food-producing animals are those of insufficiency, manifestation of sexual behavior in steers is also a problem. Approximately 3% of feedlot steers are buller steers that are mounted by other steers. Steers are implanted with various types of anabolic steroids, usually in combination; these include estrogen, progesterone, testosterone, trenbolone, or zeranol. Stilbestrol appears to stimulate bulling least.[67,256] The greater the number of steers, the larger the percentage of bullers. There is a large component of dominance-related aggression in the buller syndrome. Penile erection and anal intromission rarely occur. More aggressive animals mount, and the rate of mounting increases dramatically when new steers are added.[1232] The syndrome is seen most frequently when groups of animals are mixed, especially in crowded conditions and in warm weather. The economic losses resulting from the syndrome are due to the increased activity of the mounting steers and the harassment of the buller steer. None of the animals will gain weight as they should.[1116] The usual means of treating bulling behavior is to remove the steers involved; other solutions, including metal buller rails under which the steer can hide, electrified wire placed above the pens so that a steer that reared to mount would be shocked, avoiding conflicts over food and water, and painting odiferous substances on the buller, can be used to reduce the incidence of the behavior.[1116]

Sheep

The Ewe

Estrous Cycle

Sheep are short-light breeders, that is, they usually cycle in the fall of the year as the light phase of the photoperiod decreases. The ewe is polyestrous and will cycle several times during one breeding season if not bred; the average cycle for the ewe is 16 days (range: 14–20). The actual period of estrous receptivity is 30–36 hours in the ewe. The duration of estrus in lambs and in the first estrus of the season is shorter than that of the normal estrus. Puberty is dependent on the time of birth. Females born early enough in the year will cycle their first fall season, indicating that puberty may occur as early as four months of age. Progesterone is necessary for estrous behavior, so the first ovulation of a ewe lamb is a "silent heat."[660] Other environmental influences affect the estrous cycle of sheep. Domestic sheep raised in the tropics and subtropics are non-seasonal breeders;[1085] reproductive activity occurs all year.

Feral sheep display an even shorter breeding season than most of the domestic breeds, and it is likely that both predation pressures and the necessity of foraging over large areas for limited resources established estrous synchrony as an evolutionarily stable strategy in the ancestral forms. In feral sheep, the adult rams form a flock separate from that of the ewes and lambs and join the females only during the breeding season. Flocking tendencies are strong in sheep, and a ewe lambing after the remainder of the flock would be unable to keep up with the movements of the flock.

The Ram Effect

Most sheep breeding is still done naturally, with the rams pastured with the ewes all year or introduced in the late summer. The introduction of a ram, when the ewes have not been with one, tends to synchronize estrus in a high proportion of the ewes 15–17 days later. The mechanism is through LH, a pulse of which is released within minutes of exposure to a ram. If contact with the male is maintained, a preovulatory surge of LH at around 36 hours occurs accompanied by a rise in FSH. Ovulation occurs, but no estrous behavior (silent heat). The ram effect is pheromonally based. The pheromone is present in the wool, wax, and anti-orbital gland secretion of the ram.[1240] The pheromone probably consists of more than one component.[436]

Sexual behavior with subsequent ovulation appears 18 or 25 days after introduction of the ram. The ram effect occurs only in sexually experienced ewes. Continuous exposure to a ram tends to increase the incidence of estrus in the normally anestrous period.[1933] The presence of a ram also shortens the duration of estrus, but this depends on direct physical contact with the ram and probably on mounting of the ewe by the ram, rather than on pheromones.[1797] Rams that court more vigorously cause more ewes to ovulate than do less sexually active rams.[1797]

Estradiol-treated wethers can stimulate estrus in anestrous ewes, indicating that testosterone must be aromatized to produce the ram effect. In sheep, the odor of wool rather than of urine, which is so important in rodents, appears to be involved in both sexual and maternal recognition. There is some effect across species. Although ram wool does not stimulate resumption of cyclic behavior in does, buck hair increases LH levels and thus induces ovulation in ewes.[1744]

Farm animals do not appear to be completely dependent on odor, however; for example, the ram effect can occur even in ewes without the sense of smell.[435] Anosmic ewes exhibit the ram effect in response to a ram, but not to its fleece. Olfactory cues – the main olfactory, not the vomeronasal, organ – are not necessary, but they may be sufficient to stimulate estrus, because the synchronization of the first estrus of the breeding season in sheep can occur in the absence of direct contact or visual cues.[42] Synchronization of estrus is a desirable property of the ewe cycle for management purposes, because breeding may be accomplished in a short time and the lamb crop will be born synchronously and tend to reach market size simultaneously.

Synchronization may also be accomplished by using progesterone compounds, and this procedure is used more as the practice of AI in sheep increases. Estrus occurs 48 hours after withdrawal of vaginal progesterone sponges.[2271] Synchronization is more successful using these compounds if a male is added to the flock before the ewes come into estrus (120 hours) than if it is present only for the 48 hours after withdrawal of progesterone.[1952]

Courtship Behavior

The estrous ewe can be identified because she follows or seeks out a ram; turns her head as the ram approaches; may circle, sniff the male's body and genitals, and then thrust her head against his flanks; fans or wags her tail; and stands to be mounted. Estrous ewes will choose a ram on a two-choice test and will do so even on the basis of a photograph.[1201,2257] She may call frequently with non-specific bleats and be more active.[351] Standing occurs when the female is receptive, and she will look over her shoulder at the ram as he investigates and nudges her. Like cows, most ewes are in standing estrus at night.

The active role of the ewe in seeking the ram was demonstrated in an experiment in which two-thirds of a flock of ewes were bred even though the rams were tethered.[1388,1393] The ewes apparently use olfactory cues to locate the ram because anosmic ewes were unable to find tethered rams.[705] Ewes can be attracted to a male in the next field or to an infertile male, so ram seeking does not guarantee pregnancy. Ram-seeking behavior seems correlated with estrogen levels but does not occur without the visual and olfactory stimuli of the male.[1391]

Competition involving agonistic behavior has been observed between estrous ewes over access to a ram. Older ewes are generally more successful in gaining access to the ram; otherwise, experience does not seem to be an important factor in ewe sexual behavior, but maiden ewes should be kept in separate flocks from experienced ewes or the latter will outcompete the former for the ram's attention.[1428]

The Ram

Sexual Behavior of Free-Ranging Sheep

The sexual behavior of the primitive and free-ranging Soay sheep may give some clue as to the optimal manner of raising breeding rams. Ram lambs remain with their dams from late spring when they are born until the following fall when they begin to chase ewes. They will be rejected by most adult ewes until they are larger. Meanwhile, the adult rams have been living in separate, all-male flocks on separate feeding sites. Before the ewes are in estrus, the rams begin to move toward the ewe flocks. They will chase away strange rams but remain on friendly terms with their own flock mates. As the season progresses, however, they will begin to fight with one another. The fights consist of head clashings in these horned sheep and nudging behavior similar to that seen in courtship. All this takes place before the ewes are receptive, although young rams will have harassed the ewes already. When the ewes come into heat, the sexual contests between the males have been settled and the males can turn their attention to breeding. The winner of the most contests between males breeds the most ewes, but he does so sequentially by tending each ewe for a day, or at least half a day, grazing with her and performing the courtship activities described earlier in this chapter for domestic sheep.[864] The rams graze and rest less while courting and fighting, and they may lose weight. These observations indicate that the best way to rear breeding rams would be to leave them with females for as long as possible, certainly until puberty, and then put them in an all-male group.

Domestic Sheep

The reproductive capacity of the ram is not seasonally limited as is that of the ewe. Estrous ewes may be satisfactorily fertilized at any season, although semen quality may decline somewhat during the spring.[1792,1793] Thus, the breeding season in domestic breeds is primarily determined by the environmental input to the female's hypothalamic–hypophyseal tract. Although the ewe may seek out the ram, courtship is more elaborate in the male than in the female.

Courtship Behavior

Rams need not have exposure to females as young lambs to have normal sexual behavior, but they should have exposure during adolescence. As does the female, the male spends a great deal of time sniffing the other's genitalia and urine; the flehmen response may be noted (see Figure 4.9). The flehmen response has no visual communicative properties but may be a method of introducing material into the vomeronasal organ. Rams flehmen less frequently when ewes are in estrus, apparently because estrous ewes urinate less.[261] Urination appears to be a sign that the ewe is not in estrus. The male may also lick the female's genitalia, a form of tactile stimulation that may also be part of the testing procedure. Normally, rams can discriminate estrous from non-estrous ewe urine using olfaction.[264] Bulbectomized (no olfactory bulb) rams in a range situation show some difficulty in identifying estrous females; they are nonselective in the ewes they approach

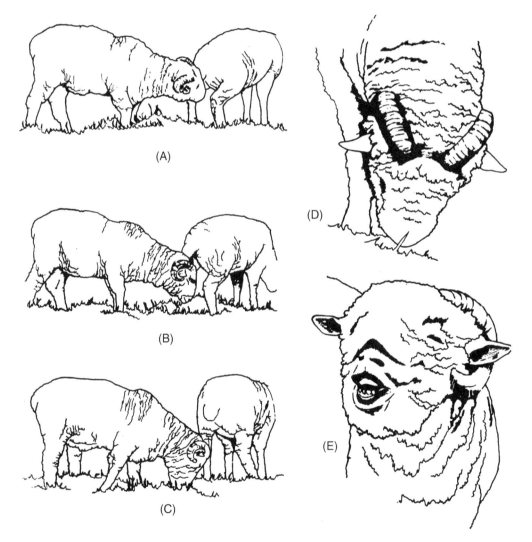

(A)

(B)

(C)

(D)

(E)

Figure 4.9 Response of the ram to urine of an estrous ewe. (A) Urination by ewe; (B–D) ram nosing urine on the ground; (E) the flehmen response. *Source:* Banks (1964).[159] Reproduced with permission of Brill Academic Publishers.

and test but are able to identify estrous ewes, presumably via visual and auditory cues.[1387] In fact, confined rams may not use any sensory cue to detect estrus; they may rely entirely on the willingness of the ewe to stand. When given a choice of restrained ovariectomized ewes, rams sniffed, nudged, mounted, and copulated with ewes with equal frequency whether or not they had received estrogen; all had received progesterone.[2122]

Perception via the vomeronasal organ is important in that intact rams mount and ejaculate more than those with blocked vomeronasal organs.[2307] Ewes do differ in their sexual attractiveness to rams. This attractiveness is stable from estrus to estrus and depends, at least in part, on wool. Woolly ewes are preferred to shorn ones, indicating that wool and/or wax is an important source of attractivity.[2257] The attractiveness of estrous ewes for rams depends, in part, on the bacterial flora present in their vagina. The bacteria may react with pheromones or themselves contribute to attractivity.[2304]

A ritualized kicking with a foreleg is performed as the ram orients himself behind the ewe; the leg is raised and lowered in a stiff-legged striking manner (see Figure 4.10). Tongue flicking accompanies the nudging. Nudging is also stereotyped: the head is tilted

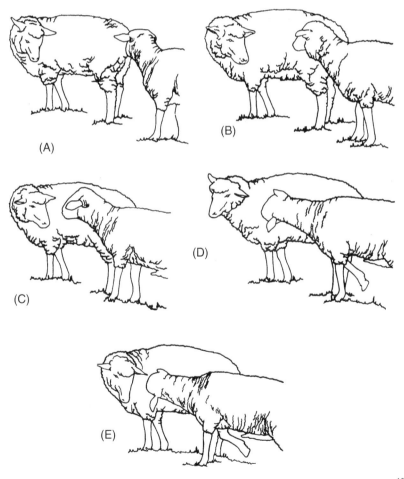

Figure 4.10 Nudging sequence in sheep courtship behavior. *Source:* Banks (1964).[159] Reproduced with permission of Brill Academic Publishers.

and lowered while the shoulder is brought into contact with or oriented toward the flank of the ewe; simultaneously, the ram utters low-pitched vocalizations or gargling or courting grunts. Six nudgings of the ewe per minute are observed at the peak of the ram's sexual interest.[2246] Several abortive mounts may be made with pelvic thrusting but without intromission. When the tip of the glans penis contacts the vulvar mucosa, a strong pelvic thrust accomplishes intromission, and ejaculation occurs immediately. After dismount, the ram may sniff the ewe's vulva, appear depressed, and stand near the female with head down; he may urinate.

The latency to ejaculation increases with the number of observed ejaculations during an observation period, but it is subject to large individual variation. The number of ejaculations that occur when a ram is presented with a large number of estrous ewes is similar to the number that occur in response to an electroejaculator, indicating that physical capability rather than libido is limiting. A ram will show a reluctance to re-mate a recently mated female, whether or not he was the male who inseminated her originally.

If rams are mated to sexual exhaustion with one ewe (usually three to six matings),[1083] rapid recovery may be obtained by introducing a new ewe, whereas a much poorer recovery rate is obtained by removing and reintroducing the original ewe.[200] This effect of novelty is the Coolidge effect. Another method of demonstrating this phenomenon is to present four receptive ewes to a ram; he mates three times as much as he does when only one ewe is in estrus.[42] There is some evidence that habituation to a sexual partner may last several weeks after a mating as measured by the degree of recovery in the sex drive following satiation. These effects make evolutionary sense to the species and are fortunate for the rancher. A ram is capable of something less than 20 ejaculations daily. If many of these copulations were repeat breedings to especially persistent ewes, the fertility rate for the herd probably would be low. This breeding efficiency allows a rancher to introduce only a few rams to service a flock. Ewes can in a single pregnancy produce lambs sired by different rams.[660] In wild or feral sheep, a dominant male can spread his genes over a much larger proportion of the population than if the mechanisms for reduced repeat breedings by either himself or subordinate males did not exist.

Serving-Capacity Tests

One serving-capacity test that is predictive of the lambs sired is to place a ram with three restrained estrous ewes and record mounts and ejaculations. The test is repeated nine times. To test for mate preference, the ram is observed with restrained rams and two restrained estrous females. When released with ewes, low-sexual-performance rams sired as many lambs as the female-oriented rams (not all rams prefer ewes; see the "Clinical Problems of Rams" section), but the high-sexual-performance ram sired nearly twice as many.[2177] Rams do not discriminate between ewes in natural estrus and ovariectomized ewes treated with progesterone and estrogen,[1856] so either may be used for serving-capacity tests. Rams show similar rates of ejaculation and mounting whether ewes are restrained or free to move in a pen; however, if copulation is prevented (by covering the perineum), there are many more mountings and foreleg kicks as well as buttings.[1860] Foreleg kicking and sniffing the anogenital area of the ewe are considered courtship behavior, whereas attempts to mount, mounting, and ejaculation are considered copulatory behavior. The courtship behaviors are a good measure of libido because when copulation or mounting is prohibited, males sniff and nudge more if they have higher serving capacity (that is, ejaculations).[1855]

Prenatal Effects

The intrauterine environment influences subsequent ram sexual behavior. Rams born co-twin to a ram have a higher serving capacity than those born co twin to a ewe. The larger the litter size, the higher the serving capacity of its male members.[700]

Rearing Effects

It seems to be important for lambs to have heterosexual experience in the period between weaning and their first birthday in order for them to prefer ewes to rams as sexual partners. Ram lambs at six months will begin to exhibit adult sexual behavior sooner if they are exposed to estrous ewes for as little as 30 minutes per day for four days. By eight months, exposure to estrous ewes does not result in an earlier onset of adult sexual behavior. This is important because the young ram lambs could be used for breeding before they are a year old. In addition to the immediate effects of exposure to females, delayed effects can occur. Exposure to estrous ewes for several hours at 10 months of age enhances sexual performance at two years in rams that were otherwise kept in all-male groups.[1855]

Dominance Effect

When more than one ram is being used to service a flock, dominance effects may influence the percentage of the flock each ram inseminates. Mature rams may dominate younger rams and almost always will dominate yearling rams. Dominance orders, as determined by the number of butts each animal delivers when the animals are confined together, also exist and may be more marked between yearling rams. Rank in a food competition hierarchy corresponds to rank in the sexual hierarchy.[720] In a confined ewe flock, a dominant ram may copulate 12–15 times daily over the breeding season, whereas the subordinate ram(s) may average only two to five copulations daily.[1149] The subordinate rams may service ewes, but this occurs mostly at times when pregnancy is not likely to result, that is, long after ovulation. In a feral population or a multi-ram pasture breeding situation, a number of rams may copulate with a ewe. The ram who copulates between the 9th and 15th hour of estrus is most likely to sire the lambs because that is when the ewe is most fertile.[1149] In less confined conditions, the monopolization of mating by the dominant ram may be restricted only to the harem of ewes he is able to hold.[1479]

When groups of rams are to be used together in a mass-mating system, the age groups should be uniform and space should be adequate.[1083] Three rams per 100 ewes or 20–50 ewes per ram has been suggested for a range-breeding situation. It is unwise to use a pair of rams to breed a group of ewes because agonistic activity may take precedence over mating behavior. Three rams served 50% more ewes than a single ram over a four-day period.[1392,1393] It is unfortunate that dominance or sexual aggressiveness does not necessarily correlate with fertility; the combination of dominance with infertility in a flock ram could be disastrous to a rancher.

In pen breeding, a teaser, or vasectomized, ram is used to mark ewes by means of a harness and crayon attached to his brisket. A ewe that is in estrus will be mounted and, therefore, marked.[1389] The marked ewes are then added to the breeding ram's pen. Problems can arise if the breeding ram is submissive to rams in nearby pens. He may be inhibited and not mount. Another problem is seen when young and mature ewes are added simultaneously. Rams prefer or are monopolized by the older ewes. For most effective pen breeding, ewes should be checked for heat at 12-hour intervals and the breeding rams should be free of disturbance from rams or ewes in adjacent pens.[1219]

The effects of the presence of the ram on the reproductive status of the ewe have been discussed already. The ram is influenced in his turn by the presence of the ewe. Testosterone levels, testis size, and levels of aggressive behavior are all higher in rams in pens next to ewes than in isolated rams,[1103] and rams thus stimulated show more sexual behavior when they have access to ewes.[1964] Rams, like ewes, prefer mates of their own or their dam's breed.[1207] The presence of lower ranking rams stimulates mounting of ewes by mid-ranked rams, but has no effect on high-ranking rams.[2303]

The effects of castration in pre-pubertal rams are extremely variable; there may be some decline in, or the complete elimination of, sexual activity.[159] Post-pubertal castration causes decreased sexual activity in rams,[42] but erection and intromission may persist for years postoperatively, albeit with a marked decrease in frequency.

Clinical Problems of Rams

Rams are often reared in large monosexual groups or individually. The isolated males show some aberrations in behavior when first exposed to estrous females, but most are eventually able to mate.[2518] The previously isolated rams were more proficient than rams raised in all-male groups.[349] Some of the rams raised in monosexual groups are sexually inhibited or show homosexual preferences and do so for long periods or permanently after maturity. In one study, after nine days' exposure to estrous ewes, some rams (17%) still had not copulated.[1086,1858] Continuous exposure to ewes eventually stimulates sexual behavior in most

rams. Six to eight percent of rams are male oriented. Even those rams who do eventually mate estrous ewes after several exposures continue to exhibit subnormal sexual performance, that is, they are not "cured."[1861] The frequency of mounting in an all-male group cannot be used to predict sexual behavior in a mixed-sex group. Homosexual rams have fewer estradiol receptors in the amygdala[26] and may have lower blood levels of estrone and estradiol.[1822] Aromatase activity, which converts testosterone to estradiol in the brain, is lower in male-oriented rams.[1967] There is a sexually dimorphic nucleus in the ovine brain, and it is larger in female-oriented (heterosexual) than male-oriented (homosexual) rams (Figure 4.11). These results indicate that male-oriented rams have not been masculinized completely.

Some individuals in the male groups learn to associate courtship and mounting activities with agonistic behavior, but the physiological data indicate an earlier neurological cause.[2518] It seems reasonable, nevertheless, to suggest not raising rams in monosexual groups in order to avoid sexual inhibition or the development

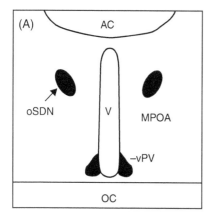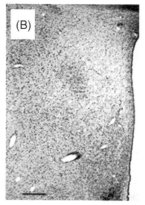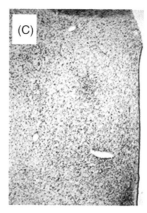

Figure 4.11 (A) Schematic diagram of a coronal section through the sheep at the level of the optic chiasm (OC) and anterior commissure (AC). The position of the ovine sexually dimorphic nucleus (oSDN) is shown bilateral to the third ventricle (V) in the central part of the medial preoptic nucleus (MPOA). The ventral paraventricular nucleus (vPV) is shown at the base of the ventricle. (B) Micrograph of oSDN from the left hypothalamus of a female-oriented ram. The third ventricle is at the right of the figure. (C) Section of a male-oriented ram comparable to that in (B). The photomicrograph is taken near the midpoint of the anterior–posterior extent of the oSDN. The scale bar is 1 mm. *Source:* Roselli and Stormshak (2009).[1966] Reproduced with permission of Elsevier.

of homosexual preferences. Mixed groups are probably ideal, with isolated rearing less preferable but acceptable.[1184] Fence-line contact (separate sexes in adjacent pastures) only partially improves sexual performance of rams, and only those that are attracted to ewes on the other side of the fence exhibit normal male sexual behavior.[1861] The sexual performance is reflected endocrinologically. High-performing rams exhibit an increase in LH when allowed fence-line contact with ewes but do not respond hormonally to rams, whereas in low-performing or male-oriented rams, no change in LH occurred regardless of the sex of the animal on the other side of the fence.[27]

Goats

Free-Ranging Goats

During the rut, feral bucks join female groups and fight for access to the estrous does. The most successful goats are five to six years old. Older males select groups in which they are more likely to be successful, that is, groups with few other males, whereas young males select the groups with the largest number of does.[591]

A detailed study of feral goats indicated that does permitted large, horned bucks to mount, but small, hornless goats were virtually excluded from breeding. When pursuing a doe, the buck would gobble, a sound produced by moaning and rapidly thrusting his tongue in and out. Courtship activity would cease when the buck exhibited the flehmen response to a non-estrous doe's urine. Although large males were usually able to chase off rivals, occasionally many males would mount a female in quick succession without regard to their position in the dominance hierarchy.[2090]

The Doe

Goats, like sheep, are short-day breeders. Does in estrus show an increase in tail wagging, vocalization, urination, and mounting of other females. This is probably proceptive behavior

in that it does not occur as frequently if males are in the same enclosure. Does are in estrus for 39 hours once every 20–21 days. There is a male effect in goats as well as sheep. Contact with bucks induces in anestrous goats an immediate increase of LH followed by ovulation. The bucks must be sexually active – that is, exposed to a light regime simulating fall – but they need be present only part of the day.[1939] Estrous does are attracted to the urine of bucks, but that produced during self-enurination is not preferred to normally voided urine.[2753] Does isolated from males during the non-breeding season begin to cycle much later in the year than those maintained with males during some part of the non-breeding season.[533] In contrast to ewes, a large proportion of does exhibit sexual behavior with the first ovulation.[660] Doe preferences seems to depend on the male's testosterone level, because they prefer castrated, testosterone-treated males to intact males during the non-breeding season when testosterone levels are naturally low.[2588] Testosterone level concentrations and courtship rate were positively correlated.

The Buck

There is a close relationship between agonistic and sexual behaviors in male goats.[442] In general, billy goat or buck behavior is similar to ram behavior, kicking at the doe with the front legs, stretching his neck toward her, and emitting the gobbling vocalization. The buck holds his tail straight up during courtship. He is stimulated sexually by observing does that are tail wagging.[940] A component of the mating sequence unique to the goat is the urination by bucks on their own forelegs and beards during courtship. This behavior is termed "enurination." Occasionally, mouthing of the penis also occurs. Although various functions have been attributed to enurination, including increasing the intensity of the buck's odor and advertising his nutritional fitness, the behavior occurs most frequently in a situation of sexual frustration when the buck is restrained from mating.

See Figure 4.7 for normal caprine sexual behavior. Observation of does mounting one another or copulation by a male and female stimulates ejaculation sooner and with more frequency.[2096]

Goats reared in a group of males from the time of birth have fewer agonistic interactions with other bucks at puberty and mount other males more frequently.[2305] The dominant goats initiate homosexual behavior toward the subordinate ones. Homosexual behavior does not interfere with their ability to ejaculate into an artificial vagina in response to the stimulation of an estrous female.[1735]

Male goats are usually sexually inactive during the non-breeding season, but can be brought into sexual activity and hormone levels by exposure to sexually active goats. This is termed the "buck to buck effect."[2713] When semen is to be collected from bucks, their libido, as measured by the number of mounts before ejaculation and latency to ejaculate a second time, was better if they had a choice of two females, whether or not the second female was mounted. Post-pubertal castration causes a decline in sexual behavior in goats, but wethers may still be sexually active, mounting half as many does as do intact bucks.[931,2266]

Clinical Problems

The Doe
Silent Heat
The first ovulation of the season is often a silent heat.[249,410]

The Buck
In contrast to sheep, bucks are unlikely to exhibit substandard sexual performance if denied heterosexual experience in their first year.[1859] Not all goats that mount homosexually in an all-male group will fail to mount heterosexually; those that do probably have a strong preference for one partner who happens to be male. The bucks that are mounted by other males are less apt to restrict their sexual activity to males. White bucks appear to be mounted more often than colored ones, which may be a function of the calm disposition of white Saanen goats rather than of coat color preference by the mounters.[1859] Homosexual behavior was more frequent during the late breeding season than during the early and the non-breeding seasons, and was more common in males isolated from females than in males housed near estrous females.[2304]

Horses

Free-Ranging Horses

Free-ranging mares will often seek out a stallion during estrus and display the normal behavioral signs of estrus in front of him.[676,2300] It is unusual for free-ranging two-year-old mares to breed (1%) and even uncommon for three-year-olds to breed (13%).[2300] Stallions generally do not exhibit much interest in the sexual displays of young mares. Yearling mares may show very exaggerated signs of estrus and may attract males from bachelor herds. It has not been established whether the yearlings are in true or psychic estrus (see "Clinical Problems") because it has been most often observed in free-ranging horses. It is rare, but not unknown, for two-year-old feral mares to deliver a foal, indicating that they can conceive as yearlings. It is hypothesized that the exaggerated signs of estrus in young mares may be a means of attracting stallions from a distance (that is, unrelated stallions). Incest is unusual in free-ranging bands; mares usually leave the band when sexually mature, but those that remain in their sire's herd have a much lower foaling rate than those who join an unrelated male's herd. Those who join a half-brother herd have an intermediate rate.[1195] Mares may breed with their fathers or sons, but this is rare.[2992] Stallions base their avoidance of incest on familiarity rather than on kin recognition.[239] Although feral stallions almost never breed their own daughters, those used for breeding before release may do so.

Human-controlled reproductive experience may contribute to incestuous behavior observed in reintroduced semi-feral Konik stallions. These stallions failed to expel their daughters as juveniles and then bred them when they became sexually mature.[2765]

The stallion is the sire of foals born in his band in 85% of the cases. In the other cases, the mare has been bred by bachelor stallions or the stallion of another band.[1182] In multi-male bands, the dominant horse sires most of the foals as determined by electrophoresis of foal and stallion blood proteins. Dominant mares have dominant colts that sire more foals than do the male offspring of subordinate mares.[672]

The Mare

Estrous Cycle

Mares show the opposite seasonality in estrous pattern to that of sheep and goats; that is, they are long-day breeders and cycle in the spring. Foaling season is late winter and early spring, and the 11- to 11.5-month gestation period has dictated a rapid recycling and rebreeding if foals are to be born to coincide with the spring grasses. Most free-ranging horses are probably bred on the first, or at latest the second, heat after foaling.[2300] If breeding does not take place, estrus recurs approximately every 21–24 days. The older the mare, the earlier she starts exhibiting estrus-positive behaviors (lowering and abducting the hind limbs, winking urinating, deflecting the tail), and ceased estrus-negative behaviors (vigorous switching of tail, biting and kicking teaser).[2951] The average length of receptivity is five to seven days, longer than most ungulates. Breed differences in the length of estrus in different localities have been noted, but are of uncertain significance, owing to the probable interplay of genetic and environmental factors, methods of testing for the presence of estrus, and statistical analysis.[2387]

Modern management usually isolates the stallion from the mares. Teaser animals are used to determine the receptivity of the mare. The teasers are usually stallions that are introduced to a mare across some form of barrier; the mare is restrained and sometimes hobbled. A non-receptive mare will react to the teaser's advances by squealing, striking, kicking, and moving away. During full estrus, the mare indicates receptivity by her immobility and by permitting the teaser to nibble her rump and withers. The mare exhibits a characteristic breeding expression in which her ears are turned backward but not flattened and her lips are held loosely (refer to Figure 1.4 in Chapter 1). She adopts a base-wide squatting stance, urinates frequently, and rhythmically exposes the clitoris with a series of labial muscle contractions known as "winking" (Figure 4.12A).[105,117] Rectal palpation or ultrasonography may be helpful to ensure that follicular development coincides with the behavioral aspects of estrus. The optimal breeding time is usually the second or third day of estrus. In a pasture situation with 10–20 mares per stallion, a mare will mate six times in an estrous period.[478]

Mares show individual preferences for stallions, and the preferences are influenced by the stallion's vocal behavior. The more the stallion neighs, the more likely the mare is to approach him.[1819] The importance of vocal stimulation is demonstrated by playing a recording of a courting stallion's vocalizations and/or manipulating the mare's genitalia. Mares will exhibit receptivity and an increased intrauterine pressure.[1425,1490,2341] They discriminate in their response, preferring the voices of stallions with lower frequency vocalization; these stallions are more fertile.[1340] This makes it possible to detect behavioral estrus in the absence of a stallion. Exposure to male odor, a procedure that is effective in sows, elicits the signs of estrus in only half of the mares tested. Mounting of mares by other mares occurs, but rarely. The mounting mares are usually in the follicular phase and have a higher plasma testosterone.[800]

Bringing a pregnant mare that had been mated away from home into a vicinity of a

(A) (B)

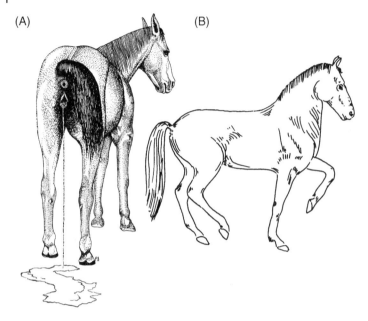

Figure 4.12   (A) The posture of the estrous mare. The clitoris is everted, and the tail deviated. (B) The prance, or piaffe, of the courting stallion. *Source:* Houpt (1977).[1042]

familiar male who was not the father of her fetus increased the probability of pregnancy disruption, so that 31% of the mares aborted.[177] This is an example of the Bruce effect.

Foal Heat

Foal heat following parturition is quite predictable, occurring usually nine days (range: 5–18 days) after foaling. Regular estrous cycles usually continue thereafter at approximately 21- to 22-day intervals, although a few mares appear to have a lactational diestrus due to maintenance of the corpus luteum following the foaling heat. Other mares are cycling but do not show estrous behavior in the presence of a stallion. Instead, the mares protect their foals. Habituation to the stallion might result in normal estrous behavior. Many mares are bred on the foal heat because it is predictable and easily detected and planned for, although the endometrial epithelium is rarely restored or complete at foaling heat and usually does not accomplish restoration until days 13–24 following the heat. The 30-day heat following foaling is a safer time to breed; a higher conception rate occurs.

Clinical Problems of Mares

The common sexual behavior problems of mares are silent heat, psychic estrus, and excessive sexual behavior.

Most of the sexual problems of mares occur at either end of the breeding season. Mares are seasonal breeders that come into estrus as daylight increases. Feral horses in the United States have a restricted breeding season. The foals are born in early summer, and the mares are bred on foal heat. No doubt, if all domestic mares were pasture bred during the late spring and summer, they would be increasing in number at the same rate as the wild horses. Mares normally are anestrous from October to February; however, mares can and do show estrus and conceive all year round, especially if artificial light is used to simulate long days and the mares are well fed and well sheltered. Despite our ability to manipulate the equine reproductive cycle, seasonality is expressed in the large numbers of abnormal heats observed in mares.

Split and Prolonged Estrus

It is at the transitional periods, the beginning and end of the breeding season, that such sexual abnormalities as prolonged estrus and split estrus are usually seen. The length of estrus can be prolonged from five to seven days to up to 90 days. This may be accompanied by aggressive behavior. Other mares may show split estrus. Split estrus may consist of one to two days of "shallow" estrus in which the mare does not react to the stallion with vigorous squatting, tail deviation, and urination, but rather tolerates him and occasionally exhibits signs of estrus. A few days later, she may show strong signs of sexual receptivity. Both prolonged estrus and split estrus may be accompanied by active ovaries in which follicles are present but do not mature. In the fall, follicles may remain on the ovaries rather than regress, and this condition may be accompanied by complete anestrus or abnormal estrus. Mares that have either prolonged estrus or split estrus may begin to have normal cycles as the breeding season progresses and daylight length increases.

Anestrus

One of the most common reproductive problems of mares is anestrus. Mares may be either physiologically or behaviorally anestrous. The former includes mares with persistent corpora lutea and those with inactive ovaries. Older mares may have inactive ovaries due to degenerative changes in the endometrium and/or degenerative changes in the ovary itself. There may be senile changes in the ovaries, including the formation of germinal inclusion cysts. The age at onset of these senile changes varies from the mid-teens to well into the twenties.

A developmental cause of anestrus in mares is hypoplasia of the gonads and the reproductive tract. This condition, which is relatively rare, is similar to Turner's syndrome in humans because it is associated with an XO rather than the normal XX pair of sex chromosomes.

Although most pregnant mares do not show estrous behavior, a few may, and these mares may be carrying female foals.[106,954] The sexual behavior is most likely to occur between days 30 and 40 of pregnancy, when accessory follicles are formed. The behavior of the pregnant mare can be distinguished from that of the non-pregnant estrous mare by the rapid tail lashing or wringing of the former as compared with the deviated tail of the latter. The pregnant mare will not usually stand for the stallion; she is not truly receptive. Her urine will be clear rather than cloudy, as is that of the estrous mare.

Silent Heat   Behavioral anestrus is also known as "silent heat." Palpation of the ovaries may reveal normal follicles. Ovulation will take place normally. There is physiological, but not behavioral, estrus because the mare will not accept the stallion. One reason for silent heat may be related to the fact that mares do show mate preferences. These preferences should be considered in teasing a mare in silent heat; more than one stallion should be used. Environmental factors can influence the behavior of the mare just as they influence the behavior of the stallion. A mare may not show estrus if she has just been trailered to a strange stud farm or handled by a strange person. If the mare does not show signs of estrus even in a familiar environment and with exposure to several stallions, she may still conceive if she is artificially inseminated or tranquilized, restrained, and forcibly mated by the stallion.

Psychic Heat

Squealing and urinating accompanied by tail lashing are aggression, not estrus. A careful examination may reveal lower genital tract lesions. Not all sexual abnormalities of mares are caused by a deficiency of sexual behavior; some result from an excess of sexual behavior. Some mares, for example, show estrous behavior without the normal physiological correlates of estrus. This abnormality is known as "psychic heat." It may occur when any horse is brought into the environment of a solitary mare. In that case, it is usually a relatively short-lived phenomenon. Much more serious is psychic heat of performing mares. A mare that stops frequently to urinate and is attracted to stallions, geldings, or mares will not be a good competitive trail horse or show ring performer. Despite posture and behavior, the mare in psychic heat may not tolerate mounting by a stallion. Before psychic estrus is diagnosed, a painful condition of the pelvic area must be ruled out.

Progestins such as altrenogest (0.02 ml/kg orally) or progesterone (0.4 mg/kg i.m. daily) have been used successfully to treat mares that show severe psychic heat. The progestins are believed to act on those neurons in the brain, probably in the hypothalamus, that control sexual behavior. Ovariectomy may be performed to treat psychic estrus or estrus-related poor performance, but about 30% of spayed mares show constant estrus. If psychic estrus persists in an ovariectomized mare, dexamethasone may be used in an attempt to suppress endogenous adrenal steroids that might be inducing estrous behavior, but serious side effects can occur.

Excessive Sexual Behavior

Two pathological conditions of the ovaries can cause excessive sexual behavior in the mare. The abnormalities are granulosa cell tumors and persistent follicles. These conditions should be differentiated because granulosa cell tumors should be treated surgically, but persistent follicles usually resolve themselves. The excessive estrous-like behavior of mares with persistent follicles is sometimes called "nymphomania." The cysts will regress in time and do not need to be manipulated as follicular cysts of cows do. The persistent follicles may also be treated with gonadotropins, LH, or an increase in artificial day length to 16 hours or more.

Mares suffering from granulosa cell tumors can show a variety of signs. Twenty percent will show continuous estrus, and 25% anestrus. About 40% of granulosa cell tumors also contain thecal cells that produce testosterone.[497] The affected mares will show stallion-like behavior, aggression, flehmen, urine marking (they straddle the urine of another

horse as a stallion would, but their urine will be deposited behind rather than on the target), arched neck threats, mounting mares, and other symptoms. The affected ovary should be removed.

Effect of Estrous Cycle on Performance

An owner who believes a mare's performance waxes or wanes with her estrous cycle should keep a daily record of her performance and have frequent veterinary examinations to determine when the mare is in estrus.

The Stallion

Stallions exhibit libido throughout the year but show peak sexual behavior in the spring. Seasonal changes are also seen in sperm number and testosterone levels.[1821] Stallions with a harem have a higher level of testosterone than those in a bachelor herd, which in turn have a higher level than stalled stallions.[1514] This variation indicates the importance of the social situation. At times of turmoil, such as after a Bureau of Land Management roundup, the percentage of foals sired by stallions other than the dominant one is 30%.[306]

Sexual behavior was seen in two- to three-month-old colts, with full penile erection during resting, play fighting, or mutual grooming,[2300] but the age at the first successful copulation varied from 15 months to three years in the same study. Stallions may actively prevent young males from mounting females.[2300] When exposed to estrous mares, stallions raised from weaning in bachelor groups did not exhibit mounting until two years old.[1555]

Courtship Behavior

Courtship behavior will vary with the management practices involved. The following description assumes that the mare and stallion have free access to each other.

Driving, herding, or snaking with a distinctive head-down position is a behavior usually elicited by the presence of another stallion. Piaffe-like prancing is also a display to other stallions (see Figure 4.12B).

Intromission may be achieved only with a full erection, and this is correlated with the degree of sexual excitement. Thus, an adequate period of sexual foreplay is essential.[2387] Males may tend a female for several days before she is fully receptive. Nipping and nuzzling begin at the mare's head and proceed gradually along the body of the mare to the perineal area. During this testing phase, he exhibits the flehmen response. As sexual excitement increases, the male calls with neighs and roars. The stallion licks the mare around her rear limbs and back. Full erection usually develops over several minutes in the mature stallion. Several mounts are usually made before intromission and ejaculation. During copulation, the stallion rests his sternum on the mare's croup and may reach forward to bite her neck. Ejaculation occurs around 15 seconds after intromission and after approximately seven thrusts,[2260] and intromission lasts less than 45 seconds.

Post-copulatory tending was not noted in feral bands in Wyoming and England.[677,2300] The male may sniff the mare's genital area and exhibit the flehmen response, but the pair soon separates. Under test conditions, sexual satiation occurs after 1–10 ejaculations (average: 2.9).[245] Although stallions usually are limited to a few hand breedings per week, a six-year-old Belgian stallion bred 20 mares in nine days, with an 85% conception rate. Prostaglandin had been used to synchronize estrus, so eight mares were in heat and were bred by the stallion on one day.[336]

Sensory Stimuli

Visual and other sensory stimuli are probably vital to the display of sexual behavior; however, their importance may be modified through learning. The visual stimulus of the mare's posture with raised tail may be important for attraction and penile erection. This reaction may be generalized so that a dummy or phantom in the general shape of a mare will be mounted by a sexually experienced stallion. Inexperienced stallions will not mount the dummy.[2448] Experienced males will also mount a mare or dummy while blindfolded. The stallion is undoubtedly stimulated by olfactory information, but the stimulation may precede the copulation by several minutes to hours. Typically, a stallion will stop chasing an estrous mare to sniff and flehmen at the small volume of urine she has expelled. Odor stimulation of the vomeronasal organ may lead to an increase in LH, testosterone, and consequently libido, so his behavior is synchronized with that of the receptive mare. Experienced males do not show any inhibition to mounting a mare or dummy when olfactory input is blocked, but inexperienced males will mount a dummy only when it has been sprinkled with urine from an estrous female.

Clinical Problems of Stallions

Ten percent to 25% of stallions presented for breeding soundness examination have some behavioral problem. Those stallions most at risk are young and/or novice breeders, frequently bred stallions, those in a new environment, and those in transition from racing to breeding.[1504] Young stallions appear to be particularly affected by exercise; as little as 30 min/day of lunging can decrease libido.[551]

Some common problems of sexual behavior in the male are as follows:

- Stallions that show sexual interest in mares but will not mount, or mount but do not ejaculate;
- Stallions that have low or no libido, that is, do not show interest in a sexually receptive mare;
- Stallions that will mount mares only when another specific horse is present;
- Stallions that injure, or "savage," mares or handlers;
- Stallions that self-mutilate;
- Stallions that mount but do not intromit;
- Geldings that behave like stallions.

Masturbation

Masturbation is normal behavior in a stallion. The stallion flips the erect penis against the ventral abdominal wall. Ejaculation rarely occurs.

Stallions masturbate four times a day, spending 30 minutes with an erect penis sometimes, but not always, accompanied by masturbation.[2259] This behavior usually occurs in the resting stallion, even one at pasture with mares available. Masturbation may occur in association with recumbency.[2451] Feral pony stallions are resting, standing quietly, grazing, or playing 80% of the time when they are masturbating.[2770]

Sexual Experience and Decreased Sexual Behavior

Too much serious sexual experience too early is very detrimental to normal libido. Many stallions overused as youngsters are presented with sexual behavior problems. The most common problems are impotence or low libido. Other stallions that are over-worked as studs may bite the mares viciously or be uncontrollable by their attendants. It is not always clear whether the young stallions have had traumatic or unpleasant experiences. They may remember being kicked by a mare, or they may simply remember that they were exhausted. The resultant loss of libido can persist indefinitely unless treated.[1820]

A typical case is that of a four-year-old Arabian stallion that showed different behaviors to different mares. He mounted without erection and bit a Morgan mare with which he had been housed as a two-year-old. His sexual behavior was normal toward another mare with which he had had no previous contact. He had been noted to display snapping (see Chapters 1 and 6) to the Morgan mare as a youngster and presumably was subordinate to her. As an adult, he showed aggressive behavior toward her, perhaps because of an approach–avoidance conflict. He was sexually stimulated, but because she was dominant, he did not want to mount. His displacement behavior was aggression.

Stallions that are used as teasers – that is, to detect estrus in mares – but are not used for breeding may eventually show a loss of libido. In addition, they may show stereotypic behavior, such as stall weaving. It has not been determined how often a teaser stallion should be allowed to copulate to prevent these abnormal behaviors, and there are, no doubt, individual differences in response to use as a teaser.

Stallions can learn to inhibit sexual behavior as easily as they learn to express it. Stallions may be fitted with stallion rings, devices placed on the penis that cause discomfort if erection occurs. They are used on stallions that are in training or in other circumstances in which sexual behavior would be inappropriate. Many stallions apparently can be fitted with these devices and learn not to respond sexually when wearing them, and yet respond normally when the rings are removed. Other stallions have learned too well and are impotent even when the ring is removed. Stallion rings and belly brushes are also used to prevent masturbation, which, as already noted in this chapter, should not be considered either abnormal behavior or a cause of infertility. Ejaculation rarely occurs, so the behavior is unlikely to lead to a drop in fertility; attempts to punish masturbation, however, do cause libido problems.

Physical Impairment

The treatment of any behavior problem must begin with elimination, or at least identification, of any physical problem. The two most common physical problems associated with breeding are genital injury or limb injury. Any lameness or limb injury will inhibit the stallion's ability to mount, so he may exhibit normal libido and penile erection but will not mount. An older stallion with navicular disease or chronic arthritis is a typical example of the effect of organic limb disease on sexual behavior. When pain is the cause of libido problems, nonsteroidal anti-inflammatory agents such as phenylbutazone and flunixin meglumine may be of value. Another factor that may be responsible for failure to mount is improper flooring. If the flooring is slippery, for instance, the stallion will be reluctant to mount, especially if he has fallen when trying to mount a mare on other occasions. He is much more likely to mount if taken to an environment with a different substrate such as grass or tanbark. A stallion with a mild loco-motor problem may mount but be reluctant to ejaculate in cold weather. In warm weather, when he is pain free, he will be normal.

Injury to the genitalia can be a cause of breeding difficulties. Naturally, a stallion will avoid intromission if his penis is painful. Stallions may be reluctant to copulate long after the injury is apparently healed because they have learned too well that copulation is painful. Any impairment of blood flow to the penis may produce behavior problems such as ejaculatory failure.

Stallions with physical impairment of the legs or back should be mounted on secure mounts, that is, sturdy mares. The flooring should be adequate, and the mare should be the correct size so that the sternum of the stallion rests on her croup. Anatomical fit is important because even normal stallions may lose their balance and slide off a mare that is too small or too large. Situating the mare in a depression can be a solution for a lame stallion. Physically impaired stallions can be trained to an artificial dummy mount that is secure when AI is permitted for the breed. At first, an estrous mare may have to be held next to the dummy, but stallions can, like bulls, be conditioned to ejaculate in the absence of the normal stimulus of the mare.

Breeding Environment

The total breeding environment must be considered because another cause of injury to the stallion can be a low roof or an overhang. A stallion rearing on his hind legs to mount a mare is considerably taller than when he is standing on all fours. If a stallion strikes his head while mounting, he may not only sustain serious injury but also be inhibited from mounting on subsequent occasions.

Perhaps the most important aspects of the breeding environment are handlers. Handlers must be familiar with the routine of breeding and experienced in controlling horses. Some handlers are better able to calm stallions than others with equal experience, and the calmer

the stallion, the less likely are accidents. Such simple arrangements as placing all attendants on the same side of the mare and stallion can facilitate communication between them and prevent difficulties. Most breeding injuries and accidents occur when an inexperienced, highly nervous, or non-receptive mare is bred without adequate restraint or judgment. Because errors in detection of estrus can be made and because the situation is unnatural, mares should be hobbled before breeding. Distractions in the form of extraneous people or animals should be avoided.

No single treatment exists for all abnormal sexual behavior in stallions. Patience and time are necessary with almost all cases. It is advisable to take advantage of the stallion's seasonal breeding pattern and institute behavioral therapy during the spring and summer. Advantage should also be taken of the stimulatory effect of the presence of other stallions. It already has been noted here that wild stallions are most likely to copulate when other stallions are present; the same appears to be true of domestic stallions. Some stallions have been known to breed mares only if another horse, even another mare, is present. The stallion may regard the second horse as a competitor – another stallion – or some other, unknown reason may be present.

The antianxiety drug diazepam (0.05 mg/kg slowly i.v.) has been used successfully to overcome impotence caused by pain associated with breeding and for the loss of libido shown in a novel environment.[1512,1513] Imipramine (500 mg i.v.) has been used to treat stallions that will mount and intromit but not ejaculate.[1506] Gonadotropin-releasing hormone may act directly on the brain of horses to stimulate sexual behavior and could have clinical application.[1511]

Finally, some stallions have definite mate preferences, and they should be allowed to exercise these preferences while recovering from loss of libido or impotence. Tease the stallion with several mares, and use the one to which he is most responsive for further treatment. A quiet mare is necessary for a stallion that has been injured by another mare. A stallion that will not mount a mare may ejaculate into an artificial vagina. He may gain confidence and overcome his fear by this process and can later be induced to mount a mare.

Vicious behavior toward the mare and the attendants is, like most other abnormal sexual behavior, most apt to occur when stallions are used for breeding outside the normal breeding season. Therefore, stallions may be unmanageable in January but well-mannered by May.

Overuse and Rough Handling

Overuse and rough handling are often the cause of misbehavior in stallions during breeding. They may bite the mare or be generally intractable. Attempts to improve the horse's breeding manners should be delayed until normal libido and copulation have been reestablished. Punishment of a horse with sexual abnormalities will retard its progress. If the stallion's viciousness is not attenuated as his libido improves, various physical devices, such as a muzzle and breeding bridle for him and a withers protector for the mare, may be used.

Self-Mutilation   Self-mutilation is a very common behavior problem. Although it occurs in horses of both sexes, it is much more common in stallions.[557] The behavior consists of biting at or actually biting the flanks or, less frequently, the chest. The horse usually squeals and kicks out at the same time. The signs mimic those of acute colic, but can be differentiated because self-mutilation does not progress to rolling or depression and is chronic. It is extremely important to eliminate discomfort as a cause of self-mutilation because penile, testicular, or urethral lesions; gastrointestinal pain; limb pain; bladder disease; or the like can cause self-mutilation.[1507] The cause of the behavior is unknown, but when self-mutilation decreases with a change in the social environment, it is probably caused by sociosexual deprivation. The behaviors observed in a self-mutilating stallion mimic those of a stallion confrontation:

sniffing and nipping at the genitalia, defecating and sniffing the feces, circling, and squealing. McDonnell[1506] has hypothesized that removing feces or skin secretion of the stallion, even his own, may reduce the arousal that precedes a bout of self-mutilation. Most breeding stallions lead deprived lives in that they are kept in stalls in isolation from other horses, particularly from other mares; however, most do not self-mutilate. The question arises as to whether stallions that self-mutilate should be used for breeding. Castration sometimes, but not always, stops self-mutilation. Preventing the behavior with the use of cradles and side poles does not remove the cause; the stallion will continue to vocalize and kick, so although he can no longer injure himself, he can still injure a bystander. A soft muzzle will prevent injury, slow down his prehension of hay and grain, but not frustrate his attempts to bite as much as other forms of restraint. Providing a stall companion such as a donkey will reduce the incidence of self-mutilation. Allowing the stallion to live on pasture with a mare will eliminate the problem in some cases. The chances that the stallion will be injured by the mare are less than the chances that he will injure himself or someone else by self-mutilating. Opiate antagonists will prevent self-mutilation.[558] Unfortunately, naloxone, the antagonist now available, is metabolized very quickly by horses and is quite expensive (see the "Cribbing" subsection in Chapter 3 for a discussion of the involvement of endogenous opiates in equine "vices"). Simply reducing the grain in a stallion's diet and increasing his exercise and roughage can reduce self-mutilation.[1496]

Effects of Castration

A horse that exhibits stallion-like behavior could be either a cryptorchid from whom the undescended testicle was not removed at castration or a gelding in which sexual behavior persists. A negligible plasma testosterone will distinguish the gelding from the cryptorchid stallion.[785] The testosterone response to gonadotropin administration is the best test for castration. Sexual behavior persists in more than one-third of geldings.[1394] The sexual behavior may be as innocuous as exhibition of flehmen or as extreme as mounting and intromission. The sexual behavior itself is usually not a problem, but aggression directed toward other geldings by the one who is acting like a harem stallion is. Another unwelcome stallion-like behavior is attacking foals, particularly newborn foals. Management can be used to prevent these problems. A gelding that acts like a stallion should be stalled alone or pastured only with other geldings, and it should not have access to foals.

Geldings may also self-mutilate. These are usually geldings that are displaying other stallion behaviors but, unlike intact males, they self-mutilate in the presence of mares. Stall confinement or pasturing without visual contact with mares usually reduces the incidence of self-mutilation. If not, progestins or cyproheptadine (8 mg increasing to 88 mg/day) may be used. Castration has been suggested as a means of controlling the population of feral horses, but gelding feral stallions does not have a large impact on population growth. The geldings who had been harem stallions kept their bands initially, but the size of their bands decreased and they kept their bands for a shorter period. Bachelors who were gelded were less apt to obtain a harem than intact ones. The gelded males marked less and were more affiliative.[2827]

Donkey Sexual behavior

An estrous donkey exhibits a behavior called "yawing" in which she opens and closes her mouth. This expression is seen in some estrous mares. Female donkeys have a distinctive tail posture. The base of the tail is raised and held out from the hindquarters at an angle of approximately 45°. This tail posture occurred whether or not males were present. During copulation the jenny exhibits the mating face as seen in mares. See Figure 4.12A.

The jack approaches the female, sniffs her genital area sometimes laying his head on the jenny's rump. He may drive the female and then mount.[2890]

Pigs

The Sow

As is the cow, the sow is a non-seasonal breeder. After regular cycling commences, the sow will cycle every 18–24 days (mean: 21 days) until bred. Puberty occurs at five to eight months. The presence of a boar leads to the occurrence of estrus at an earlier age and in more gilts.[2249] Puberty is accelerated in gilts older than 160 days exposed to a strange male for 20 or more minutes per day.

Estrous Cycle

As do females of other species, the sow also shows an increase in activity as estrus approaches.[49] The increased motor activity eventually takes the form of searching behavior, which seems vital to the initial uniting of an estrous sow with a boar.[2124] Urination is frequent, as is calling to the male. The call is a soft, rhythmic grunt. An estrous female approaches the boar and sniffs him around the head and genitals. Estrous sows attempt to mount other estrous females, but subordinate sows rarely mount dominant ones.[1780] Olfactory stimuli alone will instigate this searching; anesthetized boars readily attract estrous sows. Olfactory bulbectomy drastically impairs the ability of the sow to discriminate between males and females.[42] Bulbectomy may eliminate sexual behavior and prevent normal ovulation and estrus, but in other studies, bulbectomized females mated, conceived, and reared their litters, although there were deficits in maternal recognition (see Chapter 5, "Maternal Behavior").[1543,2123]

This proceptive behavior can be used to detect estrus in sows using electronic monitoring to detect which sows visit a boar housed in a pen adjacent to the sow. Boars and sows show individual differences in mate selection; each animal has its favorite or favorites.[2231] Boars differ in the degree to which they attract sows, but this attractivity is not related to their libido.[986] Subordinate sows and gilts exhibit fewer signs of estrus and approach the boar less often, especially in crowded conditions.[1780] Even fear of humans can suppress estrous behavior.

Searching behavior appears to be under endogenous control and requires estrogen during behavioral ontogeny for full development. Gilts reared in isolation will show this behavior upon reaching puberty.[2124] The immobility response of the fully receptive sow, however, seems to require both tactile and olfactory or auditory stimuli. The specific auditory stimulus is the courting song of the boar (see later in this chapter under "Courtship Behavior" of the boar).[2124] As with searching behavior, the immobility reaction does not seem susceptible to learned modifications. The olfactory stimuli to which the sow responds are pheromones present in both the saliva and preputial secretions of boars. The chemicals involved are metabolites of androgens and have been identified as 5α-androst(16-ene)3-one.[1556] These compounds have been used experimentally and are available commercially to elicit the immobility reaction.[1913]

Olfactory and auditory stimuli from adult boars, supplied by an aerosol spray and a tape player, will increase the proceptivity of gilts toward young boars.[1081] The presence of mature boars can advance puberty and the onset of ovulation in weaned sows.[981] The presence of a boar has a slight effect on the rate of conception and number of piglets or the size of the litter.[988]

A robot boar – even with androstenol and a recording of a boar's calls – is less effective than a real boar in stimulating immobility response, and the duration of estrus is shorter.[810] Estrus is less apt to be detected in sows with less than 1 m^2 (11 ft.^{2}) of pen space and those living in pairs. It is also easier to detect estrus if the sows are housed across an aisle from a boar rather than in an adjoining pen. This may be because the sow has had close olfactory contact with the boar when the attendants were not present; she has shown the immobility response, but no person was there to notice.[984,987,988,991]

Clinical Problems of Sows

Aberrations are unusual, perhaps because of the somewhat rigid genetic control of sexual behaviors. Breed differences in the length of estrus are seen,[2121] but these are minor and unimportant clinically. Although not quantified, some sows seem to have decided mate preferences and display strong aversions to specific males.[2124]

Failure to Reproduce in Confinement

The most important problem is failure of reproduction in confined gilts. Confinement and the social environment appear to play a role in inhibiting estrus in young gilts.[712] Puberty is delayed in regrouped or crowded pigs or roughly handled pigs,[171,430,991] but accelerated by gentle handling. The stress of trailering can also stimulate the onset of estrus. It is interesting that chronic stress of overcrowding delays puberty, but the acute stress of transport accelerates it.

The Boar

Pigs are unusual in that defeminization occurs well after birth and is under the control of estrogenic metabolites that act as late as three months postnatally.[14]

Courtship Behavior

After contact with an estrous female has been made, the boar will pursue the female, attempting to nose her sides, flanks, and vulva (Figure 4.13). Unique to the pig is the boar's "courting song," which is used during this phase of courtship. This is a series of soft, guttural grunts, about six to eight per second.[2124] Tactile stimulation of the female continues

Figure 4.13   The courtship sequence of pigs. *Source:* Hafez (1975).[679] Reproduced with permission of Elsevier.

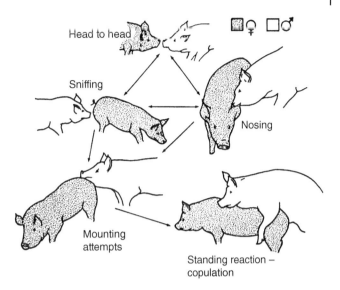

Head to head

Sniffing

Nosing

Mounting attempts

Standing reaction – copulation

and increases in intensity as the boar's sexual excitement increases. The boar usually emits urine rhythmically; pheromones in the urine may further increase the female's willingness to stand. Several mounting attempts may be made until the female becomes immobile, after which mounting and intromission follow rapidly. The boar's ejaculatory time approaches that of the dog, although no copulatory lock occurs in swine. Ejaculation occurs within 3–20 minutes, with an average of four to five minutes.[2124] Consort behavior continues for a short time following copulation. Boars mate an estrous female around 10 times over a two- to three-day estrous period.[355] Although domestic pigs are not considered seasonal breeders, libido and testosterone levels increase earlier in prepubertal boars if the day is artificially lengthened to 15 hours.[1017] Boars tend to have greater libido in a separate mating pen than in their home stalls.[992] Cortisol levels increase following mating.[1351]

Olfactory Stimuli

Olfactory cues seem unimportant in stimulating a boar to mount a female or a dummy. Olfactory bulbectomy, for example, does not prevent normal sexual behavior.[286] Some but not all boars can distinguish between estrous

and anestrous females from a distance, that is, on the basis of olfactory information.[1523] The initial contact with the sow, however, triggers a behavioral response from her: immobility, reflecting the degree of her sexual receptivity. It is this tendency toward immobility that seems to arouse the boar. As with the female response, this reaction is under fairly strict genetic control and not subject to much learned modification. Thus, what is noted by human observers as homosexual mounting or aberrant mounting of artificial stimuli is explained as being a normal response to immobile objects of approximately the correct size and shape. Although some breeds are easier to train for semen collection than others, training of a young boar to mount a dummy will usually be successful on the first few attempts.

Early Socialization

In the boar, as in most species, the early social environment is important to later sexual behavior. Boars raised in isolation from three weeks of age copulated less often with estrous sows than did boars raised in groups. Boars with visual and olfactory contact with other boars were not nearly as inhibited as the isolates, indicating that contact with other pigs, even male pigs, is important.[988] Later, contact with females is also important because boars with visual and olfactory contact with sows copulated more often and ejaculated longer than boars kept in isolation or with visual and olfactory contact with other boars.[985,992] This is probably a hormonal effect; testosterone and corticosteroid levels are higher in boars that are in contact with sows.[1400]

Clinical Problems of Boars

As with the other domestic animals, differences in the level of "sex drive" appear to be larger between individuals than between breeds. Low libido, however, has been associated with a high plane of nutrition; and, at least in the United Kingdom, is seen more frequently in Landrace than in boars of the Large White breed.[66] Libido may be impaired through mismanagement of a young boar. A young male turned in with a group of gilts may be frustrated by excessive curiosity or bullied by the gilts. This incompetence or fear may become conditioned and a permanent problem. Supervision of early matings is recommended. A quiet sow or one recently serviced by a mature boar should be used for the first mating.[66] Another common problem is aggression by the boar toward humans. This is usually resolved by culling the boar, which removes the danger and prevents an aggressive animal from reproducing.

Mounting as a welfare issue should be considered as producers move away from castration. Males mount more than females, and the frequency of mounting does not vary with the dominance hierarchy in a food competition. The recipient of mounting is usually a heavier pig, whose screams indicate that the behavior is aversive.[1014]

Dogs

Free-Ranging Dogs

Stray bitches avoid their male littermates but can be bred by a persistent brother. Estrous females attract two to seven males; they will show less proceptive behavior in the presence of many males and also less active rejection of non-preferred males. Only half of the stray male dogs are able to copulate, and those under a year of age rarely do so.[812]

The Bitch

Estrous Cycle

The domestic dog, unlike most of its canid relatives, is a non-seasonal breeder. The length of each estrous cycle is extremely variable from individual to individual, and sometimes from one heat to the next in the same bitch. One to four cycles yearly may be seen, with two being the most usual. The Basenji is an exception; one seasonal breeding per year is seen in the early fall.[768] Basenji–Cocker spaniel crosses show both monocyclic and polycyclic activity, indicating genetic control of this aspect of the reproductive cycle. The proportion of urinations that are directed (i.e., next to a conspicuous object) is higher during proestrus and estrus.[2478]

The onset of puberty also varies widely among individuals. No strict correlation of age at puberty may be made with either body size or conformation;[730] generally, however, the smaller breeds reach puberty earlier than the larger breeds. It would be very rare for a St. Bernard to reach puberty by six months, for example, but not unusual for a Miniature poodle to do so. Thus, puberty onset for all dogs ranges from 6 to 15 months, with 7–10 months being the usual for the "average" dog.

Courtship Behavior

The correlation of hormonal levels and sexual behavior in the dog is illustrated in Figure 4.2. The first proestrus and estrus of a bitch's life are shorter than subsequent ones, and the levels of LH and estradiol are lower.[403] She is less attractive to the male and less proceptive.[812] Courtship behavior is marked by play behavior in the proestrous part of the cycle, but this play behavior decreases during estrus. The female will run with the male, approach him using the typical play bow of puppies, and even whimper submissively. She will sniff and lick the male's body and genitalia. Urination becomes more frequent as estrus approaches, and the posture used will frequently be the squat-raise. She may stand before the male momentarily during proestrus, but turns before the male can mount, often with a bark or growl.[426] Attraction of males and proceptivity appear in proestrus, but receptivity occurs later, during estrus.[197] During estrus, she stands more quietly to allow male investigation and eventually intromission toward the end of estrus. When the male touches her vulva, she will flex her body laterally;[922] while he is thrusting, she will move her perineum from side to side and ventrally, a motion that increases the probability of intromission. After the lock or the copulatory tie has been established, she may roll or twist and turn (the copulatory lock is discussed in the "Courtship Behavior" subsection of "The Dog" section in this chapter). Contractions of the constrictor vestibuli muscles and the anus occur as an after-reaction.

If the male does not mount, the female will "present" her hindquarters to him and even back into him and deviate her tail. An older and more experienced bitch may mount a young male and execute pelvic thrusts.[730]

Other social behaviors, in addition to sexual ones, are influenced by the reproductive condition of the bitch. Dominance relationships between females may shift, especially during metestrus. Males may defer to females in food competitions not because they are chivalrous males but because they are more motivated to mount than to eat.

Clinical Problems of Bitches

Owners unfamiliar with canine courtship may be upset because the bitch appears to tease the male by soliciting and then threatening him if he mounts, but this is normal. Females may refuse males for any of several reasons. A bitch may display dominance over a male by not allowing the male to "stand over" her (a normal canine signal of dominance) or to approach

from behind. Dominance relationships are learned, but can be established rapidly. Thus, dominance relationships probably help inhibit mother–son matings and may prevent certain sib–sib matings, but may also develop quickly if an aggressive bitch is placed with a more submissive dog.[730] There are definite female preferences for certain males.[193,1322] Refusal can range from avoiding a particular male to actively chasing and biting him. Not all the females rejected a male to the same degree, and dominant males were not necessarily chosen as preferred mates.[190] Sexual preference could not be correlated with social affinity outside the mating period.

The Dog

Sexual behaviors may appear in five-week-old male pups, and mounting behavior becomes an important part of the male's social repertoire as it matures. As with many other mammals, mounting is used as a sign of dominance; a submissive animal will stand for a more dominant male, but standing over is not tolerated by the dominant animal. Most dogs are sexually mature physiologically long before they copulate for the first time.[730] Perhaps the lack of dominance in young dogs inhibits early mating. Social contact is vital in the ontogeny of normal sexual behavior. Dogs raised in social isolation showed abnormal mounting orientation that persisted for longer than it did in dogs with similarly limited sexual experience but more social experience.[188]

Courtship Behavior

Male dogs are attracted to estrous bitches.[195] Urine of the estrous bitch appears to be more attractive to the dog than vaginal secretions,[568,588] but a component of the vaginal secretions, methyl p-hydroxybenzoate, has been shown to induce male sexual behavior when applied to the vulva of an anestrous bitch.[842] The pheromone may be considered a "releaser" of sexual behavior in the male. Mammalian behavior is not as stereotyped as that of fish and birds, so although sexual arousal may occur in all male dogs exposed to the pheromone, the expression of that arousal may vary considerably; therefore, male courtship behavior is extremely variable. Males may show extreme interest or indifference to females, although mating may occur successfully in either case. Play behavior may be marked or absent. The male sniffs the female's head and vulva; he may lick her ears. While canids do not show the classic flehmen response of ungulates, it is possible that the "tonguing" response seen during this olfactory investigation accomplishes transport of pheromones to the vomeronasal organ in a manner similar to that postulated for ungulates. The length of the play activity and olfactory investigation probably varies with the past experience of the male and female, perceived degrees of dominance within the pair, stage of estrus, and sexual satiation of either partner. Bitches can be forced to accept copulation by a strong and aggressive male who chases her until she is exhausted and holds her with his teeth by the neck or with his paw on her back. The male mounts in response to female immobility; he grasps her with his forelegs just cranial to her pelvis.

He thrusts with his pelvis and when intromission has been achieved, the rate of thrusting increases. Engorgement of the bulbus glandis and contraction of the vaginal muscles following intromission result in the copulatory lock or tie, a phenomenon most closely associated with canids but not restricted to them. The male will usually dismount and turn around so that male and female are facing opposite directions while ejaculation occurs (Figure 4.14). The lock may last 10–30 minutes (mean: 14 minutes), after which the bulbus decreases in size and the pair separates.[921] Following copulation, recovery from sexual refractoriness may be rapid. Up to five copulations by a male dog in one day have been reported.[730]

Clinical Problems of Dogs
Impotence
Male impotence or loss of libido can be the result of organic disease. Most commonly this would be musculoskeletal disease such as hip dysplasia, arthritis, or trauma-induced pain in the hindquarters. Balanoposthitis is generally a mild disease in dogs and unlikely to affect sexual performance, although a severe form could conceivably do so.

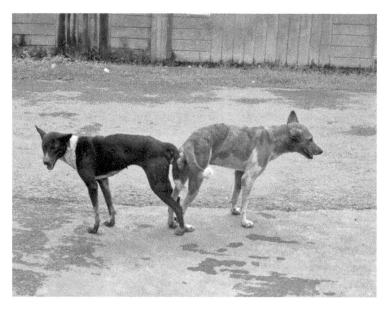

Figure 4.14   Copulatory lock in dogs. *Source:* Courtesy of S.K. Pal.

Lack of Socialization

The lack of sufficient social contacts as a puppy may inhibit successful copulation. This becomes a very real problem, not only an experimental one, when a pup is ordered from a pet shop. Pups are weaned as early as possible (four to five weeks) and shipped shortly thereafter to pet shops. The pup, if he survives transport, is kept isolated in the new owner's home, protecting him from infectious disease. When the owners finally do try to use their sheltered pet for breeding, they have great difficulty persuading the dog to perform or find it impossible to do so. Their dog has been essentially isolated from social contacts with conspecifics. Not only have the motor patterns of sexual behavior not been perfected, but also they have never been placed in a proper social context. Some dogs may overcome this void in socialization, but their sexual and other behaviors may never be normal in direction or quantity. An example of poor libido occurred in a pointer that was kept with his sister. Both the sister and his owners reprimanded the dog for sexual interest in his sister, and when presented with an unrelated estrous bitch, he had no libido and seemed frightened. With increasing age and exposure to other bitches, his libido increased.

Timidity Timidity, especially in Poodles and German shepherds, may be both learned and genetic in nature. Affected dogs may be inhibited to the point of impotence. Leaving the male and female together for several days, rather than allowing only a short breeding period, has been suggested. This prolonged period of acquaintanceship could, however, exacerbate a potential problem if the female is dominant.

A conditioned fear of any phase of the breeding program may be inadvertently instilled in a stud dog. Analysis of breeding techniques and reversal of the conditioning may alleviate the problem successfully. Thus, a young dog forced to court a very aggressive female may associate the rough treatment he received with the breeding process in general, with a specific breeding location, or with a specific color or type of female. Young dogs may make some clumsy mounting attempts and may otherwise prolong courtship, but should successfully mount a bitch within the first few exposures to a female. If the dog is a persistently timid breeder, however, he should be dropped from the breeding program. AI is recommended if the timidity is suspected to be learned, or the result of the particular dominance relationship in the attempted mating. Most dogs will breed with most other dogs; therefore, mating problems with behavioral etiologies are unusual and require serious consideration.

Environmental Disturbances

As are other male domestic animals, dogs are sensitive to environmental disturbances in the breeding process. If one member of a breeding pair must be transported to the other, the female should be brought to the male. Noise and other disruptions in the breeding area should be minimized. The rather curious insistence of some breeders on helping a male dog mount and copulate might actually cause more difficulties than it is thought to prevent. Besides the physical disruption of the observer-helper, the breeder will likely frighten the dog and, thus, be somewhat inhibitory to the male's sexual performance. A timid dog may require the owner's presence if his dominance over a female is doubtful; but, as already discussed here, the continued use of a dog this timid would be unwise. Slippery floors, such as waxed linoleum, may prevent mounting, but this problem should be easily avoided.

Masturbation

Masturbation is not an unusual problem in house dogs. Semen quality or value as a breeder is not affected, but the habit becomes an embarrassing or annoying one for the owner. Masturbation using inanimate objects is probably seen in most puppies, but will become an insignificant behavior in the normally socialized adult. Mounting of people should be discouraged. To resolve the problem, the owners should teach the dog submissive behavior by counterconditioning the dog to stay down when it attempts to mount. Castration usually eliminates or decreases the problem (see the "Sexual Behavior after Castration" section). Owners reporting homosexual behavior in their dog should also be informed that mounting of one male dog by another is probably a sign of dominance.

Sexual Behavior after Castration

Prepubertal castration greatly reduces sexual interests. Because mounting is an integral part of the dog's behavioral ontogeny and is used in agonistic interactions, all sexual behavior will probably not be eliminated (Figure 4.15). Ninety percent of the post-pubertal dogs, castrated to control roaming, showed a rapid or gradual decline in this behavior.[1027] Intermale aggression was reduced noticeably in only 60% of the dogs, and urine marking in the home in only 50%.[2859] Sixty-seven percent of the dogs showed a decrease in mounting behavior following surgery; mounting of people was reduced in seven of eight dogs castrated specifically for that problem. Mounting of other dogs was reduced in only one of four dogs castrated

for that reason. There were no reported changes in the owners' handling or attitude toward their dogs following surgery, however, which might have been responsible for some of the behavioral changes noted. Age at castration was not correlated with the noted effects. Although in no cases did the occurrence of an objectionable behavior return to its preoperative level, some behaviors appeared intermittently for long periods following castration.[1027] Castrated dogs may retain sexual mounting behavior, with intromission, lock, and ejaculation for several years post-castration or indefinitely, although the frequency of the behaviors decreases.[921]

Non-sexual Behavior after Neutering

Castration reduces aggression to people in only 30% of dogs, and the effect is independent of age at castration or duration of the aggression.[1680] Although aggression to other males is decreased, aggression to bitches persists.[1430] Castrated male dogs exhibited less mounting behavior, pulling on the leash, and roaming behavior.[2923] Spayed German shepherds are more aggressive to people and other dogs than their non-spayed littermates.[2826]

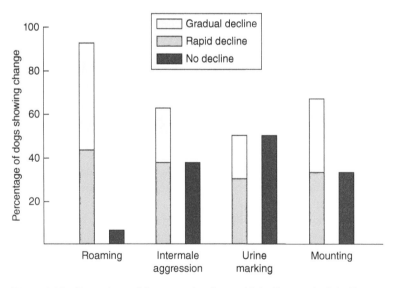

Figure 4.15 Percentage of dogs experiencing rapid decline, gradual decline, or no change in four behaviors after castration. *Source:* Hopkins *et al.* (1976).[1027] Reproduced with permission of American Veterinary Medical Association.

When owners rate their own dogs, gonadectomy had no effect on aggression to familiar people or dogs and severe aggression to strangers was somewhat more common in gonadectomized dogs.[2734,2998] Age at neutering had no effect on the incidence of aggressive behavior [2801] although there may be breed interactions because Vizslas neutered before seven months of age were more likely to have fear of storms as well as behavior problems in general.[3047] Spayed Golden Retrievers showed more frequent or more intense fear reaction in response to loud noises, unfamiliar objects approaching on or near the sidewalk, or if they were approached by unknown dogs.[2655] On the one hand, it was found that the younger a bitch was when she was spayed the more likely she was to be fearful of loud noises and overreactive to delivery people. On the other hand, the less likely she was to howl and the more likely to fetch.[2999] Early spaying significantly reduced reporting of 10 (mostly unwelcome) behaviors. Of these, one related to fearfulness and three to aggression.[2998]

Cats

Free-Ranging Cats

In a feral situation, one estrous female will be surrounded by a group of males. Tomcats will knock one another off an estrous queen or mount the tom that is mounting the female, but little overt aggression takes place during courting. A male dominance hierarchy, based on size and age, gives the dominant tom priority of access to females. Dominant males tend to be closer to estrous females than are subordinate males, but they do not mount more frequently.[1669] Fifteen copulations will occur in 24 hours.[514] Groups of cats living on farms seem to have only one sexually active tom. Although pair bonding does not occur in the domestic cat, short-term consort behavior occurs normally. A male and female may remain together for several hours or days, mating many times. Juvenile males tend to move away from their birth area before their third year.[1364]

The Queen

Estrous Cycle

The queen is seasonally polyestrous, and most cats will cycle at least twice yearly if not bred. Although population peaks occur in mid-January to March and May to June in the Northern Hemisphere, individual cats may be in estrus at any season. The nadir for reproductive output of a population is late fall, making the availability of kittens as Christmas presents very unreliable. If unbred, the cat will cycle every three weeks for several months. Actual estrus lasts 9–10 days without copulation and around four days if the cat is bred.

Most felids, including the domestic cat, are induced ovulators, thus breeding may be accomplished whenever the female shows receptivity. Owners unwilling or unable to have a pet cat neutered may use this feature of the reproductive cycle to shorten estrus; artificial stimulation of the vagina using a cotton-tipped applicator stick will induce ovulation and shorten the receptive time. This is an especially useful procedure in terminating repeated heats.[725] Females will usually reach puberty at 6–10 months, but females born in April may not cycle until the following year.[725] Free-ranging cats may not reach puberty until 15–18 months, although "barn" cats born in May to July in Ithaca, New York, routinely give birth to their first litter 12 months later.[618]

There appears to be avoidance of incestuous mating in that estrous females will travel farther from home if the closest male is related.[1364]

Catnip

Nepetalactone, a volatile terpenoid found in the catnip plant (*Nepeta cataria*), and estrus elicit similar behaviors, and there has been continued debate as to whether this is a release of sexual behaviors or a non-specific pleasure inducer.[929,938,1012,1762,1119,2265,2380] Estrous behavior is similar to, but not identical with, catnip-induced behavior.[938] Catnip does not cause vulvar presentation, vocalization, or foot treading, and cats in estrus do not head-shake as do cats exposed to catnip. Also, male cats respond in an identical manner. The body-rolling and head-rubbing behaviors characteristic of both the estrous and catnip-induced states could be induced in males and females by an extract of tomcat urine.[2264] Nepetalactone may be mimicking one of the compounds in male urine on to which an estrous female may be especially primed, but to which most or all cats are sensitive.[924] Catnip exposure results in more time sleeping, less time standing and actively exploring the environment, as well as the catnip response.[633] The response to catnip depends on the main olfactory system, not on the vomeronasal organ.[929]

Courtship Behavior

An estrous female will call and purr. She is restless and shows increased general motor activity. If she is a house cat, she may run from one room to the next, stopping to call at each door or window. She may be very affectionate toward the owners. Urination occurs frequently, and she may spray. She rubs her head and flanks on furniture; glands in these areas may produce pheromones that contain information announcing the presence of an estrous female. She crouches, elevates her perineal region, and treads with her back legs.[2430] This will usually be accompanied by a rhythmic opening and closing of the claws of the front feet. Rolling, squirming, and stretching are seen. This activity occurs whether or not a male is present but becomes synchronized with male behavior when the female is interacting with the male. During proestrus, she will roll and solicit the male's attention but act aggressively if he mounts.[1574] This may be termed "postural acceptance" and "affective rejection." When fully receptive, she becomes immobile and stands crouched in lumbar lordosis, and with her head held on the ground between her forelegs (Figure 4.16). Her tail is deviated to one side, and she allows the male to mount. This latter sequence may be stimulated

in an estrous female by scratching her over the dorsal tail base.

An estrous female may show a darting behavior in the presence of several tomcats. She will repeatedly run a short distance from the toms, and this may be her means of assessing the relative strength of the males as they chase her and try to displace one another.

Clinical Problems of Queens
Female–Female

Female–female mounting behavior is seen only rarely and usually in colony situations. Two estrous cats may try to squirm underneath each other when presenting to an inaccessible male; one may mount the other and perform male-like pelvic thrusts. There are definite examples of female mate preferences in colony cats, and the dominant members of the colony were sometimes bypassed as mates.[1361]

Effects of Ovariohysterectomy

Spaying (ovariohysterectomy or, less commonly, ovariectomy or tubal ligation) is performed quite commonly on the domestic house cat. Spaying eliminates sexual behavior but may affect other behaviors. Care must be taken not to ascribe changes in behavior to surgery, when the changes might be caused by maturational changes in the cat or changes in the cat's environment. A common behavior problem following spaying is an increase in aggression between cats in a multi-cat household, resulting from either the lowered progesterone levels of the spayed cat and/or the change in her odor that precipitated attacks by the other cat. Maternal behavior has also been observed in newly spayed cats, perhaps triggered by the fall in ovarian hormone levels – which is similar to the fall that occurs at parturition – and the presence of neonatal kittens.

The Tom

Courtship Behavior

The male probably locates an estrous female via olfactory cues deposited as pheromones in

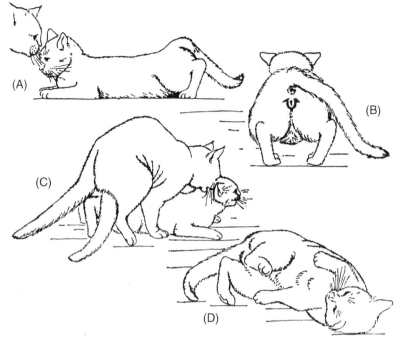

Figure 4.16 Sexual behavior of the female cat. (A, B) The typical posture adopted by the queen in full estrus. Note leg flexion, lordosis, and deflection of the tail. (C) Tom holding queen with neck grip during intromission. (D) Postcoital rolling by the queen. *Source:* Scott (1970)[2070]/Lea & Febiger.

the urine and by some sebaceous gland secretions. A male placed with a female in a mating arena will spend some time investigating and marking the area with urine and anal gland secretions before mating. The cat shows a flehmen response, or gape, similar to that of ungulates (refer to Chapter 1, "Communication," Figure 1.12). He calls to the female, circles her, and sniffs her genitalia. A non-receptive female will actively, even violently, rebuff a male. When a female is receptive, the male approaches her from the side and behind and grips the skin of her neck in his mouth. He then mounts with the front legs, then the hind, and rubs her with his forepaws. Intromission follows a forward stepping with arched back and pelvic thrusts.[725] Ejaculation occurs seconds after intromission, and intromission usually lasts less than 10 seconds. The penis is covered with numerous small spines that apparently cause an intense stimulation as

evidenced by the loud copulatory cry of the female with intromission. With retraction of the penis, the female rolls and claws at the male. The male will often lick his penis after copulation. Copulation may occur every 10–15 minutes for several hours. A seasonal variation in sexual readiness with a decline in the fall is seen in the male cat under experimental conditions.[100]

Clinical Problems of Toms

Reluctance of the male to breed a female is usually the result of the female's being nonreceptive and thus aggressive toward the male's advances. Inexperienced males may be especially intimidated by the aggressive responses of a proestrous female. In a laboratory, only one tom in three will consistently copulate with fully receptive queens. It is not surprising, therefore, that many visits to the tom are necessary before successful breeding takes place.

Estrous females may indicate a mate preference by actively rebuffing one male or staying near another.

Effects of Castration

Castration is a widely accepted procedure for the pet cat. Prepubertal (six to eight months) castration generally eliminates sexual behavior. Although testicular androgens are secreted by four months, mating behavior does not develop until eight to nine months.[725] Some owners object to a feminine-appearing male and so delay castration until 12–14 months, or the first serious fight abscess. The effectiveness of castration in eliminating mating behavior depends on the previous level of sexual experience.[1972,1973] Thus, owners should be advised to restrict the access of their cat to females until after surgery unless they do not mind the cat's continued sexual interests. Early castration when the kitten is less than four months old virtually guarantees that he will not spray as an adult. No negative side effects occur from early neutering in male cats, so it should be recommended highly.[2155]

Castration of post-pubertal cats seems much more effective in reducing or eliminating fighting, roaming, and spraying in the cat than it is in the dog. Eighty-eight percent of cat owners interviewed 23 months after having their cats castrated reported a rapid or gradual decline in fighting; 92% reported the same for roaming; and 87% responded favorably for spraying.[930]

The failure of surgery to eliminate these behaviors completely probably is due to the learned components of the behaviors. Mounting behavior, either mounting inanimate objects, other cats, or the owner, occurs in 25% of castrated male cats. It is interesting that the copulatory or consummative aspects of sexual behavior, but not the appetitive activities such as roaming, persist.

Chickens

When the chickens are familiar with one another, the rooster simply tests the hen by placing a foot on her back. Roosters have a courtship behavior toward unfamiliar hens in which the rooster waltzes (circles the hen with the outer wing relaxed) and exhibits tidbitting – picking up food and bringing it to the hen. The non-receptive hen will depart, but the receptive hen will crouch with head low and wings spread and tail held to one side. The rooster stands on her back and both evert the cloaca, the vents meet and the rooster ejaculates. Roosters will choose unfamiliar rather than familiar (brood-mates) hens, but those of the breed with which he was raised. Most mating occurs in late afternoon.[2744] Roosters can induce feather loss if they repeatedly mount a hen. Increasing the ratio of hens to roosters can solve this problem or hens can be fitted with "aprons" to protect their backs and feathers.

5

Maternal Behavior

Introduction: General Principles of Maternal Behavior

Internal Factors That Elicit Maternal Behavior

Hormonal and Neural Controls

The combination of the proper hormonal milieu and the stimulus for maternal behavior, the neonate, plus prior experience of being a mother can elicit maternal behavior. The stimulation of maternal behavior appears to be under both hormonal and neural control. Estrogen rises and progesterone falls at parturition in sheep. Estrogen appears to facilitate, and progesterone to inhibit, maternal behavior in this species.[2112] In regard to neural control, one of the sequelae of parturition is cervical stimulation. Vaginocervical stimulation for five minutes will result in the reflex that stimulates oxytocin release. Oxytocin is released not only from the posterior pituitary into the bloodstream but also from the terminals of cells whose cell bodies lie in the periventricular area of the hypothalamus, the axons of which can stimulate the neural mechanism underlying maternal activities in other parts of the brain. Brain oxytocin levels increase at parturition, at suckling, and when the vagina is stimulated,[1200] and increasing oxytocin in the cerebrospinal fluid can stimulate maternal behavior.[1199] Six weeks of treatment with intravaginal progesterone and estradiol, plus cervical stimulation at the time of introduction of the lamb, stimulated normal maternal behavior in anestrous ewes, indicating the importance of both hormonal and neural factors. Cervical stimulation will also cause a ewe that is already selectively maternal toward one lamb to be maternal toward another, alien lamb.[1206]

Hormonal priming by estrogen and progesterone, plus vaginocervical stimulation, is necessary in order to reduce aggression toward, or withdrawal from, alien lambs by ewes. Experience is also necessary for full expression of maternal behavior because only multiparous ewes would show positive maternal behavior (licking, sniffing, and low-pitched bleating) after the combination of hormonal and vaginocervical stimulation.[1197]

The fact that primiparous ewes routinely reject their lambs if they have been delivered by Cesarean section also indicates the importance of neural stimulation by the passage of the lamb through the vaginal canal. The fact that multiparous ewes will readily accept their lambs even if they have been delivered by Cesarean section indicates the importance of prior experience in ovine maternal behavior.[39]

Learning

Evidence for the role of learning in maternal behavior is found mostly in higher primates and rodents. Monkeys that had been artificially reared made very poor mothers and very reluctant sex partners.[914] Apparently, a monkey must have been mothered in order to be a good mother spontaneously. It is interesting that monkeys that neglected or even killed their first offspring exhibited normal maternal behavior after the second pregnancy. This aspect of maternal behavior has not been well investigated in domestic animals; it is worth noting, however, that most problems in maternal behavior are seen in primiparous animals. Ovine maternal behavior, in particular, seems to be more independent of physiological changes after the ewe has mothered one lamb. The quality of maternal behavior in artificially reared cats, dogs, or sheep has not been documented. When maternal behavior in beef and dairy cattle is compared, the beef cattle exhibit more maternal behavior. These animals, at least on the range, raise their calves, and adequate maternal behavior is necessary for their calves' survival. Artificial rearing of dairy calves has been practiced on many generations of cows; consequently, few dairy cows have had much experience at mothering or at being mothered.

Concaveation

The presence of neonates can induce maternal behavior in virgin females and even in males. This phenomenon is called "concaveation." When exposed to rat pups daily for seven days, virgin female rats, and even male rats, will begin to retrieve the young, lick them, and even huddle over them in the typical nursing position. Mice will show similar behavior with no latency whatsoever as long as the pups presented are only one or two days old. Maternal behavior can, therefore, be induced in these rodents in the absence of hormonal stimulation, although hormonal stimulation accelerates the appearance of maternal behavior. The phenomenon of concaveation is used to force acceptance of alien (not the female's own) or rejected young. It is used to treat lamb and foal rejection.

Recognition of the Young (Individual Signature versus Maternal Labeling)

It is not clear whether licking the neonate imparts the mother's odor to the offspring or consumption of her milk imparts a recognizable odor to the offspring's feces. If that is the basis of recognition, it is maternal labeling. Another possibility is that the mother learns the individual olfactory signature of the offspring.

External Factors That Elicit Maternal Behavior

What stimuli emanating from the neonate are important in maternal behavior? Some of these stimuli are presumably olfactory, such as the smell of a small conspecific wet with amniotic fluid. The appearance of the newborn may also serve as a visual stimulus, for Konrad Lorenz[1412] hypothesized that the short forehead, cheeks swollen by sucking fat pads, and erratic gait of the neonate elicit maternal behavior in a number of species, including humans.

Summary

To summarize our somewhat sketchy knowledge of the biological basis of maternal behavior, we conclude that hormonal priming can lower the threshold for the initiation of maternal behavior that can be brought on and maintained as a response to the stimuli characteristic of the neonate, even in the absence of the appropriate rise and fall of gonadal and pituitary hormones and cervical stimulation. Animals can learn to be good mothers both by having been mothered themselves as infants and by having been mothers previously. Vaginal stimulation and oxytocin release appear to be important in sheep and horses; otherwise, the hormonal and central nervous system control of maternal behavior in domestic animals is virtually unknown and is a field

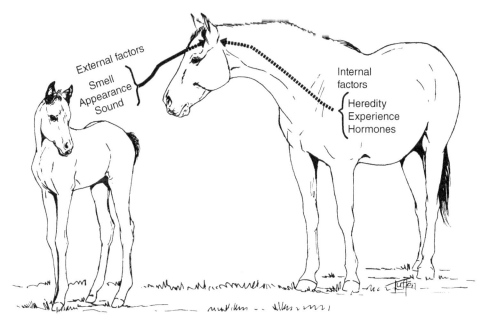

External factors
Smell
Appearance
Sound

Internal
factors
Heredity
Experience
Hormones

Figure 5.1   Factors that influence the expression of maternal behavior. The horse is used as an example, but there are similar influences on maternal behavior in all domestic animals. *Source:* Houpt and Wolski (1979)[1052]/John Wiley & Sons.

that demands more attention from biological scientists. Figure 5.1 summarizes the factors involved in maternal behavior.

Pigs

The Free-Ranging Sow

Maternal behavior in sows can be divided into two prepartum behaviors, nest site seeking and nest building, as well as the postpartum behavior of nursing. One day before farrowing, free-ranging sows will leave their herd and their normal home range, traveling as little as 50 m (153 ft.) or as far as 7 km (4 mi.). They will build several rudimentary nests before selecting a final site at which they dig a hole, which typically is 10 cm (4 in.) deep and 1.5 m (4.5 ft.) wide. They will bring grass and sometimes sticks to the nest.[1145] The nest is usually located under protective overhead cover, usually in a forested area.[1656] The sow will spend more and more of her time building her nest during the

day of parturition. Usually, four to six hours elapse between the onset of nest building and farrowing. Nest building will cease one to three hours before farrowing.[3043] Oxytocin increase may inhibit nest building.

The sow stays with the piglets for the first two days and then leaves to forage for short periods. This is reflected in the behavior of sows provided with a crate and access to a group pen. They voluntarily spend the first five days in the crate.[276] The nest will be defended against the sow's juvenile offspring and against other adults. Failure to defend the nest results in crushing of the piglets and a consequent threefold to fourfold increase in mortality.[1686] Nursing takes place every 45 minutes. Piglets do not all suckle simultaneously at first, but later their behavior becomes more synchronous. For the first two days, the sow initiates all nursing, but after that the piglets initiate at least half of the nursing bouts. On day seven, the piglets leave the nest and the sow rejoins the herd. By day nine, the piglets sleep in the herd's communal nest. The pigs are weaned at 14–17 weeks.[1141]

The Group-Housed Sow

Sows housed in group pens become more aggressive as parturition approaches.[84] Gilts, but not sows, prefer an enclosed area in which to farrow. That is probably an innate behavior related to the behavior of the free-ranging sow that leaves her herd to farrow.[1812,2168]

Nest Building

Farrowing crates prevent sows from building the elaborate nests used by wild and feral swine; all that remains of the nest-building behavior is a futile pawing at the floor of the crate. The restlessness, which increases linearly during the last 48 hours prepartum, probably represents attempts at nest seeking and nest building. If sows are introduced to farrowing crates the day before farrowing, they had more stillborn piglets, indicating that environmental changes can be detrimental.[1781]

Nest-building behavior consists of two distinct factors, gathering nest material and arranging it by rooting and nosing. Environmental factors, such as temperature and udder comfort, influence nest building.[43] Sows gather more material when no artificial shelter is available.[1142] When given access to an earth floor, sows will excavate a nest eight hours before farrowing and farrow in it.[1096] Sows begin to build nests from 4 to 16 hours before farrowing, ceasing 1–3 hours before farrowing and are most likely to build a more complex nest if straw is available. They may continue to build nests for several days after parturition.[907,1298,2443,3043] Nest building is triggered initially by endogenous factors, including prostaglandin F2 alpha[357,358] and prolactin, which stimulate nosing and rooting, but external stimuli (nest material) is necessary for pawing, carrying, and arranging; that is, pigs do not engage in carrying nothing to their nest.[400] If the pig has a preformed nest, nest building is increased, not decreased.[1142] For

example, if a hollow in the sand filled with 23 kg (50.7 lb.) of straw is available, sows begin to nest build earlier and root more but do not carry as much straw to the nests.[83] Provision of sawdust to preparturient sows increases nesting behavior, shortens their labor, and may result in fewer piglet deaths.[472]

The Confined Sow

Farrowing Crates

Modern husbandry practices have all but eliminated most porcine maternal behavior except nursing. Sows are placed in farrowing crates that prevent them from turning around or touching the sides of the pen; consequently, the piglets are protected from crushing. Most crushing takes place when the sow lies down, especially when she lies down on her side rapidly. Sows lie down in five steps: (a) one foot is lifted and placed before the other until she is kneeling on one limb, and then the other limb is advanced until she is kneeling on both limbs; (b) there is a pause; (c) the sow slides one knee forward along the floor and rotates her head and upper body until her shoulder and head rest on the floor; (d) another pause may occur; (e) the sow lowers her hindquarters, rotating slightly, causing the rear legs to slide sideways and the hindquarters to drop so that the upper thigh lands on the floor. This takes between 7 and 20 seconds. The slower the sow is to lie down, the less risk to her piglets. If she leans against the wall or a rail of a farrowing crate, she is less likely to crush the piglets.[505] Sows that lie on their sides during the immediate prepartum hours rather than nest building are more likely to crush their piglets.[1782]

Sows can be kept in an ellipsoid crate that allows them to turn around but does not result in any more crushing of piglets than does a traditional crate.[1415]

Because crushing of piglets by the sow is such a common cause of piglet mortality, it is interesting that sows do not respond to the feel or sight of a piglet under them; they do respond to the sound of a piglet squeal, although it must be loud.[1097-1098] Sows respond to only half of the calls by standing up or rolling.[1106] Sows that crush their piglets have less maternal behavior in general; they spend less time building a nest pre-farrowing and respond less to playbacks of piglet distress calls.[56] Maternal response to piglet vocalizations (both an unrelated piglet and their own) declines with parity.[975]

Sows are most responsive to piglet squeals on the first two days postpartum, the time when piglets are in the most danger of being crushed if the sow lies on them.[1099] Crushing of piglets is reduced but not eliminated by farrowing crates. Losses can be reduced further using a device that shocks the sow's belly when a piglet screams; however, the sow may also be shocked when extraneous noises trigger the device.[761] Another approach to preventing crushing is to attract the piglets away from the sow with a simulated udder, a warm, resilient, sow-scented area under the heat lamp.[1319] Because most piglets are crushed as the sow lies down, it is important that she lies down against a wall that not only protects the piglets, but also supports the sow. Sows prefer the back wall of the pen, so a solid wall with no protuberances should be available there.[506]

Parturition

Most farrowings take place in the afternoon or night.[2124] After labor begins, most sows lie in lateral recumbency. Parturition is painful in animals and, apparently, is more painful in multiparous than primiparous sows.[2807] The sow will swish her tail violently as abdominal straining takes place. Parturition usually takes three to four hours, but varies considerably with litter size and the condition of the gilt. If parturition is interrupted by moving the pig to a new pen after one piglet is born, a delay of hours occurs until the next piglet is born. Opiates released in response to the stress of moving inhibit oxytocin release; however, exogenous oxytocin will reinitiate labor.

Behavior of the Sow toward the Neonate

Maternal behavior in sows is composed of three main factors: (a) calmness, which involves low cortisol response to minor stressors, care when lying down to avoid piglets, few changes in behavior, and remaining in the nursing posture following milk ejection; (b) protectiveness (response to piglet squeals and human approach to piglets); and (c) nursing activity.[2159]

When not confined, the sow will eat the placenta. The function of placentophagia remains unknown. It may be a recycling of nutrients or a form of defense against predators by removing odors. Placentophagia enhances analgesia in rats.[1267] The question of whether this occurs in domestic animals as well deserves investigation.[1317] Parturition is painful, so the use of analgesics is warranted. In fact, piglet crushing can be reduced by treatment of the sow with butorphanol, probably because the sows were less active.[1319]

Sows do little licking of their newborns, even when not confined in a farrowing pen. Therefore, human attendance at parturition is recommended. Although most piglets begin to breathe and quickly struggle free from the fetal membranes, a few will not. The removal of membranes, clearing of the airway, and stimulation of respiration can save a piglet that would otherwise die.

Behavior of the Neonatal Piglet toward the Sow

Piglets make a most startling transition from fetal to independent existence. They may be apneic for 5–10 seconds after birth. Then they give a few gasps before beginning to breathe regularly. Their eyes and ears are open, and they are able to walk immediately, although their gait is staggering for the first few hours. The firstborn may be slow to find the udder, but later-born pigs apparently respond to the voices of their littermates and quickly begin to seek the udder. Most piglets are suckling within 30 minutes of birth.[1141] During farrowing and for some time afterward, piglets can suckle continuously, presumably because oxytocin levels are high; thus, they are rewarded for each suckle in the correct place, that is, on a teat.

Piglets are attracted to soft, warm surfaces, pig vocalizations, and the sow's odors, and they move in the direction of the sow's hair growth.[1951,2408] Washing the udder with an organic solvent delays nipple location, as does blocking the piglet's sense of smell, indicating the importance of odors.[1634] Texture may be even more important because piglets are more attracted to a cloth-covered artificial udder than to one to which sow odor has been applied.[2284] The firstborn pigs appear to use thermal, tactile, and olfactory cues to find the udder, whereas the later born probably respond to the suckling sounds of their older littermates and walk straight to it because social facilitation is strong in pigs at birth. Suckling attempts are probably stimulated by tactile contact with a protuberance (the teat). Piglets rarely attempt to suckle on a haired portion of the sow; they will suck on the snout or the tip of the sow's vulva. Piglets nose the udder and intersperse nosing with gapes, the behavior in which the piglet opens its mouth as if to grasp a teat. Larger pigs do more gaping, which may account for their success in reaching teats. The nosing behavior of lighter pigs declines more rapidly than that of heavier pigs.[1951] The piglet may find the udder, give a few inept sucks at a teat, and then make another circuit or two of the sow before it settles down to nursing.

Experiments using artificial sows have revealed that the piglets are attracted to the voice of the sow and to either end of the udder, but they avoid the middle and quickly abandon teats that give no milk.[1147] Competition during formation of the teat order is intense, and only one-third of pigs end up on the teat initially chosen. After a teat has been chosen and won by competition with other piglets, it is recognized by odor rather than visual cues.[1148]

Nursing

Nursing causes release of opiates so that sows are less reactive to painful stimuli at that time. The opiates stimulate prolactin and somatotropin release.[2004] Approximately 10 hours after the birth of the first pig, nursing becomes cyclic.[1358] Nursing bouts occur approximately every 45 minutes. The interval between nursing is longer at night than during the day. Small litters suckle less frequently than large ones.[2473] The sow ordinarily calls the piglets to suckle with a low-pitched rhythmic grunting. As the piglets begin to massage the udder with their snouts, the frequency of the sow's grunts increases from 1 per second to a peak of 10 per second. The more pigs massaging the udder, the faster the sow grunts and the less time until the release of oxytocin, which occurs at the peak of grunting followed in 25 seconds by milk letdown.[45] Piglets grunt faster and faster as they await milk letdown, but there is no increase in grunting rate preceding an unsuccessful suckling bout (no milk letdown).[1107] Sows may stretch a foreleg and rotate it toward the udder (foreleg rowing) while the piglets are massaging the udder. Rubbing of the udder of a lactating sow can induce her to lie down and begin to give the nursing call. Stimulation of the anterior half of the udder and, especially, rubbing of the nipples in that area can increase the grunting rate.[743,746,747] Rubbing of the belly has a calming effect on even immature or male pigs, and can be used to great advantage in handling swine.

A suckling bout is divided into four phases: an initial massaging of the udder for one minute; a quiet phase during which the piglets' ears go back and they stop massaging, which may correspond to the peak of the sow's grunts; true suckling for approximately 14 seconds while the milk is ejected, during which the piglets' ears are back, their tails are tightly curled, and their front legs are in rigid extension; and a final massage phase that is quite variable in length, from 2 to 15 minutes. The massage stimulates prolactin release, which will increase milk production. The less weight a piglet gains, the more it will massage the udder after suckling, indicating that hunger drives this behavior.[2159] These slow-growing piglets also suckle more between nursing bouts.[2279] Young piglets often fall asleep on the nipple or curled beside the udder, whereas older pigs will nose the udder and pull the teats for some time.

Not all nursing bouts are successful. In 22% of the nursing bouts, the sow may call the piglets, which approach and massage the udder, but no milk is ejected. Unsuccessful nursing usually occurs less than 40 minutes after a successful bout. The piglets leave the udder as they do after a successful nursing but return much sooner.[749] The proportion of unsuccessful bouts increases if sows are moved to an unfamiliar pen.[2005] Apparently, unsuccessful nursing bouts occur in free-ranging sows.[1144] Unsuccessful nursings can also occur when the sow terminates the bout by changing position. She may be responding to the vocalization of piglets fighting for a teat.[1104]

The strong social facilitation and dependence on vocal communication exhibited by pigs can be used to practical advantage. If one sow in the farrowing house calls her litter to nurse, soon all the litters will be nursing. Nursing rates and weight gain can be increased by playing tape recordings of nursing noises to the sows at more frequent intervals than they normally nurse.[2189] A talented manager can imitate the noises and accomplish the same thing.[933] Piglets can also initiate suckling by their calls and persistent nudging at the sow. If half a litter has been fasted, the hungry piglets will induce the sow to lie down, and then all the piglets will nurse, although the non-fasted piglets will consume less.[1060]

Despite the apparent low level of maternal activity in sows, piglets separated from their mother for even a short time (a few hours) exhibit considerable distress. They vocalize with either squeals or closed-mouth grunts up to 21 times per minute.[745] The vocalizations increase with the length of isolation. The vocalization changes to a higher frequency, quacking vocalization when the piglets can hear their mother's voice, which they can discriminate from that of another sow.[2103] If the piglets are in a strange pen, they will make persistent efforts to escape, they vocalize, and they often urinate. The behavioral and physiological effects of isolation are mitigated by the presence of another piglet, but the effect is stronger if the companion is a littermate.

The effect of the presence of littermates is additive with that of the sow, so a litter placed in a strange pen with their mother gives only closed-mouth grunts and a few squeals. The olfactory cues are not sufficient to prevent vocalizations because the presence of the sow's bedding alone has no attenuating effect on vocalizations.[881] If the separated litter is closely confined and provided with a heat lamp, they are much quieter, and weight losses, especially due to urination, are reduced. Similarly, cuddling of a piglet will reduce the number and volume of its squeals. Twenty-one-day-old piglets when separated from the sow will grunt, but scream only if she is in the next pen.[1101]

Mutual Recognition

Sows and piglets apparently use olfaction to identify one another but need more than one day and possibly as long as a week to learn. The piglets can identify their dam's feces, milk, and urine odors,[1033,1035,1635] as well as her vocalizations.[998] Sows respond to playbacks of piglet separation calls by vocalizing,[2397] but cannot discriminate their own from other piglets on the basis of their voices. They can identify their own piglets by the time they are a week old on the basis of olfaction.[1033] Piglets can be fostered easily onto another sow when they and the sow's litter are less than a day old. After that, the fostered piglets walk around, vocalize, and are reluctant to suckle, perhaps because they had already formed a bond to their dam.[1854] There may be prenatal perception of the mother's emotion. Piglets are influenced by sounds that hear *in utero* so that when isolated piglets were more distressed if they heard the voice that was associated with maternal negative emotional state *in utero*.[3003]

Sows will reject strange piglets older than two days. The rejection is based on olfaction, because anosmic sows will accept strange piglets.[1543]

Defensive Reaction

Sows normally exhibit strong defensive reactions when their piglets are threatened. They give a crescendo of barks, open their mouths, and attack. Only when pigs are defending their young are they really dangerous. The use of the farrowing crate has had a definite effect on the maternal behavior of sows. The sows can do nothing if their piglets are handled or hurt despite the piglets' loud distress calls. In herds in which the piglets are handled often and by many people, as in university or research institutions, the sows become accustomed to the distress calls of their pigs; therefore, a sow may even continue to sit on a piglet that is screaming loudly and eventually smother it.

Weaning

Weaning begins at five weeks when the sow begins to aggress against the piglets; however, the piglets continue to suckle for 80 days. Although the number of nursing bouts (approximately 20/day) does not change much from day 3 to day 30 of lactation, the duration of individual nursing bouts decreases from seven to five minutes. The number of nursing bouts terminated by the sow increases.[2330] When able to leave piglets behind by stepping over a barrier, sows spend increasing time away from their piglets; the amount of time varies with litter size.[1755,2396,2397] Surprisingly, those sows that spend most time away from their piglets respond most to calls of isolated piglets.[269–271,1827] Some sows that have the opportunity to leave their piglets may do so, but confining sows with their piglets

reinstates normal maternal behavior.[269] This fact indicates that contact, particularly visual contact, with the piglet is necessary to sustain the maternal behavior.

Under modern management techniques, piglets are weaned at four weeks or even younger. Early weaning (at three to four weeks old) of piglets is often practiced in order to decrease the inter-litter time.[1838] Early-weaned pigs massage and nibble on one another, yet spend less time rooting or nibbling on other objects. If placed in cages, early-weaned pigs dog-sit (on their haunches) seven times more frequently than do piglets in straw-bedded pens, which indicates that flooring type and age at weaning influence behavior.[2330] Aggression is higher when pigs are weaned at four weeks than if they are weaned at three weeks, but it decreases with time.

Because piglets eat little solid food at two weeks of age, weaning at this time is more stressful and is associated with greater inhibition of growth than is weaning at four weeks.[1571] The younger the piglets are when they are weaned, the more they squeal and "quack" and the higher pitched the squeals, declining from eight to one squeal per hour after four days of separation.[2400] Piglets weaned at three weeks are still vocalizing six days after weaning, in contrast to pigs weaned at four weeks.[446] Improvements in diet for young piglets led to the practice of segregated early weaning (SEW).[2400] One of the behaviors observed in piglets weaned at one or two weeks of age is *belly nosing*. Eighty-one percent of the piglets engage in this behavior, which occupies 2.4% of their time. The behavior gradually increases, peaking by day 26 and decreasing by day 33. It is associated with social interactions with other pigs and so may not be a suckling attempt.[1363] Piglets that spend more time suckling before weaning are less likely to belly nose.[2279] Enrichment in the form of a foam rubber mat on the pen wall decreases belly nosing, but neither a rubber teat nor soil in which to root deceases the behavior.[232] These pigs weaned on or before

14 days of age ate less, especially when first weaned, and gained less.[2494]

To prevent piglets from sucking on one another and to prevent spread of gastroenteric diseases that plague artificially raised piglets, they can be housed separately. Pigs reared without the sow would defecate in the nesting area, whereas normally raised pigs do not.[137] Piglets raised in germ-free isolators give distress calls almost continuously during handling and feeding; conventionally raised pigs give distress calls only when hurt.[1710] Piglets weaned at six days show an initial increase in cortisol. A week after weaning, their urinary norepinephrine is lower than that of pigs weaned at 28 days, possibly indicating adrenal exhaustion.[1104] Food intake of weanling pigs can be increased and aggression decreased by application of the synthetic porcine pheromone to the pigs' snouts or to the feeder.[1522]

Weaning at four weeks is also stressful, particularly if the piglets of one litter are mixed with those of another. Aggression occurs, but can be reduced by pairing enrichment, in this case a novel palatable food with an acoustic signal. This classical conditioning leads to more play and less aggression, presumably as a response to the anticipation of the enrichment. Enrichment alone was less effective.[582] Another method of reducing aggression and increasing weight gain at weaning is to allow litters in adjacent pens to interact so that they are "socialized" to one another before weaning.[1005] Little cross-suckling occurs.

In the United States, the majority of sows have been kept in gestation crates during pregnancy in order to prevent aggression among sows and to allow intake to be monitored. Because these sows cannot walk or turn around, group housing is now being considered. Effects of the sow's housing environment on their offspring's behavior have revealed that piglets of group-housed sows gain more weight, do not have to be hand fed at weaning, and are less stressed by isolation.[2153]

Clinical Problems

Cannibalism

Cannibalism occasionally occurs in sows; nervous primiparous gilts are the most likely offenders. Cannibalism is responsible for 4% of piglet deaths and occurs in 18% of litters.[471] The most common occurrence is immediately after parturition. In fact, many sows will bark at the first piglet that walks by their heads after parturition.[1891] Farrowing crates successfully prevent cannibalism unless an unwary piglet walks right in front of the sow.

Refusal to Nurse

A more common problem is seen in sows suffering from mastitis; a sow that is normally a good mother will attack her litter whenever they attempt to nurse. This early behavioral sign warns of disease before many physical signs can be detected. This type of behavior is seen in sows that become afflicted with mastitis late in lactation, after the farrowing crates have been removed. Sows that have the mastitis–metritis syndrome shortly after farrowing are usually too ill to protest when the piglets suckle. The failure of the sow to eat and of the piglets to gain weight is the best clinical evidence of the latter syndrome.

Sheep

Maternal behavior in sheep has an important clinical aspect, as most lamb mortality occurs within the first week of life in range-reared sheep. Mortality rates are from 5 to 15%, rising to as high as 50% in huge flocks in bad weather, even in the absence of predators.[1625] Ewes do use shelters more after lambing, probably as predator avoidance behavior.[1835] Abnormal or weak maternal behavior accounts for parts of these high losses and perhaps for some of the losses attributed to coyote predation. Most maternal rejection or simply poor mothering without absolute rejection occurs in young ewes and in those that had difficulty at parturition.[2378]

Lambs may be born at any time of the day or night, with peak frequencies being noted at 9–12 a.m. and at 3–6 p.m.[1383] A few days before parturition, the ewe withdraws from the flock, if on the range, and seeks some sort of shelter. Shelter seeking by the ewe improves the environment into which the lamb is born so that its chances of survival are greater; however, the ewe is responding primarily to her own thermoregulatory needs whereby shorn, but not unshorn, sheep seek shelter.[1426] Allelomimetic behavior is so strong in sheep that some of the flock may follow her. In a pen, the ewe will withdraw from social contact and seek a corner.[321] She will show restlessness, circle, vocalize, rub her head on her flanks, lick herself, and paw at her bedding 60–90 minutes before parturition.[617] Grazing and ruminating cease. The older the ewe, the shorter the lapse of time between the onset of restlessness and the onset of labor. The interval between onset of labor and the appearance of the lamb can vary, but is usually 30–60 minutes.

Even before parturition, 20% of ewes show maternal behavior toward other lambs.[90] This prepartum maternal behavior results in lamb stealing (discussed later in this section). The amniotic fluid dripping from the vagina to the ground attracts the ewe. She will sniff and lick at bedding contaminated with amniotic fluid. This attraction to amniotic fluid can be used to predict parturition because only ewes close to parturition will eat food mixed with amniotic fluid. Ovine or caprine,[1354] but not bovine, amniotic fluid is accepted,[99] indicating that some subfamily specificity exists. The attraction of the ewe to this fluid may serve to keep the ewe in the area where the birth will take place, ensuring that the lamb will not be abandoned before it can get to its feet.[2142]

Licking and Bleating
When the lamb is born, the ewe begins to lick it for 80% of the first hour after parturition.[605]

The ewe licks the trunk, head, and perianal region.[2339] Simultaneously she emits a special parturition call that is a very low-pitched gurgle or rumble, a call that also may be given before parturition. Primiparous ewes bleat more, and hill breeds, such as Cheviots, bleat more than Suffolks, perhaps reflecting the greater risks of losing lambs in the harsher hill environment.[607,610] The call is heard only at parturition in domestic sheep, but it persists in the feral Soay sheep as a close-contact call.[2109] The lamb's behavior influences that of the ewe. If the lamb is inactive, the ewe will cease licking. Licking of the lamb can be very important in cold or windy weather because it serves to dry the neonate; it additionally serves to stimulate the lamb (Figure 5.2). While the lamb is recumbent, the ewe licks its head, even restraining the lamb with a front leg to prevent it from standing.

Licking of the perianal area stimulates the lamb to rise. After the lamb is standing, usually within 30 minutes,[2378] the ewe continues to lick it, but mostly on the hindquarters. If the ewe stops licking, the lamb gives distress calls.[165] Finally, licking of the lamb by the ewe

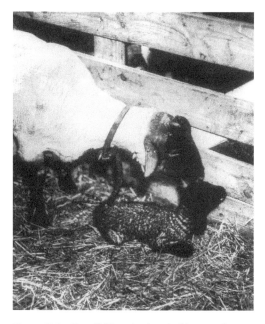

Figure 5.2 Ewe licking the head of her newborn lamb. *Source:* Courtesy of Dr. Martin Siegel.

establishes the maternal–offspring bond, for the ewe will be able to identify her lamb by smell and taste. Usually, the fetal membranes are licked off the lamb and ingested, but the placenta is not eaten.

The lamb-licking rate is correlated with estrogen levels at parturition. Circulating estrogen and the estrogen-to-progesterone ratio in late pregnancy are higher in sheep with good maternal behavior.[609] Ewes are less attentive to embryo-transferred lambs of a breed different from themselves.[611] Although mothers of twin lambs spend more time licking their offspring than do mothers of singletons, the increase is not double; so twin lambs, especially the second born, are licked less than singletons.[1719] The lack of licking is reflected in the longer interval to successful suckling in twins.

The lamb raises and shakes its head, rolls onto its sternum, and bleats. It rises to its knees and stands first on the hind limbs and then both fore and hind. Although lambs are able to stand within 30 minutes or an hour of birth, it may take two to three hours before they find the udder.[31,2378] The ewe plays a part in the search. She may either facilitate or inhibit teat seeking.

Suckling

The ewe is most attracted by the head of the lamb. As she circles to maintain head-to-head contact, she moves her hindquarters and udder away from the lamb, which hinders the lamb's attempt to find the udder. The innate pattern to which lambs appear to respond is the curved underline of the ewe. The newborn lamb moves toward the ewe's head and toward her udder: both areas appear to be attractive (Figure 5.3). After the lamb has established contact with an underline, odor, texture, and temperature probably serve to guide him.[2357] The warmest surface of the ewe is her woolless inguinal area; furthermore, the lamb is attracted by the odor and resilience of the inguinal wax.[247,248,2358,2359] Having its face contacted stimulates the lamb to push its head up and forward. Contact with the lips causes it to

open its mouth and protrude the tongue.[1428,2357] Contact with its tongue causes the lamb to curl the tongue into the suckling position.[2360] This series of innate responses serves to bring the lamb to the ewe, then to the udder, then to the teat, and finally to suckle the teat.

Lambs whose dams are stanchioned take longer to locate the udder,[31] indicating the active role the ewe usually plays. The drive to suckle is inhibited, but not eliminated, by intragastric loads of milk; consequently, hunger is not the lamb's only motivation.[32] After the udder has been located, the lamb uses visual cues to relocate it for subsequent sucklings.[164] The ewe signals when she is prepared to nurse by standing with her head up and/or vocalizing. Ewes refuse far fewer suckling attempts if those behaviors precede the suckling attempts.[608]

Advantage can be taken of the features to which a lamb responds to build a colostrum feeder from which the lamb will suckle without human aid. The colostrum feeder consists of a fleece-covered horizontal ledge through which soft rubber teats protrude at a 45° angle, 50 cm (20 in.) off the ground.[752]

After suckling has begun, it occurs with great frequency; twin lambs suckle 22 times during 16 hours of daylight, and single lambs, 6–14 times.[564,1649] Newborn lambs may nurse for as long as three minutes in one bout; later, the duration falls to 20–40 seconds. Frequency of suckling and suckling duration both decrease with age. By the end of the first week, lambs suckle hourly, and by nine weeks, every three hours.

Triplets nurse less often and for shorter duration than singletons or twins.[650,654] Probably because they are not receiving adequate nourishment from their dams, they are most likely to try to suckle an alien ewe. During the first two weeks, the ewe will allow one twin to suckle without the other. Later, the ewe will walk away when the lamb nudges her in the inguinal area and will refuse to let one twin nurse until the other is also present. If the ewe is lying down, the lambs will not only nudge her but also jump on her back and paw at her

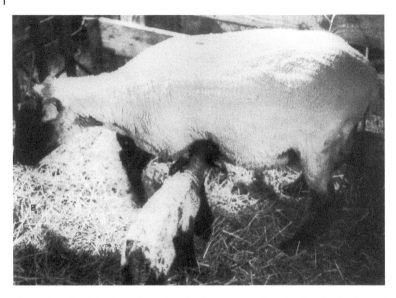

Figure 5.3   Initial orientation of the lamb to the ewe's underline, but in the axilla rather than the udder. *Source:* Courtesy of Dr. Martin Siegel.

in an attempt to make her stand. The ewes will call their five-week-old lambs to them and then refuse to let them nurse. Such behavior encourages the lambs to stay in close contact.[652] As suckling decreases, grazing by the lambs increases. Although the ewe stays within 10 m of the lamb the first few days, she will increase her distance from it as the lamb ages. During the first month of her lamb's life, the ewe will leave the flock to seek out her lamb if it has strayed. Thereafter, she will bleat but remain in the flock.

Acceptance of the Lamb

The "critical period" during which a ewe will accept a lamb is the first several hours after parturition.[442,2142] Normally, a ewe will stay within 2 m of her lamb for most of the first day.[1426] If a ewe's lamb is removed immediately after birth and before she has licked it, the ewe will accept any lamb presented to her. After the ewe has spent 30 minutes to 2 hours with a lamb, her own or a substitute, she will not accept another. If the lamb is removed four hours after birth, the ewe will continue to exhibit maternal behavior if it is returned within 24 hours.[1355] If the lamb is removed

seven days after parturition, the ewe will accept it when it is returned after 36 hours, but not after 72 hours by which time her maternal behavior has ceased.

The importance of olfactory cues in the establishment of the bond is demonstrated by the fact that ewes will temporarily accept strange lambs that have been rubbed with the ewe's placenta. Ewes can also be induced to follow their placentas.[442] Primiparous ewes will not accept a lamb whose wool has been washed free of amniotic fluid, whereas multiparous ewes will, indicating both the importance of amniotic fluid and the importance of prior experience at mothering.[1352] Olfaction is necessary for normal maternal behavior in primiparous, but not multiparous, ewes.[1355] If the ewes could not smell the lambs, they bleated less and licked the lamb less; the lambs took longer to suckle.

In hilly country, newborn lambs may roll down the hill away from the site of their birth. The ewe may neglect the lamb because the odor at the birth site is more attractive than the lamb itself. In this situation, a weak lamb, or the weaker of a pair of twins, is most likely to roll away and not be licked. A more vigorous lamb will survive and seek out the ewe. If too long a time elapses between parturition and the presentation of the lamb, the lamb may be rejected.

Mutual Recognition by the Ewe and Lamb
Recognition of the Lamb by the Ewe

Recognition of lambs depends on at least three senses: olfaction, audition, and vision. The wool of the lamb contains the odor used by the ewe to identify her own lamb.[29,36] Apparently, ewes base their recognition of their lambs at a distance on vision and hearing and at a close range (0.25 m [10 in.] or less) on smell,[35,1390] recognition cues being reinforced each time the lamb suckles. By six hours postpartum, the ewe can recognize her lamb at a distance.[1709] During nursing, the ewe sniffs at the tail and perianal area of the lamb. Olfactory bulbectomy eliminates the preparturient lip licking observed in Soay sheep, as well as the licking of the newborn and normal lamb recognition. The bulbectomized ewe will accept other lambs indiscriminately.[145] After a month of exposure to their lamb, anosmic ewes do not accept alien lambs as readily, although they still allow more contact and show less aggression than normal ewes.[680] Other senses can compensate in part for olfaction.

At least two senses must be impaired before ewes are unable to find their lambs.[1626] Visual cues may be most important, as indicated by ewes having had more trouble finding a hidden lamb than a silent one.[30] By changing the appearance of various portions of the lamb's body, it was found that maternal recognition was most impaired by altering the appearance of the head.[33] Although it represents only 12% of the body surface, the head is apparently the area that the ewe uses to identify the lamb visually. Evidence also shows that ewes use the color of their lambs to identify them. They reject their own lambs when they are dyed, and, if they do reaccept them, they will choose lambs of the same color when their own is not available.[35] Laboratory experiments (see Chapter 1, "Communication") indicate that sheep can perceive color; the studies on lamb recognition indicate that sheep use color vision.

The strong individual recognition of her lamb by a ewe, however, can break down. Multiple-birth lambings of three, four, or more lambs are not uncommon, especially in Finnish landrace sheep. As sheep are bred to produce litters, there may be changes in maternal behavior. The ewes rearing three lambs bleated less and approached a solitary lamb less often than ewes with singletons or twins.[1834] If several ewes and their litters are penned together, the ewes may not distinguish their own lambs from the others; communal suckling of all lambs by all ewes results. Multiparous ewes are better at recognizing their own lambs than primiparous ones, and their lambs are more proficient at choosing their dam from another ewe.[789]

Recognition of the Ewe by the Lamb

A signal originating from the lamb's gastrointestinal tract can be the mechanism for recognition of and preference for the dam. Lambs given their dam's colostrum by stomach tube and with no experience suckling from her chose her instead of an alien ewe at 24 hours of age.[846] The bond of the lamb to its mother is stimulated by colostrum ingestion, which leads to release of cholecystokinin and stimulation of vagal afferents (Figure 5.4).[1709] Without that stimulation, the lambs do not prefer their mother. They can learn which ewe will allow them to suckle while giving low-pitched bleats and which will butt them away while giving high-pitched bleats. They detect their own mothers faster and more accurately with age. During their first several days of life, lambs are not able to discriminate their mother from other ewes very well except at very close range. A lamb separated from its mother will rush up to the nearest ewe and attempt to suckle, only to be butted aside. Lambs can distinguish their dam from an alien ewe at 24 hours of age by approaching her pen, but, if tested again, will approach the same pen whether or not their

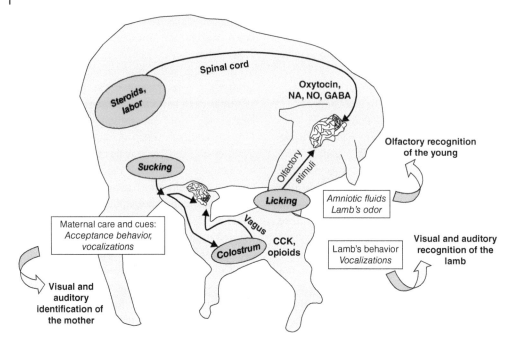

Figure 5.4 The bond of the lamb to its mother is stimulated by colostrum ingestion, which leads to release of cholecystokinin and stimulation of vagal afferents. *Source:* Nowak *et al.* (2007)[1709] Reproduced with permission of Elsevier.

dam is there. That indicates that after they have learned where to find the dam, they have difficulty finding her in a different location. By three days, they are able to recognize their dam from a distance, but they do not appear to use olfaction to recognize their dams even at close range. If isolated from their flock mates for 24 hours, lambs fail to differentiate their mother from other ewes.[2334] Hearing may be more important than vision.[1708] Lambs are not attracted to photographs of their mother, but do prefer their mother's voice to that of a ewe familiar to them.[3015] Given a choice between their own mothers, similar (same breed) ewes, or dissimilar (different-breed) ewes, they will continue to be more attracted to similar rather than dissimilar ewes.[36,2119] After being weaned at three months of age, the preference of lambs for their mother in comparison to a familiar ewe decreases within 30 days, and finally disappeared 60 days after weaning.[3109] The association of dams and twin-born lambs is significantly lower compared to the

association between dams and single-born lambs suggesting that the twin-born lambs had a greater association with their siblings compared to the association with their mothers.[3110]

The importance of hearing is indicated in the study that found that lambs were more apt to approach a ewe that was not their mother when the voices of the ewes were muffled.[93] Technical advances in reproduction have allowed advances in understanding of auditory recognition. Most Dalesbred and Jacob lambs born after embryo transfer to Dalesbred ewes could identify the ewe on the basis of her voice, whereas most of those born to Jacob ewes could not.[2107] Sonographic analysis indicated more inter-sheep differences among bleats of Dalesbred ewes than among Jacob bleats.[2104,2107] Ewes differentiate their bleat characteristics in regard to the number of offspring; ewes with one offspring produced bleats with lower formant frequencies.[3089]

Two-day-old lambs can discriminate their mother's bleats from those of an unfamiliar ewe, but only the low pitched closed mouth bleats or rumbles described above, not the open-mouth high-pitched bleats.[2073] As lambs mature, visual cues become more important. A lamb less than a week old is not affected by a change in his dam's coat, such as shearing or blackening, but a two-week-old lamb may hesitate to join a visually altered dam.[28] Blocking visual access by covering the pen in which the ewe is restrained slows the approach of their lambs.[2108]

A critical period within the first few hours after parturition may exist for acceptance of lambs by ewes; however, the lamb is not restricted in time as far as his social attachments are concerned. The tendency to follow any large moving object is most marked during the first three days of life; for the next three days, fear responses predominate, but from six days to two months, lambs will continue to follow even an artificial sheep model.[2471] Lambs tend to follow large moving objects, but imprinting in the avian sense does not occur, for a lamb's attachment can be quite impermanent. Lambs easily can become attached to a nanny goat or to a human who feeds them. Lambs that had been normally reared with ewes quickly formed attachments to dogs with which they were penned as pairs. Within eight weeks, the lamb would follow the dog, vocalize if the dog was removed, and even run a maze to be reunited.[369] After living in a normal situation for four months, the lambs no longer preferred dogs to sheep. Therefore, social attachments in lambs seem to be relatively easily formed and equally easily dissolved. This phenomenon of attachment can be used to bond sheep to cattle. The cattle deter coyotes from attacking the sheep. See the "Guard Dogs for Predator Control" section in Chapter 2, "Aggression and Social Structure."

Weaning

Maternal response (increased bleating and heart rate) to separation from the lamb declines over the first seven weeks of the lamb's life, although the lamb's response to separation increases with age – an example of classical parent–offspring conflict.[2595] It is the mother's best interest to reserve her resources for the next offspring and in the lambs to maximize the resources he can obtain from his mother. Weaning does not exactly parallel decline in milk production. Milk production falls gradually, but suckling stops abruptly when milk production reaches a threshold.[94] A study of free-ranging Soay sheep found that the ewe–lamb bond ceased just before the estrous period. The ewe lambs continued to follow their dams, but the ram lambs did not. None of the lambs slept touching their dams as they had done previously. The young sheep associated with their peer groups, the ewe lambs remained in the dam's home range groups, and the ram lambs wandered off to join a ram group.[863]

Artificial Weaning

Weaning lambs at two days causes a rise in cortisol and immune suppression. Lambs weaned at 2 or 15 days do not gain weight as quickly as unweaned lambs.[1668] When weaned at three weeks, lambs will bleat, but the bleating rate is lower if they are paired with another lamb, especially if that lamb is its twin.[1843] Lambs remember one another and are less stressed (i.e., emit fewer distress vocalizations) if they are with a lamb they lived with a week before separation from the ewe. They show a preference for familiar lambs, but treat lambs they have lived with recently similarly to those they had lived with previously; that is, they remembered the latter.[1379] Two-stage weaning, in which the lambs are prevented from suckling for a week by a udder net before separation from the ewe, results in less stress as evidenced by less agitation and fewer vocalizations than seen in one-stage weaning, in which the lamb is simply removed from the ewe.[2044] Inducing estrus in the ewes and tethering rams in the enclosure with the ewes reduce weaning stress and vocalizations by the ewes.[1796]

Cross-Fostering

The problem of cross-fostering of lambs is a common one. In general, older ewes will more readily accept lambs than will younger ones.[2142] Fortunately, if a ewe is exposed to young of its own species long enough, maternal behavior will occur. The process (concaveation) may take weeks, and the ewe should be stanchioned or somehow restrained so that the lamb will not be badly butted in the interval before maternal behavior appears. Tranquilization of the ewes with perphenazine will facilitate acceptance, but does not facilitate fostering of alien lambs onto ewes with their own lamb present.[2272] Diazepam administered after parturition will facilitate acceptance of an alien lamb by a ewe and could be used to facilitate cross-fostering as well.[684] A variety of methods have been used to facilitate cross-fostering. The time-honored method is to tie the skin of the ewe's own deceased lamb over the lamb to be fostered. There are, however, quicker and easier methods of providing olfactory cues from the ewe's own lamb that do not depend on skinning a dead lamb. These include pouring amniotic fluid on the alien lamb, washing the lamb,[38] and putting a garment worn by the ewe's own lamb inside out on the alien.[30,41] This method of transferring the familiar scent to the alien lamb also is successful in fostering a second lamb onto a ewe.

Visual cues should also be altered. Either the lamb can be tied so that it cannot stand, thus mimicking the attempts of a neonate to stand, or visual cues can be eliminated. Stanchioning the ewe is effective because the ewe cannot move away from the lamb or butt it, and if her view of the lamb is also blocked (eliminating visual cues), fostering is facilitated.[37] Advantage should also be taken of cervical stimulation, as already discussed here, to facilitate fostering.[1200] The technique of slime grafting, in which the vaginal fluid of the ewe is rubbed on the lamb to be fostered, probably owes its success to the consequent vaginal stimulation in addition to, or instead of, the transfer of her odor to the lamb.

Clinical Problems

Poor maternal behavior is often seen in ewes that have been in labor more than 30 minutes. The corticosteroid levels of such ewes are elevated, indicating that they are stressed.[321] Poor maternal behavior may vary; the ewe may reject the lamb outright, but more frequently she will lick it in a desultory fashion only and nervously avoid the lamb's attempt to nurse.

Large breed differences appear in the frequency of abandonment of one of a pair of twin lambs. Merino sheep are much more likely to abandon one of their twin lambs than are Dorset or Romney.[40]

Mismothering

Mismothering – that is, maternal behavior directed toward a lamb that is not the ewe's own – is a common problem, especially in large flocks in which ewes are not penned separately for parturition. Up to 15% of lambs may be raised by ewes that are not their mothers. Many combinations exist. A ewe's lamb may be born dead, and the ewe will steal another ewe's lamb. She may steal a lamb before parturition, have one of her own, and be credited with twins. Although stolen lambs may survive, it is impossible to make accurate statements about productivity of a given ewe under these circumstances. A shepherd might cull a productive ewe and keep one that never produces twins but often acquires them.[2410] The opportunities to mismother are increased when sheep are confined in a group pen at parturition; however, if cubicles are provided, the incidence of mismothering is considerably lower in those ewes that choose to lamb in them.[835]

Oral Vices of Artificially Reared Lambs

Artificially reared lambs suck one another's navel or scrotum and eat feces. Such behavior may cause injury or interfere with weight gain.[2183]

As parturition approaches, does, especially multiparous ones, leave the herd and seek a sheltered place, almost always near a vertical object, to kid. The does will defend this area and the kid both before and for the first day after the kid is born. A doe is usually very agitated, vocalizing, urinating, and moving, but this response disappears just before parturition.[1833] Vaginocervical stimulation can induce maternal behavior in goats as well as sheep. Parturition is most likely to occur during the day at a time when goats are generally inactive. As parturition approaches, they grunt, paw the ground, kick, and lick their backs.[1885] Does usually lie down to kid.

After parturition, the kid will be sniffed and immediately licked; the head is the primary target. The licking continues for two to four hours. Although the total time licking twins by the mother is longer, it is not twice as long; therefore, twin kids are licked less than singletons.[1886] The doe will vocalize frequently, using a low-pitched bleat similar to the rumble of periparturient sheep. Vaginocervical stimulation can be used to induce a recently parturient doe to accept an alien kid.[1954] There seems to be a critical period of an hour for acceptance of the kid; kids removed at birth and presented to the doe an hour later may be rejected.[1953] The doe must have contact with the kid for more than five minutes to become not only maternally responsive but also selective in that response, that is, accepting only her own kids.[295,867,1953] Olfaction seems to be important for selective maternal behavior; anosmic goats accept all kids, rather than only their own.[1238,1953] Within four hours after the kid's birth, the doe can recognize it by sight and sound.

The small ruminants seem unable to distinguish between species: lambs can easily be cross-fostered onto goats, and vice versa.

Intensive maternal behavior is short-lived in goats because within a day (or after three days in some goat populations) the kid will have left

the doe to hide. Hiding can last as long as six weeks. Some does are stayers, remaining close to the area where the kid is hidden, but others are leavers, traveling a considerable distance from the kid. She will approach the hidden kid several times a day and call to it. The kid will answer and emerge to suckle as infrequently as twice a day. In the absence of a proper hide, a dim area with vertical sides and a roof, hiding behavior may not be recognized, but it has persisted in domestic as well as feral goats.[1365,1998]

Goat kids should stand within 20 minutes and suckle within an hour.[46,1003,1366] The kid seeks the udder and usually searches the axilla first because the doe is turned toward the kid licking it. The kids of does with udders transplanted to the neck region located the udder as quickly as the kids of normal does.[2184]

Young kids – one week old – do not respond to doe calls until an hour after they last suckled, but then respond more to their mother's calls than to those of other does; at a month, they respond immediately.[328] Two-day-old kids can identify their mothers visually; apparently, they use their dam's pelage for recognition.[1368,2001] Twin kids are slower to learn to recognize their dam than singletons.[116] After the hiding period, if it occurs, twin kids suckle every 30 minutes the first week, but only once every hour or two by one month.[534] Kids are more apt to be farther from their mothers than is the non-hiding lamb, which develops visual recognition only slowly. Does respond more to their own kids' vocalizations at five weeks postpartum than 11–17 months later, but a year later displayed stronger responses to calls of their previous kids than to calls of familiar kids from other females.[330]

Weaning in the wild occurs between three and six months. It is interesting that prolactin release occurs in response to suckling by any kid – own or alien – but oxytocin release occurs only in response to suckling by the doe's own kid. Maternal behavior is maintained by the visual, auditory, and acoustic cues from the kid; suckling is not necessary.[1833]

Kid Rejection

The importance of olfactory identification of the young is emphasized by the following case: a week-old kid was castrated; an open castration technique was used in which incisions were made and the testes removed. When the kid was returned to the doe, she took one sniff and rejected it. The kid had to be hand raised (Dr. Mary Smith, personal observation). The smell of the fresh wound was probably responsible for the rejection response. Closed castration techniques should probably be used in suckling kids.

Cattle

Some of the signs of imminent parturition are relaxation of the sacrosciatic ligament, slackening of the tissue of the perineum and vulva, distention of the udder and teats, and mucous discharge from the vulva. Unless the afternoon body temperature is below 39 °C (102 °F), parturition is unlikely even in the presence of all the other signs.[649] The normally lower body temperature of cattle in the morning interferes with the predictive value of temperature at that time.[584,586] Cows will alternate standing and lying much more frequently in the hours before parturition.[2373]

Parturition

The majority of cattle do not leave the herd to calve. This is probably an example of flexibility of behavior that takes advantage of geography. When trees or rocks are available, the cow leaves the herd and hides, but in an open pasture the risk of predation is less if she stays with the herd.[1377] Cows choose dry, elevated areas with shelter available, so those are the areas where one should search for lost neonatal calves.[1868] Cows spent less time lying, had more lying bouts, and were more active the day before calving as compared to two to four days

before calving. The number of lying bouts and the level of activity increased throughout the six hours prior to calving. During the last two hours prior to calving, the duration of contractions and the number of times the cow turned her head toward her abdomen increased, while eating and drinking decreased.[2574]

A periparturient cow will sniff and lick an alien calf, especially if she is within 24 hours of parturition and the other calf has just been delivered, whereas after parturition all her activities are directed toward her own calf. Licking of alien calves does not cause rejection of the cow's own calf, nor does suckling of an alien mother cause a calf to fail to suckle its own dam. Other cows will sometimes push or butt a newborn calf.

Eighty-two percent of all parturitions take place between noon and midnight.[808] Parturition times are distributed throughout the 24 hours, but dystocias occur mostly at midday.[1748,2504] During the first stage of labor, heifers were more restless and pawed more than older cows. When introduced into a calving box during first-stage labor, all cows explored the pen and most sniffed. They tended to build a nest by pushing the straw into a pile and lying on it; most got up again before calving. The frequencies of lying and tail raising increase before parturition.[1578] Cows that were to have a dystocia were more likely to rub against the walls and urinate during the first stage of labor, and they spent more time tail raising.[2405]

A greater proportion of births will take place during the day if cows are fed late at night.[1417] Arching of the back and an elevated tail occur for one to three hours before the chorioallantoic membrane ruptures. When the membrane ruptures, the cow often licks the fluid and tends to stay near the spot, now attractive to the cow, where the fluid fell. Attraction to amniotic fluid begins up to 12 hours prepartum.[1823] Ninety-five percent of all cows are recumbent at the actual time of delivery.[2080] Approximately 100 minutes elapse from the rupture of the membranes to the birth of the calf. Placentophagia occurs in 82% of cattle. Parturition is longer in cows that give birth to large calves and in nervous heifers. In fact, labor may cease if nervous heifers are disturbed.[585] Handling of the cows at the time of calving appears to result in improved behavior at milking.[990]

Bonding

Contact between the cow and her calf for as brief a period as five minutes postpartum results in the formation of a strong, specific maternal bond. Cows groom their calves during the early postpartum period, concentrating on the back and abdomen. Licking the calf occupies up to half the cow's time during the first hour postpartum; heifers lick less.[621] Licking not only dries the calf, removes bacteria from its coat, and stimulates the calf but also results in analgesia in the cow.[1245] Opiates are released at parturition, and their analgesic effect is enhanced by ingestion of amniotic fluid.[1824] If contact between cows and their calves is delayed for five hours postpartum, 50% of the calves will be rejected; therefore, the critical period for formation of the cow–calf bond must be the first few hours postpartum. When the calf is removed after a brief initial contact, the cow vocalizes and is restless; however, after 24 hours, she can no longer distinguish her own calf.[1079] There appears to be a sensitive period for calves to bond with cows. If calves are fed colostrum by bottle for three days, they suckle less and rub or lick the foster cows less than do calves who had suckled their dam before being placed with a foster cow.[2311] Cows respond more quickly to their own calf's call, and calves are more likely to respond to their own mother's call than to that of another.

Cows on pasture are found further from other cows for the first three days after calving and multiparous cows are not as close to their calves as primiparous ones.[2929] Cows who are most defensive of their calves do not exhibit stronger maternal behavior to those calves.[3012]

Cows do not show kinship recognition of their calves. When twins were created by transferring an embryo into the uterus of already pregnant cows, the unrelated calf was treated just like their own calves.[2381] Maternal experience is also important in that maternal protectiveness increased with parity.[1028] Calves can recognize their dams but make many errors when trying to identify their dam from 20 other cows. They tend to choose a cow of the same coat color as their mother.[1650] Advantage can be taken of the cow's nonselective maternal behavior to foster several calves – up to four – onto one cow.

Suckling

The newborn calf shakes its head, snuffles, and sneezes. This behavior may begin during parturition as soon as the calf's shoulders are free of the mother's vulva. Some calves will remain motionless for up to 30 minutes after birth, but within an hour most calves can stand. A calf may take 30 minutes to an hour to locate the teats, and the cow's conformation may not provide the higher recess that the calf appears to seek. Passive transfer of immunity to calves is poor in cows that have had dystocias, presumably because the calves did not suckle as much or as often.[562] Most calves suckle within three hours, but up to a third of calves may not suckle within six hours of birth. This is particularly apt to be the case when the cow has a pendulous udder.[620] After the teat has been located for the first time, the calf will be able to locate it much more quickly at subsequent nursings. As the calf suckles, the cow will lick the perineum, stimulating urination and defecation by her calf. Calves that have not suckled for the first six days of life cannot learn to suckle.[690] Younger calves or those that have had suckling experience can learn to suckle from another cow.

When suckling, calves assume a particular stance with spread legs so that their shoulders are lowered, allowing them to butt upward at the udder. The butting appears to function in the stimulation of milk flow.[880] As do other young ruminants, they nuzzle and lick along the cow, especially in high recesses such as the axilla and groin, and will mouth any hairless protuberance as they seek the udder.[2080] They appear to be confused when they encounter a hairless, teat-like object that does not supply milk. They wag their tails while suckling, although not at as high a rate as that of lambs. Newborn calves normally suckle 5–10 times a day.[905] Suckling bouts are long, approximately 6–12 minutes, and do not seem to vary with frequency of suckling.[799,882,1804,2151] Brahman calves spend 13 minutes suckling per bout.[3077] Usually, the number of suckling bouts decreases with age, but beef calves may actually suckle more frequently with age, possibly because the milk supply of the beef cow is small.[1722] The most regular suckling time is at daybreak, with other bouts occurring between 9 a.m. and noon, 3 p.m. and 6 p.m., and 10:30 p.m. and 1 a.m.[2376] Most suckling takes place during the day.[2040] Dairy calves spent seven minutes suckling their dams. Older calves have longer nursing bouts and butt the udder less. The dairy calves probably differ from the beef calves because dairy cows produce more milk. Calves only suck on one or two teats.[1376]

When housed in groups, calves will sometimes allosuck (suckling on a cow that is not their dam), usually from behind rather than in reverse-parallel position. The calves that do so may not be obtaining adequate nutrition from their dam because they tend to be lighter weight.[2351]

It is now possible to produce twins in beef cattle by embryo transfer. These twins, like triplet lambs, suckle more often and are more apt to suckle from an alien cow. They usually approach the udder from the rear rather than in the normal antiparallel position. The smaller of the twins is the most likely to suckle from an alien cow, and the cow suckled usually has a single calf.[1857] The twins are groomed less than single calves.[1853]

When calves are raised artificially on a nippled feeder, they show similar rates of nursing when the milk is similar in concentration to cows' milk, but nursing increases in frequency when the milk is diluted. The calves often stand touching the wall while sucking from the feeder, just as they would touch the side of the cow if they were nursing. Calves weaned from a milk diet to solid food call less if the transition is made by supplying water rather than milk from the nipple feeders[354] or by reducing the amount of milk they receive in proportion to the amount of grain they consume.[1982]

Most dairy cows do not suckle their calves, but they are still physiologically responsive to calf stimuli. Playing tape recordings of hungry calves during one milking increases milk production in the following milking.[1500] Artificially reared calves butt as they would butt the udder when milk flow is slow from an artificial teat.[886] One result of the increased popularity of organic products is that dairy calves may be raised more naturally, that is, with their mothers. Calves allowed to suckle for 20 minutes twice a day grew as well as calves fed milk and cross-suckled less.[763] Calves allowed to remain with their mothers in an automatic milking system lay down more and ruminated more but ate solid food, moved, socialized, and explored less than calves fed from an automatic milk dispenser. They did not exhibit stereotypic tongue rolling as the artificially fed calves did.[762]

Weaning

Cows do not break the bond with their yearling calf when their next calf is born; they may even allow the yearling to suckle, although they are more aggressive toward the yearling than they were before the birth of the younger calf.[2344]

In Brahma (*Bos indicus*), bull calves are weaned at 11 months, but heifer calves are weaned much earlier, at eight months.[1920] The cow apparently invests more of her resources in a son that can produce many offspring per year than in a daughter that can produce only one.

The shorter the time that a dairy cow and calf have been together, the less the effect of weaning; weaning at six hours results in fewer vocalizations by both the cow and the calf than if they were separated later.[2395] Cows that are allowed to suckle their own calves for 10 weeks produce more milk than do cows whose calves are removed. Although the suckled cows produce a large supply of milk, some of the total goes to the calf, and they do not compensate with marketable milk for all that the calf consumes. Calves allowed to nurse only twice a day gain more weight than those fed from buckets and those with continuous access to their dams.[648] Beef calves are weaned at 200 days, much closer to the natural weaning age, but still show a reduction in growth. Allowing the calves fence-line contact with their dams reduces the negative effects of separation. The calves spend nearly half their time within 3 m (10 ft.) of the fence separating them from their mothers.

When calves are weaned from a foster cow, the process can be done in two steps. In the first step the calves are fitted with a nose flap to prevent suckling, and in the second step they are separated. They are less stressed as measured by behavior and cortisol levels than abruptly weaned calves.[1406,1407]

Clinical Problems

Sucking Problems

Non-nutritional inter-suckling is a very frequent problem when calves are raised in groups, especially if they are pail, rather than nipple, fed. Some calves raised by cows inter-suck even before weaning and will continue to do so afterward. An inadequate diet increases the frequency of inter-suckling.[1188] The hungrier the calf before a meal, the more it will try to suckle after the meal. They will suckle on one another, particularly on one another's udder, mouth, ears, or scrotum or rarely the prepuce. Nonnutritive inter-suckling can occur 78–300 times a day, most frequently in the 15 minutes after a milk meal.[882] Weaning from milk to grain

reduces the frequency. Nonnutritive suckling is observed in calves following a milk meal drunk from a bucket. The motivation to suckle after drinking milk lasts for less than an hour. Calves that are hungrier before they drink will suckle more afterward.[2002]

Skin irritation or even hernias can result from prolonged sucking by one calf on the umbilicus or sheath of another. Calves that engage in nonnutritive sucking often fail to thrive.[218,248] The incidence of inter-suckling on British dairy farms is 13%. If the problem exists on a farm, as many as 30% of the calves and 11% of the adult cows may be affected; there is apparently social facilitation of the behavior.[2248] Most dairy farmers solve the problem by penning calves separately, but they may still suckle on buckets or themselves. Various harnesses and even surgical procedures, such as splitting of the tongue, have been devised to deal with the problem.

Nonnutritive suckling on inanimate objects or self-suckling may be decreased by providing a dry teat for the calf to suckle. The component of milk that stimulates nonnutritive suckling is not fluid, fat protein, or calories *per se*, but lactose.[522] Calves that can suckle dry teats are calmer.[2344] When this is not feasible, however, other procedures are available that may prevent the behavior, such as muzzles, or application of unpalatable substances to the part sucked, and changing to dry food rather than milk. To reduce inter-suckling, serrated rings are placed on the suckler's nose so that the suckled animals will be prodded and rebuff the suckler. None of these methods reduce the calf's motivation to suckle. Most nonnutritive suckling occurs immediately after feeding, so provision of nipples in the feeding area will decrease self-, or auto-suckling, and allo-suckling.

Calves weaned after six days are more apt to suckle one another than are calves weaned earlier. A related problem is that of self-suckling.

Cross-Fostering

Cross-fostering can be accomplished by draping the calf with the skin of the cow's dead calf, if that is available. A more difficult problem is convincing a cow to accept a foster calf in addition to her own offspring. Fostering calves onto dairy cows is fairly easy because they have not been selected for maternal behavior that includes rejection of alien calves. Beef cows have been selected for these traits, so it is much more difficult to foster additional calves onto them. There are practical reasons for wishing to do so; a well-fed beef cow has a milk supply large enough for two calves. Dairy calves can be fostered onto these beef cows and will, when raised in this manner, suffer far less from maternal deprivation and from the respiratory and enteric diseases to which artificially reared calves are susceptible.[1078,1212]

Persuading the cow to accept the dairy calf presents difficulties. Although the cow–calf bond is presumably formed when the cow first encounters the fetal fluids and the newborn calf, a beef cow may reject a dairy calf even when its own calf has been removed immediately after birth and when the foster calf is rubbed with fresh amniotic fluid. The cow apparently still can discriminate between a newborn and the older, larger, more active foster calf, probably on the basis of visual cues; blindfolding the cow may help.[1212] Substituting one calf for another is possible by removing the cow's own calf 48 hours postpartum, leaving the cow with no calf for three days, and then returning her own calf plus the alien calf. The bond to the original calf has been broken, but maternal responsiveness persists.[1204] Placing a jacket worn by her own calf inside out on the calf to be fostered is helpful; the same technique is used in sheep.[999]

Much obviously remains to be learned about the basis of maternal bonding in cattle. Some cows will grudgingly foster the dairy calf and mother their own calf. Others will become promiscuous mothers that allow four or more calves to suckle.[1216] The maternal bond has been broken in these cases and replaced by non-discriminative tolerance. The promiscuous mother may suffer teat or udder damage when too many calves suckle. There is also the danger that mastitis may be passed from nurse cow to nurse cow by the calves. It is not necessary to find a foster mother who has recently calved; cows will accept foster calves as long as 178 days after separation from their own calves, but their milk production will be lower.[1408] Cows that live in a group with their foster calves continuously present are more likely to be maternally selective than those cows that are exposed to the calves only for nursing periods twice a day.[2608]

Horses

Parturition

The onset of parturition in mares is heralded by waxing of the udder, but the length of time between the appearance of udder waxing and the appearance of the foal may be quite variable, up to 21 days. The calcium level of the milk increases as foaling approaches and can be used as a predictor. Body temperature is lower the day prior to parturition.[2091] The mare will walk more and stand less the evening of parturition. Mares may begin to weave, paw, lie down, and stand up 30 minutes before foaling.[3074] In the free-ranging situation, only primiparous mares leave the herd to foal; multiparous mares remain with the herd.[239]

In the first stage of labor, which lasts for about four hours, the mare is restless and will crouch, straddle, and urinate. The smell of fetal fluids is attractive to parturient mares. The mare will exhibit the flehmen response to any amniotic fluid she has expelled. Sweat will appear on her elbows and flanks.[742]

During the second stage of labor, the mare will lie in lateral recumbency. This second stage is very violent and very short in horses, lasting less than a half hour. For that reason, it is important to have a veterinarian in attendance when complications are expected. There will not be time for professional help to reach the mare if problems develop in the course of labor.

Mares are notorious for their ability to thwart observation of their parturition. Although most mares foal at night, some will wait until they are released from their stalls in the morning in order to foal in the solitude of the pasture. Thus, parturition appears to be under some type of voluntary control in such mares, but the evidence is all anecdotal.

The most exciting findings in equine maternal behavior is that lactation can be induced using the dopamine antagonist sulpiride and that maternal behavior to an alien foal can be stimulated by vaginal stimulation of those mares induced to lactate. The process of inducing lactation takes a few weeks, but could be used to produce nurse mares without producing unwanted foals.[1667]

Postparturient Behavior

Ordinarily, the foal is delivered in such a way that the mare need only turn her head to meet her foal muzzle to muzzle. The establishment of the selectivity of maternal behavior is still uninvestigated in horses. It may be based on olfaction, because the mare licks the fetal membranes and then the newborn; licking behavior usually is confined to a few hours after parturition.

Licking, as well as sniffing, is concentrated first on the head of the foal and later on the hindquarters, particularly the perianal area. The rate of licking decreases markedly during the first hour postpartum. Although the period for bond formation has not been identified in horses, the first hour is probably critical for the mare to learn to recognize her foal selectively. The foal appears to take much longer, perhaps as long as a week, to recognize the mare. The foal will follow any large, moving object. The mare is usually very aggressive toward other horses and sometimes toward people for the first day or two after foaling. This behavior serves to keep away other horses that the foal otherwise might follow. Mares show pronounced circadian rhythms until the day of parturition. They and their foals have no discernible cycle during the first day postpartum, but the mares return to a circadian rhythm while foals are active both day and night, presumably because they suckle several times an hour.[814]

Suckling

Standing and suckling occur within the first hour after birth for pony foals and within the first two hours for Thoroughbred and Saddlebred foals.[393,1979,2385] Many managers of brood mares guide the foal to the udder and place a teat in its mouth in order to ensure the foal obtains colostrum. This appears to have a detrimental effect on the foal because it will remain closer to the dam and play less months later.[945]

Foals suckle four times per hour at one week of age and gradually decrease the frequency to once per hour by five months (Figure 5.5).[392,393,475,2300] Mares spend approximately two minutes nursing, during which the foal spends less than half the time actually suckling. The rest of the time is spent in nuzzling the teat and butting the udder.[163] The mare usually flexes her hind leg on the side opposite the foal, possibly conserving energy by shifting her weight to the stay apparatus (Figure 5.6).[2468] Subordinate mares have shorter nursing bouts because dominant mares aggressively disrupt nursing and nursing attempts.[2009] High-ranking mares are closer to their foals and in late lactation allow their foals to suckle more.[971] Nursing also occurs after any separation, even a very brief one, or after the foal has been frightened. When a foal approaches its dam to nurse, it often shakes its head and nickers or crosses in front of the mare. Foals turn their heads sideways to nurse, especially as they grow larger.

Fillies suckle longer, but obtain no more milk than colts.[374] Colts may suckle more frequently than fillies when food is a limiting factor.[239,596] There appears to be more investment in a colt by mares in good body condition and more in fillies by mares in poor condition,

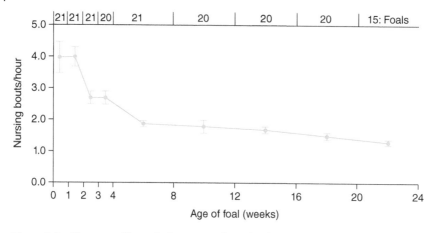

Figure 5.5   Changes with age in frequency of nursing by pony foals. *Source:* Crowell-Davis (1985)[475] Reproduced with permission of Elsevier.

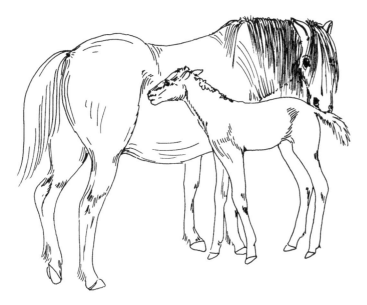

Figure 5.6   Identification of the foal. The mare sniffs the anal area of the foal. The hind leg on the side opposite the foal is flexed to facilitate nursing. *Source:* Houpt (1977).[1042]

which is explained by Trivers'[2289] hypothesis that a surviving son will father many or few offspring depending on his success, whereas a daughter always reproduces a small number of offspring.[373] Nursing is often terminated by the mare, not by aggression but by simply walking away from the foal. This behavior occurs most frequently during the first month of the foal's life.[475] The foal may be forced to practice following the mare as a result of her behavior.

The more skilled the foal is at identifying and following his dam, the more likely he is to survive. Mares do aggress toward their foals during nursing, but the aggression appears to be a response to bunting of the udder and does not prevent or shorten suckling bouts.[476] Pregnant mares allow their foals to spend more time suckling than nonpregnant mares.[2658]

Weaning occurs at 40 weeks when the mare is about to foal, but is prolonged beyond a year if the mother is not pregnant.[596] Under domestic conditions of abundant food, foals continue to suckle for three or four years, even when they are larger than their mothers. Orphaned or newly weaned foals will often attempt to nurse from non-lactating mares, suckle the sheaths of geldings, and investigate the inguinal area of any horse.

The Mare–Foal Bond

Mares seldom venture far from their foals throughout the first few months and foals still prefer their dams five months after weaning, indicating that the mare–foal bond is still present.[2843] The distance between a mare and her foal is proportional to the age of the foal, that is, young foals are closer to their dams than are older foals. Foals spend several hours per day lying down. During these periods, the mare remains with the foal, either grazing in circles around it or standing next to it. This behavior, the recumbency response, which probably functions to protect the foal both from predators and from becoming lost, wanes as the foal matures. When the foal is awake, it is responsible for maintaining contact with its dam.[476] The mare is within five yards of the foal 94% of the time during the first week and 52% of the time the fifth month of the foal's life. The other circumstance in which the mare follows the foal is when the young foal ventures more than 10 m (33 ft.) away.[476] The typical equine family group will travel in the following order: mare, most recent foal, yearling foal, and then the other offspring in the order of increasing age.[2039]

Mares are very protective of their foals, especially during the first few days of a foal's life. Mares may be dangerous to humans, even familiar ones, at this time. Good maternal behavior including protecting a foal from aggression by other horses as well as predators is important for foal survival, especially in the first month. Older mares spend more time defending their foals during this period, which may account for their greater reproductive

success.[373] Mares are more protective of their foals in multi-male bands than in those with a single stallion, presumably to protect the foals from infanticide by non-parental stallions. Stallions, on the other hand are more protective of foals when a canine predator was present.[3024]

Mutual Recognition

The roles of the three senses, vision, audition, and olfaction, in the mare–foal bond is complex. The neighs (or whinnies) of the separated mare and foal are impressive, and horses make use of these calls to locate one another. The more frequently a mare neighs, the more quickly her foal will find her. The mare's neighs are not specifically recognized by the foal, but the mare neighs more often to her own foal.[2484] Changing a mare's or a foal's appearance by hooding, blanketing, and bandaging does not interfere with recognition, yet visual cues must be involved because both foals and mares have difficulty finding each other when one is in a closed stall. They orient toward whinnies but need visual confirmation of the dam's or foal's presence.

Olfaction is also important. Mare and foal sniff each other's heads, and the mare sniffs the anal region of the foal (see Figure 5.6). Masking olfactory cues with a strong odor greatly retards location of mares by foals, especially in the absence of visual cues.[2484] Thus, olfactory and possibly vocal cues (nickers) are used for close-range identification, whereas other vocal cues (whinnies) and visual cues are important for more distant communication of identity or presence (Figure 5.7). Visual cues are probably not of vital significance; many blind mares have successfully raised foals even in semi-naturalistic conditions.

Artificial Weaning

At least five different methods of artificial weaning are available: (a) removal of the foal from the mare and confinement of the foal by

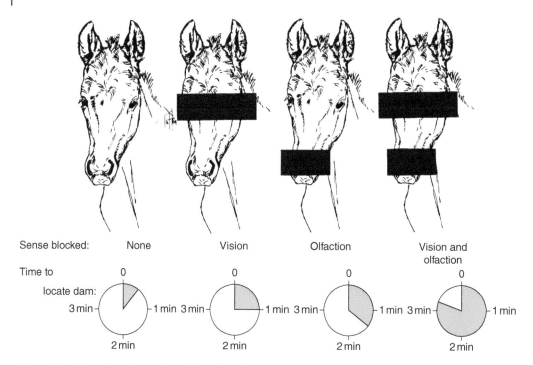

Sense blocked: None   Vision   Olfaction   Vision and olfaction

Figure 5.7   The effect of masking vision, olfaction, or both on the time that a foal takes to locate its dam. *Source:* Houpt and Wolski (1979)[1052]/International Veterinary Information Service.

himself; (b) removal of the foal from the mare and confinement of the foal with another foal or foals; (c) interval weaning, in which the mare alone is removed from the pasture while the foal remains with the other younger foals and their dams (the other mares are removed gradually in order of their foals' ages); (d) separation of mares and foals into adjacent corrals for one week, and subsequent removal of the mares; and (e) feeding mares and foals separately and gradually increasing the duration of separation. This latter method is particularly valuable for the owner of a single mare–foal pair. Although pony foals seem less stressed when weaned as pairs rather than singly, Thoroughbred foals are more stressed, apparently because more aggression takes place between members of the pairs.[1046] Feeding concentrates before weaning appeared to reduce stress.[1021] In addition, separation of the two foals may also be stressful. Weaning by the fourth method, in which the

foals can see and hear their mother but cannot make direct contact (or suckle), appears to be less stressful than methods in which the mother cannot be seen, probably because weaning is more gradual.[1493] Weaning from the mother as a food source occurs before weaning from the mother as a social companion. Interval weaning is associated with fewer gastric ulcers and less cribbing than weaning into a stall and feeding of concentrates.[2391] Creep feeding foals a high-fat and high-fiber diet decreased activity in newly weaned foals.[1691] Weaning foals at five to six months leads to an increase in fecal corticosteroids for several weeks and a change in resting postures from recumbency to standing.[2712]

The optimal age to wean is also debatable. From the foal's point of view, the later the better. From the mare's point of view, the sooner the better. One study found that weaning foals from the same mare–foal group by placing them in a barn together seemed to be less stressful for six month old foals than for seven- and eight-month-old foals, but those foals may have been simply less active and thus bit and kicked less than older foals. Drinking and urination increased in all age groups, while moving slowly and rolling decreased.[2499] Mares separated from their foals were slightly less anxious and agitated if a painted image of a foal is present.[1948]

Clinical Problems

Mismothering

Mismothering can occur in equids, although it is much rarer than in sheep. A female mule adopted and successfully raised a foal; only examination of the foal's karyotype revealed that the foal was a Shetland pony, one of a pair of twins born to a pony mare in the same pasture as the mule.[625] Mules may be particularly prone to this behavior; in another case, a mule stole a calf from its mother and raised it.[2094] Mules have successfully raised Thoroughbred foals born to them after embryo transplant, but a donkey foal was rejected.[2094]

Foal Rejection

There are three types of foal rejection that occur immediately after foaling: (a) rejection of suckling, (b) fear of the foal, and (c) attacking the foal. All three forms are more common in the primiparous mare, but the third form may occur again and again.

In the first type, many mares lick the foal and appear attracted to it but will not tolerate suckling. They will kick the foal if it persists. These mares can usually be treated successfully either by tranquilization and/or by milking the mare while holding the foal next to the mare and feeding the milk to the foal from a bottle held in the inguinal area. The newborn foal normally nurses every 15 minutes, so this exercise should be repeated many times to nourish the foal, transfer colostrum antibodies, and teach the mare that milking relieves tension on the udder. Gradually, the foal should be encouraged to suckle the teats, and

less and less restraint should be applied to the mare until the pair can be left alone safely.

Some mares resent manipulation of the inguinal fold – not the udder itself. These mares can be treated quickly by negative reinforcement. The mare is made to trot on a lead line until she will allow rigorous manipulation of the inguinal fold (Jeannine Berger, personal communication).

In the second type of foal rejection, the fearful mare tries to escape from her foal and may injure him by running over him. She will kick when the foal approaches her. Several behavioral methods can be used to stimulate maternal behavior. Turning the mare and foal out in a paddock so that both the mare and the foal can avoid each other may lessen the mare's fear. Adding another horse may stimulate the aggression that periparturient mares normally show, and this may be followed by acceptance of the foal. A large dog has been used for the same purpose, that is, stimulating maternal defensiveness.

In the third, and most dangerous, type of foal rejection, the mare actively attacks her foal, usually biting him in the withers and throwing him across the stall. These mares act toward a foal as foal-killing stallions do. She will not have licked the fetal membranes or the foal. She will also kick if the foal approaches her. Tranquilization with acepromazine, passive restraint for as long as three weeks, and administration of oxytocin and progestins can result in acceptance. For milder forms of rejection, the prolactin-stimulating tranquilizer domperidone and alprazolam can be used to facilitate foal acceptance.[2485] This problem can be seen in any breed of mares but is most common in Arabians that reject 5% of their foals in comparison to less than 2% of Paints, indicating a genetic component.[1165] Passive restraint is best obtained by placing a pole across a box stall so that the mare cannot move sideways, forward, or backward. She can still bite, but the foal can escape and soon learns to avoid her head. She can kick forward, that is, cowkick, but a persistent foal can suckle. Usually, the mare will accept the foal after a week or two of restraint. These mares tend to be merely tolerant of their foals, and some may relapse after a few weeks. Mares that reject their foals have lower levels of progesterone before parturition than normal mares.

Pain, such as that associated with passing the placenta or with uterine contractions caused by suckling-induced oxytocin release, may result in aggression toward the foal. Removing the source of pain eliminates the aggression. Maternal rejection may occur after foaling. Too much disturbance of the mare and foal has been implicated, as has changing the odor or appearance of the foal. A common clinical problem is rejection of the foal that has had to be separated from its mother for treatment of a medical problem. The foal is changed in odor and may have had its appearance altered by clipping and bandaging. Allowing the mare to have visual contact with the ill foal may help to prevent rejection even if the foal is too weak to suckle for many days.

Redirected aggression also occurs. A mare may be aggressing against another horse and then bite or kick her foal. More frequently, the foal is simply kicked accidentally during a fight. Occasionally, a mare may aggress against her own foal when an alien approaches or due to failure of recognition.

Some mares do not reject their foals but do not respond vocally to them when they are separated. This can lead to injury to the foal because it will approach other mares and be attacked, or will try to jump a fence or gate to return to the stall where it last saw the mare. Although this would be presented clinically as accidental trauma to the foal, it is the result of poor maternal behavior.

Mares can be vicious when protecting their foals, but they can also be vicious when weaning them. When the foal attempts to nurse, a mare may bite not only the foal but also a nearby person. This behavior also may be caused by mastitis or injury to the udder, or may have an unknown cause.

Donkeys

Jenny appears to separate itself before parturition. Nursing duration for free-ranging feral donkeys was about 255 sec/h (bout length 85 seconds and an average of 3 bouts per hour[2891]:whereas domestic donkeys nursed every 3–10 minutes for the first 5 days and by 10 days only every 20–30 minutes.[2752,2891] Nursing bout frequency and total nursing duration, but not bout duration, decreased with age. Low nursing rates were still observed in 11- to 12-month-old foals.[2835]

Cats

Parturition

Gestation is 63–66 days in cats. Births have a seasonal distribution, with the greatest number of litters being born in the summer and the least in autumn and early winter.[1848] Cats rarely deign to use the boxes carefully provided for parturition by their owners. Most cats will choose a cave-like place, such as a closet or a linen cabinet. A cat is attracted to the smell of the amniotic fluid at the birth site, so moving the kittens to a more suitable location will not entice her from her chosen spot. Parturition in the cat is characterized by a great deal of licking by the queen: self-licking mostly directed at the belly and genital area, licking of the fetal fluids from her body or the floor, and licking the kittens. The queen is responding to the fluids, rather than to the kittens, at this time.

The queen is typically very restless, and a normal protocol will list lying down, sitting up, licking of the vulva, squatting, bracing lordosis, circling, walking around the cage, lying down again, rolling, licking of a kitten, and so on. No consistent pattern emerges, and the behavior of the queen varies with the endogenous stimuli (from the uterus) and exogenous stimuli (from the birth fluids and kittens). The uterine contractions of labor can be distinguished from fetal movements because the raised hind legs of the queen usually flex when she is in labor.[2050]

Most cats prefer solitude, though some highly socialized ones seem to be content only when the owner is present. Cats, with the exception of Siamese, are usually quiet during parturition. The restless behavior of the queen serves to stretch the umbilical cord of the newly delivered kitten. When the placenta is delivered, the queen will eat it and part of the cord with the same tilt of the head and pronounced chewing motions that she shows when consuming prey. In the process of eating the placenta, the queen stretches the umbilical cord so that little bleeding occurs when the cord is severed. It is rare for the eating to extend to cannibalism of the kitten. The interval between kitten births can be as long as one hour, even in normal births, but is usually much shorter. The queen seems unaware of the kittens despite her bouts of licking them, as demonstrated by her inadvertent stepping on them in the course of her pacing, as well as her ignoring of their cries. The bursts of activity are interspersed with periods of fatigue.

When the last kitten has been delivered, the queen directs her attention to her litter. She lies down with an encircling motion, positioning her legs in such a way as to form a U around the kittens. For the next 12–24 hours, she rarely leaves the newborns and then only for brief intervals to eat, drink, and eliminate. Each time she returns, she arouses the kittens by licking them, after which she encircles and then nurses them. Queens emit a specific call, the chirp, when they are approaching the nest. Her kittens will respond more to her chirps than to those of another cat.

Suckling

Finding the Teat

Most kittens are suckling within an hour or two of birth. Kittens with anesthetized tongues can find the nipple but cannot suckle; kittens with anesthetized lips cannot locate the nipple but can suckle.[2114] Olfactory bulbectomy also eliminates the ability of kittens to find the nipple,[1257] but damage to the olfactory bulb eliminates more than the sense of smell alone. Newborn kittens with no suckling experience respond to the ventrum of lactating females, but not of non-lactating females, with search behavior, and they attach to nipples within minutes. Even in older kittens, nipple attachment depends on females' reproductive state: some attach on pregnant females, the greatest number on early-lactating females, followed by a decline on late-lactating females. Kittens can locate their particular, most used nipple on their mother but not on a female of similar lactational state, even after eye opening. Kittens respond from birth with efficient nipple-search behavior to inborn olfactory cues on the mother's ventrum. Kittens also quickly learn olfactory cues specific to their own mother and to their own particular nipples.[2615]

Kittens locomote by pulling themselves along with their front limbs while paddling with the weaker hind limbs. As they crawl forward, they turn their heads from side to side. When they encounter the nipple, they pull their heads back and lunge forward with open mouths. Eventually, the nipple is secured in the mouth. The position of the mother facilitates locating the mammary region. The responses of the kittens to the areola and nipple appear to be innate, almost reflex in nature.[2263]

Experiments conducted on artificially reared kittens revealed that before their eyes were open, they followed a path produced by their own body odors to find the nipple of the brooder. The kittens could also make tactile discriminations under these experimental conditions, learning to choose a nipple with bumps on it over one with concentric ridges when the former was associated with milk reinforcement.[2050]

Prolonged experience (one to three weeks) with suckling from an artificial teat delays, but does not abolish, the kitten's ability to initiate natural suckling.[1971] Milk reinforcement is not necessary for suckling, because intragastrically fed kittens will initiate suckling on the teats of a non-lactating cat as rapidly as on a lactating cat, even on repeated trials.[1244] The ability to initiate suckling disappears after 22 days of age if the kittens have been fed intragastrically.

Teat Order

Within 12 hours of birth, kittens have a teat order determined that is usually but not always followed. There is no relation between kittens' use of particular nipples and their weight gain, milk intake, or involvement in contests during suckling, but the kittens do push one another off nipples at least once a day. The kittens ingest 1.4 g per nursing for the first week and 4 g by four weeks.[657,1077]

In some litters, no regular teat order is formed. After the teat order is established, a kitten can use the presence of its sibling on either side to help guide it to the proper nipple, although sometimes the kittens obstruct more than facilitate one another's progress. Kittens massage the udder with treading motions of the paws. Treading on soft surfaces persists in the adult cat, presumably as a pleasurable activity or in pleasurable social situations. Cats do not tread when alone.

The feline nursing period has been divided into three stages: stage 1, 1–14 days: mother initiates nursing; stage 2, 14–21 days: both mother and kittens initiate nursing; and stage 3, 22–35 days: kittens initiate nursing. In the hormonally primed queen, the suckling of kittens is probably tactilely pleasant. However, as kittens grow older and their feeding demands become more persistent, the female develops an approach–avoidance type of behavior toward her kittens; she discourages their attempts to suckle from the third week onward by moving away. Although in a home situation she could easily escape from the kittens, in a cage she can only jump to a shelf to which the kittens can soon gain access as their locomotor skills improve. Another ploy by the mother is to lick the kittens vigorously, thus preventing them from attaching. Figure 5.8 illustrates the change with time in the queen's relationship with her kittens. In a two-kitten litter, the time of weaning occurs later.[1471] In the single kitten, these stages are not as discrete. The queen spends less time with a single kitten initially (30 vs. 70% of her time), but she continues to allow it to nurse long after a larger litter would have been weaned. Apparently, a single kitten is less attractive than several kittens but also less aggravating. From the fourth week on, "barn" cats will begin to bring live or dead prey to their kittens (see Chapter 6, "Development of Behavior"); however, these females sometimes allow intermittent nursing until the next litter is born.

Homing and Retrieval

Even before the opening of their eyes, kittens can return to their nest from several feet away. Apparently, they use olfactory cues; a washed floor between the kittens and the nest prevents them from finding their way back.[2050]

Feline retrieval behavior is quite different from the canine form. Queens retrieve their kittens in response to auditory, not visual, signals. The more the kitten vocalizes, the more apt the queen is to retrieve it.[937] The queen usually picks the kitten up by the scruff of the neck, although occasionally she grasps the skin of the back of the head or even the kitten's whole head. Queens are able to lift and even jump several feet carrying large kittens. In fact, the peak of kitten carrying occurs when they are three weeks old.

Communal Nests

Cats frequently move their kittens to new nests, moving four to nine times before the kittens are weaned, a phenomenon many cat owners have observed. Various hypotheses have been put forth, such as avoidance of predators or infanticidal males. In a seminatural situation, the nests are moved closer to the food source.[678] A queen may share a nest with another lactating female where the kittens are suckled

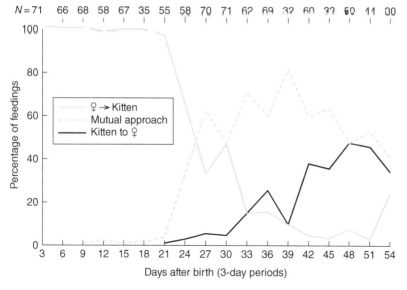

Figure 5.8 Approach of the queen to her kittens and kittens to the queen during the first eight weeks of life. *Source:* Schneirla *et al.* (1963)[2050]/American Psychological Association.

communally and where one cat can remain with the litters while the other hunts. The cats that share litters are members of the same group but might not be related. Communal nesting has advantages to the kittens; they leave the nest earlier (20 days) than do kittens in single-litter nests (30 days). Kittens in communal nests are moved to different nest sites more often than those in a one-litter nest.

Grooming

Grooming plays as important a part in feline maternal behavior as in most other species. Queens lick their kittens frequently and in particular lick the perineum to stimulate urination and defecation for the first two to three weeks of life. Female cats ingest the kittens' urine and feces for several weeks postpartum, thereby keeping the nest clean.

Acceptance of Kittens

Cats will accept alien kittens that are not too much older than their own at the time of parturition. Maternal behavior persists much longer in cats than in ungulates, so a queen whose kittens were removed at birth will accept one kitten weeks later and encircle it. Three kittens will be avoided or actually attacked under the same circumstances.[2050] In general, species that produce litters are more willing to accept foster young than are those that produce singleton or twins, probably because the mothers of litters do not discriminate between individual offspring.

Clinical Problems

Few clinical problems of maternal behavior arise in cats. In fact, the efficiency of feline reproduction is much more of a problem. Occasionally, a queen may reject her litter, but this happens less frequently than in other species.

Infanticide

Tomcats may kill kittens, an abnormality of paternal, not maternal, behavior. Infanticide by males is rare in cats; there is only one authenticated case. There is no particular reproductive advantage to the male from infanticide in feline society, where many males can mate with each female[1670] (see Chapter 4, "Sexual Behavior").

Infanticide and cannibalism by the queen, although infrequent, do occur, usually at parturition or shortly thereafter.

Mismothering

Cats sometimes care for one another's kittens or nurse communally.[1432] An interesting variation of this behavior occurred in a newly spayed cat that stole the kittens of another cat in the household. The problem was easily solved by shutting the natural mother in a room with the kittens. This case indicates that maternal behavior is independent of ovarian hormones and/or is stimulated by a dramatic decline in estrogen and progesterone levels as occurs at spaying and at parturition.

Overgrooming

Some primiparous cats trim their kittens' whiskers; others chew their claws.[622] Overgrooming to the point of removing the kitten's fur in spots can occur.

Nonnutritive Suckling

The nutritional, but not the social, development of orphan kittens will be adequate if they are artificially fed. Because cats socialize with one another almost exclusively as kittens, orphan kittens should probably be placed with the litter of another lactating queen, if possible. Sometimes, older kittens will show suckling abnormalities. They may suckle on one another, on a human skin or hair, on cloth, and on wool. The latter is particularly likely to occur in Siamese (see Chapter 8, "Ingestive Behavior: Food and Water Intake"). Occasionally, this behavior can be related to early weaning, but more commonly, no explanation is immediately obvious. The suckling is usually not injurious to the kittens' health and will gradually diminish in frequency.

Dogs

Parturition

The pregnant bitch gives little indication of her condition for the first 30 days. Late in pregnancy, her activity decreases and her appetite increases. In the last weeks, she may wish to eat small, but frequent, meals as abdominal pressure increases. She may grunt each time she sits, especially if she is carrying a large litter. The slow development of the fetuses during the first half of pregnancy allows the bitch in the natural state to hunt and forage as well as ever. She is encumbered for only the last two weeks of the 60- to 63-day gestation period. During that time, she may even urinate or defecate in the house unless she is taken out frequently.

In contrast to the more independent feline behavior, when a nest box is provided, bitches usually will use it. If nesting materials, such as strips of rags or paper, are provided, the bitch will make a nest. Like the sow, she will make digging attempts in the absence of nesting material. Restlessness, inappetence, and a drop in body temperature are the cardinal signs of impending parturition. After labor begins, the bitch usually lies in lateral recumbency. As labor progresses, her hind legs twitch and she shivers; several strong abdominal contractions are visible just before the puppy is expelled. The fetal fluids appear to be attractive to the bitch. She licks herself, any soiled bedding, and, almost incidentally, the puppy. The pup's head, umbilicus, and perineum are the areas most frequently licked. The bitch cuts the umbilical cord with her molars and then licks the stump. She may recut the cord if it is too long. If the placenta has not been delivered, she may extract it by pulling on the cord. The placenta is then nearly always eaten. She is usually silent as labor progresses, unless dystocia occurs. Adult male dogs, if present, often whine.[263]

Pups are usually born at 30-minute intervals, but delays of a few hours are not pathological. Labor can be interrupted if the bitch is disturbed; the disturbance can be as mild as the entrance of another human observer. If she is resting between deliveries, the birth interval will be lengthened; if she is in the middle of labor, it may stop. Depending upon the temperament of the dog, 15 minutes to an hour are required for normal parturition to proceed.[263]

Amniotic fluid is very important because if pups have been cleaned, the bitch will not accept them.[1] Although the bitch licks the neonatal puppy dry, she pays little more attention to it until all the puppies are born. In fact, she may step on the puppies and ignore their cries at this time. After all the puppies are born, she lies quietly and allows them to nurse. She helps to orient the puppies to her by licking.

Suckling

The puppies move forward by paddling and turn their heads from side to side, as they cannot lift their bodies from the floor yet. If they encounter a wall or any cold object, they will change their direction. After they encounter the mother's body, they nuzzle through the fur, usually attempting to burrow beneath her. High-chested breeds such as Shetland sheepdogs present much more of a challenge to the pup seeking a nipple than do flat-chested breeds such as Cocker Spaniels. When the pup locates a nipple, it does not immediately grasp it but rather noses it from beneath. Unless the pup opens its mouth at the same time as the nipple moves past, it will not succeed in grasping it. Puppies improve markedly in the first two or three days of life in their ability to locate nipples. After it locates the nipple, the pup jerks up with its head, pushes at the mammary gland with its front feet, and arranges its hind feet to support itself against the mother.[1929] All this is not proceeding in a social vacuum; the other pups are also struggling for positions. The efforts of one will dislodge the other, and whining and scrambling will ensue. The supposedly serene maternal scene is, in fact, noisy and tumultuous. Puppies do not appear to have as definitive a teat order as cats or pigs. Puppies frequently switch nipples, seldom fight over a teat, and show a mild preference for the middle teats.[2652]

Puppies have two vocal signals, the whine and the grunt. The whine is emitted whenever the puppy is cold, hungry, or separated from its litter or mother. Whining stops immediately if the puppy's head and neck are covered with a warm towel or if it is again placed with its litter. Puppies show a distinct preference for soft surfaces; they spend more time on a cloth-covered versus a wire-covered artificial mother.[1102]

Textural, as well as olfactory, cues may help puppies locate their mother and her mammary glands. The grunt is apparently a pleasure communication that occurs when sought-after warmth or reunion is obtained. Despite the puppy's loud vocal response to separation, the bitch appears to notice that a puppy is missing when she sees it rather than when she hears it.[263]

Licking

Bitches lick their puppies a great deal. Licking serves three functions in puppies; two are common to other species, and one is unique to dogs. The licking arouses the pups to eat, and, when it is directed at the anogenital area, it stimulates urination and defecation that would otherwise not occur spontaneously. The bitch keeps the nest area clean by consuming the urine and feces of her puppies for at least the first three weeks of their lives. The third function of licking is retrieval. Bitches seldom carry their puppies. Instead, they lead them back to the nest by licking the pup's head. The pup will orient toward the bitch and move toward her. The bitch will back toward the nest, continuing to lick the pup that follows until the nest is reached. Licking can be reinstated by substituting young (two- to three-day-old) puppies for older ones.[1254]

Differences in maternal behavior, especially licking, can lead to differences in stress response and fearfulness. The more an offspring is groomed, the less fearful and reactive to stress it will be. Increased grooming causes an increase in hippocampal glucoreceptor number and, therefore, greater negative feedback sensitivity of glucocorticoid secretion.[2028] Furthermore, rats groomed often by a foster dam as pups will groom their own pups more, indicating the behavior is transmitted epigenetically.[733] German Shepherd pups from litters provided more maternal dams care scored higher for social engagement, physical engagement, and aggression than those brought up by less attentive mothers, but puppies raised by more maternal dams were less successful as guide dogs.[2672,2751]

Weaning

During the first few days, the bitch spends most of her time with the pups (22 nursing bouts per day). Nursing reaches a peak at the end of the first week. The amount of time that she spends with them decreases with time (Figure 5.9). The undisturbed litter is weaned gradually by the bitch; weaning usually is complete by 60 days by the well-fed laboratory bitch but is delayed by three weeks among stray bitches in India who remain with the puppies for 13 weeks. Males, presumably the sires, remain with and actively guard the puppies for six weeks.[1757]

During early lactation, the bitch always approaches the puppies to initiate a nursing bout. By three weeks, the puppies have opened their eyes and can locomote well. They then approach the bitch and initiate most of the nursing bouts. Bitches rarely punish their puppies until the third week. Even during the weaning process, the punishment is mild enough that it may momentarily deter the pups' attempts to nurse but will not inhibit them from trying again. The punishment may consist of a growl, a snarl, or an inhibited bite. The level of aggression of the bitch toward her puppies increases and the number of nursing bouts per hour decreases after the puppies' third week.[2464] Exposure to the canine-appeasing pheromone Adaptil® resulted in bitches more likely

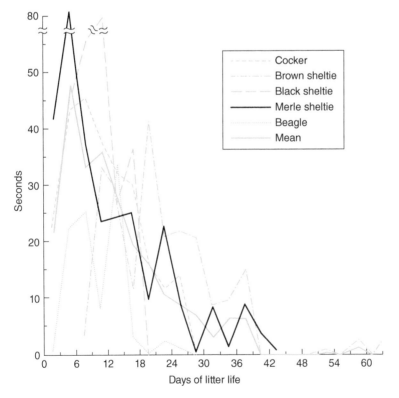

Figure 5.9   The decrease in licking of the puppies by the bitch as the puppies mature. *Source:* Rheingold (1963)[1929]/American Psychological Association.

to lie in lateral recumbency, rather than sitting when the puppies suckled.[2967]

Some bitches, and all stray Indian dogs, may regurgitate food for their pups during the weaning process at four to six weeks.[1448,1449,1475,1757] Pet dogs and feral dogs show alloparenting with nearly 50% of breeders indicate that another dog in the household regurgitated food for puppies.[2922,2933] Among feral dogs the lactating mothers were observed to nurse less by the third week and at that time, there was more alloparenting, that is, nursing and regurgitation for the pups done by other kin-related females.

This behavior, commonly seen in wild canids, helps to maintain adequate nutrition in the young during the transition from a milk diet to a raw meat diet, when their powers of mastication and digestion may not have matured enough to enable them to survive on the raw meat.[612] Wolf pups beg for regurgitated food by licking at the mouth of the adult. This behavior is occasionally seen in domestic dogs and may be the basis of face licking and licking intention movements directed toward people by adult dogs.

Clinical Problems

Pseudopregnancy

Pseudopregnancy in the intact, nonpregnant bitch during the luteal phase of the canine reproductive cycle is so common that it may be normal behavior. Bitches do vary, however, in the severity of the behavioral signs. Some dogs show only slight enlargement of the mammary glands, whereas others go through pseudoparturition at 49 days post estrus and actually lactate. The pseudopregnant bitch becomes less active, mimicking the slowing down of the truly pregnant animal. She may make a nest, usually either in her own bed or in some cave-like environment, under a table, or in a dark corner. She may adopt a toy, a leash, a shoe, or some other object to mother. She will not only place it in her nest and assume a nursing posture next to it but also often defend it. Serious problems with aggression can arise in the pseudopregnant bitch. She may be generally aggressive but, more commonly, she attacks only when her nest is invaded or her "offspring" are threatened. Mibolerone, an androgenic anabolic steroid, will relieve the signs of pseudopregnancy, but ovariohysterectomy should be recommended. The bitch that shows recurrent cycles of pseudopregnancy is prone to uterine infections, pyometra in particular. It is advisable to wait until after the behavioral signs of pseudopregnancy have passed before performing the ovariohysterectomy, as protective behavior persists if the animal is operated upon while pseudopregnant (B.L. Hart, personal communication). Pseudopregnant bitches can adopt and successfully raise foster puppies.[721] A bitch spayed during late metestrus may also exhibit lactation and maternal behavior, including maternal aggression, for a few weeks.

Maternal Rejection

Some bitches will kill and eat their puppies, and this may be associated with subnormal oxytocin levels. Because oxytocin prevents the behavior in bitches that had killed previous litters.[2830] Maternal rejection is most common in dogs that have undergone Cesarean section and have been anesthetized during the time they would normally be licking and smelling the neonatal puppies. It rarely happens if the bitch has delivered a puppy normally before surgical intervention was necessary. She may lick the puppies if amniotic fluid or even water is applied to them; this will improve chances of acceptance. The bitch may tolerate the first nursing better if some milk is expressed from the engorged glands before the pups suckle. She can be restrained while they nurse for the first time and sedated lightly if necessary. Attacking of puppies at some time after parturition is less common but does occur.

Moving Pups

A nervous bitch, especially one housed with other dogs or in an area with too much commotion, may repeatedly move her puppies.

They will not be nursed often enough. Providing a nest box in a quiet room with no other animals and minimal visitors can solve the problem.

A related problem is continued carrying of pups in circles and without much other maternal behavior. Isolation and tranquilization may be helpful.

Chickens

Laying behavior is triggered by the release of estrogen and progesterone at ovulation which occurs 24 hours before laying. Hens choose a nest site, usually an enclosed area and often build a nest if straw or other material is available by arranging the substrate in a circular pattern around their bodies Once the egg is laid the hen may incubate them. This behavior is termed "broodiness." It is stimulated by prolactin and has been selected against in egg-laying breeds. Broody hens can be quite aggressive. When after the 21 days incubation period, the chicks hatch, the hen continues to brood them by sheltering them with her wings. This behavior can be stimulated by distress (cheep) calls of the chicks. Hens give a distinctive call to attract the chicks to a food source, one to attract them to her and one to warn of danger. She leads them to safe places and indicates food by pecking the ground.[2678,2906]

An example of avian maternal behavior is that hens did not show any significant physiological or behavioral response to air puffs in their own cage. However, when they observed their chicks receiving the air puffs, there was a demonstrable response on the part of the mother hens, with physiological and behavioral changes indicating emotional distress. Their responses included increased heart rate and lower eye and comb temperatures (indicating vasoconstriction and increased body core temperature) as well as standing alert and maternal clucking.[2870]

6

Development of Behavior

Introduction

One of the most pleasant aspects of owning animals is watching the young develop. Even in a world overpopulated with cats, kittens have not lost their attraction. The gangly foal and the playful kid are also very appealing. The veterinarian or animal scientist will find that more questions are asked about normal developmental behavior, when to take a puppy home, and when to start various types of training than are asked about adult behavior. To answer these questions correctly, the clinician should be familiar with the neurological development and behavioral maturation of various species because owners spend more time observing infant than adult animals.

Dogs

Critical or Sensitive Periods

During the past 40 years, the behavioral concept of critical periods has emerged, a concept that has had a strong impact on practical dog handling. Recently, the term "sensitive period" has replaced "critical period." Nevertheless, socialization can occur in older animals, albeit with difficulty. For that reason, the adjective sensitive, rather than critical, is now used for these periods.[181] A *sensitive period* is a time in the life of an animal when a small amount of

experience (or a total lack of experience) will have a large effect on later behavior. The developmental periods for dogs are defined as the neonatal period (one to two weeks), the transitional period (third week), the period of socialization (4–14 weeks), and the juvenile period (14 weeks to sexual maturity).[755,2065,2067] The sensitive periods are not sharply defined and may vary among breeds that are fast or slow to mature. Cocker spaniel puppies appear to mature more slowly than do Basenjis, for example. Marked neurological changes appear during development.[723] See Figure 6.1 for a canine development chart.

Neonatal Period

The neonatal period, during which the puppy is deaf and blind and able to find the nipple only through tactile and olfactory cues, is described in Chapter 5, "Maternal Behavior." Most of the puppy's time is spent eating and sleeping. The sleep is characterized by a high proportion of rapid eye movement (REM) or stage IV sleep. Urination and defecation do not occur spontaneously but can be elicited by stimulation of the anogenital area; usually such stimulation is supplied by the mother's licking. Puppies locomote with their front legs, pulling their hind legs along.

During this period, several reflexes are present that will gradually disappear as the central nervous system matures. One can use the presence or absence of these reflexes to determine

Domestic Animal Behavior for Veterinarians and Animal Scientists, Seventh Edition. Katherine A. Houpt.
© 2024 John Wiley & Sons, Inc. Published 2024 by John Wiley & Sons, Inc.
Companion website: www.wiley.com/go/houpt/7e

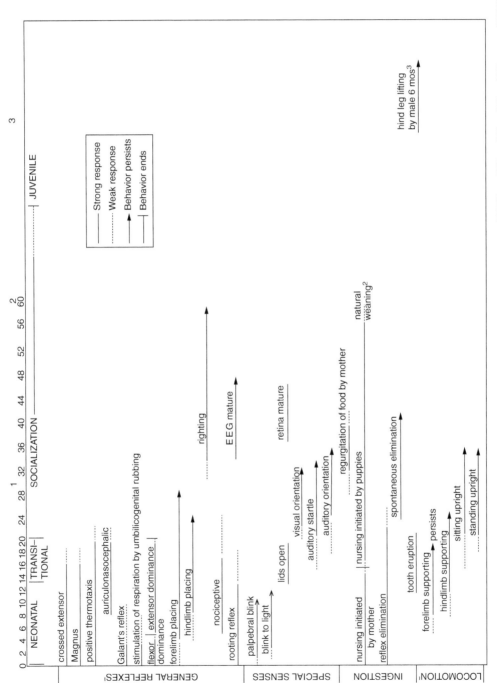

Figure 6.1 Behavioral development of the dog. Superscript numbers refer to the references: (1)[723,730], (2)[1929], (3)[236], (4)[263], (5)[2066], and (6)[726,728].

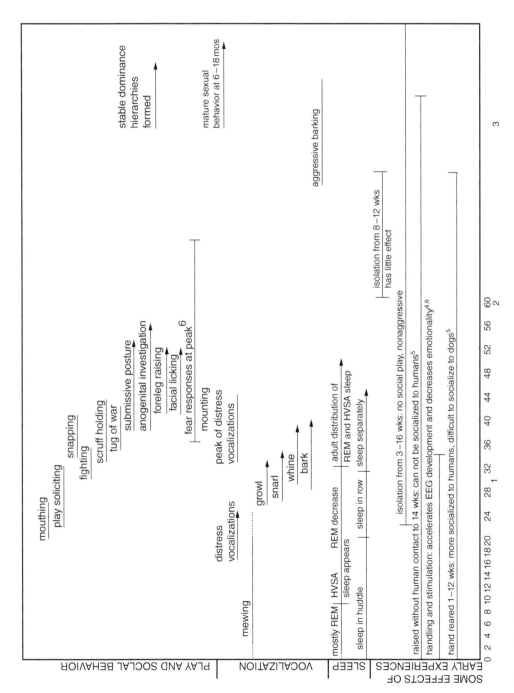

Figure 6.1 (Continued)

the age of a normal puppy and to assess development if pathology is suspected in a puppy of known age. For the first three days, puppies show flexor dominance; that is, when picked up by the scruff of the neck they will flex their legs. From three days until the fourth week of life, extensor dominance occurs; that is, the puppy will extend its legs when it is picked up. Gradually, normotonia appears.

The Magnus reflex is present for the first two weeks. The reflex is demonstrated by turning the pup's head to one side. The front legs and hind legs on the side toward which the head is turned are extended; the legs on the opposite side are flexed. The crossed extensor reflex is also demonstrable for the first two weeks. The reflex is elicited by pinching on a hind foot; that foot is withdrawn while the opposite leg is extended. The rooting reflex is best demonstrated after the puppy is a few days old. The puppy will push its face into a cupped hand and crawl forward. This is the reflex utilized by the mother to retrieve a puppy (see Chapter 5). Like the Magnus and crossed extensor reflex, the rooting reflex will wane by the fourth week.

Transitional Period

During the transitional period, the puppy begins to be bombarded by many more stimuli as his sensory organs develop. The eyes open between 10 and 16 days, although visual acuity is poor and puppies will not follow visual stimuli when the eyes first open. As vision improves, the puppy no longer swings its head from side to side as it locomotes. The ears open, and a startle response to auditory stimuli can be elicited at 14–18 days. By day 16, sound can be localized.[108] The crossed extensor reflex disappears from the front legs first, as does the Magnus reflex. Urination and defecation occur spontaneously; the bitch continues to ingest the excreta for several weeks. When kept in a kennel, the puppies will begin to leave the nest to eliminate and will use the same area as that of the bitch. If the bitch is paper trained, this is the ideal way to train a puppy, long before it can follow its mother outdoors. The puppy can

support its weight on all four legs by 12–14 days, although normal adult sitting and standing will not be seen until 28 days. Tooth eruption begins to take place during the transition period, and the pups will chew on one another, begin to play clumsily, and growl.

Socialization

The third period, socialization, is the most important from a behavioral viewpoint. During this time from the 4th to the 14th week, pups learn about their environment, about their littermates and mother, and about humans. Play begins and has its highest frequency in the socialization period. Canine play is discussed in more detail later in this chapter. Dominance hierarchies are formed. Strong avoidance behavior develops, and by eight weeks, fear reactions are seen. There are breed differences in the first appearance of the fear response. German shepherds show fear at 39 days, Yorkshire terriers at 44 and Cavalier King Charles spaniels at 55.[1632]

This period is also most important from a clinical standpoint. Puppies weaned and removed from the company of other dogs before the period of socialization will, as adults, often be difficult to handle in the presence of other dogs. They will be either frightened of other dogs or, less commonly, too aggressive. They will not be able to play with other dogs and will be difficult to breed. A dog that has not had the opportunity to interact with other dogs will be too human oriented. Male dogs may direct their sexual attentions toward humans. Unfortunately, playing with other puppies and being handled by other people ("socialization") in the puppy socialization classes will not change the dog's innate response to social stimuli such as strange dogs or people.[2079] Puppies from pet shops and those ill as puppies are more apt to have behavioral problems.[2087]

Normally, pups are not weaned before four weeks of age, but they may be weaned even earlier if the bitch has died and the puppies must be hand fed. The nutritional requirements of the orphan puppy can be met, but many of the tactile and social requirements may not be. Hand-fed puppies usually will suck more on fingers and other objects than will normal puppies, indicating that the need to suckle has not been met, despite scheduled bottle feedings.[1975] It would be best to foster a litter of orphan pups onto another lactating bitch. If this is not possible, the litter should be kept together and separated only for an hour after feeding, when suckling on one another is most apt to occur. A similar situation may arise if the bitch has lactation tetany, in which case the litter may have to be weaned quite early.

Again, the litter should be kept together at least until the puppies are six weeks old.

The importance of social contact to the puppy during this period is demonstrated by the emotional reaction to separation from the litter. Six-week-old Beagle puppies yelp 1,400 times per 10 minutes when placed in a strange pen. Older and younger dogs are less disturbed and, therefore, less vocal (see Figure 6.2).[630] Human contact is more effective than canine contact in alleviating separation distress in four- to eight-week-old puppies.[1805,1978] By seven to eight weeks, a fear posture, tail tucking, is first seen in Beagle puppies.

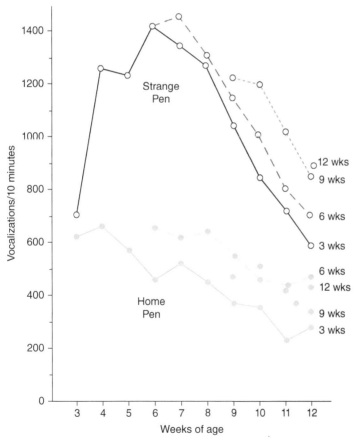

Figure 6.2 The average number of vocalizations by puppies at different ages and in two environments. Note that vocalization of a puppy alone in the home pen is consistently lower than that of one in a strange pen. Puppies whose tests were begun when they were older than three weeks showed a slightly higher rate of vocalization, but the curves are parallel.[1667] *Source:* Elliot and Scott (1961).[630] Reproduced with permission of Taylor & Francis.

Socialization to humans is equally important. A dog that has had little contact with humans until 14 weeks rarely becomes a good pet.[2065] This is, of course, typical of kennel-raised, rather than family-raised, dogs and is sometimes called "kennelitis." Such a dog is well socialized to other dogs but has had limited experience with humans. The dog, depending on his genetic background, may be overly timid or most difficult to control. Although normal dogs find contact with a human rewarding,[2170] the dog that has not been socialized with humans will not; it will, therefore, be a much more difficult animal to train.

A substantial amount of experimental evidence supports the sensitive period hypothesis. Most impressive is the effect of early isolation.[16] If puppies are completely isolated from the 3rd to the 20th week of life, they are markedly disturbed. Their learning ability is impaired.[1557,2250,2251] They are socialized to neither humans nor dogs, and their response to either species is fear. Even a week in isolation will produce changes in the canine electroencephalogram (EEG), although the changes are transient.[723]

Complete isolation is rarely, if ever, imposed on puppies except for experimental purposes, but exclusive human, dog, or cat contacts do occur. Dogs raised with cats prefer the company of cats to that of dogs and fail to recognize a mirror image.[723] Hand-raised or early-weaned (by 3.5 weeks) puppies will approach a human much more quickly than will dogs that were weaned at eight weeks with little human contact before that time. Puppies are often left in their home without human or canine contact during the working day. Puppies left alone vocalize, lip lick, yawn, and scratch, and those younger than three months were most apt to exhibit these behaviors. Over time, they will be inactive more often, and explore and play less. The signs of stress decrease over time.[385]

Not only the presence or absence of human contact but also the quality of that contact will affect the puppy's later behavior. It has been shown in many species that early handling can influence emotionality in later life; the dog is no exception. Dogs were subjected to varied stimulation (exposure to cold, vestibular stimulation on a tilting board, exposure to flashing lights, and auditory stimulation) from birth until five weeks of age. The stimulated pups differed from controls in several physiological and behavioral parameters. They showed earlier maturation of the EEG, larger adrenal glands, and lowered emotionality, which enhanced problem-solving ability in novel situations, than the non-stimulated pups. Most interesting was the finding that they were dominant over non-stimulated controls in a competitive situation.[724] Some effects of early stimulation are not permanent. Development is accelerated, but the non-stimulated animal eventually catches up. Not only social deprivation but also food deprivation during early life can affect later canine behavior. Food-restricted puppies were more attached to their handlers during the period of deprivation and later showed increased eating rates and increased intake of highly palatable food.[629] Puppy socialization classes, usually held as soon as the dogs have had at least one vaccination, are useful in that dogs learn obedience easily at that stage, but it has no effect on their later behavior toward strange dogs or people.[2079] It does indicate owner motivation, and, therefore, puppies taken to socialization classes are more likely to remain in that home. Other factors important for retention are being female, wearing a head collar as a puppy, sleeping on or near the owner's bed, and living in homes without children.[603] German shepherds that attended a puppy class were more likely to be confident and less likely to be nervous.[764]

Juvenile Period

During the juvenile period, a dog increases in size and in competency at adult activities. Although dogs can follow pointing gestures as puppies, they become better at finding objects using olfaction rather than human pointing gestures as they mature from 3 to 11 months during training for explosive detection. In fact, dogs that are poorer at following human gestures become better scent detection dogs.[3082]

Puppies begin to show adult sexual behavior at four to six months, when they begin to show greater attraction to estrous bitches than to spayed ones. This attraction increases with age until they reach two years old, at which point dogs are fully mature.[190] Dogs (retrievers) at eight months were less likely to obey a command from their trainer (but not from a stranger) than they were before or after that age. Bitches that showed more attachment to humans came into heat sooner.[2653] Although considered to be adult at puberty, most dogs do not mature socially until 18 months or later.

Conclusions

The conclusion to be drawn from the experimental studies and clinical observations of the sensitive periods of the development of dogs is that dogs should be exposed to both dogs and humans during the period of socialization. The exposure to both species should be pleasant because fear responses are also strong during this period. The effects of isolation are most pronounced in dogs that have been isolated during the period of socialization; however, isolation, or even partial isolation, in a boarding kennel for several weeks during any portion of its first year can reduce the sociability of a dog and increase its fearfulness. The importance of human socialization to canine training is exemplified by a study in which 90% of the dogs (mostly German shepherds) that were home raised from the 12th to the 52nd week of life were trainable as guide dogs for the blind. Dogs that remained in the kennel for the same period failed the training program.[1806] Properly socialized dogs will be much more willing to work for a reward as simple as verbal praise or even reunion with the human handler.

Neurological Development

There is an old adage that "One can't teach an old dog new tricks," but it is equally difficult to teach a very young one. As discussed in Chapter 7, "Learning," six-week-old puppies could not solve a barrier problem, nor could four-week-old puppies (even after 13 days of training) remember the location of hidden food for more than 10 seconds, although 12-week-old puppies could remember for 50 seconds. Puppies younger than 21 days old cannot learn to pull food into their cage with a ribbon, and five-week-old puppies took twice as long to learn a visual discrimination as 12-week-old ones.[723] Neonatal puppies, however, can learn to avoid an aversive stimulus.[2170]

The poor performance of the young puppy is not surprising in light of the stage of development of its nervous system. The brain consists of only 10% dry matter at birth. The adult percentage (19%) is not reached until the fourth week of life.[723] Myelin is almost completely absent from the newborn puppy's brain and appears gradually over the next four weeks. Conduction speed along nerves is related to the presence of myelin, and the more rapid reactions of the month-old puppy attest to the myelinization of its central nervous system. At birth, the length and width of the canine brain are nearly equal. The increase in length of the brain with age is due to an increase of the frontal and occipital areas. A great increase in the complexity of the gyri and sulci also occurs.[723]

Placing measures the ability of a dog to put its paws onto a table when held up to it, usually without visual contact. Placing reactions mature in the following order: chin placing (if the dog's chin makes contact with a surface, he will reach for it with his paws), visual placing (if the dog sees a surface, he will put his paw out), contact forelimb placing (if the dorsal surface of the paw is touched to the lower surface of the table, the dog will place the paw on the upper surface), contact hind limb placing, and tail placing (if a dog's tail makes contact with a surface, the dog will reach toward that surface with its hind legs). By six to nine weeks, all these reflexes are functional.[495]

Sleep

Sleep shows many changes in duration, type, and posture with development. The newborn puppy spends most of its time (96%) sleeping except for brief nursing bouts. Most of the sleep in the neonate is REM or stage IV sleep. Only 1% is slow-wave sleep (SWS). REM sleep is associated with dreaming in the adult human, but one wonders what the newborn puppy dreams of, given that its experience is limited to intrauterine life. Owners are often concerned about the twitching exhibited by puppies during the neonatal period, but this is normal.

Newborn pups sleep in a heap, which may serve to prevent heat loss. A puppy removed from its littermates will waken and whine until it is either returned to the litter or placed on a soft, warm surface. Holding a puppy will often calm it, probably because of the warm body contact. As puppies mature, the percentage of time spent in REM sleep drops from 85% at seven days to 7% at 35 days. Meanwhile, the percentage of time that the dog is awake has increased to 62% by day 35, and SWS occupies another 31% of the 24 hours.[728] By 3.5 weeks, puppies sleep in a row with side contact only. Later, they will sleep apart but may sleep against a wall for contact.[1929] Even adult dogs often try to maintain contact while sleeping by curling against their owner or simply lying on the owner's foot. Much of the nocturnal distress of the newly weaned or separated puppy can be alleviated by providing it with a warm "companion" such as a hot water bottle or even an old, and preferably dirty, sweater with lots of olfactory stimuli.

Play

Puppies, kittens, lambs, and even foals are attractive both because their foreshortened faces and awkward gaits inspire maternal, or at least protective, attitudes in humans[1412] and also because they play. Play remains an enigma not because we do not know how animals play, but because we do not know why they play. Play appears to be important in the development of the social organization of animals, but that does not explain solitary play. Play may be important simply as a form of exercise or perhaps as a means of practicing and perfecting

the skills necessary for the hunt, in the case of carnivores, or the escape, in the case of herbivores. None of the preceding reasons explains adult play and why it persists more in some species and in some individuals than in others. Finally, play is presumably pleasurable and may, therefore, be its own reward whatever the ultimate value to the organism may be.

Characteristics of Play Behavior

It is important to the participants, as well as the observer, that play be distinguished from serious behavior. This is particularly true of fighting behavior. By 3.5 weeks, puppies can effectively signal that "what follows is play." The signal most often used is the play bow, in which the dog lowers its forequarters and often paws at its own face while wagging its tail (refer to Figure 1.11 in Chapter 1). The play bow is an innate, not learned, display, for it occurs in hand-raised puppies.[223] In adult dogs, the play bow is used to reinitiate play.[366] The play face is distinguished by an open mouth and erect ears. Other signals are the exaggerated approach, repeated barking, approach and withdrawal, and pouncing and leaping. Dogs are aware of the direction of a play partner's attention and will use fewer visual signals such as the play bow and more attention-getting behaviors such as barking or jumping on the other dog.[1032] A submissive dog is more successful in soliciting play than is a dominant one; perhaps this is because the dominant dog usually is taken seriously by its subordinates.[222] In another demonstration of theory of mind, dogs rarely give play signals to an inattentive dog, for example, one that is facing away. Instead, they make exaggerated approaches or retreats, pawing, presenting the rear quarters to, bumping, leaping on, or even biting the inattentive dog. When that dog turns to face its tormentor, play signals ensue.[1032]

Higher ranking and/or older dogs generally showed higher proportions of attacks and pursuits and lower proportions of self-handicapping than their disadvantaged play partners. Furthermore, there is rarely role reversal of mounts or muzzle bites (dominant gestures) or muzzle licks (submissive gestures).[184] Dogs often roll over on their backs during play, but this is a defensive move to protect their necks from their partner, not a submissive signal. The rollover can also serve as a play signal.[1705]

Play in the dog, as in all species, is characterized by actions from various contexts (aggressive, sexual, etc.) incorporated into unpredictable sequences in which the actions are repeated and performed in an exaggerated manner. A typical sequence would begin with a play bow, followed by an exaggerated approach, veering off, a chase, general biting, head shaking while biting, rolling and wrestling, reciprocal chasing, more wrestling, inhibited biting, rearing, and pushing with forepaws. Typical bouts last for 5–15 minutes in puppies between the ages of three and seven weeks. There are breed differences in play in puppies. For example, Fox terrier puppies showed higher interest in racing and chasing among siblings, whereas Beagle puppies scored higher in play behavior associated with competition, such as pulling and winning objects.[1255] Adult dogs will also play; they habituate to (will no longer play with) a toy after five 30-second presentations of the same toy (independent of the toy's color or odor).[1872]

In feral puppies, play increases from three to nine weeks, then abruptly decreases.[1758] Play in puppies begins with mouthing of one another. The mouthing is concentrated on the head region of the opponent. This should not be surprising because it is the cranial nerves that are most myelinated in the suckling animal. The biter and bitten will get maximal sensory input from play that involves the puppies' heads. As the puppies' strength improves and as their teeth erupt, the mouthings become genuine nips. Four-week-old pups may nip painfully, but the violent reaction of their littermates and, in particular, their mother to painful bites soon teaches them to inhibit the force of the bites. The early-weaned or orphaned pup will not learn to inhibit its bites;

it is up to the owner to discourage the painful nips. The worst disfavor one can do a puppy is to wear heavy gloves when playing with it; the dog will not learn to play gently. Safe chew toys should be substituted for human hands.

Play Fighting

By four to five weeks, play fighting becomes more skilled as the puppies' motor and perceptual skills improve. Male puppies play more than females.[1758] Scruff holding and shaking or worrying appear. Pouncing, snapping, and growling occur in the course of play. The facial expressions of the adult dog replace the mask-like expression of the younger pup. Tug-of-war is a favorite game with littermates. Wrestling bouts occur, with the puppies alternating the standing-over and lying-on-the-back positions.

Sexual Play

Elements of sexual behavior appear at six weeks, but the frequency of sexual play never equals that of social play and – like social play – decreases in frequency from week 10.[1758] The puppies will mount, clasp, and perform pelvic thrusts without regard to the sex of the partner. Male puppies, in particular, exhibit this behavior. Dogs deprived of all play experience and social contact as puppies can mate but are often misoriented when they mount and, consequently, achieve fewer intromissions.[188] The poor sexual performance of socially isolated dogs indicates the importance of play in puppyhood to normal adult behavior.

Play is valuable not only for the development of normal behavior but also for its diagnostic use. Play occurs most often in the warm, well-fed, healthy puppy. The absence of play behavior in three- to nine-week-old puppies is an indication of pathology. Social play is the most common form in dogs, but solitary play does occur. The dog's pouncing upon and carrying a stick is an example. Tail chasing occurs in the absence of another puppy to chase. Games of fetch between owner and dog are the outgrowth of chasing play. If the game is not initiated during the period of socialization, it is very difficult to teach, especially to a dog that is not genetically a retriever.[2065]

Exploratory behavior may be classified as a thrill-seeking type of solitary play. Exploratory behavior increases with age, in contrast to social play, which decreases after 10 weeks of age. By six weeks of age, the puppy has mastered many of its social skills. It can signal play and aggression. It approaches another dog and investigates the inguinal area. It is beginning to form a dominance hierarchy. It eliminates in the same area as its mother and littermates do. It can eat food and sleep alone. In the next week or two, it should be ready to become socialized with novel humans.

Toys are important to adult dogs, who spend 24% of their active time using toys, but this can actually result in a decrease in time spent playing with other dogs.[1074] Nylon bones are used longer than rawhides, although the latter are preferred initially. Dogs prefer toys that can be chewed easily and/or make a noise.[1873]

There are dogs that prefer to play tug-of-war and those that prefer to retrieve a ball. They do not differentiate between their owners and an unfamiliar person as a play partner. Dogs that prefer tug-of-war are more reactive, but no matter which game they prefer, dogs highly motivated to play are not fearful.[184,2285]

Cats

See Figure 6.3 for a feline development chart.

Sensitive Periods

The feline sensitive period for socialization, occurring at two to seven weeks, is earlier than that of dogs.[2298] A litter of kittens isolated for the first month will be reluctant to approach people even if they are genetically friendly (see Chapter 9). Handling for 15 min/day from two to six weeks will result in friendly kittens.

Kittens were separated from their mothers at two days, six weeks, or 12 weeks, and those weaned at 12 weeks did not cry upon separation, even though they had been living on their mother's milk alone. Kittens weaned at six weeks cried for a day or two. Those weaned at two days and fed by dropper cried for one week.[2078] As adults, the early-weaned kittens showed the most random activity, such as trying to escape from a carrying cage, and were most disturbed by novel stimuli. When tested with food, they were most persistent in trying to obtain food secured under a wire cover but least successful in competing with other cats for food. The early-weaned cats were also the slowest group to learn to associate the sight of a light with food. Early-weaned (less than 12 weeks) cats are more aggressive.[3048]

In another experiment, kittens were weaned at two days of age. The kittens were fed by nipple and handled as little as possible. When tested in an unfamiliar room, the cats raised in the restricted environment explored, played, and approached less than conventionally reared cats.[1251] Kittens raised in isolation from 40 days of age spent more time close to another cat than did kittens raised communally, but all the cats spent more time with another cat as they grew older.[384]

Handling kittens each day for the first month accelerates eye opening and EEG synchronization. Such cats are more active and aggressive when confined and are quieter in a novel environment.[1549] Cats that had been handled and raised in a stimulating environment made fewer errors in a visual discrimination task.[1550] Kittens raised with their mothers and without handling were very slow to approach humans. Handling of the kittens appeared to impair their ability to learn some tasks several weeks later.[2462] Handling of the kittens also affects their personalities: more handling before eight weeks increases boldness for the first year, but thereafter the genetic component is more important, a trend seen across species.[1416]

It appears to be difficult to slow a kitten's development. Neither limitation of food nor severe hypoxic episodes affected kittens' development, although treatment with a goitrogen

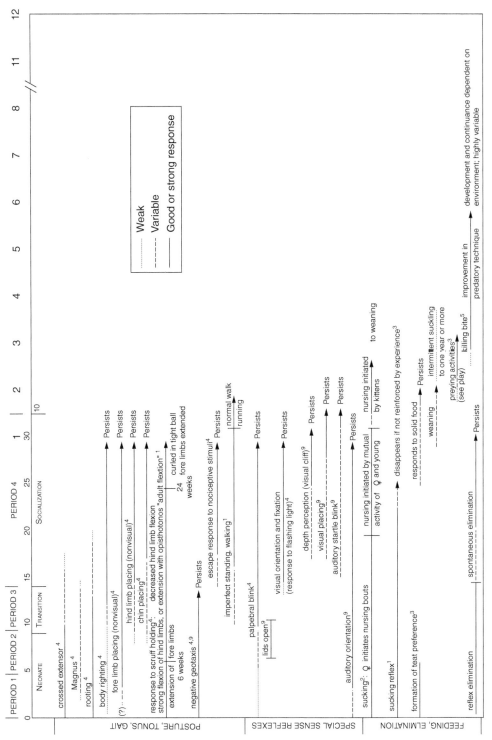

Figure 6.3 Behavioral development of the cat. Superscript numbers refer to the references: (1)[1234], (2)[1974], (3)[725], (4)[722], (5)[1361], (6)[2426], (7)[2078], (8)[441], (9)[2353], anc (1⁊)[2298].

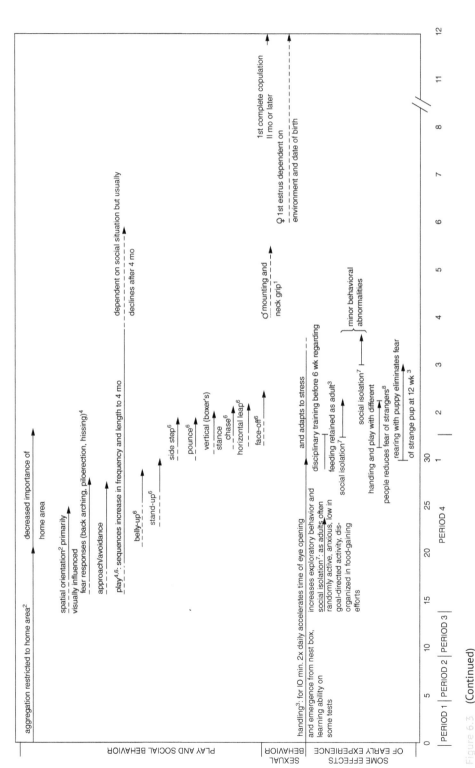

Figure 6.3 (Continued)

did delay development of solid food ingestion and locomotor skills, and resulted in slow physical development.[242]

There are breed differences in development: Norwegian Forest cats exhibit earlier thermoregulatory ability, but Orientals open their eyes sooner and are more active.[2868]

The physiological basis of the behavioral abnormalities seen in early-weaned kittens may be inferred from the changes in the function of the visual pathways observed in cats reared either in the dark or in an environment in which they had no, or very limited, visual stimuli, such as horizontal or vertical lines. Both behavioral and neurophysiological evidence demonstrated that the visual system, especially the cortical components, does not develop normally; cats exposed only to horizontal lines show little response to vertical lines.[260] Kittens raised without the opportunity to see their front paws because they were either in darkness or wearing Elizabethan collars have difficulty in visual placing. They extend their paws appropriately, but may miss a small target that normally reared kittens reach 95% of the time.[968] Kittens must learn to match paw position to target position. Similar changes occur in more complex behaviors: a cat that never had the opportunity to play as a kitten does not respond to the appropriate play signals as an adult. Kittens have adequate genetic capabilities to form the neuronal connections necessary for normal vision or social behavior, but the complex connections between cortical neurons form with visual or play experience during a critical period.

Relationships with Humans

Handling of kittens during their sensitive period of socialization from two to seven weeks is important.[1181] Handling kittens for less than 30 minutes twice a week from the time the kittens are five weeks until they are eight weeks does not increase their friendliness.[1923] More handling beginning at an earlier age does, especially if the kittens are genetically inclined to be friendly.[1502] Handling by humans may increase friendliness, but weaning before 12 weeks of age increases aggression and overgrooming in cats.[3048]

Neurological Development

The neurological development of the cat has not been studied as systematically as that of the dog. The kitten shows a dominance of flexor tone for the first two weeks of life and then a dominance of extensor tone for the second two weeks. The motor cortex involved in forelimb movement develops during those first two weeks, and cortical control of the hind limbs in the second two weeks. This is reflected in the locomotion of the kitten. It drags itself by its forelimbs at first, but later the pushing movement of the hind limbs grows stronger.[725,1930] The eyes open at seven days (range, 6–10 days), and orienting responses to auditory stimuli develop a day or two before.[717] The ear canals are fully open by four weeks. Between the third and sixth week, cats develop the ability to land on their feet (air righting).

Visual acuity improves 16-fold between 2 and 10 weeks of age. The development of the cytoarchitecture of the sensory cortex is interesting in that the cortical layers of the kitten brain are arranged in an orderly fashion with few dendrites linking the cells. The adult cat brain possesses disordered layers with many dendritic processes on the cells, which apparently pull the cells out of the original orderly alignment. It is hypothesized that the interconnecting dendrites form with increasing sensory experience.

Adult cats and dogs will respond to a silhouette of their own species as they would to a real animal. Five-week-old kittens do not even orient themselves to a cat silhouette, but six-week-old kittens do, and the frequency approaches the adult level by eight weeks. Adult cats are apparently threatened by silhouettes and will show piloerection toward a silhouette on its first presentation. Five-week-old kittens show no piloerection, and six-week-old kittens show very little, but eight-week-old kittens show the adult response to silhouettes.[1247] Their adult personality emerges at weaning. Hypothalamic stimulation does not elicit adult-like affective response with piloerection and enlarged pupils until three weeks, although sensory motor responses, such as arching and jaw movements, can be elicited at four hours.[1233]

Adult cats show a unique expression, the gape, to conspecific urine (refer to Figure 1.13). It is equivalent to the flehmen response of ungulates. This response is not seen in kittens younger than five weeks old and is essentially similar in frequency and performance to adult gaping at seven weeks.[1247] Kittens can make ultrasonic vocalizations. In general, the frequency limit and range fall with age. Deafened kittens produce vocalizations similar to those of normal kittens, indicating that learning is not important; however, their calls are louder than those of normal kittens, indicating that feedback through the auditory system normally occurs.

As kittens mature, they become more proficient at finding their way back to their home area. They also vocalize less when placed on a cold surface (30 cries per minute at one day of age as compared with 17 cries per minute at 15 days). After the eyes have opened, the kittens use visual cues to find their nest; prior to that time, they use olfaction. Very young kittens will become less active and less vocal when placed on a warm rather than cool surface, but the calming effect of thermal stimuli is lost after the first week.[756,757,1971] Isolation produces most vocalizations (four cries per minute) at three weeks of age; younger and older kittens vocalize less. Response to restraint remains high and unchanged (five cries per minute) throughout development.[937]

Sleep

Sleep in kittens also shows a developmental pattern. For the first three weeks, the EEG cannot be correlated with the other behavior defining the different sleep stages, such as eye movements and muscle quiescence. Although the percentage of time that kittens are awake remains constant, the percentage of active REM sleep decreases and that of quiet sleep increases. Muscle twitching, which is characteristic of REM sleep, also decreases with age. The kitten's sleep cycles are also much shorter than those of the adult cat. Kittens also pass directly from the awake state to REM sleep; adult cats almost always pass through SWS sleep before entering REM sleep.[1518] Not until three months of age do forebrain maturation and environmental influences mediate a mature sleep–wake cycle.[1029]

Play

Play in kittens is first seen at the beginning of the third week at the same time that the queen begins the process of weaning by repulsing the kittens' attempts to nurse (see Chapter 5). Play in cats has been thoroughly studied.[387–389,1472,2425,2426] Although severe malnutrition leads to a suppression of play, less severe restriction of the food of a lactating queen leads to more play, especially more contact play, by her kittens. This is presumably in response to milk deprivation of the kittens and may be a form of early weaning or preparing the kitten to hunt for its own food.[182] Perhaps some of the kittens whose play is too exuberant for their new owners were deprived while suckling. Certainly, this appears to be true of hand-reared kittens.

There is a play face in kittens – a half open mouth.[3060] Play in kittens begins with gentle pawing at one another. As kittens improve in coordination, biting, chasing, and rolling replace simple pawing.[2714] One kitten is usually in the belly-up position (the kitten lies on its back with all four limbs held in a semi-vertical position). Social play increases from 4 to 11 weeks, and then declines relatively rapidly (Figure 6.4). At first, three or more kittens may play together, but by eight weeks, almost all play is between pairs of kittens. A reliable sign of play is the arched back and tail, but a definite play signal has not been defined in

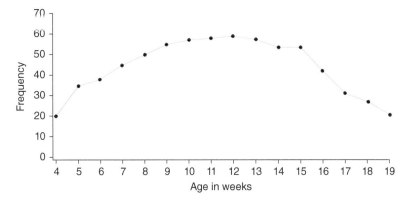

Figure 6.4 The change in playing behavior of kittens with age. Social play reaches a peak at 12 weeks and then declines. *Frequency* refers to the percentage of the daily 90-minute observation period in which play was observed.[2003] *Source:* West (1974).[2426] Reproduced with permission of Oxford University Press and Meredith West.

cats, although tail position and movement have been suggested.[2367] Differences between kittens in general activity are observable at one week, and these differences persist as the kitten develops.[2615]

Play Periods

Usually, four play periods occur per day. Almost an hour a day is spent in play at nine weeks of age. Most kitten play bouts begin with a pounce and end with a chase. In between, the kittens frequently face off, hunching forward with tails arched out and down. They may bat at one another. Kittens also assume a vertical stance in play, rearing back on their hind limbs, sometimes standing up by extending the limbs. Various leaps are also seen. Kittens are much more apt than puppies to paw rather than bite at one another. The prevalence of pouncing, stalking, and chasing in feline play may be evidence that it is practice for hunting. Play bouts may have one chase per minute. Play may occupy 9% of the kitten's total time and only 4–9% of its energy expenditure, indicating that play may be important, but it is not calorically costly.[1470]

Predatory Play

The mother plays an active role in the development of her kittens' predatory behavior. Mothers not only attack and eat prey in front of their kittens but also vocalize to attract the kittens' attention to these activities. These behaviors occur when the kittens are four to eight weeks old. After that, the mother defers to the kittens in that she rarely kills and almost never eats the prey. The kittens are more apt to interact with the prey if the mother has just been interacting with it than if a littermate has, indicating that the mother has a greater influence.[387–389] Kittens also learn other tasks better from watching their mother than from watching another cat.[413]

A very definite increase in predatory activity occurs around eight weeks. At that time, most kittens will kill and eat mice, and more of their behavior is directed toward prey than toward playing with one another. After the prey is dead and eaten, the kittens return to playing with one another, indicating that the motivation to play is still present but is overridden by the motivation to hunt. Social play and predatory play are not correlated and probably are controlled by different systems.[388] By two months of age, those kittens that will be frightened rather than aggressive toward prey and toward other cats can be identified; these same kittens are reluctant to explore and to relax with people in a new environment.[7] This is unfortunate because some people prefer that their cat does not hunt, and many wish their cats to be less aggressive toward other cats; but almost all owners want their cat to be friendly, even in a novel environment. Play can be encouraged in adult cats by a pause of five minutes after a two-minute play bout and by changing toys.[2426]

Sexual Play

Elements of sexual behavior are not seen in kitten play, but one sex difference appears in feline play. Males show more object contact than females; females with male littermates play with objects more than do females with no male littermates.[173] Play may be more important for intraspecies socialization in cats than it is in other species because the ancestral species are solitary for much of their adult lives.

Solitary play in kittens also begins to decline at four months, but the decline is much more gradual.[2426] Kittens will chase small rolling objects or even a moving string. They particularly like to bat at suspended objects, such as window shade pulls or tassels. Many of the pounces and face-offs of social play may be performed by solitary kittens with "imaginary" playmates, a mirror, or their own shadow. Solitary play persists in many adult cats. Playfulness is a factor for which breeders should select because it enhances the pleasure a cat gives to its owner as well as to itself. Social play may also occur between species. Cats will often play with dogs with which they are familiar. Interspecies play consists mostly of chases by the dog and pounces by the cat.

Several factors may contribute to the decline of play in kittens. Subadult cats begin to sleep more during the day. Older cats tend to spend more time sitting quietly but alertly. Male kittens show sexual activity by 4.5 months and attempt to mount and bite the scruff of females that will reject these attempts until they reach sexual maturity a few months later. Young feral cats may also devote more time to finding their own prey. When canine and feline plays are compared, dogs are found to chase (especially in a group), mouth, wrestle, shake, and indulge in solitary play more than cats. Cats stalk and ambush more frequently.[24]

Horse

The Foal's First Day

First Hour

The perinatal behavior of American Saddlebred, Thoroughbred, and pony foals has been described.[1979,2386] The foal can move its head and legs immediately after birth. The suckling reflex appears within the first few minutes and is elicited by anything put into the foal's mouth. Righting itself to sternal recumbency and the first attempts to stand occur within the first 15 minutes, but the foal will fail in a dozen attempts, so an hour may elapse before the foal stands. Pony foals can stand at a younger age than those of the long-legged breeds (Figure 6.5).

The foal begins to use all its senses within the first hour. It experiences tactile stimulation from its mother's licking and will begin to respond and orient to visual and auditory stimuli within the first hour. Within the first hour, it will begin to communicate by nickers to its mother and by snapping at any fearful object. The foal can walk soon after it can stand, although it will not be well coordinated for another few hours. As soon as the foal can walk, it begins to search for the udder. It may attempt to suckle from the walls of the stall or from inappropriate parts of its mother, as well as suck when no oral contact has been made (vacuum suckling). The feature that the foal innately seeks is an underline, so it will attempt to nurse from the axilla as readily as the inguinal region. Defecation also occurs within the first hour. Dysmaturity is a common problem in foals. A Brainstem Auditory Evoked Response (BAER) can be used to detect brain damage; the response will be asymmetrical in the neurologically abnormal foal.[1326]

The Rest of the First Day

Successful suckling is the major event of the foal's second hour of life. Although pony foals suckle within the second half hour of life, a further 30 minutes is necessary before

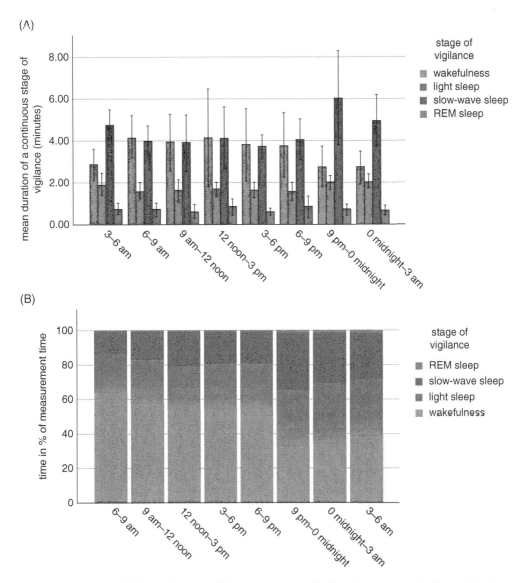

Figure 6.5 Stages of vigilance. Duration (A) and percentage (B) of the four stages of vigilance in foals (n = 10) during the three-hour periods of a one-day cycle (total measurement time 48 hours). The x-axis shows the three-hour periods of the 24-hour cycle. The y-axis shows the sequence duration in minutes (A) or the percentage (B) of each stage of vigilance and percentage (B) of the four stages of vigilance in foals (n = 10) during the three-hour periods of a one-day cycle (total measurement time 48 hours). A sequence represents a single continuous vigilance stage. The stages of vigilance are shown in different colors (green: wakefulness; orange: light sleep; red: slow-wave sleep; blue: REM sleep). *Source:* Zanker *et al.* (2011)[3100]/Springer Nature/CCBY 4.0/Public domain.

Saddlebred and Thoroughbred foals are able to suckle. By the second hour, the foal has also begun to follow its dam or any other large moving object. Lying down is another difficult task for the foal to master but is usually accomplished within the second or third hour. The foal will then sleep; a few foals will sleep standing up if they have not been able to lie down but will fall down if they go into REM sleep. By the third hour, the foal can also groom itself and gallop. Within the first day, the foal can play, urinate, flehmen, and graze as well as communicate, suckle, and locomote; in other words, it is already a well-coordinated, functional horse. See Figure 6.6 for the behavioral development of the foal.

During their first week foals spend half their time awake, 25% of their time in light sleep, 20% in SWS, and 1% in REM sleep.[3100]

The First Year

The behavior of foals is well illustrated in McDonnell and Poulin.[1508] The ontogeny of the foal has been extensively studied in Welsh ponies,[476,483,484] New Forest ponies,[2300] Camargue horses,[307] Thoroughbreds,[1289,1290,1292] and Belgians.[163] Little difference appeared in the time budgets and rate of development among these five types of horses, even though the environments varied considerably in the degree of confinement and amount of forage available. Thoroughbreds and other horse breeds are more apt to be managed intensively than ponies; therefore, differences in time budgets are more apt to reflect artificial feeding and stall restraint rather than breed differences in ontogeny. For example, Thoroughbred foals lay down more often while stalled at night than during the day on pasture, whereas foals on pasture 24 h/day distribute their lying time more evenly.[1292]

Grazing

Foals at first must spread and flex their legs in order to graze, especially if the grass is short; later, their necks lengthen in relation to their legs and they can graze more comfortably. Foals gradually increase the length of time that they spend grazing, from 4 to 16 min/h during the period from birth to four months. Thereafter, the increase is more rapid, reaching adult levels (60–70% of the time) at natural weaning (40 weeks).

The development of feeding behavior is interesting because social facilitation plays such an important part. Foals graze only when their mothers are grazing (Figure 6.7).[483] This fact illustrates the importance of providing creep feed for a foal in a location from which the foal can watch his mother eat. Drinking may not occur in foals on lush pasture. They obtain all their water needs from their dams' milk and moist grass, and although they follow their dams to water, they do not drink. In arid areas, foals do drink.[309]

Adult horses normally will avoid feces,[1721] but coprophagy is a normal ingestive behavior of foals, although its function is unknown. Both negative and positive consequences may occur: the foal may ingest ova of parasites, but it may also ingest bacteria and protozoa that inoculate its gastrointestinal tract with the proper flora. The dam's feces are consumed in preference to those of another horse.[479,480,734]

Sleep

Foals rest either standing or lying. As foals develop, they spend less time lying down and more time resting upright.[477] During their first week foals spend half their time awake, 25% of their time in light sleep, 20% in SWS, and 1% in REM sleep.[3100] They spend a great deal more time lying than adult horses. The percentage of time spent in lateral recumbency decreases with the age of the foal from 15% (first month) to 2% (after weaning).[307] Resting in sternal recumbency does not change very much throughout the foal's first six months (averaging about 15% of its day) and is still higher than adult levels in two- and three-year-olds. Standing and resting also occur in foals. The foal usually stands beside the mother, often facing in the opposite direction to take advantage of her tail to ward off flies.

Play

As the foal matures, it spends less time resting; it suckles less and grazes more. In between these activities, it plays. For the first two weeks, play is solitary. Foals gallop away from and

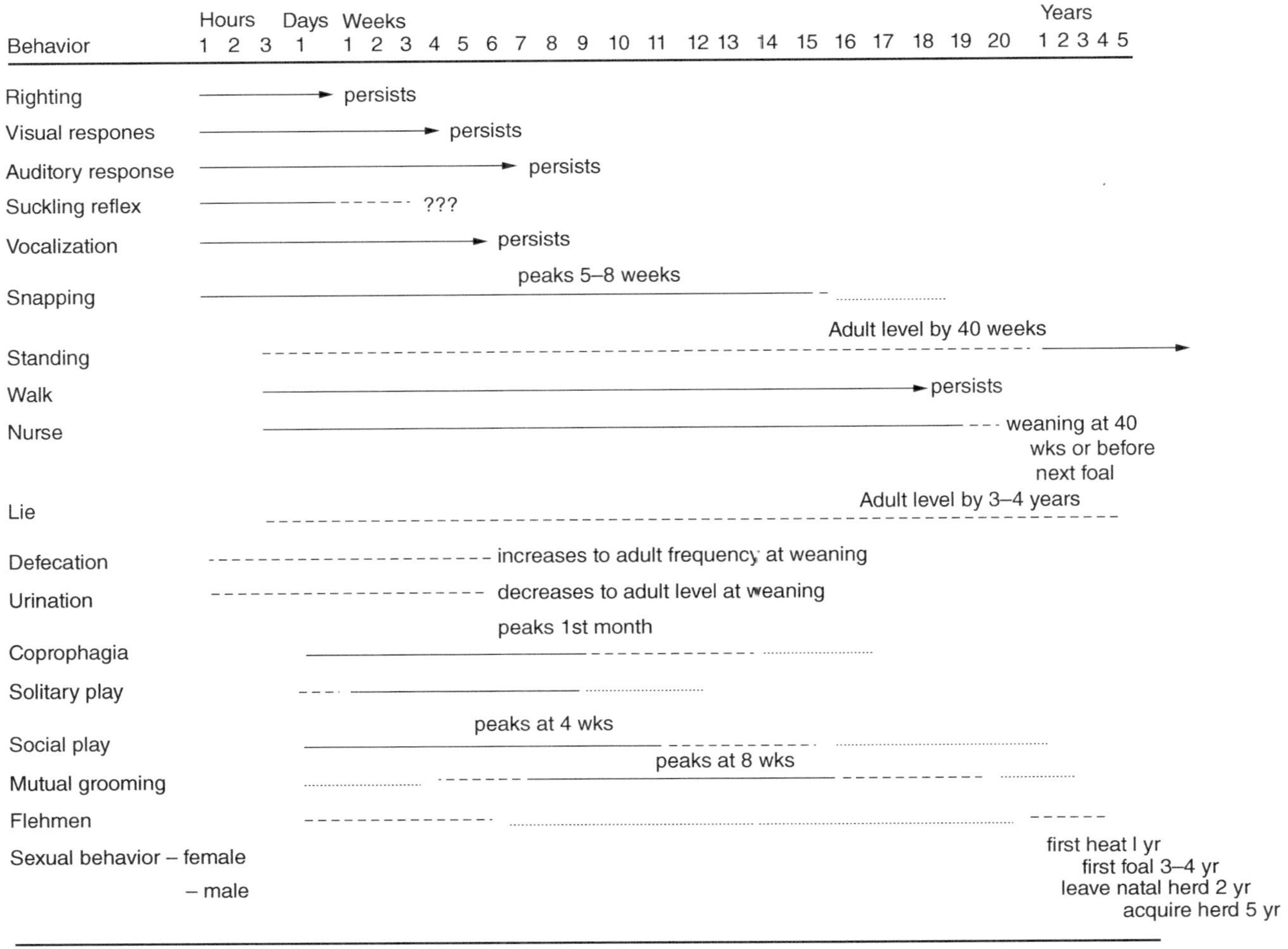

Figure 6.6 Behavioral development of the horse. References:[239,480,483,484,593,2386].

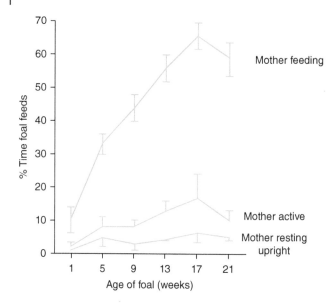

Figure 6.7 The mean percentage of time the foals spent feeding when their mother was feeding, active, or resting upright. *Source:* Crowell-Davis *et al.* (1985).[483] Reproduced with permission of American Society of Animal Science.

toward their mothers, which may be a form of exploration or even thrill-seeking behavior.[24] Play in foals is one of the best examples of play as exercise. Seventy percent of locomotion in foals is in a play context.[663] Foals at first play with their mothers by nibbling at their legs and mane. Later, this will become true allogrooming. Social play with other foals gradually increases with age, and solitary play declines; by eight weeks, solitary play is rarely seen (this,

of course, would not be true of foals that do not have companions available; see Figure 6.8). In lone foals, solitary play persists and social play may include dogs and humans.[2039] Foals may also play with inanimate objects, such as twigs, by tossing them into the air.

Although at 20 weeks of age foals still spend more than half of their time within 5 m (16.4 ft.) of their mothers, they are most apt to leave her to play.[476] Definite sex differences appear

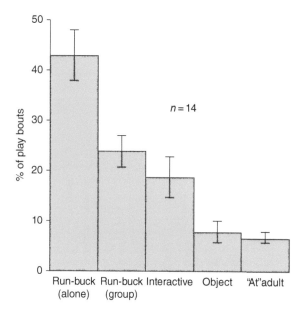

Figure 6.8 Relative frequency of various types of play. The mean percent of total play bouts by 14 foals in which the type of play was running and bucking alone, running and bucking as a group, interactive, manipulation of an object, or play at an adult. Standard error of the mean is shown as a vertical bar. *Source:* With permission Dr. Sharon Crowell-Davis.

in play: colts mount and fight; fillies chase and mutually groom one another. Play in foals often centers about the head. Nipping of the head and mane, including gripping of the crest, accounts for the greatest number of play sequences. Rearing up and mounting are frequently seen, especially in colts. Properly oriented mounting is seen even in very young colts. Chases are a common play sequence.[2051] Side-by-side nipping can progress to circle fighting in which each foal attempts to bite the tail and legs of another. When colts do mutually groom, they tend to groom fillies rather than other colts.[482] Grooming the mare is part of the courtship behavior of the stallion. These sex differences in play may prepare the animals for their adult roles. Adult horses, especially geldings, play, but the horses that play most are more likely to be aggressive to people and to appear depressed in their stalls.[773] Play in adult horses may be a reaction to confinement in their environment; free-ranging horse almost never are observed to play.[2664]

Aging

The response to short separation (15 minutes) from the dam was studied in Azteca horse (a breed created by crossing Quarter Horses with Criollos and Andalusian horses in the 1970s) at the first postnatal week and repeated until the foals were six months old. The individual's number of vocalization and locomotion as well as changes in heart rate variability during separation were consistent across ages of the foals, indicating that attachment is a trait that manifests early and can be used as an indicator of adult behavior. When the same horses were separated from their companions after weaning, the behavioral changes were still consistent, but the physiological changes were not.[2867] Similarly, horses that neigh frequently when separated from conspecifics at eight months will show the same reaction at three years, indicating a stable reaction.[3080] Foals reactivity to novelty is also stable over development.[3080]

When comparing horses aged 5–20, younger horses showed a higher frequency of avoidance as well as greater exploratory activity, while the older subjects were less behaviorally responsive and lower heart rate variability.[2657]

Figure 6.8 illustrates the types of play seen in pony foals on pasture. Play in horses reflects their dam's investment: colts of feral mares in good body condition play more and are larger at one year than colts of mothers in poor condition. In contrast, fillies of mares in poor condition play more. In either case, the mother of the foal that plays more loses more body condition, reflecting her investment in the foal.[375] This may be an example of the sociobiological hypothesis that the mother should invest more in a son when she has plenty of resources because he can sire many offspring, but should invest more in a daughter when resources are scarce because a daughter is likely to foal at least once if she survives for a year; whereas a stunted colt may never sire a foal because he cannot win mares from stronger stallions.

Foals have a dominance hierarchy that is related to their age and their dams' rank. The effect of birth order disappears postweaning when foals are all about the same size. Colts receive more aggression than do fillies. Fillies are more likely to kick; colts, to bite.[72,2404] Foals are most likely to have as a preferred associate the foal of their dam's preferred associate.

Flehmen and Snapping

Flehmen behavior is also much more frequent in colts than in fillies. It is probably investigatory behavior. Flehmen peaks during the colt's first month, possibly because his dam will be in estrus then and/or because he is still somewhat precocially masculinized owing to his prenatal hormonal environment (Figure 6.9).[481]

The facial expression of snapping (also known as "tooth clapping" or "champing") occurs almost exclusively in foals and subadult horses (Figure 6.10). This expression persists in zebra and donkeys as yawing, the mouth movements associated with estrus. In fact, the facial

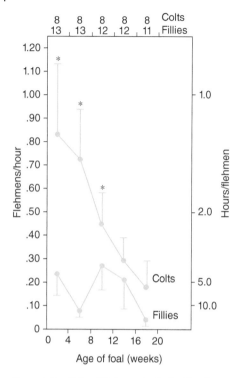

expression of snapping and that of yawing occur in the same circumstances, that is, an approach–avoidance situation. A colt is most apt to snap when approaching a stallion to whom he is apparently attracted, but who is also frightening. Estrous donkey and zebra mares and, rarely, a submissive, estrous mare[2493] may be attracted to the stallion but may also be frightened and exhibit snapping behavior. Snapping in foals is likely to occur when a stallion is courting the mare. The rate of snapping falls rapidly with age from one every three hours during the first month to one every 20 hours during the sixth month. The peak of snapping is during the foal's second month of life.[484]

The Juvenile Period

Play and activity in general decrease with age; two-and three-year-olds are more active than adults. The age at which colts leave depends on whether there are colts of the same age in the band; if so, the colts stay longer. Ninety-seven percent of colts and 81% of fillies leave their natal band.[2009] Fillies leave their herd and tend to join bands with familiar females but

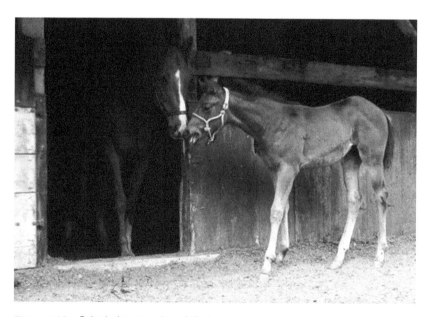

Figure 6.10 Submissive snapping of the immature horse. Foal approaches its dam while snapping. *Source:* Wolski *et al.* (1980).[2484] Reproduced with permission of Elsevier.

unfamiliar (i.e., unrelated) males.[1617] The first male offspring of a mare may leave and return several times, indicating a particularly strong bond.[1209] Colts also are influenced to leave by scarcity of food as well as by the birth of siblings. Bachelor males spend much time playing, half of which is play fighting.[419] Those colts that remain in their natal herd do not have this experience and appear to be slower to mature. The peak of colt play occurs at three years. At five years, he will begin to show adult male behaviors such as marking of urine and feces, true aggression toward other stallions, and driving of mares.[1020]

Donkeys

Jennys form what appear to be permanent bonds with their offspring, often mutually grooming.[2752,2958]

Pigs

Pigs are intermediate in their development at birth. They can walk, albeit unsteadily, within a few minutes of birth; they can see and hear. Their brain development is not complete at birth, however, and some homeostatic mechanisms, such as temperature regulation, are not yet mature.

The neurological development of the pig has not been extensively studied despite the considerable clinical application such a study would have. Piglet mortality is very high, approaching 20%. Some of this mortality is due to infectious disease, but a considerable number of deaths are "accidental." The piglets may wander out of their pen and drown in a gutter or simply become chilled and die from exposure, or they may wander in with older pigs that maul them to death. Other piglets are crushed by the sow, even though she is in a farrowing crate. Normal piglets do not wander; they stay close to their littermates, the heat source, and the sow's udder. Piglets, especially

those among the last delivered, may suffer various degrees of brain damage as a result of hypoxia during birth. If these brain-damaged pigs could be identified and hand reared or otherwise given extra protection, piglet mortality would fall.

Piglets coordinate their behavior with the sow, resting when she does and moving around when she is standing. They spend most time lying (75%), about 10% suckling, and another 10% nosing.[2318]

Piglets have some unique physiological problems that affect their behavior. Piglets are born almost hairless and with little subcutaneous fat for insulation. Their small size, lack of insulation, and low energy reserves leave piglets very vulnerable to hypothermia.[1640] Piglets solve the problem of heat conservation behaviorally rather than metabolically. They huddle with their littermates, thus decreasing their surface area and, in effect, making one large animal from 12 small ones. If a heat source is provided, they lie next to it. Unless the environmental temperature is over 26 °C (79 °F), a heat lamp should be provided.[2262] Piglets prefer a higher temperature, including 42 °C.[2337] A quick inspection of the farrowing house can enable one to determine whether the temperature conditions are correct: if piglets are sprawled on the floor in extension, they are warm enough; if they are crouched on their sterna with their legs drawn under them, they are too cold.

Sleep

As with most newborns, piglets tend only to eat and sleep. Piglets sleep for 16 minutes of every hour. The number of REM bouts decreases with age, but each bout remains of similar length.[1283]

Teat Order

Nursing behavior has been described in Chapter 5. The teat order is formed on the first day. The peak of aggression occurs one hour after birth. On day 2, there is only one fight per nursing and even fewer of the screaming fights. There are more fights pre- than post-milk ejection, but sows would change posture, thus endangering the piglets, when there was screaming post-milk ejection.[312]

By day 6, only 10% of the piglets change teats.[983] To reduce injuries to the sow's udder or to the piglets that may occur during the formation of the teat order, it is common to clip or grind the incisors and canines of day-old pigs.[748]

Feeding

Piglets rest for most of the day during the first week but are active most of the time by their eighth week. Piglets begin to eat creep feed around day 12; their intake is less than 5 g/day, but within a week they are eating 10 times as much.[1754] Intake can be increased by providing more feeders so that advantage can be taken of social facilitation.[70] The time spent eating the creep feed was greater when the feed was available on flat trays rather than troughs.[2394] Piglets that start consuming solid food earlier will consume more.[71,272] Piglets that had access to the most productive teats gained less weight when first weaned, probably because they had not learned to eat solid food as soon as their hungrier littermates.[44] Piglets are more apt to eat solid food if the food is sweet, because suckling piglets possess a well-developed sweet taste preference.[1050]

Piglets will begin drinking from a bowl at 15 days of age and drink mostly right after suckling.[535] Pigs weaned at 27 days did not eat for almost 20 hours, although they spent more time drinking than they did on the second day.[612] When pigs are weaned and housed with other pigs, there is considerable fighting. One method of alleviating that problem is to mix the litters before weaning. This also results in fighting, but may not be as serious when not combined with the stress of separation from the sow.[1769] In a semi-naturalistic environment, piglets begin to graze by four weeks, and

the percentage of time spent in this activity rises from 7 to 42% by eight weeks.[1802]

Play

In a Seminatural Environment

When sows leave the maternal nest and rejoin the herd, the piglets are gradually integrated into the social life of the older animals.[1801]

In a Confined Environment

Piglets begin to explore their environment by rooting, biting, and chewing within the first days postpartum. They also play alone, jumping and running. Play with the sow – nudging, climbing, and biting as well as naso-naso contact – begins in the first two days of life. Social play with littermates begins at three to five days.[255] Male piglets play more frequently than females, and play occurs more frequently between same-sex pairs than mixed-sex pairs. Play can be object play, locomotor play (scamper, running, head tossing, pivot, hopping, and flopping to the floor), or social (nudging, pushing, mounting, and fighting).[346] These fights are usually head-to-head confrontations in which each piglet chews and roots at the other's shoulders and neck. Piglets engaged in play fighting when the danger of being harmed was lowest and their chance of winning was highest.[3059] Increased play-fighting experience was linked to contest success in female pigs while the opposite pattern was found in males.[3026]

In older piglets (three to four weeks old), chases and gamboling can be observed. Pigs increase play after weaning at 28 days – especially non-harmful fighting.[3053] At about the same age, the typical porcine startle reaction (a woof and freezing behavior) can first be elicited. The amount of play is positively correlated with birth weight and rate of weight gain. Failure to play is of diagnostic value in determining the seriousness of neonatal pig disease. Pigs may be weaned as a litter or mixed with pigs from other litters. There is more mounting between pigs in the mixed groups as compared to littermate groups.[2685]

Exploratory behavior is very pronounced in piglets and consists of rooting and mouthing anything that is new in the environment. Pigs in an environment enriched with straw, logs, and branches spend less time manipulating the sow's udder and later spend less time nudging or tail biting.[1803] In the absence of manipulable objects, piglets chew the floor and walls of their pens and one another; therefore, toys should be provided. Pigs prefer hourglass-shaped rubber dog toys to chains, ropes, or rubber hoses.[68] They prefer shredded paper to rope as toys.[1356] Hanging toys are preferred to the same toys on the floor of the pen.

Straw bedding seems to be the most effective enrichment in that pen-mates are not manipulated. The piglets will spend 18% of their time in straw-directed behavior. Piglets will choose to investigate a novel object, and other forms of play, such as scampering, increase in the presence of novel objects.[2492] The novelty of an object wanes with exposure after two days.[821]

Elimination

Pigs begin to eliminate only at the edges of their pens as they mature.[2431] In pet minipigs, this behavior can be used to facilitate housebreaking. Defecation is more frequently performed in brightly lit areas,[2235] so a darker rest area might encourage elimination away from the bedded area.

Relationships with Humans

An investigation into the effect of early handling revealed that piglets handled daily were not larger than non-handled littermates but were more aggressive when penned with strange pigs.[2052] The effects of human handling depend on the quality of the handling and can have economic importance. For example, pigs treated pleasantly (stroked) grew more rapidly and had better feed conversion than those treated unpleasantly (pigs were shocked if they approached the handler).[989] Handling of pigs from zero to three weeks or from 9 to 12 weeks

reduces their fear of humans.[982,991] Gently handled pigs not only were less afraid of humans than harshly handled ones, but also came into estrus sooner. More intensive handling by an individual resulted in pigs spending more time with humans, avoiding them less, and being easier to catch.[2230] Unfortunately, few farmers would be able to spend 10 minutes a day with each pig. Boars handled 10 min/day for the first 14 days gained less weight in the following seven months and had a greater adrenocorticotropic hormone (ACTH) response at slaughter. In contrast to handled rats, handled pigs did not have an increase in hippocampal glucocorticoid receptors.[2401]

Ruminants

Very few behavioral studies of development in ruminants have been done. Despite the detailed knowledge we possess about growth rates in these food-producing animals, next to nothing is known about the daily activity of young ruminants or how their relationship to their environment and their peers changes with maturity. The change in suckling patterns with age is discussed in Chapter 5. Some general statements can be made. Young ruminants are born in an advanced state of development; they are true precocial animals. They can stand and walk within a few hours of birth and can apparently see and hear.

Lambs

By 30 days of age, young lambs will spend 60% of their time with other lambs, but for the first few weeks they stay quite close to their dams. This behavior is to be contrasted with the behavior of the kid, who is much more apt to stray. The lamb may depend on its proximity to its mother for protection, whereas the kid uses its own behavioral pattern, that of freezing, to protect itself. Handling by humans seems to affect artificially raised lambs more than ewe-raised lambs in that the artificially raised lambs investigate more.

Play

By a month of age, play is well developed in lambs.[1625] Play begins with investigation of one another when the lambs are only a few days old. Play consists of intentional butting; vertical leaps; rearing up on the hindquarters, which may be a play signal; and twisting the forequarters and kicking. Play may be centered around rocks or mounds so that one lamb can butt others from above. The lambs push one another, lay their heads on one another, and mount each other. Male lambs mount much more than females and are the only ones to "nudge," raising a foreleg under the belly of another lamb while standing close behind it. The sex differences in lamb play are mediated by prenatal testosterone.[1734] Male lamb behavior is less synchronized with that of their dams than female lamb behavior, and, therefore, the males are at greater risk of predation.[1480]

Lambs form groups by a few weeks of age and rest, graze, and play together. Disportive or solitary play also occurs in which lambs gallop and leap. Adults may join the lambs in play. Lambs are especially playful in the evening. By four months of age, play begins to wane.[863]

Feeding

Lambs tend to prefer foods their dams eat, rather than avoiding what she rejected.[1603] Lambs will eat less of a shrub avoided by their dams,[1602] but this may not apply to more palatable foods.[2253] They will eat low-quality roughage diets if their dams have done so.[553]

Grazing times of lambs that had had a week of experience with pasture prior to weaning were twice as long as those of naïve lambs. Exposure to a novel flavor (onion and garlic) from a month of age for three months resulted in only a temporary preference for those flavors.[1703]

Social Relationships

The social relationships of sheep are formed in the first few weeks and appear to persist for life in the undisturbed flock, but this may vary with breed and environment. Twin lambs are less upset if their twin is visible, indicating that they use vision and olfaction to identify each other.[1844] Whether a yearling ewe associates with her mother may depend on environmental factors such as high population density. The yearling that remains with its dam may gain more weight, and the ewe will incur no costs. The ewe is followed by her lamb, and the lamb is submissive to her. Even as adults, daughters will follow the mother, and their lambs will be close at the heels of their respective dams.[2060,2064]

Sexual Behavior

Sexual behavior develops gradually in ram lambs. Despite the sexual elements of play, six-month-old lambs rarely even investigate a ewe in estrus. At 10 months, they investigate ewes in estrus, and at 13 months will mount; but only at 17 months is the complete mating sequence, including copulation, seen in all rams.[2469]

Sleep and Activity Patterns

Sleep can occupy up to 40% of the lamb's day, but only 15% of the adult's.[1996] Grooming behavior, scratching with the hooves or teeth, occupies as much as 9% of the lamb's time, but far less of the adult's.[864]

Relationships with Humans

Restraining lambs in a head gate (stanchion) and handling them did not increase their tendency to approach people; allowing the lambs to approach on their own did.[1478,1843] Lambs that had been bottle fed for their first three weeks, after three weeks with no visual contact with humans, could recognize the shepherd who fed them at six weeks of age but not later at 14 weeks.[281] Apparently, it is the tactile contact with humans that is important because lambs held separately from feeding were as likely to approach the handler as bottle-fed lambs, although bottle-fed lambs interacted more than lambs that were only held.[2225]

Kids

The activity patterns of goat kids change as they develop. Lying decreases markedly around four weeks from 60 to 70% of the time to 30% for the next few months.[1367] Ruminating begins at about four weeks as they begin to graze. It is apparent that the change to a herbivorous ruminant accounts for the biggest change in behavior during development. Presumably, this is true of all ruminants and contrasts with the more gradual changes that can be seen in the foal. Standing increases somewhat at the time that lying decreases. By 15 weeks, grazing is the predominant activity, and behavior of the kid is synchronous with that of its mother.

Play

Kids appear to be much livelier than lambs. Even in the confined environment of a pen, they will play a game that can only be described as "king of the mountain," as each kid leaps onto the highest available horizontal surface, which may be an overturned bucket or even another animal. Other types of play consist of short bursts of running (less than 15 seconds), leaping into the air, kicking, butting and mounting (more in males than females), mouthing objects, and standing on the hind legs with the forelegs against a vertical object. Play occurs mostly at dawn and dusk in one-hour periods separated by a period of rest. Restraint in a pen or other forms of play deprivation are followed by a rebound of play in which play may last for three hours.[412]

Vocalizations

The call of the kid changes during development. The fundamental frequency falls from 600 kHz on the first day to 250–350 kHz on the fifth day. By four weeks, sex differences appear, with the male voice being three octaves below the female voice. Call lengths vary. The orienting call is 1 second in duration, and the distress call is 1.5 seconds.[1341] Kids living in the same group develop more similar vocalizations than kids living in different groups.[330] This probably functions to enhance group cohesiveness because herd mates can be identified by voice at a distance. Full sibs have more similar calls than half sibs, indicating a genetic component, but half sibs growing up in the same group have more similar calls than those raised in different groups, indicating a learned component.[332]

Social Relationships

The pattern of older animals being dominant over younger ones is true of a stable herd of goats, but not if strange adult animals are mixed.[2188] The dominance that an adult nanny shows over an alien kid is apparently never challenged by the kid, even when it is itself adult.

Calves

The development of calves has not been studied in great detail. In particular, beef calves have not been studied, so most of the descriptions of play and ontogeny are based on Brahma or Masai cattle (*Bos indicus*) or on the primitive Maremma cattle (*Bos primigenius taurus*).

Calves, as with other ruminants, must change in a few weeks from simple-stomached milk-drinking animals to grazing ruminants. Rumination increases to occupy 7 h/day by seven weeks of age in calves kept on pasture. Sleep time declines to 4 h/day. Calves tend to sleep in groups or "kindergartens." This attraction of calves for one another results in the calves spending more than half of their time or more away from the mother. The mothers leave their usual sleeping areas to rest near their calves.[1919] When calves that had been suckling were separated from their mothers, they spent more time with other calves. This effect is due to social rather than nutritional needs; if the dams remained, but nursing was prevented by cloth placed around the udder, the calves did not shift their social contact to their peers but instead maintained close contact with their mothers.[2343]

Feeding

Most female dairy calves are weaned at birth, given colostrum, and raised in single-calf hutches with milk replacer as their diet. Calves are normally fed 10% of their body weight per day, but would consume twice as much and gain four times more weight. The restricted calves stand more, engage in more nonnutritive suckling, and make more unrewarded visits to the feeder.[523] Group housing of calves allows more normal social interactions, but problems can arise when calves less than two weeks old cannot compete for access to an automated milk dispenser.

Play

Calves play most in the morning and at feeding times, and are active about 20–30% of the time, but only a fraction of that time is spent in play.[1137] Calves, as well as older cows, have a special play vocalization, the "baa-ock."[347] Calves play in a variety of ways, often trotting or galloping with the tail elevated. They often buck, kicking up and to the side with both hind legs, but these kicks are not aimed at anything in particular. Directed kicking, which is playful rather than aggressive, may be aimed at a stationary or moving target. Calves also play by making noise with inanimate objects, such as buckets or latches. They may be increasing their auditory stimulation level, just as children increase their vestibular stimulation level on slides, swings, and merry-go-rounds.[24] At seven weeks, about 3 min/day is spent in play.[1986] This type of play, solitary play, is more commonly seen in young calves. Social play, especially frontal butting and mounting, predominates in the older calf. Play tends to occur during grazing bouts.[2368] Calves head butt with each other or with inanimate objects. This is the same action used by adult cows in dominance interactions. They may prance, paw the ground, or gore as adult bulls do, and even threaten human attendants. Soft snorting noises may accompany play. Mounting behavior is also seen in calves. Mounting and pushing play decrease with age, whereas butting increases.

There are sex differences in bovine play. Male calves play more than females, the same pattern that is seen in most animal play. Exploration peaks later than play; yearlings are more apt to investigate a novel object than older or younger cattle.[1651] Males mount, push, and exhibit the flehmen response more than females, but butting and social licking are seen equally in both sexes. Mounting and pushing by bull calves are usually directed toward other males, but the flehmen response is directed toward females.[1920]

As in other species, play can be used as a diagnostic criterion, for calves play more when well fed and healthy than when malnourished or ill. They also play more often in fine weather than in foul. Play is stimulated in calves by any change in the environment. They play most when let loose from confinement, after gaining access to new terrain, or even when new bedding is placed in their stalls. A new pen-mate, the arrival of a human attendant, or even the stimulation of scratching their backs may set off a play bout in calves.

Activity Patterns

Weaned calves raised in individual pens spend their time in the following manner: standing, 40%; ruminating, 28%; feeding, 22%; grooming, 5%; and drinking, 2%. When calves fed from a teat were compared to those fed from a bucket and those suckling from their dam, the artificially fed calves had more sleep bouts and more fragmented sleep than dam-fed ones. The calves spent 70% of the day and 80% of the night resting, and they lay in lateral recumbency more often at night.[905] Such calves quickly learn to anticipate feeding times and become restless at those times.

Many calves are able to make contact despite being penned separately, by making tongue contact through the opening where they are fed.[1223] Calves raised in single pens are most likely to associate with the calves that had been in adjacent pens when they are released in pasture. The singly raised calves rarely associate with group-raised calves. There is no difference in weight gain between the groups.[340] Dominance hierarchies are not stable even though artificially fed calves may compete fiercely for access to their feed.[383] Calves raised in isolation for the first 10 weeks of their lives had higher cortisol values when stressed as yearlings than did calves raised with the opportunity to interact with other calves,[467] indicating the long-term effects of stress during development.

Social and Sexual Behavior

Bulls mount females by nine months of age but do not usually achieve ejaculation until they are a year or older. Aggressive behavior increases markedly among bulls from 9 to 18 months, but stable hierarchies have not formed by two years.[1851]

Free-ranging cattle remain in the same general vicinity (less than 1 km) that they experienced as sucklings, although drought can cause them to travel elsewhere.[1072]

Relationships with Humans

Handling influences cattle more if the breed has not already been selected for docility.[280] Handling in the first 10 days, or for 10 days when the calves are six weeks old, or just before or after weaning at eight months, all seem to eliminate aggressive behavior. Handling six weeks after birth and again after weaning appears to be most effective.[279] Calves raised artificially are friendlier to humans if they were handled (fed milk and stroked) on the first four days of life than if they were handled later (days 5–14) or not handled.[1270] Ninety seconds a day of stroking was enough to cause calves to be easier to load and to have a smaller increase in heart rate, but not all studies have found an effect of handling.[1123,1124] Calves are easier to handle when they are out of visual and auditory contact with other calves.[860] Calves raised in isolation are more friendly to humans and

learn more quickly; they are not handicapped in achieving dominance but may initially be fearful of other calves.[1138,1876] Calves change with age in their latency to interact with a startling object. They become less willing to approach a novel object.[1312] The older calves are slower to learn which teat to suckle from in an array of two blind and one open nipples.

Chickens

As birds age they show less avoidance of novel objects and Tetras, though not ISA Browns, showed progressively shorter tonic immobility.[2791] Play in chickens consists of sparring (play fighting), worm running (rapidly carrying food or even a nonfood item away from the other birds), and frolicking (running with raised or flapping wings). As birds age they show less avoidance of novel objects. Sparring replaces frolicking by 25 days of age, peaks at 32 days and then decreases as true fighting appears.[3072] Play behavior is reduced by environmental enrichment in fast-growing broiler chickens.[3083] Play then is replaced by aggression which peaks at 10 weeks when sexual behavior interactions begin to occur.[3093] Chicks increase the time they spend preening and at the same time down is replaced by juvenile feathers. They spend less time resting and more time foraging (pecking and scratching) between 0 and 31 weeks of age, and were less afraid of novel objects. Tonic immobility lasted for a shorter period, which also indicated that the chickens were less frightened as they aged. Chickens at 12 weeks spent a large proportion of time standing idle whereas this time was filled by foraging behavior after the onset of lay. They increase the time they spend preening and at the same time down is replaced by juvenile feathers. The social organization is stable by 7 weeks in males and 3 weeks later in females (Figure 6.11).[2770]

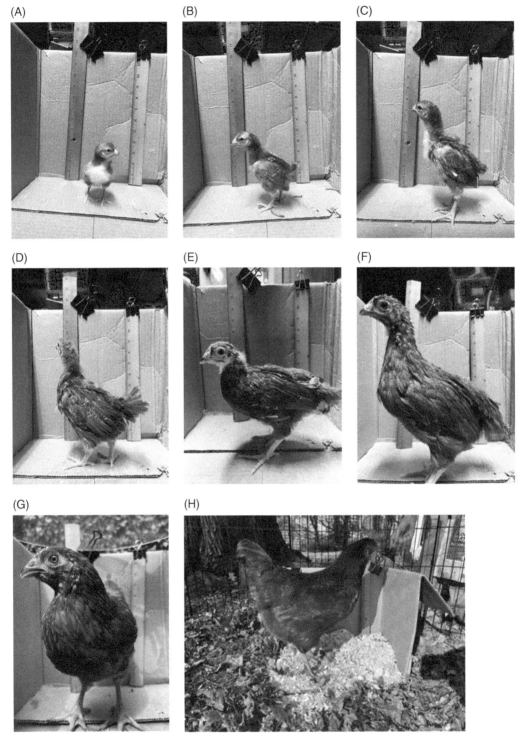

Figure 6.11 Ontogeny of a Rhode Island Red chicken.
A) 4 days
B) 11 days
C) 18 days
D) 24 days
E) 32 days
F) 39 days
G) 46 days
H) 234 (adult).

7

Learning

Introduction

Types of Learning

Learning in animals can be classified into various types. Horses are used for most examples.

Habituation

Habituation, considered the simplest type of learning, is the long-term, stimulus-specific waning of a response, or learning not to respond to stimuli that tend to be without significance in the life of the animal.[1872] Horses habituate to the feel of a halter on their heads just as we habituate to the feel of glasses on ours. We make use of habituation when we try to desensitize horses to the sound of crowds at a horse show. Another example of habituation is a horse's response to traffic on a road beside its pasture. When first put in the field, he will react to traffic on the nearby road; later, he will not. Other examples of habituation are found in pigs that soon ignore a sparkler over their feed trough,[518] sheep that become more willing to approach humans within and across tests[641] and dogs that are not repelled after a few exposures to a dog olfactory repellent. Dogs habituate to toys rapidly. Apparently, dogs habituate to visual and olfactory signals equally, so an identical but untouched toy will disinhibit as much as a different toy.[1872]

Shying by horses from objects, often innocuous objects, is a common cause of rider injury. Horses can habituate to novel objects after exposure to several simultaneously. Habituating horses to potentially scary objects is valuable, and horses so trained generalize to other novel objects, making the horses less likely to shy.[422]

Classical Conditioning

Classical conditioning or signal learning was first demonstrated in dogs by Pavlov. An unconditioned stimulus (UCS), such as the sight of meat, which produces a response (R) by the animal, such as salivation, is paired with a conditioned stimulus (CS), for example the sound of a bell. The stimuli are paired repeatedly until the CS alone elicits the R; the dog salivates when the bell is rung. Because horses do not salivate at the sight of food (the food must be in their mouths before salivation is stimulated), it is interesting to speculate on what might have happened to the field of psychology if Pavlov had used horses rather than dogs.

Perhaps the best illustration of classical conditioning is the release of oxytocin in response to the jangling of milking equipment; oxytocin causes contraction of the myoepithelial cells of the mammary gland, or milk "letdown." Cows normally release oxytocin in response to

Domestic Animal Behavior for Veterinarians and Animal Scientists, Seventh Edition. Katherine A. Houpt.
© 2024 John Wiley & Sons, Inc. Published 2024 by John Wiley & Sons, Inc.
Companion website: www.wiley.com/go/houpt/7e

suckling on their teats by the calf or squeezing of the teats by the negative pressure of the milking machine or the hands of the milker. When a cow has been milked in the same environment a number of times, the sounds of the approaching machinery and milk cans will have been paired with the milking process, and those noises alone will elicit oxytocin release.[637] This type of classical, or Pavlovian, conditioning reduces the time required to milk a herd of cows.

A pet animal's fear reaction to the smell of a veterinary hospital or, these days, in surgical scrubs is often a classically conditioned response. The dog or cat responds to a painful stimulus (UCS) with the fear or escape response. The hospital and the professional staff are the CS. It does not take many pairings of these stimuli to produce a fear response whenever the animal encounters the CS. It is somewhat disheartening for veterinarians to discover that many of their patients turn tail and hide whenever they approach, sometimes even outside the veterinary clinic. The behaviorally oriented clinician will make every effort to reduce the painful and frightening incidents,

especially during a young animal's first visit, so that a conditioned fear response will not develop and hinder future patient–veterinarian (not to mention client–veterinarian) relationships. This is the goal of the Fear-Free Initiative. Figure 7.1 shows classical conditioning of the goat.

Operant Conditioning

The third type of learning is called "operant", or "instrumental", learning. Operant conditioning was first demonstrated by Thorndike,[2254] using cats as experimental animals. Hungry cats were placed in slatted boxes. Food was available outside the box within sight and smell of the cats. At first, the cats struggled vigorously to reach the food. Eventually, some of them, by chance, pulled a latch string that opened the box door. The cats were then free to consume their reward. Each time a cat was replaced in the box, it took a shorter time to escape, making fewer and fewer extraneous motions, until eventually it pulled the latch string immediately upon being placed in the box.

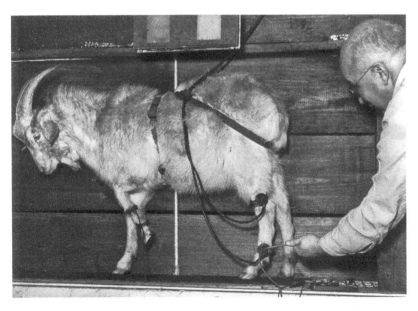

Figure 7.1 Classical conditioning. Pairing the sound of the metronome with shock to the foreleg conditions a goat to lift its leg when a metronome ticks. Also shown is the late Professor Liddell, who compared the rate at which various species of farm animals learned a classically conditioned response.

Operant conditioning is also called "instrumental learning" because the behavior is the instrument by which the reinforcement is obtained. A laboratory example of instrumental learning is a rat in a *Skinner box*, named for the psychologist who popularized the technique,[2136] in which an animal presses a bar to obtain food, water, or electrical stimulation of its brain. Figure 7.2 demonstrates a dog using a Skinner box to feed itself.

Operant conditioning is also used on the farm. Swine use electronic feeders. Horses use automatic waterers, and cows can be taught to enter an area to be milked by a robot, that is, the cows milk themselves.[2477] Operant conditioning devices that dispense food when a cat or dog presses a switch are sold as novelty items.

Chaining

A fourth type of learning is chaining. Chaining is the performance of a series of operant responses in sequence. A good example is goats who were trained to jump three hurdles, walk on a raised walkway, pass through two barrels, and press a lever 10 times.[2100] Many dog owners inadvertently chain obedience commands, with the result that the dog sits, shakes, lies down, and rolls over when the owner says "Sit." The owner always gives the commands in the same order, and the dog has chained the responses.

Discrimination Learning

A fifth type of learning is discrimination learning. Animals can learn to discriminate between various visual, auditory, or tactile cues. One of the simplest tests of visual discrimination in horses, cattle, and sheep was done by Gardner.[792-796] Her studies revealed that all three species could learn to choose a feedbox covered with black cloth instead of two uncovered feedboxes. With increasing trials, the number of errors decreased. The animals retained the discrimination when tested over a year later.

Spatial working memory (delayed response) is seen as a form of short-term memory that typically holds information relevant within a spatial test trial, such as a list of holes in a board that have been visited recently; whereas reference or long-term memory holds trial-independent information about the rules and solution of a spatial task, for example which holes in a board were not baited in the last trial.

Imprinting

As defined by Lorenz,[1413] imprinting is a special process that (a) can occur only during a definite and short period of the animal's life; (b) is irreversible; (c) involves an attachment to an object that will later evoke adult behavior patterns, including sexual behavior; and (d) involves reactions to a particular object that can be generalized to all objects in that class,

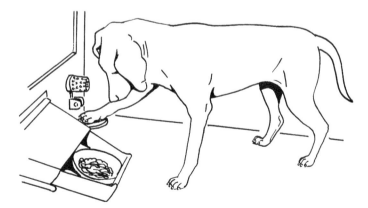

Figure 7.2   Operant conditioning. The dog pushes a pedal (operates on the environment) to obtain a dish of food.

for instance all humans or all duck decoys. For example, a hand-raised lamb subsequently showed abnormal social and maternal behavior.[2064] The lamb's situation was quite comparable to that of the geese that were hand-raised by Lorenz.[1412] Subsequent laboratory studies have revealed that in ducks, imprinting does not appear to be irreversible or to influence any adult patterns of social behavior.[1609]

Imprinting is often misused and confused with socialization. Imprinting occurs most commonly in birds and involves a following response. Ducklings will follow their mother because she is the first moving object they see. If a red ball is the first moving object they see, they will follow that.

Imprinting begins before hatching because the chicks can hear their mother's clucks. Once hatched the chicks will follow their mother (or various approximations of a chicken, even a red ball, in the absence of the hen).[2728] The period in which this type of learning can occur is three days before to seven days after hatching. The chick that is properly imprinted will be close to its mother and thus be led to food and water, sheltered by her wings from cold wind and predators and defended from other dangers. They will follow a moving object and, with repeated exposure, form a sexual attachment to that object.

Neonatal foals will follow any large moving object. That is the reason they may follow a human if the mare has not yet risen after foaling. Imprinting occurs more rapidly in frightened animals, which explains why a newborn foal may follow a horse that has been biting him. Mares may have developed the tendency to guard their foal against any animal or person who approaches, not only to defend the foal from predators but also to prevent the foal from following the wrong animal.

The few studies done to date indicate that the following tendency is not irreversible. Normally reared lambs, who presumably followed their mothers, began to follow dogs when the two species were housed together, but lost the response after returning to the company of other sheep.[369] In order for goats, pigs, and other domestic animals to direct sexual behavior toward humans, the animals must have been isolated from conspecifics and been in close association with humans.[2019]

Dr. Robert Miller[1589] has popularized "imprint training" in foals. His technique involves habituation and probably learned helplessness when practiced on a foal too young to stand or otherwise resist. The foal is not really imprinted on humans. Foals handled for 10 minutes twice a day during their first week and then weekly until weaning at four months of life were no more likely to approach people than were foals that received only routine and emergency veterinary care.[1400] Imprint-trained foals were calmer and friendlier to humans (would approach sooner), but did not accept hoof handling and other management techniques any better than untrained foals.[2126,2457] Both these studies employed mare–foal pairs that were pastured soon after birth of the foal. Whether imprint training would be more or less important to foals that were raised in box stalls has not been determined. Foals handled for 10 min/day (alternating rubbing, touching, and picking up feet) five days a week beginning at two weeks of age were easier to catch and handle than those reared in a stall but without intensive handling, which in turn were easier to handle than those who had been running free for 10 months.[1150] Even more extensive training beginning within seven hours of birth and continuing for two weeks resulted in easier handling of the foals. They were tested at 16 days and at 3, 6, and 12 months, and their behavior was compared to unhandled foals. The handled foals were easier to handle (halter, pick up hooves, and lead) at 16 days, but by one year there was no difference between handled and unhandled foals. As yearlings, there were no differences in discrimination and spatial learning between the handled and unhandled foals.[1310] See Table 7.1 for the results of imprint training on foal behavior.

Table 7.1 Results of imprint training.

Imprint age	Repetitions	Test	Age	References
14 days	Until 24 weeks	Hoof[a] lead[a] approach[a]	6, 12, 18, 24 months	1150
24 hours	Daily for 42 days	Halter, lead[a]	85 days	1445
10 minutes	24 hours	Restrain halter	90 days	2626
		Worm		
		Vaccinate hoof		
Birth	Daily for 7 days	Approach responses to stimuli	120 days	1446
2–8 hours	Daily for 5 days	Approach[a] stimuli	4 months	2126
45 minutes	12, 24, 28 hours	Approach stimuli	1, 2, 3 months	2457

[a] Significantly better performance by imprint-trained foals.

One of the most interesting findings is that interacting with the mare, not the foal, is as powerful as, and much less difficult than, imprint training. Grooming the mare for 15 min/day minutes per day for five days after the foal's birth had long-lasting consequences. At one month, the foals whose mothers had been brushed accepted a saddle pad on their back more quickly, tolerated it longer and were more likely to approach a person. The reaction to humans persisted in those foals as yearlings.[996]

Foals exposed weekly to potentially frightening objects with their dams who had been habituated were less frightened of these objects than unexposed foals. This is apparently learning safety by observation.[417] Later handling can, of course, be used to increase tractability and reduce fear. If weanling horses are stroked for five minutes twice a day for two weeks, they are more likely to approach a strange person than those unhandled or those stroked only when they approached a person voluntarily. Most important, they were much less apt to kick when approached and haltered four months later.[1378] Thoroughbred yearlings were tested before and after a six-week training period of 45 minutes' duration daily in which they were haltered, groomed, and received veterinary examinations. It is not surprising they were less nervous and more likely to approach an unfamiliar human if they had been handled daily.[1600] Genetics are important too. Foals from certain sires and dams are easier to halter train than from others.[2665]

The pre-pretraining environment is important because pastured horses were more easily trained using a round-pen technique than were stalled two-year-olds.[1940]

Conditioned Taste Aversion

Taste aversion, or bait shyness, is the process by which an animal learns to avoid a food not because it tastes bad, but because it associates it with illness, particularly gastrointestinal malaise. This form of learning has long been recognized by those attempting to rid farms of rats. When first used, a poison usually kills many rats; but after the first application, very few rats are killed. The animals that survive will no longer eat the bait. The same phenomenon occurs when rats are exposed to radiation and at the same time offered a novel food. They soon avoid the food that they associate with radiation sickness.[790]

Three unique characteristics of taste aversion differentiate it from classical and operant conditioning. One is that it appears to be specific for taste and olfaction; other stimuli such as visual or auditory cues will not be avoided. Rats will learn to avoid the taste of saccharin, which they normally like, but not a blue solution. On the other hand, birds readily learn to avoid novel-colored foods; avian species, which possess few taste buds, apparently depend more on sight than on taste for food identification. Second, the illness must be of internal origin, a general or gastrointestinal malaise. External injury, as from electric shock to the feet, is not a sufficient stimulus. Third, the novel taste and the illness can be widely separated in time, and learning will still take place. This is in contrast to both operant and classical conditioning, in which the stimulus and the response must be close together in time for learning to take place. Sheep and cattle can form taste aversions to a particular food even when the illness follows the ingestion by as much as eight hours, but the aversion is weakened if the food is present in an unfamiliar location or in the presence of conspecifics that are consuming the food.[359-362,1271] Taste aversions can be formed even if the animal is anesthetized during the time illness was present. Anesthesia blocks other forms of learning, so taste aversion may be noncognitive learning.[1870] It is always difficult to know how an animal feels, particularly when the sensation is something subtle, such as nausea in an animal that cannot vomit. Whereas anesthesia does not prevent taste aversion, an antiemetic does, indicating the critical importance of nausea.[1870] The higher the doses of toxin and, presumably, the sicker the animal, the stronger the conditioned taste aversion. The concentration of the flavor is not important, but sheep will generalize from one food to another if the flavor is the same.[1313] Sheep seem to generalize the categories of plants to which they have a taste aversion. They will eat less legume if conditioned with a different legume or less grass if conditioned with a different grass.[825] Horses form taste aversion only if the illness occurs soon after the food is tasted.[2800] Even when hay is fed *ad libitum* horses do not sort poisonous *Senecio* from harmless hay probably because the toxin does not act immediately.[2894] Taste aversion has four uses, one experimental and three practical. Experimentally, taste aversion can be used to determine what substances an animal can taste or perceive. An animal will show an aversion to a substance at concentrations far below those at which it would show preference or aversion if the taste had not been paired with illness.

Practically, taste aversion has been used to teach coyotes to avoid lamb. Repeated pairing of lamb infused with lithium chloride, which produces nausea and vomiting, resulted in a definite aversion to live or dead lambs by the coyote.[872] Taste aversion techniques have not been successful on a large scale to reduce livestock predation by wild coyotes. The second practical use is to teach livestock to avoid a poisonous plant. Many poisonous plants, such as larkspur, do not make the animal nauseated, but instead are chronic poisons. The cattle or sheep can be taught using another emetic to avoid that plant before they encounter it on the range. Finally, taste aversion can be used to prevent wildlife from eating agriculturally or ornamentally important plants. Four important factors arise in teaching a flavor cue: novelty of the cue; dose and pharmacology of the toxin used as the unconditioned stimulus; availability of alternative foods; and social facilitation, that is, other animals avoiding the plant.[1225]

Chickens can form aversions to food, but unlike mammals, they base this learning on color not taste of the food .

Formation and Strengthening of a Learned Task

Shaping

In teaching an animal an operant task, one can wait until the animal performs the desired activity or one can speed up the process by shaping the behavior. If, when teaching a dog to heel, the trainer first rewards the dog for staying within a yard of his side, then a foot, and finally only when the animal walks quietly exactly beside the trainer, he is "shaping" the dog's behavior.

Animals that are trained to perform complicated and relatively unnatural tricks are usually reinforced with food rewards and reinforced for each correct response at first. The same techniques are used to teach chickens to play baseball or to teach pigs to put giant coins in a bank.[322]

Autoshaping

Autoshaping is a phenomenon whereby an animal makes a response directed toward a stimulus that precedes a reinforcement. If a light signals that food will be delivered in a few seconds, pigeons will peck at the light, and dogs will lick the response keys. An attempt to autoshape horses failed.[570]

Reinforcement Schedules

When operant conditioning is employed, a variety of schedules of reinforcement can be used. The animal can be rewarded, for example, after every response, every ten 10 responses, or every 20 responses. These schedules are called "fixed ratios" or FR1, FR10, and FR20, respectively. This technical detail is important because the higher the fixed ratio, the faster the animal will respond; even more important, the longer it will take for the response to be extinguished or forgotten. The animal will go on responding for some time after it is no longer rewarded. Many situations arise in which owners inadvertently put their animal on high-FR schedules. Take, for instance, the dog that barks while its owners are eating. They may have given him food once or twice when it barked, until they became annoyed at the behavior. The dog continues to bark while the owners try to ignore him. Finally, they relent and give it some food; they have just increased the ratio. Dog and owner may adjust to this new level, but often the adjustment is temporary and the level of response (barking) needed for reward increases again. Dogs have been trained in the laboratory to bark 33 times for each small food reward and cats to meow 15 times.[1608,2017] The problem dog at the dinner table may continue to bark hundreds of times even though its owners do not give it any more food.

Another type of reinforcement is called "fixed interval." In this case, the animal is rewarded for a response that occurs after a certain period of time has elapsed since the last reward. Animals do have a good time sense, and their rate of responding will slow down after a reward and then increase sharply just before the end of the time interval. If animals can learn to respond in this manner, it is not surprising that they learn to expect their owners to return home at a given hour. Another variant of reinforcement ratios is the progressive ratio (PR) in which, for example, the animal must respond once for the first reward, twice for the second, four times for the third, and so on, until the break point, which is the number of responses (the price) that are too high for the animal to make (pay). The number of responses per reward increases progressively. This technique is used to measure the strength of preferences for food or other commodities.

A longer lasting response (i.e., more difficult to extinguish) follows a variable interval–reward (VI) schedule. Here, the reward follows the first response after one minute has elapsed, then after five minutes, then after three minutes, and so on. The highest response rate follows a variable ratio–reward (VR) schedule. The owners of the barking dog may find themselves rewarding their dog on this type of schedule if they inconsistently reward the barking, depending, perhaps, on their own mood on any particular evening or on which family member gives in to the pet. A high rate of barking may contribute to the owners giving in sooner, but the owners are probably not counting barks; they are merely "holding out" for as long as possible, a war of nerves that the dog invariably wins.

Obviously, however, a VR schedule is to be recommended in routine animal training; after a task has been learned using continuous reward, owners should supply verbal or food rewards sporadically during a training session rather than after every trick.

One of the most difficult tasks for the animal trainer is to get the animal to understand the experimenter's instructions.[827] Dogs, for example, have remarkable olfactory acuity and can be taught to detect gas leaks, hidden narcotics, and fatty acids at very low concentrations, but it is extremely difficult to get dogs to learn to turn right in response to an olfactory cue.[215] Dogs can learn to make the correct response using verbal cues or hand gestures and some dogs respond better to one than to the other, but best response was to a combination of verbal and hand gestures.[2759] It is also important to know what is rewarding for an animal. Dogs learn faster when the reward is simple contact with a passive person than when the reward is stroking or picking up and learn better if the reward is petting rather than just praise.[2741,3063] Stroking a dog lowers its heart rate and the area of the body stroked is not important.[2879] Dogs (Labrador Retrievers) perform better for a food reward than for a ball.[2836]

Tool Use in Animals

Some species, especially crows and monkeys, use tools, but domestic animals rarely do. When horse owners were surveyed as to examples of tool use, some horses were found to use tools, mostly to move food closer.[2837]

Influences on Learning

Drugs

Dantzer and his colleagues have studied the effects of various drugs on learning in pigs.[510–513,1627,1628] For example, pigs treated with diazepam will press a panel more times for food than untreated pigs;[510] diazepam stimulates feeding (see Chapter 8, "Ingestive Behavior: Food and Water Intake"). The muscarinic receptor antagonist scopolamine slowed maze transit by sheep;[1332] cholinergic mechanisms have been identified as part of the learning process. Administration of a tranquilizer facilitated operant conditioning of a genetically nervous pointer. Petting has a physiologically demonstrable calming effect and can be used to facilitate learning. For example, dogs classically conditioned to expect a shock following a tone have a higher heart rate during the tone,[781] but heart rate declines if the dogs are petted during tone presentation.[1427] Young dogs can learn faster when given the drug selegiline, which increases brain dopamine, but only if a food lure is visible; otherwise, they actually learn slower than placebo-treated dogs. This indicates that dopamine enhancement helps only rewarded behavior.[1597]

Diet and Supplements

Puppies supplemented with docosahexaenoic acid learned reversal tasks and visual-contrast discrimination more rapidly than unsupplemented puppies.[2519] Alpha-casozepine facilitates acceptance of handling techniques, including ear clipping and being led through novel environments.[1510]

Avoidance learning has been used to study the effects of malnutrition on brain function. Pigs previously malnourished, but subsequently rehabilitated for several months, show poorer avoidance learning than well-nourished pigs.[167]

Effect of a Barren Environment on Learning and Memory

Pigs raised in a barren environment – the typical pig pen – could learn a maze as easily as those raised in an enriched environment (larger pen with straw), but 10 weeks later they did not remember the maze as well.[521] The performance of pigs on various cognitive tasks depends on each pig's specific experience with particular stimuli rather than general experience with a wider range of stimuli.[19]

Emotions

Anxious dogs solve a simple problem slower than normal dogs, indicating the influence of emotion on ability.[1775] Learning itself can result in cortisol release; shelter dogs that were clicker trained to touch a bucket had higher cortisol than those who could not learn the task and who were depressed.[257]

Sex

Intact females dogs learn faster than spayed ones and females learn faster than males.[2893,2969]

Positive and Negative Reinforcement

An animal will learn for both positive and negative reinforcement. Positive reinforcement is a reward, usually food but sometimes social interaction, for performing a response. Negative reinforcement is something aversive applied until the animal makes the response. One pulls on the horse's mouth until it stops, or the rat is shocked until it moves to the other side of the cage. Dogs in a class using negative reinforcement displayed lowered body postures and signals of stress such as lip licking and yawning, whereas dogs in a class using a positive reinforcement–based method showed increased attentiveness toward their owner. However, neither method affected avoidance behaviors.[687] Of course, the type of positive reinforcement matters too. Dogs learn more quickly for food than for petting or praise, and they prefer petting to verbal praise, but this applies only to the initial sit-stay training.[766] Successive negative contrast effects are characterized by exaggerated reactions shortly after a stimulus is downshifted in magnitude, when compared with control animals that have always been trained to receive the stimulus at the downshifted level. Dogs downshifted from dry liver to pellets rejected food more frequently than nonshifted controls. Gaze duration also decreased in downshifted dogs below the level of a group always reinforced with pellets. In addition, downshifted dogs tended to move away from the experimenter, adopting a prone posture.[3111]

Many field dogs are trained using negative reinforcement varying from a skin pinch to a shock collar. The use of electric shock to train animals is controversial. There are definitely correct and incorrect ways to use shock. The best way is negative reinforcement in which the aversive stimulus (pain) is applied until the animal does the desired action. For example, cattle can learn to avoid a trough of hay if the shock ceases as soon as they turn away. When the shock continues regardless of what the animal does, they don't not learn as well.[1331] When Beagles were able to clearly associate the electric stimulus with their action (i.e., touching a rabbit), they were not stressed, but Beagles shocked randomly or for failure to come on recall were stressed.[2041] When dogs were trained using positive reinforcement by instructors who were accustomed to using shock, they learned no faster.[2699,2996]

A practical application of negative reinforcement (shock avoidance) learning is now commercially available as "invisible fences." Dogs, goats, and cattle can learn to avoid shock from a collar by heeding an auditory warning signal.[1328,1329] Some dogs become fearful of the boundary or even of the yard when improperly trained; others tolerate the shock to reach the target of their aggression.

One of the most difficult concepts for owners to understand is the difference between negative reinforcement and punishment.[291] Punishment is something that occurs after an action as a consequence. The dog chews the slipper, and the owner hits him. Timing is very important. Punishment will not decrease the frequency of the behavior unless it occurs when the animal is misbehaving or within a second or two of the termination of the behavior. Most owners feel that they can punish a dog hours after it has chewed a slipper or eliminated in the house, and they are surprised when the dog does not learn.

Clicker Training

Clicker training is a technique used widely to train dogs, horses, and, especially, zoo animals. The principle is that the click serves as a secondary reinforcement, usually a food reward. The clicker, a plastic device, can be used to produce the click, but any sound would do. The advantage of the clicker is that it is a unique sound. After a dozen to 20 pairings, the animal usually knows that the click means a reward is coming, an example of classical conditioning. Then the operant conditioning phase begins. When the animal makes the desired response, either by chance or by shaping, it hears a click and receives a reward. No verbal command has been given. After another 20 pairings of response, click, and reward, the animal should make the movement in response to the verbal command. The advantage is that the animal is signaled when it does the correct thing, a real advantage when working with a nonverbal species.

Learned Helplessness

A phenomenon that has considerable application to practical animal training has been discovered in dogs and cats. This phenomenon is learned helplessness. Normal, naïve dogs, when first placed in an active avoidance situation in which impending shock is signaled, at first escape the shock after it has begun, and later avoid the shock by performing the necessary task, such as jumping over a barrier during the signal before the shock begins. Dogs that previously have been exposed to unavoidable shock act in a quite different manner. They not only fail to learn to avoid as naïve dogs do, but also fail to escape; they simply sit and take the shock. These experimental findings indicate that the same form of aversive

stimulus should not be used first as inescapable punishment and then later as negative reinforcement that the dog should learn to avoid. Improper use of the popular shock collars or invisible fences may produce learned helplessness in dogs, and any form of inescapable punishment may inhibit later learning. Pigs apparently do not suffer from learned helplessness as dogs do.[1628]

Comparative Cognition

Brain Weight to Body Weight Ratio

An anatomical approach to intelligence can be used. There may be a correlation between brain size and intelligence.[1927] The brain weight to body weight ratios in decreasing order are: human, 2%; cat, 1%; mongrel dog, 0.5%; rat, 0.3%; goat, 0.3%; horse, 0.1%; and pig, 0.05%.[516,2689] [2798], [2810,2832] Figure 7.3 illustrates the brains of domestic animals.

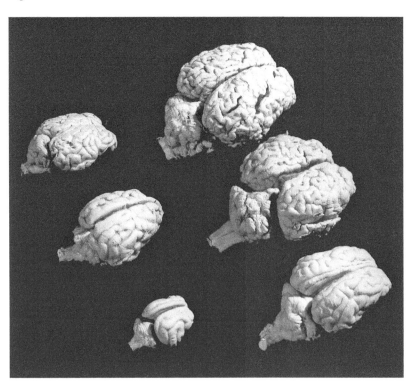

Figure 7.3   The relative brain size of various domestic animals. Right row, from top to bottom: horse, cow, and pig; left row: dog, sheep, and cat.

Cognition research includes perception, object permanence, memory, physical causality, quantity and time discrimination, sensitivity to human cues, vocal recognition and communication, attachment bonds, and personality. We have discussed perception and communication in Chapter 1, and will discuss personality in Chapter 9. In this chapter, we will consider social cognition, including following the human gaze, social referencing and eavesdropping, use of mirrors, numeracy, inferential reasoning by exclusion, object permanence, learning by observation, and theory of mind as measures of cognitive abilities. Inequity aversion and jealousy are also discussed.[2798] Perhaps different methods should be used in studies of canine intelliegence.[2919]

Social Cognition

Dogs

Following Human Gaze or Pointing

Communication between animals and humans occurs frequently, especially between dogs and their owners and cats and their owners. Dogs and cats can determine where hidden food is when a person indicates the hiding place by pointing to it momentarily or dynamically from as far away as 80 cm (30 in.).[2775,2776,2864] Trained working gun dogs are better than pet gun dogs. Pet dogs kept inside alternate gazing at the human and the unreachable food item more than outdoor pet dogs or shelter dogs.[2766] There may be a degree of associative learning rather than attribution of intent of the person pointing because dogs that learn to follow simple proximal pointing are more likely to follow distal cross pointing.[626]

Much has been made of the fact that dogs will respond to human pointing gestures, but if the pointer gives false information the dog will not choose at all or will choose the other alternative on the next occasion.[2219] There are interesting results when the human points to the wrong one of two bowls when the dog has witnessed the reward being moved from one bowl to another. Border Collies are more likely to

approach the wrong bowl than the terriers.[2855] Labrador Retrievers followed human referential gestures, that is, pointing, better than German Shepherds.[3001] Genetic selection and lifetime experience both influence human-guided task performance.[3012] Social cognition in dogs has been reviewed.[234]

When the animals know where the food is but cannot reach it, dogs are more likely to look at the owners sooner and for a longer time than cats. This is called "social referencing."[1580] Dogs owned by blind people apparently do not realize the owner is blind because they also look at unobtainable food, then at the owner, then at food, but they have added a sound, noisy mouth licking (licking their chops).[803] Dogs will watch a human, whether owner or stranger, searching for, manipulating, and eating a hidden treat longer than they watch familiar dogs. They spend the least time observing feeding behavior.[1897] A single dog has been trained to use arbitrary signs to communicate. She would press a striped symbol for a walk, a toy, or water. Best of all, she would touch a sheet of newsprint to signal that she wanted access to her urination area.[1980] Now, devices like Dog SpeechTraining Buzzers® are available commercially.

Despite their ability to communicate with humans, dogs do not seek help for their owners in an emergency situation, such as when the owner has a heart attack or is pinned under a bookcase.[1437] Dogs prioritize looking forward over looking back so may miss cues from owners.[2816]

Dogs are able to determine whether a human is likely to give them food by observing that person's behavior toward another person. This phenomenon is called "social eavesdropping." A dog observed two people, each with a bowl. A third person begged for food from each. One person would say "Take it" and share the food, and the other would say "No" and gesture the person to retreat. The dog would approach first and spend more time with the generous person. Vocal cues were more important than visual ones.[1464] A confounding factor is that the dogs may have been choosing the side on which the people sat rather than their relative generosity.[1698] Another example of social eavesdropping occurs when dogs observe a person turning away from their owner rather than assisting her when she has asked for help in opening a jar; they will not take food from that non-helpful person, indicating that food does not have to be involved. The dog will take food from a person who opened the jar, or from a neutral person who sat beside the owner but was not asked for help. This indicates that dogs are sensitive to human interactions and apparently make judgments as to whether a person can be trusted.[414]

Puppies are less likely to look to humans, and, as adults, hunting breeds are more likely to look at humans for longer than molossoid breeds (Bulldogs and German Shepherds) or primitive breeds (Akitas, Huskies, and Malamutes).[1776]

Dogs looked back at their owners more (social referencing) when the owners had previously encouraged them. Dogs flexibly adjust their human-directed behavior to the actions of their partners. In proof of this, dogs observed two people, a Filler who rebaited an empty food-dispensing apparatus and the Helper who unblocked the blocked apparatus. Dogs learn to recognize the ability of the Filler, who rebaited-baited the empty apparatus, and spent time close to her when the apparatus was empty. Independently of the problem, however, they always first approached the Helper, who unblocked the blocked apparatus.[1030]

The training a dog receives determines how often he looks to a human for help. When faced with an unsolvable task, agility-trained dogs are most likely to look at their owners, and search and rescue dogs the least. Pet dogs were intermediate.[1465] Dogs respond to their owners' emotions and respond appropriately to an object the owner appears to like rather than one the owner appears to find disgusting.[1565]

Canine intelligence has been a subject of much interest recently, as more and more human-like abilities are discovered in dogs.[2650,2651] There are two hypotheses: dogs have lost intelligence during domestication; or they possibly have gained the ability to understand the minds of humans (social cognition), but certainly have gained the ability to read very subtle signals.[2698,2702,2788,2838,3012] The evidence for the first hypothesis is that dogs that live with their owners don't solve problems – such as gaining access to food by manipulating a bowl – as well as dogs that live outdoors.[2702] In addition, dogs selected for independent behaviors, such as pointers, do better than other breeds.[2276] The evidence for the second hypothesis is that dogs do better than chimpanzees on finding a human-cued reward. The ability to interpret human gestures and a human gaze is innate, not learned, in domestic dogs; kennel-raised puppies perform as well as family-raised puppies. Puppies do not improve with age in these tasks between nine 9 and 26 weeks.

Horses

Horses are more limited than dogs in their ability to interpret human gestures. Of the four horses tested, three could respond to touching the correct of two buckets; only one responded to pointing by approaching the correct bucket.[1536] In another test, horses did respond to pointing by approaching one of two buckets, if the pointer was close to the bucket or the pointing gesture was longer than a second, but only if the pointing gesture was sustained (dynamic).[1462] Horses do show social referencing, looking to a human when food is visible but not attainable.[2866]

Goats

Goats rival dogs in their ability to follow human pointing and gazing and could follow human pointing gestures to find a food bucket, provided the pointer was close to the bucket.[1169,2904]

Cats

Cats show social referencing in that they look at their owners when faced with a novel object (in this case, a moving fan). If the owner acted frightened of the fan, the cats were more likely to alternate looking at the fan and at the escape route.[1566] When encountering an insolvable task cats will look to a human (social referencing), but only if the human is paying attention to them.[3118]

Pigs

Pigs have been bred for larger bodies, so wild boars tend to have larger ratios of brain weight to body weight. The fallacy of using so labile a parameter as body weight to judge intelligence is manifest when one realizes that the malnourished pig, which shows definite intellectual impairment,[167] has a greater brain weight to body weight ratio than the well-nourished pig. This occurs because the brain appears to be spared when the rest of the body is stunted by malnutrition. Despite these anatomical differences, wild boars are no better than domestic swine in finding food identified by a physical cue, but they were actually better at following human pointing than their domesticated counterparts.[19] Pigs also show some preference for a person who is looking at them.[1675]

Jealousy and Fairness

Dogs appear to feel jealousy if their owners pay attention to another dog or human. The dogs try to insert themselves between the owner and the other person (or dog). In formal testing, the owners petted and spoke to a stuffed dog; their dogs not only pushed at the stuffed dog, but also a third of them snapped at it.[918] Dogs are also aware of inequity because they will refuse to "give paw" when they are not rewarded but another dog is.[1898]

Object Permanence

Cats, dogs, chickens, and goats have been shown to comprehend object permanence. They will watch the place where an object disappeared from view and go to that place to find the object.[782,2247] This means that these animals have the ability to represent objects in

their brains when they are not visible. Out of sight is not out of mind. This is the level of insight usually obtained by 12- to 18-month-old children.

Mirror

Self-recognition of a mirror image has been used to assess self-awareness in animals. There are three stages of mirror recognition: (a) exploratory and social interaction, (b) contingency behaviors, and (c) removing a mark visible only in the mirror. No domestic animal has reached stage (c).

Sheep certainly show social interaction both positive and negative with a mirror, some butting the mirror. They do saccade between looking at the image of another sheep in the mirror and that sheep (contingency), but they cannot seem to use the mirror to locate food. Welsh mountain sheep show all of these behaviors more often than Norfolk horned or Borderdale sheep.[1488] Pigs also show social interaction with a mirror, and they are able to locate food based on its reflection in a mirror,[341] as can dogs, but dogs raised with cats prefer a cat companion and fail to recognize a mirror image.[723,1071]

Theory of Mind

Pigs

Pigs can learn that one of them knows where food is hidden and will follow that pig to the food source. If the follower is dominant, it will "scrounge" – take the food from the subordinate pig. That pig will learn to avoid approaching the food source if the dominant pig is close enough to take the food from him. Both pigs seem able to interpret the intentions of the other.[976]

Pigs will increase their foraging speed as a way of responding to exploitation by dominants.[977]

Dogs

Dogs do not inform humans of the location of hidden objects unless they, the dogs themselves, are interested in that object.[1134]

Horses

Food was hidden from horses in an unopenable bucket in the presence of two experimenters. One experimenter witnessed the food-hiding process while the other did not. Horses showed significantly more interest (gaze and touch) toward the witness. This has been interpreted as inferring what others witnessed – theory of mind.[3008]

Conceptual Learning

The highest type of learning – that is, the one that demands the most intelligence – is conceptual learning. The simplest form of conceptual learning is the ability to respond to a common quality or characteristic shared by a number of different specific stimuli.

Dogs

Dogs can form the concept of dog and no dog. They were trained using pictures projected on a touch screen, and they could discriminate a novel dog in a landscape from a landscape.[1899] Unfortunately, dogs can also learn that there will be no drugs in a given area and will fail to detect drugs there.[805] This phenomenon is called "context specificity" and is analogous to the superior response to commands that many of our dogs show in the kitchen. Dogs are aware of their own height. For example, when they are taller than an opening in a barrier, they will approach it more slowly.

Cats

Cats are able to form learning sets, that is, to form concepts. Cats can learn to solve a problem, such as choosing the object on the left when identical black squares were the stimulus, and would learn much more quickly on the next problem to choose the object on the left when white triangles were presented.[2389] After four problems, the cats' errors fell to 36% of the original errors, and only 58% of the trials originally necessary were needed to reach criterion. Cats seldom show insightful behavior; they do not learn to move a light box under a suspended piece of fish in order to reach the fish.[8] Captured feral cats learn discrimination more quickly than cage-reared ones.[2451] These findings indicate that a varied environment or experience may lead to an increased learning ability in cats. When trained in a progressive elimination task in which there are many sites with food, but once the food has been consumed the cat must look elsewhere (win shift); in these tests, cats choose the site closest to the start point.[565] When cats can see two food sources, they will choose the one at the smaller angular deviation, but when they cannot see them because an opaque barrier has been interposed, they choose the closest one. This is called the "distance factor."

Horses

We are most familiar with this from the children's shows on TV in which toddlers are asked, "Which of these is not like the others?" In that case, difference is the concept. Horses can form that concept. They were taught to touch two cards with the same symbol rather than a card with a different symbol even when the symbols were novel.[703]

Apparently, horses can form the concept of triangularity. The experiment was an operant conditioning task. The horse simply had to push one of two hinged panels. The correct panel was unlocked, allowing the horse access to a bowl of grain. The incorrect panel was locked, but a bowl of grain was locked behind it to ensure the horse did not choose the panel because it could smell the grain. The correct choice was not always on the same side. The first problem was a simple discrimination between a black panel and a white panel. Next was a discrimination between a cross and a circle. The third problem was to distinguish a triangle from a rectangle, and the next was to discriminate triangles from half circles and various other patterns. In the true test of conceptual learning, the horse had to choose between two shapes it had never seen before, one triangular and the other non-triangular. It learned the task quickly but was not correct on the first trial.[2029] Horses can also categorize by learning the concept of filled versus empty symbols (such as circles, squares, triangles, and trapezoids) as well as the concept of larger.[899,901–903]

Learning by Observation

Animals can learn by imitation, that is, by observing others. This form of learning has been most thoroughly studied in dogs, cats, cattle, chickens, and horses.

Dogs

The demonstrator can be a human[1839] or another dog. Puppies can learn complex tasks such as narcotics detection by observing their mother from six 6 to 12 weeks of age, despite the fact that they were not trained until three months had elapsed.[2137] When observing another dog using its mouth rather than its paw, they are more likely to reproduce an irrational behavior (i.e., using the mouth instead of a paw) than the more rational one. The mere presence of a ball causes dogs to use their mouths rather than their paws.[1171] The dog will learn from a dog that is dominant to him, but not from a subordinate. Dogs can learn by observation of a human demonstrator, but it is the subordinate dog in a household that learns, not the dominant one.[1840,1841] There are limits to dogs' ability to learn by observation. They can learn only transitive tasks (involving an object), but not intransitive ones (lying in lateral recumbency).[2239] After observing a dog go to one of four corners for a hidden food reward, a dog is more likely to go to that location if he had snout contact with that dog. It appears that they need to smell or taste the food before believing that it is where they saw the demonstrator go.[962] The most interesting finding, albeit in only one dog, is imitation of human action – carrying bottles across a room and putting them in a cabinet.[1579] Dogs appear to form memories of specific events, so-called "episodic memory," but it is short lived (minutes not hours).[2755]

Chickens can learn by observation and learn better from a socially dominant chicken.[2907]

Horses

Three unsuccessful attempts have been made to demonstrate observational learning in horses. In two cases, the horses, young quarter horses, watched another choose one of two feed buckets. In neither case did the horses that observed perform any better than those that had not had the opportunity to observe.[124,133] In the third case, horses watched a demonstrator horse step on a pedal to open a feed bin. Observers did no better than naïve horses.[1384] This is particularly interesting because horse vices, in particular cribbing, are believed to be learned by observation. Horse do poorly at solving detour problems and do no better if they watch a demonstrator horse being led through the detour.[1963] Perhaps if the demonstrators were free to walk through the detour alone, the observers would have been more attentive. Even when observing the horse who led in their respective herds, horses did not improve and could not solve a detour problem, but may learn by social transmission (social facilitation, local, and stimulus enhancement).[2954,2955] In a carefully controlled study of detour behavior, horses did not learn by observation to solve a detour problem.[2881]

There has been a successful demonstration of observational learning in horses. Horses learn "join up" (approaching the person in the center of the ring) more quickly if they observe a horse dominant to them perform; watching a subordinate confers no advantage.[1273] This is similar to the interaction of social rank and learning by observation in dogs. About half of horses tested can learn to pull a rope to access food by watching another horse demonstrate the task. The learners in the social learning test were significantly younger, lower ranking, and more exploratory than the non-learners, but not lower ranking or more exploratory than the demonstrator horses.[1277] Although they do not often learn by observing another horse they seem to be able to learn to press a handle to open a feed box by observation of a human demonstrator.[2974] There is a difference between social transmission (social facilitation, local, and stimulus enhancement) and social learning (goal emulation, imitation).

And horses may use social transmission rather than social learning.[2953]

Cognitive Bias

Cognitive bias is based on the premise that subjects in a negative affective state perform more negative judgments about ambiguous stimuli than subjects in a positive affective state. It is usually measured by teaching an animal that he will be rewarded for going to a bowl on the right but never for going to the bowl on the left. The test is the animal's response when the bowl is in an ambiguous position, for example halfway between the left and right. The speed at which the animal approaches the bowl is used as the measure of optimism. The analogy is the "glass half full" attitude. Although the judgment bias test is powerful test, it should probably only be used once because the animal learns that approaches to the ambiguous location is not rewarded.[3034]

Dogs

When dogs are rewarded for touching a target containing either milk or water signaled by different tones, they show longer latencies to approach the target if the tone is ambiguous. This negative cognitive bias increased with experience of the tests.[2173] Dogs also show a cognitive bias in that they are less optimistic if they suffer from separation anxiety, but become more optimistic if they have been treated with fluoxetine, a specific serotonin enhancer.[1175] See Figure 7.4.

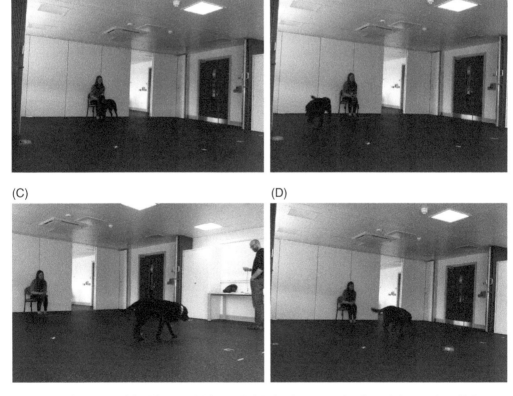

(A)   **(B)**

(C)   **(D)**

Figure 7.4 Canine cognitive bias test. (A) Owner holds dog in preparation for training session. (B) Dog learning that the bowl on the right always contains food. (C) Dog approaching the bowl on the left by a circuitous route. He has learned that there will be no food there. (D) The cognitive bias test. The speed of the dog approaching a bowl midway between the always-rewarded side and the never-rewarded side is a measurement of his optimism. *Source:* Courtesy of Dr. Daniel Mills.

Calves

Calves were taught to touch a red screen for a food reward, but if they touched a white one they were punished with a loud noise and no food. The test of cognitive bias was whether the calves would touch a pink screen. Following hot-iron disbudding, calves were less likely to touch the pink screens, meaning that they were less optimistic.[1677]

Pigs

Normal-birth-weight pigs are more optimistic than low-birth-weight pigs.[1653]

Horses

Horses are more optimistic if kept on pasture with other horses than when kept in box stalls.[1409] See Figure 7.5.

Sheep

Sheep are stressed by isolation and restraint. Release from that restraint influences their choice behavior – a cognitive bias. They are more optimistic approaching a bucket in a location farther from the rewarded location than they normally would.[574]

Numeracy

Dogs

Dogs have numeracy: they are able to assess quantities[79] and will choose the greater number of pieces of food. Dogs may be able to discriminate numbers of kibbles, but when given a choice between different amounts of sausage they cannot discriminate, even though they find it easier to detect a larger amount.[2739] If

(A)   (B)

(C)   (D)

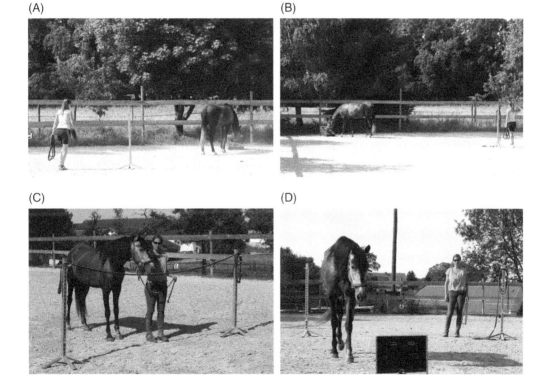

Figure 7.5 Equine cognitive bias test. (A) Horse learning that the bowl on the right will never contain feed. (B) Horse approaching the feeder on the left that always contains food. He has learned that there will always be food there. (C) Handler holds horse in preparation for cognitive bias test. (D) The cognitive bias test. The speed of the horse from the time she is released and the rope is dropped until she reaches the feeder midway between the always-rewarded side and the never-rewarded side is a measurement of her optimism. *Source:* Courtesy of Drs. Anna–Caroline Wöhr and Sandra Lockener.

the owner seemed to favor the smaller quantity by exclaiming over it, most dogs will choose the smaller over the larger. When the two choices are of equal size, more dogs choose what the owner favored, but older dogs and highly trained dogs were more likely not to choose the owner-favored bowl.[1846,2385]

If dogs are shown two bones that are then hidden by a screen, they are surprised if one or three bones are there when the screen is removed. Surprise was measured by how long the dog looked at the bones – the same method used for assessing surprise in preverbal infants.[449,2428]

Cats

Cats can discriminate two dots from three dots, although they may use the total area of the dots rather than the number of dots to make the discrimination.[1825] They can spontaneously discriminate between the number and size of potential prey choosing three mice over one mouse, but choosing a mouse rather than a rat.[2692]

Horses

Horses have numeracy in that they can discriminate one from two objects, two from three objects, or three from four, but not four from six.[779,2302] Ponies did not remember a matching to sample or a quantity discrimination task (3 vs. 2) after one year, even though they remembered how to enter the testing stall and that panels had to be pressed.[2757]

Chickens

Chickens can distinguish one versus two and two versus three, but not larger numbers.[2870]

Inferential Reasoning by Exclusion

Dogs and children can learn to choose a symbol as positive and another as negative (no reward). If a novel stimulus is presented with the negative stimulus, half of the dogs and all the children will choose the novel stimulus, having learned the significance of the negative one. When given a choice between the formerly novel stimulus and another stimulus they have not seen before, they chose the formerly novel stimulus. This ability is called "inferential reasoning by exclusion," demonstrating that they understood that the formerly novel stimulus belonged to the class of rewarded stimuli excluding the new stimulus.[112] Some individual sheep and goats can solve inferential by exclusion tasks.[2726] Horses are able to communicate referentially with humans.[2866]

Dogs can make discriminations between our verbal commands so that they can retrieve objects by name: "spoon," "brush," and "pin."[2508] The record is a Border Collie that could remember over 1000 objects by name,[1167] and, when an unfamiliar word was used, he would fetch a novel object, possibly because dogs prefer to interact with novel toys[1185] or because of reasoning by exclusion. The same dog knew not only the names of toys, but also the category of objects (toy, ball, or Frisbee) and commands such as "Paw," "Nose," or "Take."[2609] When dogs are asked to retrieve a toy they take longer to retrieve it in the dark indicating that they preferentially use vision to find the object.[2724] Dogs sometimes tilt their heads in response to human voices, but only those dogs that can learn the names of objects for retrieval do so consistently.[2988] The ability of dogs to learn the names of objects and retrieve them has been well studied. Although most animal learning experiments use food rewards, many of the most successful dogs at learning names of objects are rewarded with play. And those dogs are rated as more playful than other dogs of their breed (Border Collie).[2756] Labrador Retrievers, on the other hand, perform better for a food reward than for a ball.[2836] Cognitive traits are heritable.[2702,2760,2796]

Goats, but not sheep, seem to be able to learn by exclusion. Goats and sheep were able to use direct information (presence of food); but in the object choice task, goats rather than sheep were able to use indirect information (i.e., the absence of food) to find a reward.[1673]

Delayed Response Method

The length of time an animal can remember which of three boxes identified by a brief illumination holds the food reward can be measured.[1090] This technique, called the "delayed response method," revealed that a rat could delay its response for 10 seconds; a raccoon, 20 seconds. Children two years old could delay their responses for 25 minutes; dogs, five minutes.[1515] In other experiments, it was found that cats can remember for 6 minutes, adult dogs for 18 minutes, and goats for 30 minutes, although the goats had a more intensive signal to remember than did the other species.[2150] Of two horses tested by Grzimek,[865] one could remember for only 15 seconds, and the other for 60 seconds. Chickens can remember for 15 seconds.[2870] The delayed response time is quite variable; for cats, it varied from 18 seconds to 16 hours, depending on the test and the investigator.[1444]

Horses working memory for the location of obstacles on the ground is as long as 15 minutes. And can remember which of two buckets have been baited with food for up to 20 seconds, but not if they have been stressed by a series of frightening sights and sounds just before the test; in that case, their working memory falls to 8 seconds.[2314]

Maze Learning

Maze learning has been used to assess species differences in learning ability. Dogs learn a double alteration maze better than cats.[1179] In a series of maze tests using the Hebb–Williams maze (in which different configurations are made and in some of which the animal can see the solution, whereas in others it is hidden from view), children made the fewest errors; dogs, cows, goats, and sheep made approximately the same number of errors; pigs and cats made more; and horses made more errors than pigs or cats.[1217,1494]

Episodic Memory

Episodic-like memory requires the hippocampus and involves simultaneous recall of three aspects of a past event – what, where, and when. Pigs exposed to various objects in a different position or a different context (room) would explore them more, indicating that they remembered the object, its position, and where it had been last seen.[1256] Dogs, or at least one dog, could remember in which room one of six toys was.[1168]

The remainder of this chapter deals with our understanding of the learning abilities of domestic animals. See Table 7.2 for a list of the various types of learning that have been demonstrated to occur in domestic animals.

Table 7.2 The types of learning that have been demonstrated in domestic animals.

Pigs	Classical conditioning[1372,1373,1459,1458,1616,1701]
	Avoidance learning[896,1261,2453,2454]
	Maze[896,1217,1657]
	Massed versus spaced trials[1176]
	Operant conditioning[157,144,146,151,142,1261]
	Place preference[528]
	Conditioned anxiety[142]
	Visual discrimination[668,1236,2424]
	Auditory discrimination[1454]
	Reversal learning[636,2424]
	Taste aversion[2511]
Horses	Avoidance learning[877,2364]
	Maze[877,1217,1262,1494]
	Massed versus spaced trials[1991]
	Operant conditioning[1491,1658,2364]
	Visual discrimination[792,795,818]
	Reversal learning[1474]
	Taste aversion[1808,2512]
	Delayed response[2314]
	Long-term memory[904]
	Observational learning[124,133,1273]
	Classical conditioning[1346,1779]
Dogs	Avoidance learning[2149,2171]
	Maze[1179,1217,2066]
	Operant conditioning[1682]

(Continued)

Table 7.2 (Continued)

	Auditory discrimination[604]
	Delayed response[695]
	Observational learning[1839,2138]
	Classical conditioning[637,1779]
Cattle	Avoidance learning[1329,2438]
	Maze[1217]
	Operant conditioning[1180,1617]
	Visual discrimination[793]
	Auditory discrimination[2095,2446]
	Reversal learning[1541]
	Taste aversion[1881,2513]
	Observational learning[2342]
Cats	Avoidance learning[119]
	Maze[1217]
	Operant conditioning[2254]
	Visual discrimination[1704,2510,2511]
	Auditory discrimination[604]
	Delayed response[694,1444]
	Observational learning[413,1152]
Sheep	Classical conditioning[1370,1373]
	Maze[369,575,1217,1371,2025]
	Operant conditioning[149]
	Visual discrimination[140,2517]
	Auditory discrimination[2024–2026]
	Taste aversion[1807,2513]
Goats	Classical conditioning[1372,1373]
	Maze[1217]
	Operant conditioning[1799]
	Visual discrimination[138]
	Taste aversion[592,844,1934]
	Chickens
	Operant conditioning
	Taste aversion

Pigs

Difficulty was encountered in teaching pigs a concept such as "center"; they could choose the middle of three, but not five, doors.[2507]

Pigs have been the subject of many, many learning experiments: appetitive conditioning tasks, aversive conditioning tasks, operant tasks, lever-pressing tasks, spatial and auditory discrimination tasks, barrier tasks, avoidance tasks, choice tasks, spatial tasks, water mazes, Y-mazes, spatial arenas, multi-access mazes, choice tasks, object recognition, social tasks, and awareness tasks.[282,820]

Although season of testing, body weight, and age of dam do not account for variation in avoidance learning, pigs from large litters ran a maze more quickly than pigs from small litters.[2454,2445] Apparently, when the reward for completion of the maze was a return to the company of littermates (social reinstatement), two-month-old pigs learned a much more complicated maze for the same reward.[1134] Social isolation was more severe and the reward of reunion greater when the litter size was greater. Twelve-week-old pigs can learn which way to turn in a T-maze for a chocolate milk reward and learn the reversal.[636] Reversal learning is an example of a learning set – in this case, the ability to learn the rule underlying repeated reversals of a discrimination task and to develop a learning strategy (e.g., win-stay or lose-shift).

Operant Conditioning

Pigs will perform an operant response for some types of sensory reinforcement such as light[156] and brain stimulation.[150] Older pigs (40 to 150 days) learn to avoid shock less well than do younger pigs (three weeks) (Figure 9.6A and 9.6B).[1261]

Operant conditioning of pigs is used for a variety of purposes: on the farm, in animal acts, and in the laboratory. Feeders with hinged covers that the pig must open with its snout are a good example of a very simple operant response that pigs learn rapidly, and they can learn to use electronic feeding stations. In a more complicated system, pigs can be taught to approach whichever feeder emits a certain sound that indicates that food is available for that pig alone. Such a system reduces competition at a feeder and also reduces fearfulness.[1875] Sows in the lower third of the hierarchy learn the response – they approach the feeder when a certain sound is heard – less well than dominant ones.[1454]

Pigs prefer the place where they received a reinforcement after a delay in comparison to a place where they received an immediate reward. This conditioned place preference indicates that pigs find anticipation of the reinforcement rewarding.[528]

Consideration of the anatomy and normal behavior patterns of pigs indicates that it would be much easier to teach them to manipulate their environment with their snout than with their feet. Consequently, pigs have been taught to push a panel with their snouts for either a food reward or for heat in a cold environment.[142,144] To measure a pig's motivation for various sweet solutions, a progressive ratio technique has been used.[1202]

A conditioned anxiety reaction can be produced in pigs by training them to press a panel for a food reward and by then adding a tone that signals a shock if the animal presses the panel.[142] The pigs learn to inhibit panel pressing; although experimental neurosis is sometimes produced,[491] tranquilizers do not reduce the inhibition of responding.[512] Conditioned anxiety does lower heart rate[511] and increase endogenous levels of corticosteroids, but the rise in corticosteroids is not as great as when the pigs are exposed to cold or chased with a goad.[143,]

Visual Discrimination

Pigs are better at spatial (right versus left) than at visual discrimination tasks and must be taught to make visual discriminations before 20 weeks of age.[1236] A discrimination task can be used to show that pigs do have color vision.[2424] Pigs have difficulty in reversal learning of either a visual or spatial discrimination; they abandon the original correct response, but their performance remains at chance levels for many trials. Overtraining, or training carried beyond criterion on the first task, does improve reversal learning.[2424]

Dogs

There appears to be a general intelligence factor (g) in dogs as in people. Border collies who did well in detour tests did well in

following human pointing and in choosing a larger amount of food in a two choice test.[79] Dogs understand contact causality. When a ball rolls toward another ball, but does not contact it (violated the dog's expectations) the dog's pupils were larger in the no-contact condition and they looked longer at the object initiating the launch after the no-contact event compared to the contact event. Dogs understand contact causality.[3022]

Navigation

Dogs usually relate environmental information to their own body in space (egocentric) rather than by the relation of two environmental objects to one another (allocentric).[695] They seem to be able to determine the direction in which they saw an object disappear rather than the distance. Dogs can find their way back to a target when deprived of visual and auditory cues, presumably by direction and speed of travel on the outward journey.

They can be taught to use landmarks – for example, a wooden rod demarks which cup holds the food, but as soon as the landmark is moved away from the cup, performance falls.[1583] This type of learning is called "allocentric" (two things relative to each other) as opposed to "egocentric" (things relative to the dog) learning, and it involves the parietal not the frontal cortex as egocentric learning does.[696]

Dogs have difficulty in generalizing from one situation to the next. For example, if a target is inside a V-shaped barrier, they have more trouble reaching it than if the target is outside.[1579] Dogs do not do well in delayed gratification tests (wait longer for a better reward).[2679] When trying to solve a detour problem, low-arousal assistance dogs showed the most inhibition in a detour task when humans eagerly encouraged them, while more highly aroused pet dogs performed worse on the same task with strong encouragement.[2670,2671]

Model Rival Learning

Dogs can learn by the model rival technique in which the trainer and a colleague call the object by name and ask one another for it. This method was used to train the African grey parrot Alex a large number of words and colors. The dogs may actually be responding to stimulus enhancement because they will retrieve an object if they watched a person handle it just before they are asked to retrieve it.[464] Because social facilitation is strong in dogs, slow dogs tend to run faster with another dog than they do alone.[2369] This is in contrast to cats, who run slower for a food reward in the presence of another cat.

Global versus Local Cues

Dogs learn global not local cues. The test involved shapes formed by smaller shapes. Examples were a circle formed of small circles, an X formed by small X's, and a heart formed by small hearts. Dogs would choose an X even if it was composed of small hearts.

Incidental Memory

If dogs are allowed to inspect four bowls but eat from only two, they will visit the bowls from which they have not eaten the next time they have the opportunity.[765] This is called "incidental memory."

Effects of Age

Puppies can learn *in utero*. If their mothers were fed anise-flavored food, their day old puppies would approach that odor, rather than that of water.[3028] Dogs improve in their ability to make a delayed response. If puppies were trained for 13 days beginning at 4, 8, 12, or 16 weeks, all increased the interval over which they could remember during testing, but the 4-week-old puppies could never remember longer than 10 seconds, whereas the 12-week-old dogs could remember for 50 seconds. Sixteen-week-old

dogs did not perform as well; they made many errors, possibly because they lack inhibition at that age.[729] In another study, puppies less than a week old could be conditioned to suck more from a nipple when milk was the reward and to inhibit sucking when a quinine solution was the aversive stimulus.[2171] Earlier studies had found that puppies less than 18 days old could not be conditioned.[770] Puppies less than a week old can learn to escape from a cold stream of air and will even move from a comfortable, carpeted surface to a hard, cold one to do so (Figure 7.6).[2172] Puppies less than two weeks old could also learn to choose a wire or cloth model that contained a nipple for a milk reward if given five tests a day, two hours apart.

Dogs (retrievers) at eight months were less likely to obey a command from their trainer (but not from a stranger) than they were before or after that age. Bitches that showed more attachment to humans came into heat sooner.[2653] Both dogs and horses that are more interested in interacting with people are slower to solve problems.[2276,2853] Dogs' selective attention and sensorimotor abilities peak in middle age (3–6 years).[3023]

Older dogs – senior dogs – are significantly impaired in accuracy and reaction time compared to younger animals in a visual search task with distracters.[2987] In a social version of this task, the owner and a stranger simultaneously presented to the dog, forcing it to be selective as to whom it observed. Older dogs discriminated between the owner and the stranger to a lesser extent, because they oriented longer to the stranger compared to adult dogs.[2892] As dogs age they take longer to find food on the floor and to orient to a stimulus like a toy and they look at it for a shorter period of times indicating inattention, although these changes can be ameliorated by training.[3058] Older dogs can exhibit serious cognitive issues changing in sociability, orientation, activity, house breaking, and sleep patterns.[1037,1302]

Training is easier if the innate responses of dogs to auditory signals are used. Dogs will

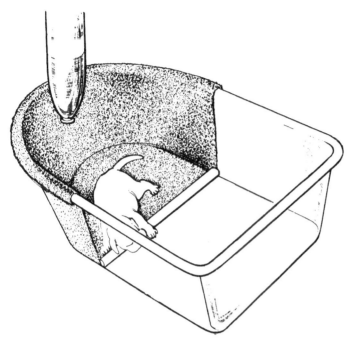

Figure 7.6 Learning in neonatal dogs. The puppy learns to avoid the textured side, for which puppies have an innate preference, if that side is associated with a blast of air.

increase their activity to high, rising tones and inhibit it to low, falling tones, and this is reflected in the signals shepherds use to signal their dogs.[1498,1499] This type of learning is another form of allocentric learning, involving the parietal not the frontal cortex as egocentric learning does.[696]

Inhibiting oneself requires energy, even though the dog does not move when asked to stay. After staying for 10 minutes, dogs would not attempt to retrieve food from a tug-a-jug toy for very long, but this effect disappeared if the dogs were allowed a sugary drink after staying and before the toy was presented.[1587] Dogs can exchange a low-value treat for a higher value or larger treat and are willing to delay – holding the treat in their mouths for almost a minute.[1345] Spatial discounting is a test in which two rewards are present – one large and one small. Initially the dog will choose the larger reward, but as the large reward is moved farther away the dog may choose the closer, albeit smaller, reward. More

impulsive dog traveled shorter distances to gain the larger reward.[2668]

Military dogs are trained fairly forcefully with leash corrections. Pats were the only rewards, but those rewarded dogs perform better than those only corrected. Perhaps they were rewarded more because they performed better, but it does indicate the value of rewards.[949]

Geriatric Cognitive Dysfunction

Dogs' selective attention and sensorimotor abilities peak in middle age.[3023] Old dogs may have physical problems such as deafness, cataracts, heart disease, or arthritis, but many otherwise healthy old dogs exhibit behavioral changes. Old dogs are also slower to learn new things. Older dogs have learning deficits that can be measured in objective laboratory tests or in simple two-session place-learning tests.[1661] At least some of these changes may be due to oxidative damage to the central nervous

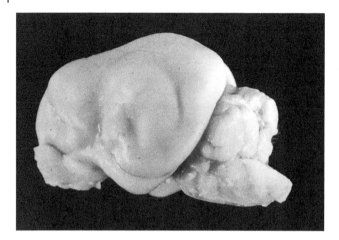

Figure 7.7 An example of a learning deficit associated with organic disease of the central nervous system, showing the brain of a Lhasa Apso that suffered from lissencephaly and could learn neither bowel nor bladder control.

system (Figure 7.7). Beta amyloid plagues are present in some, but not all, dogs with cognitive dysfunction. Owners complain that old dogs are less affectionate, are less active, lose housetraining, pace and vocalize at night, and may seem disoriented (getting lost in their own yard). Old dogs may be euthanized because of the age-associated behavior changes, especially if the owner's sleep is interrupted. The age of onset varies between 7 and 11 years, depending on the speed of aging in the particular breed.[2216]

Causality is the relationship between causes and effects. Dogs understand contact causality. When a ball rolls toward another ball, but does not contact it (violated the dog's expectations) the dogs' pupils were larger in the no-contact condition and they looked longer at the object initiating the launch after the no-contact event compared to the contact event.[3022]

Cattle

There have been few studies of learning ability in cattle, and most of those published described attempts to increase production or reduce labor on the farm.

Operant Conditioning

Cows have been trained to come in to be milked when an automobile horn connected to a timer and the electric fence was sounded.[1215] Cows were also trained to come into the barn in a given order, but the cattle reverted to their original order, probably based on dominance, as soon as the trainer was absent.[22]

Cattle have been conditioned to eat in response to an auditory stimulus and then attempted, unsuccessfully, to increase food intake when they were free-feeding by playing the auditory stimulus.[1725] Dairy cows have also been taught to press a handle with their muzzles to obtain food and to make right- and left-handle discriminations. The most difficult task was to accustom the cows to lifting, rather than lowering, their heads for food because they were accustomed to eating from the floor.[2437] See Figure 7.8 for an example of taste aversion learning.

Cattle can be clicker trained to touch a target, but teaching the same animals to eliminate on concrete rather than their bedding using a clicker was not successful.[2435]

Conditioned Avoidance

Many farmers teach their cattle to defecate in the gutter behind their stanchions rather than on the stall floor by running an electrified wire (cattle trainer) that shocks the cow whenever it arches its back to eliminate in the wrong place. Because cattle defecate seven times a day, the cows learn quickly, and the average fecal output of 60–80 pounds is deposited in the gutter.

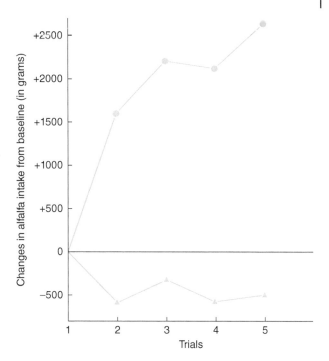

Figure 7.8 Taste aversion learning in cattle. On day 1 (trial 1), the experimental cows (circles) were offered alfalfa pellets. After they had eaten the food, apomorphine was injected. The control cows (triangles) were injected with 0.9% NaCl. Four days later (trial 2), when all cows were offered alfalfa pellets, the cows that had been treated with apomorphine ate almost nothing, whereas the controls ate more than they had initially. The experimental cows learned to avoid a feed associated with illness. *Source:* Zahorik (1990).[2513] Reproduced with permission of Elsevier.

Cattle sometimes receive shocks through milking machines. Cows were taught to press a bar for food in order to determine how large a shock had to be before it disrupted a cow's feeding and other behaviors. They stopped bar pressing when a shock greater than 7 mA was applied to one teat or 6 mA to all four teats.[2438] This type of conditioning can be used to determine what is painful to cattle.

A practical application of bovine avoidance learning is to train cattle to respect electric fences by confining them in a pen with a sturdy fence beyond the electrified wire. The cattle will then respect an electric fence even in a new environment and will not be in danger of breaking through it.[1503]

Effects of Age

When the ability to remember the location of a feeder was tested over a period of five days, heifers learned more quickly than older cattle, but cows after the second calving remembered the location best when tested six weeks later. In both tests, primiparous cows were intermediate in performance.[1258] Stress appears to enhance learning because newly weaned calves learned a T-maze more quickly than those weaned a month before training.[1343] Cattle can learn to shift from one arm of a maze to another (win-and-shift strategy) if they ate all the food in the initial arm on the previous trial.[1039] It is interesting to compare the behavior of cattle in the very artificial maze situation to that on pasture. When tested in a pasture with high-quality forage, they display the win-and-shift strategy, but on a poorer pasture, they display the win-and-stay strategy.

From a practical point of view, cows can be "trained" to use cubicles to rest as adults by providing experience with cubicles as heifers.[1718] Cows can learn to activate a robotic milking machine for "on demand" relief of mammary pressure. They are variable in their requests to be milked but averaged three times a day.[2477] No milking was done from midnight to 6 a.m., and the system was timed so that a cow could not be milked more frequently than every four hours.

Calves that were more exploratory, but not those that were more fearful, were slower to learn a complicated operant conditioning task in which they had to determine which panel, when pressed, led to a larger hay reward.[2402] Calves living in groups learned a reversal task better than those housed alone.[783,1541]

Sheep

Sheep can be classically conditioned to flex a front leg in response to a ticking metronome that had been paired with an electric shock, although the small ruminants did not learn as quickly as pigs or dogs.[1372] Sheep can learn simple mazes[1371] and will run a maze to be reunited with a cohabitant, whether the animal was another sheep or a dog.[369] The less they interact with other flock members the better they are at solving problems.[3054]

Sheep can learn to make fairly fine visual discriminations between different shapes and different orientations of the same shape. For example, they can learn to discriminate not only between a circle and a square but also between a triangle pointing right and one pointing left.[140]

Operant conditioning techniques have been used to study thermoregulatory behavior. The sheep learned to activate a heat lamp by sticking their muzzles through a slit to break a photoelectric beam. Unshorn sheep did not learn to turn on the heat at 5 °C (41 °F), but shorn sheep, deprived of the thermal insulation of their fleece, did.[149] Sheep have also learned to press a bar for reward in response to a tone signal and to refrain from pressing the bar for 30 seconds after each reinforcement.[2024–2026]

Sheep will learn to move faster through yards (chutes and alleys) with experience and will do better than inexperienced sheep months later, but training in moving a different way through the same yard is worse than no training.[1094] Apparently, the sheep have to forget their previous experience. Giving the sheep a food reward at the end of a yard is an efficient way of speeding their movement, although it will not help if an unpleasant experience, such as restraint, is also associated with the same movement.[1095] Barking and the sight of a dog will slow sheep performance in a maze, but only on the first day; apparently, they habituate quickly.[575] The ability of sheep to perform operantly conditioned tasks has been used in experiments with sodium-deficient sheep.[2139] These sheep learn to press a bar for sodium bicarbonate in proportion to their sodium deficiency. Sheep can also learn to discriminate which of five feeders contain food.[2517] Sheep have the ability to form spatial memory so that they can locate food faster after several days of experience. The sheep appeared to learn better when the resource density is low. When it is high, the sheep need not try to relocate the food, but rather find another location.[1959]

Goats

Goats can be classically conditioned to flex a foreleg when a tone signals shock (Figure 7.1). They can learn to press a bar for the reward of electrical stimulation of their brain[1799] and press more than 1,000 times in 45 minutes for a food reward.[2100] Goats can learn to make fairly fine visual discriminations between different shapes and different orientations of the same shape. For example, they can learn to discriminate not only between a circle and a square but also between a triangle pointing right and one pointing left.[139] Their learning rate improves with additional discrimination tasks, indicating that these ruminants form a learning set, or can learn to learn.[1303] In addition, goats can learn categories (filled versus unfilled symbols).[1573]

Goats can learn which food is associated with illness – which food makes them sick; but if both foods and illness occur on the same meal, the goat will respond by eating a little of each food.[592] Learning a conditioned taste aversion has been used to prevent goats from eating *Leucaena*, a palatable but poisonous plant that is a goitrogen and a depilatory.[844]

Unfortunately, conditioned safety, taught by feeding increasing percentages of sagebrush in the diet before goats were released on the range, did not cause the goats to eat any more sagebrush than inexperienced goats when they were free to select a diet on the range.[1934]

Horses

The horse is, like the dog, a species that is useful to humans only if trained. In fact, despite their aesthetic value, few horses are kept as pets unless they can be ridden or driven. Myriad volumes have been written on the training of horses, and it is appropriate to mention only a few of the basic principles. Nicol[1690] has reviewed the subject.

Horses and probably most animals learn better if a different reward is given for each separate task. For example, a sugar cube is given for taking the bit and an apple slice for standing in harness. A more complicated example was teaching horse to choose blue when it was on the right for a carrot piece and yellow when it was on left for a pellet.[2889]

It is easiest to teach a horse a natural response; consequently, horses can be trained to race at a very early age. Two-year-old horses on the racetrack are very common; a horse under age five in a dressage class is a rarity. Most horse training is based on negative reinforcement: applying an aversive stimulus until the horse performs the response. The best approach to horse training is to try to substitute conditioned stimuli (a voice command or subtle pressure from the rider's legs) for unconditioned stimuli (the painful flick of a whip). In this manner, neck reining can replace direct reining. When punishment must be given, it should be applied as soon as possible after the misdeed. A slap on the pony's muzzle 30 seconds after it has nipped will only serve to make it head shy; a blow one second after the nip may inhibit further aggression.

Round-pen training or natural horsemanship has become very popular. It is another form of negative reinforcement in that the horse is chased and learns that if he does not move in response to subtle movements of the trainer's body, a more aversive stimulus such as the lash of a whip may occur. The response of running away seems to be avoidance of a predator. The reward for the horse is not having to move quickly. The trainer must keep behind the horse's withers in order to stimulate it to run and can move ahead of the shoulder to slow the horse. Horses can be taught quickly to reverse to the outside or to the inside. An untrained animal can learn to tolerate a saddle and then a rider in one day. Pastured horses learn in a round pen more quickly than stabled ones, perhaps because they are more respectful of humans when they do not see them daily. When the trainer stops driving it forward, many horses will approach the trainer, especially if he or she avoids eye contact and backs slowly away from the horse. This is the phenomenon of "Join up."[1273] There has been a study of the relative value of this type of training over conventional training. In a modification of the round-pen technique, ponies were trained in a pen with no restraint until they could be haltered, groomed, and allowed their hooves to be examined. It took four times longer to train horses using this method than by training ponies in a stall, restrained on a lead line, but the ponies were more likely to approach people and had a lower heart rate when groomed than the more forcibly trained horses.[160] When comparing "natural horsemanship" to traditional training, which included some food rewards, natural horsemanship horses approached a human sooner, but both groups were less emotional after four 50-minute sessions of training.[776] See the "Types of Learning" section in the introduction to this chapter for examples using horses.

The basis of most horse training is negative reinforcement, but positive reinforcement also can be used to train horses to lead and to load. When ponies were taught to back up for positive reinforcement (carrot-flavored treat) or negative reinforcement (a whip waved in front of them), the positively reinforced ponies not only learned more quickly but also were more likely to approach people five months later.[2027] The methods are equally successful in training, but the positively rewarded ponies appear more eager and interested in the trainer, tenser,[1114] but no more optimistic than negatively reinforced horses.[327] Horses trained to trailer load with positive reinforcement learned the task faster and remember it better than horses trained with negative reinforcement.[2705] Horses that received positive reinforcement training, in addition to their regular negative reinforcement, were friendlier to strangers than those trained using negative reinforcement only.[2848] Horses classified as more fearful and active performed better on an avoidance task using negative reinforcement, whereas horses classified as more sensitive and less fearful performed better on a backward–forward leading task using positive and negative reinforcement.[2840] More fearful horses, however, performed poorly when tested on the negative reinforcement task in a novel environment.[2695] Less reactive or fearful horses show greater cognitive flexibility.[2748] Horses who showed more affiliative human-directed behaviors (touching the trainer) during training had an increase in salivary oxytocin while horses who showed more behavioral indicators of discomfort during training had a decrease in salivary oxytocin.[2912] Horses show reduced fear of a novel object in the presence of the trainer after training whether negative or positive reinforcement was used.[2782] A horse's response to a novel object varies with whether he has had multiple owners, and handlers and short relationships.[2853] Horses appear to "miss" people more when separated if they have been trained using positive rather than negative reinforcement.[2857]

Some people will not use positive reinforcement because they think it will lead to nipping, but giving a horse food by hand is significantly associated with investigative behaviors, licking hands, and searching but not nipping hands or clothing.[1018] Furthermore, food is a better reward than scratching the withers in that the horse learns to stand sooner.[1945]

Operant Conditioning

A single horse was taught to make a typical operant response, pushing a lever with its muzzle for a half cup of grain. After the horse had been shaped using continuous reinforcement, the schedule was changed to 3 and then to 11 responses for every reinforcement. The horse increased its rate of responding as the FR (fixed ratio of responses per reward) increased. When a fixed-interval schedule was imposed, the horse at first "sulked" by refusing to turn toward the lever, but later responded with the scalloped pattern typical of laboratory rodents on fixed-interval schedules.[944,1658]

In fact, when a larger number of horses were tested, most horses learned not to respond at all until the last quarter of the fixed interval.[465] Operant conditioning is used to evaluate drugs in equine pharmacology.[2489] The horses are usually conditioned to break a beam with their head for a food reward. The rate of responding will be lower if a depressant, such as acepromazine, is given and will be higher if a stimulant, such as methylphenidate (Ritalin), is administered. The action of an unknown drug can be tested by comparing its effect on responses to that of other, known drugs. Using this technique, one can determine whether the horse is being stimulated or depressed, that is, whether the horse's performance is being improved or worsened. Operant conditioning has also been used to measure environment preferences of horses for such things as food and exercise.[627,1051,1334] A common misbehavior of horses is pawing while restrained by crossties. Differential reinforcement of another behavior has been used to reduce pawing of crosstied horses.[2750]

Horses can learn matching to sample, even when the task is to touch a button under the correct symbol rather than the symbol itself, but ponies did not remember a matching to sample or a quantity discrimination task (3 vs 2) after one year, even though they remembered how to enter the testing stall and that panels has to be pressed.[779,2757]

A secondary reinforcer (click) did not improve learning or retention of a visual discrimination task, but was very effective in improving the learning rate of a second visual discrimination task.[2455]

Horse that exhibit stereotypies (see Chapter 3) such as weaving and cribbing are slower to learn the task of lifting the cover of a feed box, and a greater proportion never learn.[944] There also appear to be other learning deficits in cribbing horses. They do not learn to choose a reward that will be delivered more quickly (10 vs. 20 seconds), but this may be because they pause to crib for 10 seconds or more between rewards.[1767]

Fearful horses do not learn an operant conditioning task as well as non-fearful ones, but a calm companion improves their performance.[1306] The importance of a calm companion is emphasized because training two young horses to tolerate separation from their group is no more efficient than training one horse alone.[934]

Visual Discrimination

Fat horses make more errors on a simple visual discrimination test than do thin ones, which is probably a result of poorer motivation for the food reward rather than intellectual deficit.[1489] Male horses have superior visual-spatial ability.[1655]

Horses seem to be able to learn spatial (left–right or one of three positions in a row) discriminations better than visual discriminations (patterns on buckets or light on or off).[1040,1474] Horses can remember 10 years later which of a pair of visual stimuli was rewarded, and one horse could remember the concept of larger (the larger of two novel symbols was correct) 7 years later; see Figure 7.9.[904] They can also learn to recognize three-dimensional objects no matter what their orientation.[903] Despite the persistent rumor that horses cannot remember something learned with the right

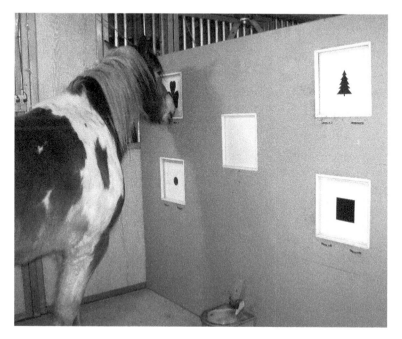

Figure 7.9   A horse demonstrating that he understood the concept of larger by choosing the largest symbol seven years after he was originally taught the discrimination. *Source:* Hanggi (2009).[904] Reproduced with permission of Springer.

eye when the object is presented to the other eye, they are perfectly capable of interocular transfer.[902]

There was no correlation between avoidance learning (negative reinforcement) and learning for positive reinforcement in a study of Warmbloods.[2364] Horses will work for food rewards and their performance on learning tasks such as clicker training and two-choice tests does not vary with their appetite.[2916] Horses that had been operantly conditioned to push one of two levers for a food reward when a particular stimulus (a striped piece of wood) indicated which lever was associated with the reward were no quicker than naïve horses in learning that the same stimulus indicated the correct side of a maze.[1491]

When young horses were trained to choose a particular patterned bucket in a particular location, they tended to choose the location rather than the pattern when the two were in conflict.[1040] Horse can learn that choosing one side of a maze will lead to being ridden in the Rollkur (extreme neck flexion) posture, whereas the other side leads to being ridden in an ordinary bridle. They avoid the Rollkur.[2372] Horses can solve barrier problems and learn to open a chest with their noses when a human demonstrates the task (but not if a horse demonstrates), and the offspring of some stallions are more successful than the offspring of others.[2484] Horses can also learn to form taste aversions,[2513] and practical use of this has been made to teach horses not to eat locoweed (*Oxytropis sericea*).[1808] But even when hay is fed ad libitum horses do not sort poisonous *Senecio* from harmless hay, probably because the toxin does not act immediately.[2993] Horses do not appear to innately or experientially reject the high colchicine plant meadow saffron (*Colchicum autumnale* L.).[2894]

Long-term memory seems to be excellent for simple tasks. Horses trained to back on command for a food reward were perfect in their responses 22 months later, as were horses trained to avoid a puff of air by crossing a small barrier. The horses differed in their response to

extinction; fearful horses were more resistant to extinction of the backing task, whereas less touch-sensitive horses were less likely to extinguish the task of avoiding a puff of air.[2314]

Influences on Learning

Environment

There was no effect of bedding or light or spatial learning, even though sleep was affected.[2769] The presence of another horse is important. Naïve horses grouped with a habituated horse showed reduced fear reactions in response to a startling stimulus (umbrella opening) and this method can be used to reduce reactivity in young horses by using a habituated adult horse to help attenuate fear reactions.[2955]

Personality

Horses classified as more fearful and reactive performed better on an avoidance task using negative reinforcement, whereas horses classified as more sensitive and less fearful performed better on a backward–forward leading task using positive and negative reinforcement.[2840] More anxious horses were reported to complete a test utilizing negative reinforcement more quickly than their counterparts.[3061] More fearful horses, however, performed poorly when tested on the negative reinforcement task in a novel environment; less reactive or fearful horses showed greater cognitive flexibility.[2748,2696]

Effects of Handling

Early handling (imprint training) does not influence trainability, but extensive handling for the first six weeks is more beneficial than the same amount of handling later in the foal's life.[1445,1446] A moderate, but not an extensive, amount of handling improves a young horse's performance in a maze-learning test.[969] Perhaps the most useful information is that handlers can predict trainability after working with a horse for 10 days, and although another interpretation might be that handlers determine performance, these scores are correlated with trainability under saddle as judged by different people. The more emotional a horse, the poorer its learning ability.[699,969,1439] The more a horse reacts to a frightening stimulus, the poorer its performance in a novel environment, but not in a familiar one.[421]

Effects of Age

Weanling foals learn to make the correct choice in the maze with fewer errors than adult mares, but the latter move faster, so despite entering the wrong side, they reach the food just as quickly as the foals. Orphan foals do not appear handicapped in their learning ability but move even more cautiously than normally reared foals.[1058]

Frequency of Training

In general, pauses between training bouts result in faster learning, apparently because the biochemical processes involved in learning do not happen instantaneously. Learning must consolidate – a process that involves formation of new protein in the relevant part of the brain. The problem is that, although the horse spends less time in training to learn optimally, more days have elapsed. Nevertheless, as demonstrated with avoidance learning, spacing training bouts is more efficient than crowding them into a few days.[1991] When given 17 days of training to lead, to lunge, to be driven, and to be ridden, yearling Thoroughbred horses that were trained every day learned better – with fewer errors – than those trained for four days, then given a three-day break, then trained for four days, and so on.[1291] How many repetitions of a task should each training session contain? Sixteen seems to be the optimum when negative reinforcement is used.[1492] When training foals to lead and stop, incorporating a rest day between daily 15 minute sessions improved recall.[2792,2856]

Donkeys

Donkeys' cognitive abilities are heritable.[2901] Donkeys were taught to cross an oil cloth for a food reward plus negative reinforcement (pulling on the lead rope). The success rate was 0.1–0.38 heritable.[3065] When donkeys were operantly conditioned to press a colored (green) button for a food reward, male and older donkeys did worse than females and younger donkeys.[2711,2975]

Mules are superior to both ponies and donkeys in visual discrimination learning. They learn more pairs and are more accurate.[1867] Mules are also better than either of their parental species in solving detour problems; they do not persevere as both dogs and horses do at trying a previously correct location.[1740]

Cats

Whereas dogs were the animals used in the earliest experiments on classical conditioning,[1779] cats were studied in the first experiment in operant conditioning.[2254] Cats learned to operate on their environment in order to escape from puzzle boxes.[2255] Cats can be classically conditioned.[913]

Discrimination

The cat's ability to learn discrimination has been used to great advantage by psychophysicists in studying vision. For example, color vision can be studied by teaching cats to discriminate between two symbols and then to discriminate between the symbols when they differ only in hue. Cats can, in fact, make this discrimination but only after 1400 trials; they do have color vision, as both behavioral (see Chapter 1) tests[2074] and electrophysiological studies attest.[437,2074] The color stimulus must be large (i.e., a big object) before the cat is able to make use of the hue.

A two-cue discrimination was used to measure the salience or importance of various sensory modalities to cats. The animals were taught to feed from one of two feeders, which emitted a buzzing noise and a flashing light associated with it. Later, one feeder flashed and the other buzzed; the cats went to the flashing feeder, indicating that auditory stimuli are less important to cats than visual ones when both are carefully equated for intensity.[1704] Cats can learn a task in which they must choose one of two pairs of visual and olfactory stimuli. When presented with mismatched combinations of visual and olfactory stimuli, they chose the visual one.[1482]

Cats can predict the presence of an unseen object from hearing the noise; it makes a good strategy for a predator.[2218]

Navigation

Cats can learn position discrimination in a T-maze and its reversal.[2099] A landmark discrimination learning test was used to assess visual-spatial learning. The egocentric spatial ability task involved determining whether the cat preferred to eat from the left or right of two wells. Once that was determined, the cat was presented with three wells – right, left, and center – and rewarded for choosing the side the cat originally preferred. In the reversal phase of the task, the opposite side was rewarded. Reversal learning provides a measure of executive function. The third test protocol examined performance on a size discrimination and reversal learning task. Then the cats had to learn to choose the cup next to which the landmark, a yellow rod, stood. Once the cat learned to choose that cup, the landmark was moved somewhat farther away.

Rewards

Unlike dogs, cats will not usually perform in order to be reunited with the experimenter. They will perform for food rewards. Feline finickiness can even interfere with the reward value of food, but in general, cats will work harder for food rewards if the experimenter is the one who feeds them in their home cages. It is even more difficult to teach a cat to press a bar for water; water must be withheld for a week.[130] Kittens will learn more quickly when the reward is freedom to explore a room than when the reward is food.[1582] Kittens learn to make a light-dark discrimination more slowly than do 35-day-old cats.[443]

Discrimination

Both cats and dogs can be taught to make auditory discriminations and to lift the lid on a food pan when one pitch but not another is sounded. When the two sounds are too close to be discriminated (less than one-third or one-quarter tone apart), the animals exhibit experimental neurosis. The cats respond to all tones as positive, and most dogs refuse to respond to any.[587] Early visual experience can influence a cat's performance on visual discrimination tasks.[2510,2511]

Cats cannot remember the location of a disappearing object very well, with a rapid decline between 0 and 10 seconds, despite visual cues; whereas dogs show a gradual decline between 0 and 30 seconds. Nevertheless, the cats' accuracy remained above chance at 60 seconds.[694]

Effects of Age

Old cats (10–23 years) do not learn as well as younger cats. They are most apt to fail to learn, even after 1,000 trials, if the CS begins too far in advance of the unconditioned stimulus; but they did well in a spatial learning task.[919]

Cats do show changes in behavior when older than their late teens. The signs are a decrease in activity; an increase in vocalization, especially at night; and house soiling, in particular defecation, outside the box. These changes may be a result of the development of amyloid plagues.[959]

Illness or age affects feline learning abilities. Cats infected with Feline immunodeficiency virus (FIV) make more errors on a learning test.[2175] FIV-infected cats showed a higher activity level and more distractibility than healthy cats. They explored more, but were more likely to return to previously baited cups, and they had more difficulty traversing a narrow plank.

A final note on performance of cats: whereas dogs tend to run faster when competing with other dogs, cats do not; in fact, they may refuse to compete for food in a runway situation.[2476]

Chickens

Chickens can be classically conditioned; for example, they will avoid a light they have associated with a puff of air but some strains (Rhode Island Red) were better than others (Leghorn).[2961] The species is also capable of complex learning tasks.[2757,2870] Chickens can be easily operantly conditioned and are often used to teach "Clicker training" to naïve students. They can learn mazes, form association, and make visual discrimination.[2870] They use local more than distal cues.[2740] They are able to anticipate differentially a positive, neutral and negative event announced by different sound cues.[3045] When experiencing an unexpected downshift in reward, chickens' food consumption decreased and heart rate increased immediately after the downshift.[2707] Domesticated chickens (Leghorns) can learn by observation to peck at a puzzle box feeder faster than the ancestral Jungle fowl.[2960] In another study, domestic hens of high social status were found to be more salient demonstrators.[2908] Chickens with fractured keel bones learn to associate an environment where they received a pain killer (buprenorphine) from an environment where they received saline.[2900] Chickens do seem to be poor at detour problems even with repeated experience. An excellent film on learning abilities of chickens is the film *Stimulus Response* by Christine Nicol, Association for the Study of Animal Behaviour (Great Britain).

8

Ingestive Behavior: Food and Water Intake

Introduction

General

Animals typically show a growth curve that includes a short, dynamic phase in which weight gain per day is large and a much longer, static phase in which there are no major gains or losses in weight but rather oscillation around a mean or set point of body weight. Most domestic animals grow rapidly for several months or the first year following birth, and then plateau at a mature body weight.

Animals treated by veterinarians fall into two general categories: either food- and/or fiber-producing animals, or companion animals. The problems of ingestive behavior of animals differ from category to category. Animals used for human food rarely survive much beyond the dynamic phase of weight gain. The objective of the producers and the veterinarians who advise them is to maximize weight gain per unit of time. The dairy cow presents a special case. She must be a good producer of milk and, therefore, must increase her food intake, yet she should route that increased energy intake, not to body fat, but to milk production.

A quite different problem is presented in some companion species, especially household pets and horses. In a semi-naturalistic setting, such as a pasture, a horse can eat *ad libitum*, but when presented with an energy-rich concentrate diet, which it would not have encountered in the wild, the horse may overeat. Acute problems such as colic or laminitis (founder) may result. Chronically, with a simple shift upward in body weight, obesity or metabolic syndrome may result. Dogs and cats face a similar problem. They can maintain their body weights on relatively unpalatable, dry-chow diets but may succumb to obesity or digestive upsets when offered a highly palatable diet *ad libitum*.

The physiology of the controls of food and fluid intake has been studied extensively by such diverse scientific groups as nutritionists, physiologists, animal scientists, and psychologists. Knowledge of the physiological mechanisms involved in hunger and satiety will enable us to stimulate intake for maximum yield or to control body weight without inducing hunger in an animal that tends toward obesity. The physiology of hunger is reviewed here, using the pig as an example; next to the laboratory rat, the domestic pig has been more thoroughly studied in this regard than any other animal. What is known about ingestive behavior in other species is then discussed, and the unique control of food intake in ruminants is described.

The central nervous system controls of feeding are complex. Neuropeptide Y (NPY) and agouti-related protein (ARP) stimulate

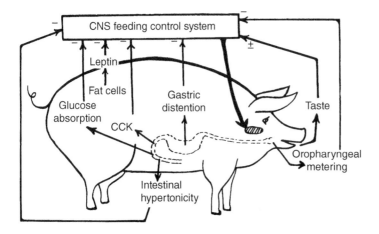

Figure 8.1   Integration of physiological factors that stimulate and depress food intake in the brain. *Source:* Courtesy of Dr. T. Richard Houpt.

feeding, whereas cocaine- and amphetamine-related transcript (CART) and melanocyte-stimulating hormone (MSH) suppress feeding by their actions in the hypothalamus. From the molecular perspective, the neuropeptide orexin-A (OX-A) promotes wakefulness, α-MSH promotes satiety, and the endocannabinoid 2-arachidonoylglycerol (2-AG) promotes appetite.[2603] A deletion in the POMC gene is associated with obesity in Labradors Retrievers.[2942]

Consideration must also be given to the mechanism by which these influences are integrated, in order that animals not only survive but also maintain an optimal and nearly constant body weight. The question is how the animal "knows" that it is becoming fatter. There is an obese strain of mice (obob) that differs from lean controls (Ob_) in one gene. The product of the gene produced by the fat cells of normal mice is formally termed "ob protein," but popularly called "leptin." Leptin is carried in the blood to the brain, and as a result, feeding signals are inhibited (NPY and ARP) and food intake decreases. In addition, the sympathetic nervous system is stimulated, with resultant lipolysis, via ß-adrenergic receptors. In this way, less food is taken in and more fat is broken down, thus decreasing fat stores. Advantage has already been taken of ß-adrenergic effects on fat stores. Pigs are fed ß-adrenergic drugs such as clenbuterol to decrease fat deposition, thus sparing calories for lean meat, that is, muscle growth (see Figure 8.1), but they tend to be more aggressive and nervous than untreated pigs. Another system is that of PYY, a peptide released from intestinal cells when ingested fat enters the cells, suppressing feeding.

Finally, feeding – or, rather, reduced or absent feeding – is one of the clearest signs of illness in animals.[2399] One of the first signs of illness is lack of appetite (see Figure 8.2). For example, pigs infected with porcine reproductive and respiratory syndrome virus (PRRSV) reduced the time spent on eating and food intake while lying more often in ventral recumbency.[643] This lack of appetite or anorexia is caused by cytokines, which are polypeptides produced by one cell that influence other cell factors. Cytokines such as interleukin-1 (IL1) can reduce food intake and rumination in goats without producing fever.[2328]

Control of Food Intake in Pigs

Meal Patterns

Pigs are essentially diurnal animals; therefore, most feeding takes place during the day.[111] Feeding behavior is a circadian rhythm modified by environmental temperature. Pigs avoid eating when daily temperatures are highest,

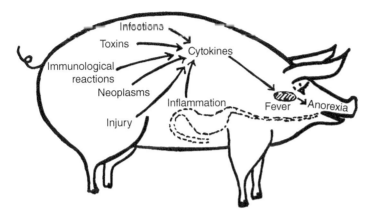

Figure 8.2 Integration of pathological factors that depress food intake. *Source:* Courtesy of Dr. T. Richard Houpt.

and therefore eat early in the morning and late in the evening.[671] They tend to eat every 45–90 minutes during the day and every 2.5 hours at night.[1623] Pigs eat meals in which eating bouts are interrupted for short periods when the pig may drink. The meals are separated by long intervals (90 minutes) from the next meal. When meals of individual pigs were recorded, the pigs were found to eat 8–12 meals/day, with the number of meals decreasing as the pig grew larger. Many "snacks" of less than 50 g are also eaten.[246] Meals are usually determined for confined pigs, and they learn to anticipate delivery of food by vocalizing and an increase in heart rate, but these changes are minimized in pigs fed twice a day on a predictable schedule.[1443] Seventy-five percent of feeding takes place during the day in lactating sows. They consume eight meals a day.[572] Younger pigs eat about 14 meals a day.[1623] If food is available from a ball that dispenses it only when the pig moves it, foraging in the bedding decreases. This means of obtaining food results in a more natural feeding behavior in which the appetitive behavior is combined with the consummatory behavior, ingestion of food.[2509] When deprived of rooting for 24 hours, sows will compensate by rooting more. If pigs have access to a substrate for rooting, such as spent mushroom compost, they spend 3–4% of their time rooting, but if food had been hidden in the

substrate previously, they root less when the food is consumed.[201]

Pigs (specifically, wild boars) will wash sandy apple slices in water by manipulating them with their snouts, but never wash clean apple slices, indicating that they can delay gratification in order to enhance the palatability.[2152] Electronically controlled feeders have enabled animals, especially cattle and swine, to be kept in groups; all have access to feed, and their individual intake and meal patterns can be evaluated. No consistent rank order of entrance into electronic feeders exists, but groups of sows that have been in a pen longer eat before more recently added sows.[325] Higher ranking pigs make fewer visits to an electronic feeder, but stay longer and consume more food.[1073] Few pigs forage for their food under domestic conditions, but they have preserved the ability to forage optimally. If they have to work harder to move from one patch of food to another, they spend longer at each patch.[871] They also can remember and prioritize food sites of different value, choosing the site with the larger quantity of food.[976]

Social Facilitation

Social animals tend to do things as a group; therefore, when one pig goes to the feeder, all the other pigs also go to the feeder. Group-penned pigs eat more than separately housed pigs.[440] The same phenomenon, social facilitation, leads all pigs to attempt to eat from one set of feeders while ignoring other feeders. Social facilitation of eating begins early; all members of a litter nurse together. Observation of a familiar pig – a pen-mate or a littermate – eating a novel food stimulates the observer to eat that food. Even contact with the pig that has eaten the novel food, in the absence of that food, still encourages intake of the novel food later by the observer pig, presumably because the odor or taste of the food was detectable.[689]

Social facilitation may increase food intake, but this tendency can be offset by the opposing tendency of subordinate pigs to eat less in the presence of dominant pigs. Pigs may refrain from eating, even in the absence of overt aggression by the dominant pig.[148] When housed in groups, the pigs tend to eat at separate times, probably to avoid competition at feeders, whereas individually housed pigs tend to eat at the same time as their neighbor.[837] Physical separation of food sites affected aggressive interactions (lower frequency and longer meal duration) compared to minimal separation. Time spent eating, number of feeding bouts, number of shifts to a new site, and food intake decreased with increasing distance between food sites.[2252]

Piglets housed in groups eat more if more feeders are available, because they are socially facilitated to eat but need not compete as much for a feeder. They will eat more of a flavored food if they have observed their mother eat it, whether or not they can eat the flavored food at the same time.[1732]

Palatability

The adult set point of body weight (see "Defense of Body Weight" later in this section) applies to an animal on a given diet. An increase in palatability can result in a shift upward in body weight set point. More simply put, animals eat more and gain weight when their food tastes good. Sows prefer high-concentrate to

high-fiber diets in short-term, two-choice feeding tests despite the findings that higher fiber diets are associated with lower levels of stereotypic behavior.[868]

Pigs show a marked preference for sweet substances,[1177,1202] consuming up to 17 l of sucrose solution per day. Advantage has been taken of this preference to increase intake.[23] Pigs initially prefer a solid diet containing glucose to one containing fructose, but over time eat more of the fructose diet.[1717] The intake and weight gain of pigs are not affected by the addition of a substance that tastes very bitter to humans, indicating a species difference in taste perception.[259] Pigs appear to separate sweet-tasting (to humans) flavors into two groups, with the first consisting of almond, raspberry, and peach, which are highly preferred, and the second consisting of vanilla and strawberry, which were not as attractive. Carrots are a preferred food, and pigs will work as hard to obtain carrots buried in sand as for easily accessible ones.[1024] Some bitter compounds such as caffeine and sucrose octaacetate are consumed, whereas eugenol, benzaldehyde, and anise are not.[259] In contrast to anosmic rodents, anosmic pigs ate with the same meal pattern as that of intact pigs, indicating that odor is not too important.[153] Although palatability is important, pigs choose cereals based on digestible nutrients.[2148]

Newly weaned pigs often show a drop in weight gain, and sweet pig starters are used in an attempt to stimulate intake. Although suckling neonatal pigs show nearly as strong a preference for the various sugars as do adults, these attempts are not always successful.[1050] A more rewarding approach may be to add to the sow's feed a flavor that will appear in her milk and then add the same flavor to the pig starter. Pigs will learn to associate a given flavor with a familiar food (in this case, sow's milk), and they will ingest that flavor more rapidly in solid food than they would a strange flavor.[377] When 129 flavors were tested, only one, a cheesy flavor, would increase intake of newly weaned pigs.[1537]

Environmental Temperature

Food intake is inversely related to environmental temperature; therefore, in hot weather animals eat less. The classic explanation is that "animals eat to keep warm and stop eating to prevent hyperthermia."[337] Certainly, inhibition of food intake in hot weather reduces specific dynamic action and other metabolic heat as further heat loads to the animal, and when body temperature rises to pathological levels, as in fever, food intake also decreases.

Food intake is stimulated by cold environmental temperature. This thermostatic control of food intake is part of body temperature regulation. When more energy must be applied to maintain body temperature, more energy is taken in.[1111] Changes in temperatures of the brain are not correlated with the initiation and termination of meals; and thermostatic eating is a response to changes in ambient or environmental temperature, not to changes in body temperature within the physiological range (Figure 8.3). If cold temperatures are too extreme, the animal will not be able to compensate for the energy lost by increasing its intake and will lose weight.

Gastrointestinal Factors

Gastrointestinal fill alone is not important. High-fiber diets do not suppress intake or motivation for food.[1887] The most likely candidates for the meal-to-meal controllers of intake are those factors that are closely associated with the act of eating, and ghrelin stimulates intake and growth hormone release when the stomach is empty.[2176]

Following a meal, changes occur in the gastrointestinal and plasma levels of various constituents, any one or several of which might influence food intake. Food intake ceases before intestinal absorption is complete. If it did not, animals would consistently overeat because food would continue to be ingested during the lag between ingestion of food and its absorption.

Gastrointestinal hormones are released as soon as food is present in the upper gastrointestinal tract; they may be satiety signals. The hormone is released from the mucosa of the upper gastrointestinal tract. CCK has several physiological actions: it stimulates contraction of the gallbladder; it stimulates release of pancreatic enzymes; and it has been shown to inhibit food intake in hungry animals,

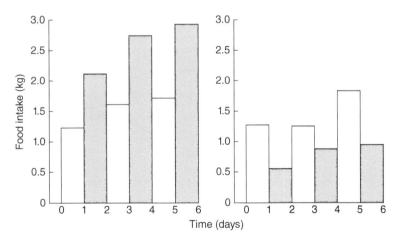

Figure 8.3 Daily food intake of pigs fed *ad libitum*. Pig on left was subjected on alternating days to temperatures of 25 °C (white) and 10 °C (green). Pig on right was subjected on alternating days to temperatures of 25 °C (white) and 35 °C (green). *Source:* Ingram and Legge (1974).[1111] Reproduced with permission of Elsevier.

including pigs.[1061,1070] More recently, the GLP1 agonist liraglutide has been found to inhibit eating in obese Göttingen minipigs.[3119] Although similar compounds like semaglutide are used for human obesity, they have not been used clinically for obese dogs and cats (Figure 8.4).

Fat in the intestine suppresses intake out of proportion to the caloric value of the fat,[856] and a CCK antagonist prevents that suppression.[1586] Immunizing pigs, but not lambs, against CCK results in a significant increase in intake and weight gain.[1909]

Removing the gastric contents before a meal has little effect on pigs' meal size. There are gastric influences on feeding, but they do not act instantly. Satiety after meals high in protein or fat is probably mediated through the release of gut peptides, but another satiety mechanism may exist for high-carbohydrate foods. Suckling pigs show a depression of food intake following gastric loads of isotonic glucose solution, but not following gastric loads of isotonic sodium chloride solutions, indicating that there may be glucoreceptors in the gastrointestinal tract[1060,2181] that produce satiety. Hypertonic solutions of either glucose or sodium chloride depress intake of both suckling and more mature pigs.[1060,1067,1068] As food is being digested, the osmotic pressure in the intestine rises, and stimulation of osmoreceptors in the intestine may be part of the basis of pre-absorptive satiety (Figure 8.5).

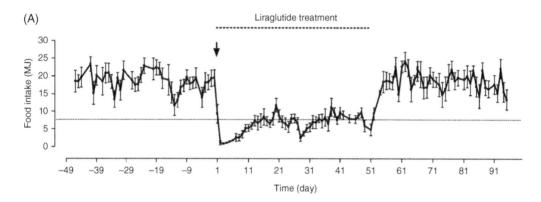

(A)

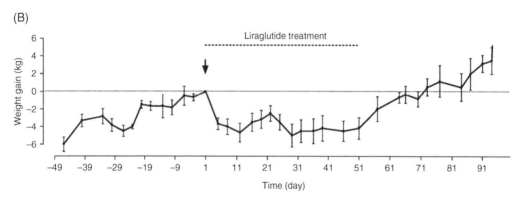

(B)

Figure 8.4 (A) Mean food intake (MJ) and (B) body weight change in obese, hyperphagic, Göttingen female minipigs fed *ad libitum*, during seven-week periods before, during, and after treatment with liraglutide (data presented as mean ± standard error, *n* = 6). The dotted line in A is the energy intake level for maintenance of normal body weight in minipigs. The dotted line in B is the body weight at start of treatment. *Source:* Raun *et al.* (2007)[3119]/John Wiley & Sons.

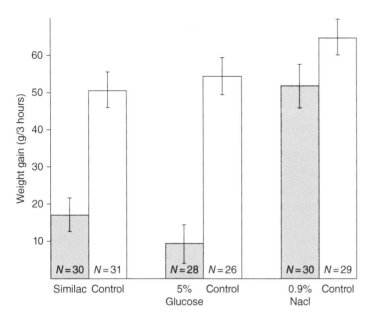

Figure 8.5 Effect of various gastric loads on three-hour intake of suckling pigs. Note that milk (Similac) and isotonic glucose, but not isotonic saline, depressed intake.[1050] *Source:* Houpt (1977)[1061]/John Wiley & Sons.

Hormonal Effect

When female pigs are in estrus, food intake is depressed and activity levels rise. Gilts eat 4 kg (9 lb.) less during a week in which they are in estrus than in weeks when they are in another stage of the reproductive cycle.[760] The increase in activity has been quantified: sows in heat walk 14,000 steps per day, whereas sows that are not in heat walk 5,000 steps per day.[49] Observation of the food intake and general activity of a sow can assist the producer in identifying a female in estrus.

Feeding at Parturition

Sows fed *ad libitum* during gestation have almost complete anorexia on the day of parturition, and although their food intake increases during lactation, it does not reach gestation levels for several weeks. In contrast, sows fed half of their *ad libitum* intake eat on the day of parturition ate more than previously *ad libitum*-fed pigs during lactation when feed was available *ad libitum*.[2410] This could be a result of depleted fat stores and decreased leptin

production in the restricted sows, or increased insulin resistance and reduced mobilization of nonesterified fatty acids in the *ad libitum*-fed pig. Unfortunately, this has led to feeding pregnant sows even less – one-third of their *ad libitum* intake – resulting in increased aggression in grouped sows and stereotypies in crated sows.[1932]

Imbalance of Dietary Amino Acids

Animals generally show nutritional wisdom in that they select an adequate amount of protein. For example, growing pigs given a choice of a protein-free or an adequate-protein diet ingested sufficient protein for maximal weight gain.[545] In certain circumstances, however, nutritional wisdom is not shown, and pigs will choose a non-protein diet over a protein diet.[1943] This occurs when the protein contains an imbalance of essential amino acids. The explanation for the marked depression of food intake seen when the imbalanced diet is the only one offered, or for the selection of no protein rather than an imbalanced protein, is unknown. It is speculated that an imbalance in essential amino acids leads to an imbalance in central nervous system neurotransmitters. Accumulation of a neurotransmitter might depress intake.

Glucose Utilization

Animals increase their food intake when the rate of glucose utilization in the brain falls. Experimentally, this phenomenon can be demonstrated by administering a competitive inhibitor of glucose, 2-deoxy-D-glucose (2DG), which decreases glucose uptake in the brain.[2182] Similarly, food intake can be increased by administering an agent that markedly lowers plasma glucose (Figure 8.6), such as insulin. Although eating in response to a lack of utilizable glucose (glucoprivation) can be readily demonstrated in a variety of species, it is probably not a practical method for stimulating intake because the dosage necessary to stimulate food intake is perilously close to the dosage that produces hypoglycemic convulsions. Eating in response to glucoprivation is an emergency mechanism the animal uses when its endogenous energy supply is approaching exhaustion. It probably is not involved in initiation and termination of meals in the free-feeding animals.

Defense of Body Weight

The constancy of body weight in the adult animal is believed to be the result of an innate set point for body weight or, perhaps and more likely, a set point for total body fat stores. The set point is most easily detected when body weight is artificially manipulated. For example, if an animal is starved for a few days it will, when food is again freely available, eat more than it did before the fast and rapidly regain the weight lost during the fast. In some cases, pigs show compensatory increases in intake after food restriction; in other cases, they do not increase their intake over that of nonrestricted controls, but their weight gain is greater, presumably owing to increased efficiency or decreased energy output (Figure 8.7).[1568] When diets are diluted with noncaloric bulk, intake rises so that caloric intake remains constant.[1586,] Conversely, if the animal is force-fed, it will gain weight but will decrease its voluntary intake while being force-fed.[1785] Similarly, animals that have gained weight while being injected chronically with insulin will, when

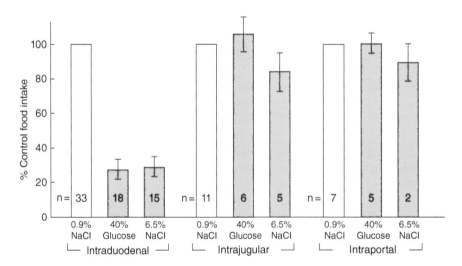

Figure 8.6 Effect of hypertonic injections administered into the duodenum (left), the jugular vein (center), or the portal vein (right) on subsequent food intake of pigs. Only intraduodenal injections depressed intake relative to saline-injected controls.

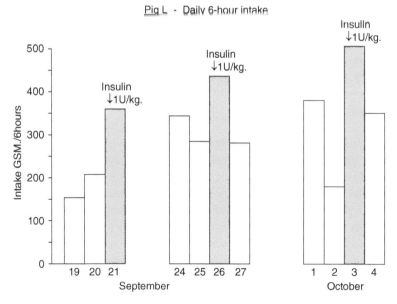

Figure 8.7 Intake of a pig following injection of saline (white) or insulin (green).

treatment ceases, decrease their intake, losing weight until their weight is at the preinjection set point. The glucagon-like peptide system (described in this chapter) is probably the mechanism in pigs, but has not been studied in that species. Set point is also maintained by adjustments in energy output that can be varied both by changes in motor activity and by metabolic changes in heat production.

The set point of body weight is more difficult to determine in the young, rapidly growing animal because it is being adjusted upward. The set point can be changed by manipulation of the neonate's nutrition. The starved piglet may remain stunted for the rest of its life.[2442] Similarly, overfeeding of piglets, as may occur in a small litter, may result in a permanently higher set point of body weight. If a young growing pig is fed 120% of its normal intake intragastrically, it will grow faster, indicating that appetite, rather than genetic growth potential or gastrointestinal fill, limits the rate of growth.[1785]

In response to changes in consumer preferences, pigs are now selected for leanness, so the set point for body fat is low and an obese pig is rarely seen on the farm. There are,

however, genetically obese strains of pigs maintained for experimental purposes.[1010,1473] Obesity can also be produced by dietary manipulation in young, meat-type pigs.[870] The number of fat cells did not increase in these pigs exposed to a palatable, high-carbohydrate diet, but the fat cells were larger, that is, they contained more fat. Pet minipigs must be maintained on an amount of food far below their *ad libitum* intake to prevent obesity. As a result, they may become destructive and aggressive in their efforts to find food.

In general, intake can be stimulated in the adult animal by any manipulation that lowers body weight or body fat stores beneath the set point. The neonatal piglet can respond to fasts of short duration with an increase in food intake, but longer fasts may produce irreversible hypoglycemia, coma, and death.

Integration of Factors That Stimulate and Inhibit Intake in the Central Nervous System

Central nervous system stimulants, in particular amphetamines, have been used extensively in human medicine to treat obesity. Less stimulating and less abused but less effective drugs, such as phenylpropanolamine, are also used as over-the-counter aids to dieting. Amphetamines apparently have their effect on neurons or neurotransmitters that mediate satiety or determine a set point. Stimulants increase satiety and lower the body weight set point.

Domestic animals' weight is controlled by the owner, and in rapidly growing meat-producing or lactating animals, depression of food intake is generally avoided. Unlike insulin, central nervous system depressants – in particular, the benzodiazepine tranquilizers that affect the γ-aminobutyric acid (GABA) receptor, such as diazepam and elfazepam – can probably be used to stimulate food intake when given as food additives to pigs, cattle, and horses.[345,1538] Elfazepam, for example, has been shown to increase pigs' mean intake from a control level of 220 to 570 g/h.[1538] A GABA-A receptor agonist increases feeding, and GABA receptor blockers decrease feeding.[154]

Whether the effects of barbiturates and tranquilizers can be used to increase food intake of food-producing animals economically and safely remains to be seen. All those interested in manipulating serotonin (5HT) function as a means of decreasing aggression should also be aware that agonists of the 5HT receptors increased spontaneous feeding in pigs, although intake may be suppressed by the same drug when food-deprived pigs are again offered food.[141,615] Kappa opiates increase feeding in pigs, and opiate blockers inhibit feeding.[151,157] It is somewhat confusing that there is a post-feeding opiate-mediated hypoanalgesia.[2004]

The controls of feeding in pigs have been reviewed.[1065] All the factors that have been discussed here – environmental temperature, rate of glucose utilization, palatability, social factors, estrus, gastrointestinal hormones, and the presence of glucose or hypertonic substances in the gastrointestinal tract – are operating at the same time. The information is integrated in the brain, and the animal eats more or stops eating accordingly. The roles of the various neurotransmitters remain unclear.[1120] Such

factors as social facilitation and avoidance of protein-imbalanced diets are mediated through the cerebral cortex. Changes in food intake in response to temperature are mediated through the anterior hypothalamus.

Polydipsia

Scheduled, induced polydipsia has been produced experimentally in pigs; that is, when food is available only intermittently and in small quantities, the pig will overdrink.[2185] Pigs that are fasted or on a severely limited ration, such as sows in gestation crates, may also increase their water intake (i.e., show polydipsia) perhaps to allay their hunger.[2002,2501,2502] Notice that in the free-feeding pig or one that is food deprived for only a few hours, drinking accompanies eating, but in a very hungry one drinking occurs as a compensation for lack of food.

Effects of Diet on Stereotypies

Adding fiber does not decrease motivation for food at 4 or 23 hours after the meal,[1887] but it does appear to reduce psychogenic polydipsia and stereotypic behavior in sows.[1941] High-fiber diets reduce rooting behavior, whereas low-protein diets increase rooting.[343] There is considerable evidence that feeding sows *ad libitum* will reduce or eliminate stereotypic behavior.[2242] Feeding the limited ration all at once (drop feeding) results in more oral–nasal stereotypic behavior in crated sows than providing the same amount of food over 30 minutes.[1082] Bar-biting behavior often alternates with drinking, a behavior the sow may substitute for eating when fed only one-third of voluntary intake, which is the standard diet for gestating sows.

Dogs that have free access to foods 24 hours a day eat many small meals a day, mainly during daylight hours.[1643] This meal frequency indicates that dogs are diurnal, rather than nocturnal, and that once-a-day feeding is not "natural," or at least not preferred, by dogs. Beagles living in individual kennels with dry food freely available tend to eat three times a day: at dawn, at dusk, and whenever fresh food is given.[1901]

Dogs differ in how they forage for food in that male dogs will widen a gap in a food container, whereas females will rip open the container. The former method is more efficient; pregnant and lactating bitches use the gap-widening technique.[1451]

Social Facilitation

Many animal owners have noted anecdotally that the addition of another animal to the household increased the original pet's interest in food. At times, the increase can be a pathological hyperphagia or excessive food intake.[721] Social facilitation of food intake has been quantitatively measured in puppies.[1127]

Palatability

Taste preferences must be determined for each species; one cannot assume that because something tastes good to humans, it tastes good to animals. Dogs prefer meat to a high-protein, nonmeat diet. This is true of feral dogs in India as well.[2537] Dogs show preferences for one meat over another: these preferences, in order, are beef, pork, lamb, chicken, and horse meat.[1056,1411] Determining a dog's food preference is not simple because dogs show preferences for different foods when tested by multiple-stimulus-without-replacement in comparison to a simple two-choice preference test, but in general dogs will eat more of the food they chose first in a two-bowl preference test.[2773,3056] Not only flavor, but also the form in which the food is offered are important in palatability. Dogs prefer canned or semimoist food to dry food.[1231] They prefer canned meat to the same meat freshly cooked, and prefer cooked to raw meat, despite the claims made for the "Bones and Raw Food" diet.[1411] Dogs do not prefer

familiar food; in fact, they prefer a novel flavor of canned food. Puppies also tend to prefer novel food, but palatability and maternal effects may outweigh these (Figure 8.8).[1643] Dogs familiar with semimoist food eat only a little canned food at first, when both are available, but soon show a preference for the canned. Dogs also have an innate preference for sucrose in liquids or solid food.[686,847] They are unusual in preferring fructose to sucrose (humans and pigs prefer sucrose). Lactose, but not maltose, is also preferred.

Palatability does not depend on taste alone because elimination of olfaction (anosmia) eliminates preference for one meat over another, although anosmic dogs still preferred meat or a sucrose diet over a bland cereal diet.[1056] Such major preferences as that for meat over nonmeat and for sucrose are not affected. Odor is most important for locating food, and it is used for detecting minor differences between foods, as in distinguishing lamb from pork; but taste is most important for identifying food.[1949]

The food preferences are reflected in dogs' attraction to the odors of meats. The odor of cooked meat is preferred to that of raw meat, and that of fresh meat to that of three-day-old meat.[212] It is important to consider taste preferences when selecting the vehicle for oral rabies vaccine. Dogs preferred, in descending order, dog food (Iams), bacon, cheese, sardine, peanut butter, hazelnut, and sugar-vanilla.[235] Taste is important in a long-term sense as well. Dogs that have been adequately nourished but deprived of taste will overeat when food is again available, indicating that deprivation both of the taste of food and of calories is important.[1318] The practical application of this is that provision of a calorie-free, but tasty, food might be less stressful than fasting.

Environmental Temperature

Food intake is believed to be controlled, in part, by the regulation of body temperature. Consequently, animals tend to eat more in the cold and less in the heat. This has been

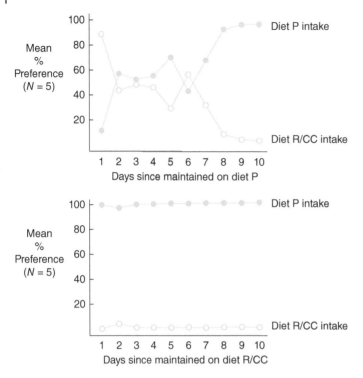

Figure 8.8 Effect of novelty on food preferences. Dogs normally prefer diet P to diet R/CC, but will show preference for either R/CC or P if it is a novel diet. Preference for P is sustained (lower graph), but that for R/CC is reversed in a week (upper graph). *Source:* Mugford (1977).[1643] Reproduced with permission of Elsevier.

demonstrated in environments as diverse as Alaska and Florida, and with breeds as different as Huskies and Beagles. Food intake doubled in the winter as temperatures fell from a summer high of 20 °C (68 °F) to a winter low of −17 °C (1 °F).[601] Indoor dogs eat less than those housed outside, probably due to the warmer indoor environment.[1281]

Gastrointestinal Factors

Oropharyngeal factors alone are not sufficient to induce satiety. Dogs surgically prepared with esophageal fistulas can swallow food, but if the fistula is open, the food will drop from the esophagus and not reach the stomach (sham-feeding). In this case, dogs will sham-feed for hours, stopping only to rest. It has also been found that gastric loading immediately before a meal does not markedly inhibit food

intake unless more than half of the normal meal is placed in the stomach. It is interesting that placing food into the stomach at the same time that the dog is eating and swallowing food does inhibit further sham-feeding.[1132] Apparently, in dogs at least, both oropharyngeal and gastric stimuli are necessary to induce satiety.

Food placed in the stomach just prior to a meal does not inhibit food intake, but a gastric load given 20 minutes before a meal does.[1133] The delayed effect of a gastric load indicates that either food must be absorbed or some humoral factor must be released by the presence of the food in the upper gastrointestinal tract to inhibit food intake.

Food intake of dogs is suppressed by CCK and glucagon, and it is markedly depressed by the opiate blocker naloxone.[1347] Neither intraduodenal fat nor peripherally administered

CCK suppresses sham-feeding in dogs, although intracerebroventricularly administered CCK does.[1765] The difference in the effect of CCK on sham-feeding and normally feeding dogs indicates the importance of integration of gastrointestinal and humoral events for satiety. Food intake can be stimulated by the ghrelin agonist capromorelin.[2641]

A drug that inhibits microsomal triglyceride protein, which assembles lipids with protein to form chylomicrons (the structures that carry fat in the bloodstream), was marketed to increase satiety and, therefore, decrease hunger in dogs. Although effective in suppressing appetite, the side effects of steatorrhea (fatty stools) led to its withdrawal from the market.

Hormonal Effect

During estrus, bitches tend to eat less; conversely, removing the source of estrogen stimulates food intake. Both cats and dogs have a lower metabolic rate following castration or spaying, which also accounts for their tendency to gain weight.[1055] Therefore, one of the side effects of ovariohysterectomy is a tendency for the spayed bitch to eat more and gain weight (Figures 8.9 and 8.10). Presumably, this is due to the removal of the estrogen source. When a dry diet is available to dogs for only an hour a day, neutered dogs do not gain weight – a strategy owners could use.

Glucose Utilization

Glucoprivic eating is seen in dogs. Dogs treated chronically with insulin eat more and gain weight,[861] and eating in response to glucoprivation produced by an inhibitor of glucose utilization has been demonstrated in dogs.[1066] A lack of glucose stimulates intake, and an excess usually does not inhibit feeding. Neither intraportal nor intrajugular glucose suppresses intake.[230,231]

Defense of Body Weight

Dogs can defend their body weight against both decreases and increases. Dogs neither gain weight when force-fed nor lose weight

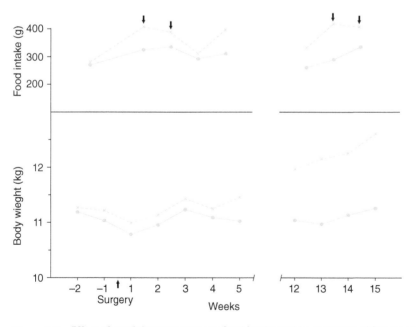

Figure 8.9 Effect of ovariohysterectomy on food intake and body weight of Beagle bitches. Solid lines = intact. Dashes = spayed bitches. *Source:* Houpt *et al.* (1979).[1055] Reproduced with permission of American Veterinary Medical Association.

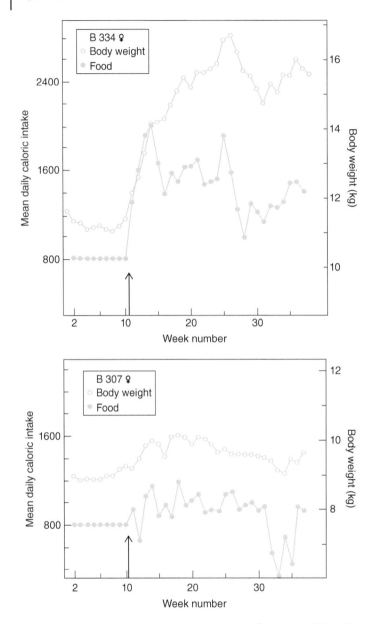

Figure 8.10 Food intake and body weight of two Beagles. *Ad libitum* feeding began at arrow. Lower graph is of a dog whose intake and body weight remained normal. Upper graph is of a dog that overate and became obese. *Source:* Mugford (1977).[1643] Reproduced with permission of Monell Chemical Senses.

when placed on calorically dilute diets. When dogs were given additional food each day through gastric fistulas, they decreased their oral intake, but not enough to prevent weight gain.[2092] The lack of caloric compensation may be due to the intragastric route of force feeding; oropharyngeal signals (i.e., taste and texture) were not elicited by the food, so satiety was not achieved.

Dogs can increase their volume of intake when their diet is diluted.[1132] Dogs deprived of food will eat more when food is again available and, thereby, defend their body weight. Different breeds of dogs defend different body weights and different degrees of adiposity. A casual comparison of Bulldogs and Salukis makes this clear. Dogs can also select some dietary components to obtain sufficient nutrition. For example, dogs can regulate their protein and energy intake when offered diets differing in protein content. When offered such a choice, they chose a 30% protein diet.[1956]

Dogs lesioned in the ventromedial hypothalamus show hyperphagia and weight gain.[1660,1989]

High dosages of amphetamines have been shown to depress food intake in dogs.[458] Their use as a treatment for canine obesity has not been evaluated carefully.

Grass Eating

This behavior is so common that it should not be considered a true pica. Young dogs are more likely to eat grass than older ones, but dogs are no more likely to vomit after eating grass.[253,2202] Puppies of grass-eating bitches eat more grass than those of bitches that do not eat grass. It may be a means of obtaining roughage. Grass eating in some situations may not be ingestion, but rather tasting and smelling substances left on the grass. This mouthing of grass is particularly common after a rain.

Control of Food Intake in Cats

Meal Patterns

As do dogs, cats eat many small meals (12) per day when given free access to food, but unlike dogs, cats eat both in the light and in the dark.[1643] One might argue that this intake pattern is not natural, yet the caloric intake per meal is approximately equal to that contained in one mouse.[701] A feral cat with good hunting skills might easily catch 12 mice (or three rats) per day.[2298]

Palatability

Cats are notoriously finicky. This reflects the strong influence of palatability on food intake in cats. There is one striking peculiarity of cats: they do not prefer sucrose, as most animals do, because of a deletion in the sweet receptor gene.[1362] Cats do not show a sucrose preference for aqueous solutions of sugar, but they do prefer sucrose in salt solutions.[178] Cats will not eat diets containing medium-chain triglycerides or hydrogenated coconut oil. This may be because they break down the triglycerides to fatty acids in their mouths (cats possess lingual lipase) and are peculiarly sensitive to bitter tastes. They will avoid as little as 0.1% caprylic acid or 0.000005 M quinine. In comparison, rabbits and hamsters avoid quinine only at 0.002 M.

Preferences of cats can be examined using a two-bowl test in which the food approached and eaten first and the amount of each food consumed can be measured. A one-bowl test can determine acceptance of the food. When testing dry food, the size and shape of the addition to taste can be measured. Some of the factors to be considered are: brittleness, firmness, grittiness, and hardness as well as odor and flavor (meaty, bitter, metallic, painty, etc.).[3095] See Figure 8.11 for the facial expressions of cats eating preferred and non-preferred foods.

Cats prefer fish to meat and, as do dogs, prefer novel diets to familiar ones.[966] Cat food manufacturers no doubt take advantage of both of these feline preferences. If the new diet is not more palatable than the familiar one, the cat will, after a few days, begin to choose the familiar food.[1643] While cats are drinking milk, their electroencephalography (EEG) reading is synchronized as it is when they are drowsy.[402,427] Observation of cats' behavior can be an indication of palatability. Cats lick their noses after encountering unpalatable food, but groom their face (licked paw over ear) after eating palatable food.[2224]

When presented with a choice between a food frequently made available to them and one that is rarely offered, cats will choose the scarcer one, even if both foods are dry

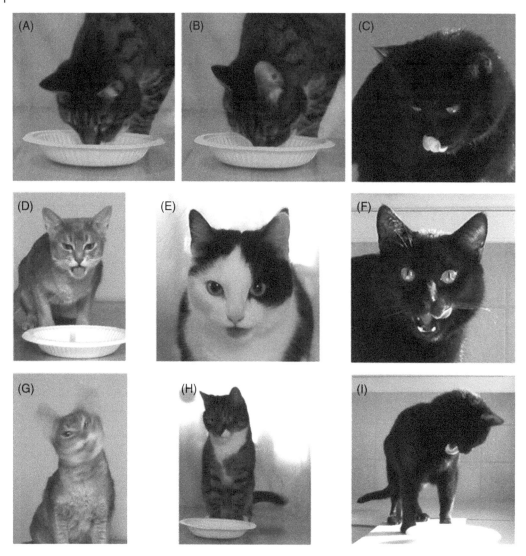

Figure 8.11 Examples of eight behavioural indicators in still images captured from video clips. (A, B) "Flick ears backwards," which involves a rapid ear movement from position (A) to position (B) and back. (C) "Lick nose." (D) "Drop item"; the cat drops the piece of food and/or the mini-tablet hidden inside it, from the mouth. (E) "Smack"; the behaviour pattern involves "smacking" the tongue with the mouth partly open, accompanied by rapid movements of the mouth that are not chewing. (F) "Flick lip." (G) "Shake head." (H) "Flick tail"; the behavioural pattern involves moving the tail sideways in rapid, wide sweeps. (I) "Groom body."

commercial cat food. Experience may modify the choice of a novel food. Farm cats avoid dry food, which is difficult to ingest, whereas pet cats avoid raw beef.[317] Aging cats prefer warmer food (37 °C) probably because more volatile products are released.[2731]

Cats avoid diets with high calcium or phosphorus and ash. They also avoid high-fiber diets which can be a problem if the cat is prescribed a weight loss diet, which may be high fiber.[3049] Cats may alter their food choice if a preferred meat is present but unavailable (tuna inside a sealed bowl); they will choose the food closest to the sealed bowl. The presence of the "phantom" food influences their choice.[2038] Cats do not indulge in contra-free loading, that is, they prefer freely available food to that for which they must work in a puzzle toy, for example.[2715]

Environmental Temperature

There has not been a complete study of the effect of temperature on food intake in cats, but one demonstration showed that cold environmental temperature, rather than changes in brain or body temperature, affects feeding. This study found that cats drinking milk not only show a decline in brain temperature but also cease to eat.[13] If brain temperature was the factor affecting feeding, one would expect the cat to eat even more as its brain temperature fell.

Gastrointestinal Factors

Gastrointestinal depressants of feeding have been studied to some extent. Glucoreceptors that suppress feeding in cats appear to be present in the liver.[2007] CCK and bombesin, a peptide related to CCK, suppress food intake of cats.[122,123]

Hormonal Effects

Ovariohysterectomized and castrated cats have a lower metabolic rate,[1961] and if the cat is fed all it wants of a very palatable food and is not very active, obesity can result.[2037]

Glucose Utilization

In contrast to most other species, cats have not been shown to respond to glucoprivation with an increase in intake. The glucose analog 2DG failed to stimulate feeding in cats,[1126] but the failure to stimulate may have been a result of species differences in the effective dose of the drug rather than species differences in the control of food intake.

Defense of Body Weight

The most important determinant of body weight in cats appears to be cyclical in nature.

Cats lose and gain body weight in cycles of several months' duration.[1893] For this reason, it has been difficult to demonstrate defense of body weight. There have been two studies in which it appeared that when their diet was diluted, cats did not eat more and, therefore, lost weight.[1015,1172] In both studies, the diet, a dry food, was diluted with a dry diluent, either kaolin or cellulose. The cats actually ate a smaller volume than they ate of the undiluted food, indicating that it was unpalatable. In contrast, when cats' food is diluted with water, they do compensate by increasing the volume of intake and maintaining a constant caloric intake.[399,1643] Because the cats were consuming more of a diet when it was diluted with water, their water intake was increased. A watery cat food may be used to increase water intake when clinically indicated, that is, in cats with urolithiasis or hypernatremia.[395]

Drug Effects

The role of endogenous opiates in feeding has not been well investigated, but the opiate blocker naloxone suppresses intake in cats.[718] The antidepressant mirtazepam stimulates food intake in cats as does the ghrelin agonist capromorelin.[2612,3036]

Obesity

The incidence of obesity in cats has increased in the past 20 years from 10 to 29%.[2037] Some of the risk factors for obesity in cats are neutering, confinement in an apartment, and free-choice feeding of a prescription diet.[2037] Feeding a limited amount of a high-fiber diet results in a greater weight loss than an equicaloric low-fiber one. Owners reported that the cats were more affectionate while their intake was limited.[1349]

Wool Chewing and Other Picas

Wool chewing is a behavior problem that occurs with greater frequency in Siamese or Burmese cats than in other breeds.[314] It should be differentiated from nonnutritive suckling that many early-weaned kittens will perform. Pica is directed most commonly at shoelaces or threads, followed by plastic, fabric, rubber bands, paper, cardboard, or wood. The cats that ingest these items are more likely to vomit. Free-choice feeding seems to be protective.[538]

Control of Food Intake in Horses

Meal Patterns

The normal feeding pattern of horses, as detailed in Chapter 3, "Biological Rhythms and Sleep and Stereotypic Behavior," is to graze continuously for several hours and then to rest for longer or shorter periods depending on the weather conditions and distances that must be traveled to obtain water and sufficient forage. It is interesting that, whether the horse is grazing or eating pellets, the statistical definition of a *meal* (feeding with breaks of no more than 10 minutes' duration) is the same.[1315,1481] When fed free-choice hay, horses chew 40,000 times/day.[627] The performance horse is rarely on pasture and is given only limited amounts of hay. When given no long-stem roughage, horses will work to obtain it.[627] In short-term tests, horses offered six different forages were not as restless and did not sift through their bedding as much as horses fed one type of roughage.[840] The frequency of oral stereotypies in stalled horses on low-roughage diets is probably a reflection of the oral activity seen in a natural environment.

One method of slowing hay intake to mimic the rate of consumption while grazing is to provide hay in a hay net. If the opening in the net is only 3 cm (1.2 in.), the rate of consumption falls by half, meaning that the horse takes six hours rather than three to eat its hay.[830] Multilayered 2.5 cm (1 in.) hay nets can increase foraging time even more from 27 min/kg of hay to 78 min/kg hay.[632] The problem with hay nets is that the hay net must be positioned high enough that the horse does not step in it, and,

therefore, the horse is forced to eat from forage much higher than grass would be: inhalation of particles is more likely to occur, and musculoskeletal problems may arise from holding the head higher the normal in order to eat and the horse may be frustrated.[2951] Intake of pellets can be slowed by putting a grazing muzzle on the horse.[2347] Wastage can be prevented and time spent eating increased with a feeder containing a cup-shaped depression.[394]

Social Facilitation

Horses eat when other horses eat, and they eat more if they can see another horse eating.[2210] This is important when creep feeding a foal and when encouraging an anorexic horse to eat. Horses appear to prefer to eat from the floor and from shallow buckets or mangers. This enables the horse to see in all directions between its legs and may have evolved as an antipredator strategy. Grazing is, of course, from the ground rather than from the usual chest height of a manger. The problem that arises when feeding confined horses is to prevent ingestion of parasite ova or sand while still encouraging intake. Horses fight less and spend more time eating from tractor tire feeders where several horses can eat at once than from single feeders or from a long manger where horses can eat side by side.[1637]

Palatability

When the basic taste preferences of immature horses are examined, they show a strong preference for sucrose, but no preferences for sour (hydrochloric acid), bitter (quinine), or even salt solutions.[1892] At high concentrations, all the solutions except sucrose were rejected. In a study of adult ponies, 9 of 10 showed a strong preference for sucrose.[950] Horses exhibit specific facial expressions in response to specific tastes. They open their mouths and protrude their tongues (gape) in response to quinine, but bob their heads in response to sucrose.[1131]

Ponies tend to prefer hay flavored vanilla and milk protein + sugar.[3099] They did not exhibit significant differences in preference for spearmint, banana, cinnamon, and coconut. They did prefer foods with sweet aromatic odor (banana and coconut) odor. Color of food can make a difference. Horses preferred yellow to white oats.[3068] Nutrient content appeared to be the main driver for diet choices. Taste appeared secondary to nutrients in determining the diet selected. A nonnutritive sweet taste or a new odor appears to encourage diet intake by horses.[3017] When used as a reward during clicker training a variety of commercial equine diets are equally effective as rewards.[3090]

The interest in adding fat to equine diets has led to a comparison of various oils. Corn oil is the most preferred of the vegetable oils, which are preferred to tallows.[1023] Horses can respond to dietary macronutrient content and will choose protein and hydrolyzable carbohydrate-rich diets rather than lipid-rich diets, especially after a few days of experience with a diet.[1911] Sensory-specific satiety exists in that horses spend longer eating flavored foods when several flavors are available simultaneously.[839] Variety itself is important.

Horses prefer pelleted feed to hay and will work harder in an operant conditioning test to obtain the former.[1697] If horses have to work hard (i.e., press a lever) to access food they eat more quickly.[2915] Timothy hay is preferred to reed canary grass and has a better calcium-to-phosphorus ratio.[1733] Alfalfa is preferred over wheat, teff, and oat hay in that order.[1946] Timothy hay is also preferred to teff, but when only one type of hay is fed; intake of the two hays is equivalent.[1501] When fed round bales, horses are less aggressive and spend more time eating if the bale is enclosed.[2883]

Grazing

Horses evolved to graze, spending the majority of their time with their heads down moving slowly from patch of grass to patch of grass.

Most grazing occurs during the day.[2744] Grazing behavior is selective; that is, unless the pasture is composed of only one species of plant, the animal has the opportunity to be selective as to the species ingested. For example, in the Mediterranean climate of the Camargue, horses consume graminoids in the marshy areas, moving to the less preferred long grasses in the winter.[1481] On Shackleford Banks, an island off the eastern US coast, the ponies eat primarily sea oats, smooth cordgrass, and centipede in the summer and fall, but eat a more varied diet in the winter, including more forbs. Availability and palatability determine their choices.[1847] Similarly, meadow and shrub land are the vegetation types grazed by feral horses in the Great Basin of Nevada, but food preferences and nutritional needs have to be weighed against the dangers of exposure in the winter and the irritation of insects in the summer.[239]

There have been several studies of the plants that ponies and horses choose to eat on pasture. The New Forest Ponies of England eat eight different species of plants but avoid the poisonous *Senecio*.[2300] These ponies will eat acorns, an overconsumption of which leads to acorn poisoning. Of 29 species of grass, horses and ponies preferred timothy, white clover (but not red clover), and perennial ryegrass. Dandelions were the most preferred herbs.[77] Horses also avoid fecally contaminated grass and long grass.[706]

Horses prefer mixtures containing tall fescue, perennial ryegrass, and Kentucky bluegrass; these preferences may change the distribution of species in the pasture.[1476] Kentucky bluegrass, perennial ryegrass, timothy, and white clover are preferred forages, and arrowleaf clover and ryegrass are the least preferred forages, with wheat and oat being intermediate in preference. In an extensive evaluation on forage palatability of 38 mixtures grown in Pennsylvania, Kentucky bluegrass, timothy, and meadow fescue were preferred to orchard grass, tall fescue, reed canary grass, and meadow foxtail. Kentucky bluegrass, timothy, meadow fescue, and perennial ryegrass had higher nonstructural carbohydrate concentrations than other grasses, and nonstructural carbohydrate concentration was positively correlated with horse preference.[2646] In another study of 29 species of grass, horses and ponies preferred timothy, white clover (but not red clover), and perennial ryegrass.[2874] Pastures are not homogeneous, so there are patches of varying nutritive value. Horses show dynamic averaging in which they return to the last patch they grazed after a short absence but a different one after a long absence – matching the long-term average of the patches.[544]

Horses prehend at a rate of 25 bites/min (prehending bites should be differentiated from chewing). Intake rate depends on bite size and rate. The larger the horse, the larger the bite size, but intake also depends on the handling rate (i.e., the time to chew each bite). Ponies may be constrained in intake when the grass is fibrous and requires more handling time. The intake rate of grass is 36 g dry matter/min for ponies and 76 g dry matter/min for horses.[706] The grazing horse chews at a rate of 30–50 bites/min for 8–12 h/day. Use of a grazing muzzle decreases the amount of forage consumed by an average of 30%.[831]

Horses, sheep, and cattle each have different modes of prehending grass: horses use their lips; cattle, their tongues; and sheep, their teeth. Presumably, the ability to be selective varies with the method of prehension as well as with the size of the muzzle. Sheep should be more selective than horses. The reason selectivity is important is that the grazer can choose a more nutritious plant or plant part, or can avoid a toxic one.

Horses vary considerably in their selectivity, which may account for deaths of only a few horses on a pasture where poisonous plants grow.[1460] Horses can spend the same amount of time grazing, but differ their intake by choosing more nutritious and shorter plants.[2838] Horses graze during the night as well as during the day and their food choice does not differ between those two periods Horses do not appear to innately or experientially reject the high colchicine plant meadow saffron (*Colchicum autumnale L*).[2894] Horses spend more time grazing and take more bites from swards with taller grass.[1672]

Gastrointestinal Factors

The horse appears to depend more on pre-gastric signals to satiety than other species. When horses sham-feed – that is, when most of what they have swallowed falls out of an esophageal fistula – they do not eat more than they do when the food reaches their stomachs.[1882] This is in contrast to dogs, which will eat very large meals under the same circumstances. Eventually, the sham-fed horses compensate for the lost feed by eating sooner than normal, but apparently the signal for satiety is some form of oropharyngeal metering; that is, 25 swallows means enough has been eaten. The importance of pre-gastric (oral) factors to horses is confirmed by the finding that prolactin levels increase after a meal is consumed, but not after the constituents are administered intragastrically.[542]

Another indication that chemoreceptors in the gastrointestinal tract are not important controls is that when administered either intragastrically or intracecally, neither glucose nor cellulose, the main digestible constituent of grass, and its breakdown products, the volatile fatty acids solutions, depress intake until they have been absorbed. Intake is suppressed, but only after a long latency. There is a mechanism for controlling caloric intake, but it appears to be postabsorptive.[1883,1884]

The first sign of colic in most horses is anorexia. This clinical observation, as well as controlled studies, indicates that pathological distention of the gastrointestinal tract inhibits feeding in the horse as in other species. This anorexia is probably mediated through pain receptors that travel in the sympathetic nerves. Analgesics intended for use in horses are often tested by determining whether a horse with a dilated cecum will eat when treated with the drug. In this case, the drug is probably working peripherally, so pain signals are not relayed to the brain.

Central Nervous System Depressants

In a preliminary study, the central nervous system depressant diazepam stimulated food intake in horses, and the commonly used tranquilizer promazine had a similar effect.[345] Horses, in common with other more thoroughly studied species, increase their food intake when the brain, presumably the areas involved in satiety, is depressed (Figure 8.12).

Defense of Body Weight

Horses can regulate their energy balance by controlling the amount they ingest. In other words, horses do not eat a fixed amount or eat until they are ill, but they increase or decrease the amount they eat to compensate for caloric dilution or enrichment.[1355] The pony gradually shifted to *ad libitum* feeding does not colic but does gain weight and is, therefore, in danger of laminitis; the body weight reaches a plateau.

Many horses, particularly ponies, are overweight, but the problem is how to reduce caloric intake, but still allow the horse to forage for half his time. Some approaches that have been used are muzzles, hay nets, and various "slow feeders." Use of a muzzle is not stressful to ponies.[2708] The type of hay in the net is also important. Shorter, finer chops of hay will encourage more normal grazing behavior, due to the ease of prehension and limited grams of intake per bite, resulting in lower average pull pressures, more bites, and longer average intake rates.[2792]

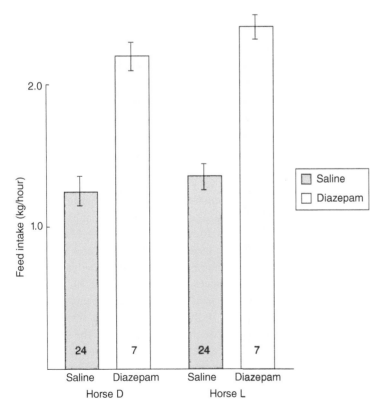

Figure 8.12 Intake of two horses following intravenous saline (dark) or diazepam (light).

Geophagia

Horses sometimes exhibit pica, including geophagia. When soil from the site where the horse was eating is compared to soil from other areas of the same farm, it is found to be higher in iron and copper. This indicates an attraction to those elements.[1530] A more serious problem is ingestion of stones, the cause of which is unknown.

Control of Food Intake in Cattle

Meal Patterns

The time cattle spend grazing on pasture and eating in feedlots or loose housing has been reviewed in Chapter 3. Defining the difference between an intrameal and intermeal interval requires measuring many feeding bouts. An *intermeal interval* for a cow is defined as more than five minutes without eating.[1957] Cattle kept in the confinement of a feedlot or barn eat approximately a dozen meals a day.[408] They show individual cyclic patterns of intake.[2197] Eating rate varies with the physical form of the feed. Cattle can eat 2.72 kg (6 lb.) of hay in an hour.[262] Meal is eaten more slowly than pellets, which, in turn, is eaten more slowly than a slurry. Dilution of the meal with water actually increases the amount consumed per minute. Silage is eaten more slowly than hay, probably because of illness produced by consuming the fermented product too quickly.

In some dairy parlors, the cows are fed grain only while they are being milked. An important consideration for dairy farmers, therefore, is the speed with which cows can consume concentrates. It takes a cow one to two minutes to eat 0.5 kg (1 lb.) of grain; slightly less time is required if the grain is cubed.[1158] If a high-producing cow is milked in too short a time, she will not have time to consume the grain that she needs; another arrangement must be made to feed her. If cows are not fed grain in the milking parlor, however, they will not be as eager to enter. All these factors must be considered when planning a milking parlor and feeding system.

Rate of chewing in cattle has been studied by direct observation or by recording jaw movement using either a balloon under the jaw or a strain gauge on the halter.[203,543] These studies have led to the conclusion that cattle that eat fast also chew fast; by so doing, they ingest more and, therefore, produce more. Cows should be selected for rapid intake both to solve the problem of eating enough while being milked and to help reduce negative energy balance during early lactation.

Feeder design is important. Cattle that have to reach under a horizontal bar to obtain feed may injure their necks. In other designs, such as a post and rail, wastage of feed may occur.[1800]

Social Facilitation

Cattle will also eat more in groups than they will individually, and first-calf heifers will eat more if grouped with older cows, but production may not be increased, because these increases must be balanced against the negative effects of dominance disputes. The more agonistic encounters, the more hay is wasted. Feeder design is important in reducing waste; a ring or cone is better than a trailer or a cradle for offering round bales to cattle.[363]

Another effect of the social hierarchy during group feeding of grain is that subordinate cows eat faster than dominant ones, probably because they have less time to eat before they are displaced by a dominant cow and must compensate.[711] Transponder-activated feeding devices are, theoretically, an excellent way to feed group-housed animals and still record individual intake, but several problems arise. Intake decreases as the number of cattle per feeding station increases, especially when there are more than five animals per station.

When limited amounts of concentrates are fed in that manner, the cows' activities are disrupted as they test the station to determine whether they will be fed. Dominant cows can displace subordinate ones after the door has opened for the subordinate.

Ruminants appear to have a definite sweet preference, but what tastes sweet to people may not taste sweet to cattle. Based on electrophysiological recording from the chorda tympani and glossopharyngeal nerves, cattle can taste saccharin but do not respond to aspartamate.[979,2075]

Cattle reject 20% sucrose, 0.08% acetic acid, and 2.5% quinine.[833] Twin cattle show similar rejection responses, as well as similar sweet preference responses.[229] With regard to the more usual feed substances, factors in addition to taste and odor must be considered. Texture and ease of prehension may explain why cattle prefer pelleted to un-pelleted feed. Unchopped silage is preferred to chopped silage,[581] in part because more bites are necessary to collect the chopped silage.

Palatability is affected by secondary plant compounds – those chemicals produced by the plant to reduce predation, that is, eating of the plants by herbivores. A common secondary plant compound is tannin, which browsers, such as deer, but not domestic ruminants have evolved to tolerate. Tannins reduce palatability because of their astringent properties;[1300] they also cause illness. There is, however, interest in adapting cattle to diets containing tannins to take advantage of many tannin-containing tropical forages.

A good example of the complexities of preference testing is that dairy heifers will choose a mean ratio of 40% grass silage and 60% corn silage, but the individual preferences ranged from a 34 to 75% preference for the corn silage.[2412]

The preferences of ruminants for plant species vary and depend on a number of factors. These include: (a) the growth stage of the plant – most ruminants prefer fast-growing, succulent species; (b) the mixture of species – clover, for example, may not be eaten if it is growing in a pure stand but will be eaten if grasses are growing with it; (c) the season of the year – ruminants will consume species that are green during the winter, although the same species will be rejected in the summer when other species are green; and (d) the relative abundance of herbage. These factors are particularly important in determining when a ruminant will ingest a poisonous plant. Many poisonous plants are bitter in taste or harsh in texture and are, therefore, avoided by ruminants; but when the poisonous plant is the first green plant to appear in the spring (hemlock or skunk cabbage) or the only forage available on a pasture, it will be consumed. In addition to these factors, the location of the plant, in particular its distance from water (in arid regions) or shelter, will influence the amount of it consumed.[89] Cattle avoid fecally contaminated areas.

Various methods have been devised for determining preferences of grazing animals. The most accurate and most direct is to collect the food eaten by sheep or cattle through open esophageal fistulas. Another method is to observe the animals closely. This method is more accurate if the forages are planted in narrow pure stands from which the ruminants may choose. A third method is to sample the plant species and heights of the plants before and after the pasture has been grazed. A fourth method is to measure the alkanes in the feces, which will differ depending on the plant species ingested and which appear in the feces 24 hours after consumption. Studies using these methods have revealed that cattle graze selectively; that is, they do not necessarily eat plants in proportion to the number of each plant species in a pasture.[998] For example, cattle most prefer meadow fescue and timothy; perennial ryegrass and cocksfoot were the next most preferred plants; and *Agnotis* and red fescue, the least preferred.[462] Ruminants are less likely to graze on plants that contain old growth or cured material. Rapidly growing plants are the most palatable, provided that they are high enough in fiber.[797]

Cattle wrap their tongues around grass and pull to prehend it. This method of foraging limits them to plants higher than 10 mm. On a fresh ryegrass pasture, dairy cattle graze at a rate of 50–60 bites (prehension) and 14–20 chews/min. Although they prefer longer swards, they will graze shorter swards at a higher bite rate of 70/min.[891] They are the least selective of the domestic ruminants. Sheep can graze much closer to the ground because they use their teeth to prehend, a fact that may have led to antagonism between cattle and sheep producers on a shared range.

Cattle eat most of their meals during daylight but may graze at night if short days or hot weather precludes obtaining the nutrient requirements during the day. Grazing time is 400–650 min/day at a bite rate of 60/min.[642] Cattle prehend a gram or two at a time, taking in 30–50 g in a minute. As bite size increases, the cattle are both prehending and chewing with the same jaw movement.[1294] Stems interfere with the process of grasping leaves and, therefore, decrease bite size and rate. Clustered leaves can be prehended more efficiently.[578] Fasted cattle spend more time grazing than non-fasted ones, and although bite size was unaffected, they chewed less, swallowing larger particles.

Do animals forage optimally? Do they increase the time spent at patches of high-density food and spend longer at patches that were hard to obtain, that is, a longer walk from water or resting areas? These questions are only partially answered. Cattle apparently graze those patches that give them the largest bite weight and instantaneous intake. For example, cattle will select short, dense patches over short, sparse ones but will select against short, dense patches when tall, dense patches are available. Selecting for maximum bite weight and rate of intake seems to occur, but they overmatch, that is, select those patches more than proportional to the reward (herbage) they contain. At the pasture level, cattle will avoid grazing in wet areas where plants have lower protein and higher fiber concentration.[1007]

Cattle can be taught to eat or at least eat more of a novel forage by first associating a visual cue (an orange traffic cone) with a palatable feed and then placing that cone on the patch containing the novel plants.[1926]

One must consider the effect of adding concentrates to supplement cattle on pasture or range. Cattle that eat concentrates rapidly differ in their grazing behavior from cattle that eat more slowly. The fast eaters have a smaller search area and spend less time near the water source than the slow eaters, and they also gain more weight.[2425] Supplemental food blocks are used frequently for delivering extra calories, vitamins, minerals, or medication to cattle. Placement of these blocks is important because cattle will not use blocks placed close to the watering site as much as blocks placed in grazing areas.[398] Neophobia is also a problem. Short-term food deprivation does not decrease the latency to eat a novel feed.[1004]

Environmental Temperature

Cattle eat less when environmental temperatures are high. In addition to the direct effects of heat on intake, there are also effects on plant growth that may render them less palatable. One of the problems of raising cattle in the tropics or other hot environments is that food intake, and therefore production, falls. The use of tropical breeds and crosses with tropical breeds of ruminants helps alleviate the problem because these cattle eat more in the heat or eat more at night when the temperatures are lower.

Cold ambient temperature increases food intake in ruminants as in simple-stomached animals. This can be observed not only when environmental temperature falls but also when the animals' heat loss is increased. (See Baile and Forbes[126] and Forbes[711] for reviews of all aspects of the controls of food intake in ruminants, including thermostatic factors.)

Flies can also influence feeding. Cattle actually eat more when face flies are present in large numbers.[569]

Rumen Fill and the Products of Rumen Fermentation

The anterior gastrointestinal tract of the ruminant (the rumen) is an anaerobic fermentation chamber in which bacteria that produce cellulase can release the energy that the animal can use. This energy is otherwise unavailable to the animals and enables cattle, sheep, and other ruminants to survive on grass and roughage diets. In the case of grazing ruminants, the time necessary to collect food and fill the rumen is probably the limiting factor in food intake. For example, when cattle are grazing on the open range, they spend 56% of their time grazing and another 21% of the time ruminating (see Chapter 3).[879] In the case of cattle fed diets high in grain for fattening, and in the case of lactating dairy cattle eating concentrates, other factors inhibit food intake. For example, cattle fed a 75% concentrate diet spend only 11% of their time eating.

The end products of bacterial digestion in the rumen are the volatile fatty acids: acetic, butyric, and propionic. When acetic acid is added to the rumen, food intake is depressed; similar amounts injected via the jugular vein

have no effect on food intake.[127] Therefore, it seems likely that acetic acid may stimulate receptors located in the rumen epithelium or in the portal circulation, or the effect may be osmotic. These receptors may, through central nervous system connections, inhibit food intake. Above and below approximately 50% forage in the diet, intake is reduced. On low-roughage, high-energy diets, production of volatile fatty acids is probably the most important satiety factor. On low-energy, high-roughage diets, rumen fill or abdominal fill is probably a satiety factor (Figure 8.13).

Humoral and Central Neural Factors

Food intake falls in estrous cattle.[1093] The decrease in intake can be used to identify cows that are ready for breeding (see Figure 4.4, Chapter 4). Stilbestrol is an estrogenic drug that has been used to fatten steers. In the doses given, it does not suppress intake, and the anabolic effect of stilbestrol leads to weight gain.[972] Since stilbestrol was banned, other estrogenic compounds have been used to improve weight gain in feedlot cattle.

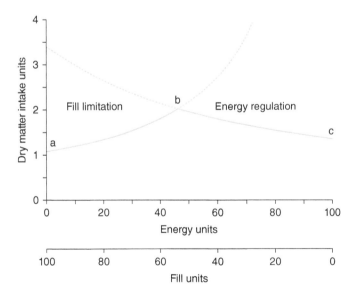

Figure 8.13 Reciprocal relationship between dietary characteristics and dry matter intake. Line a to b represents intake limited by the fill effect of the diet. Line b to c represents intake limited by the energy demand of the animal. Dashed lines represent unattained intake predicted by extrapolating the theoretical equations. *Source:* Mertens (1987).[1569] Reproduced with permission of American Society of Animal Science.

Plasma ghrelin, produced in the abomasum, is positively associated with body fat, liver fat, and milk fat after parturition and can increase food intake.[297,2634] GLP1(glucagon like petpide) decreases intake of dairy cows.[2176]

Corticosteroids increase food intake in cattle, but increase fat deposition, whereas ß-adrenergic agonists such as clenbuterol decrease fat deposition and increase muscle growth without increasing food intake.[711]

Defense of Body Weight

Although cattle can vary their intake with availability of feed, there are constraints. When concentrates are available 24 h/day, cows eat 80% more than when they are available for only five hours. Hay intake increases only 20%. This is strong evidence that rumen fill is not the only influence on satiety.

Cattle can, within limits, decrease their food intake as caloric density increases. Even young calves demonstrate this ability by decreasing their intake of milk replacer as the percentage of water in the replacer falls. The ability of cattle and other ruminants to respond to dietary dilution, that is, to increase their volume of intake as the nutrient density decreases, has been reviewed by Baile and Forbes.[126]

Low-protein content of the diet suppresses food intake in ruminants as well as in simple-stomached animals, but because of the rumen microbial production of protein, the level of protein in the diet can be much lower before anorexia occurs. Furthermore, non-protein nitrogen, particularly urea, can substitute for protein if enough carbohydrate is available to the bacteria for protein synthesis. Offering concentrates can decrease forage intake, but the decrease varies with quality of the forage. Intake of low-quality hay will be less affected than intake of high-quality hay (refer to Figure 8.14).

Parasitism

Ruminants must weigh the cost–benefit of grazing nutritious but parasite-infected (i.e., fecally contaminated) forage; generally, they

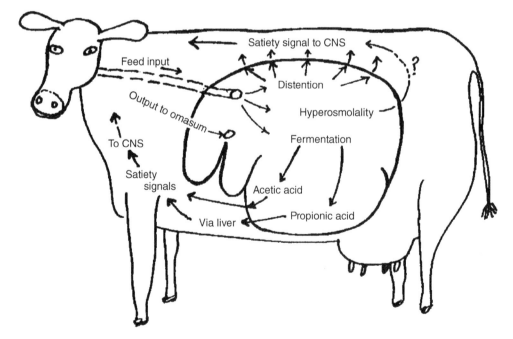

[Distention] = [Feed input] − [Fermentative digestion] − [Output to omasum]

Figure 8.14   Controls of feeding in a ruminant. *Source:* Courtesy of Dr. T. Richard Houpt.

will avoid fecally contaminated sites and deplete the noncontaminated sites. Gastrointestinal helminths stimulate the release of their host's gut hormones, including CCK. Therefore, the heavily parasitized ruminant loses weight not only because the parasites consume some of the food that their host ingests but also because the host ingests less. There are two possible explanations for the survival value of anorexia in parasitized animals: an effective immune response is stimulated by anorexia and later allows the hungry animal to select foods that will minimize the risks of infection or select foods that are high in antiparasitic compounds.

Clinical Problems

The Fat Cow Syndrome

An abnormality of feeding behavior that is being seen with increasing frequency is the fat cow syndrome.[1631] Under some types of management, dairy cows may be fed in a group that includes both lactating and dry cows. The dry cows may overeat, gain weight – consisting mostly of fat – and later at calving or during lactation become ill or even die. The pathogenesis of the syndrome remains unclear, but the initial problem is that the cow overeats. High-producing dairy cattle have been bred to eat large amounts in order to supply the metabolic fuel for lactation. When lactation ceases, the increased food intake may persist and the fat cow syndrome may result. It is interesting that lactating cows respond more precisely to food deprivation by walking farther to obtain food than dry cows.[2058]

Control of Food Intake in Sheep

Although more studies have been conducted on the effects of rumen manipulations in cattle than in sheep, most of the other physiological studies of ruminant intake have been conducted on sheep, probably because of their size.

Meal Patterns

Sheep eat approximately a dozen meals a day in a laboratory. Sheep can eat at a rate of 15–30 g of pelleted feed per minute, but only 9 g of hay per minute. Sheep eat a kilogram more if feed is available free choice rather than for a limited period of 3 h/day.

Social Facilitation

Confined, isolated lambs eat less than grouped ones. Sheep eat less when in metabolism cages, which may be due to a lack of social facilitation in a gregarious species, as well as to confinement itself.[709]

Palatability can affect flocking behavior. When grazing sheep remain within 30 m of one another, but an individual sheep will move 60 m away to obtain pellets, palatability overcomes social desires.[2116]

Palatability

Sheep do not appear to have a very marked sweet preference. Nevertheless, only 5% sucrose and glucose were preferred; higher concentrations produced no preferences or aversion. Lactose was rejected at a concentration of 2.5%. Sheep also showed no preference for molasses, for which cattle show a strong preference.[832] Sheep will learn to prefer flavored straw that is associated with nutrients, whether the nutrients are consumed or delivered intraruminally. Similarly, lambs will gradually eat more hay with added sucrose, apparently because of the post-ingestive consequences of the sugar, not the taste.[362]

Sheep are particularly neophobic, so it is best to present novel foods in a familiar environment and familiar foods in a novel environment for optimum intake.[361] Offering novel foods with a familiar flavor and frequently introducing novel foods can reduce neophobia.[1313] Similarly, offering lambs low-quality roughage early in life will stimulate them to eat low-quality roughage as adults.[553] Lambs will avoid poisonous foods better if an alternative food is available, particularly if the alternative is nutritious.[1225] Lambs prefer flavors paired with nutrients to flavored saccharin solutions, a form of nutritional wisdom.[360]

Sheep are much more sensitive to unpleasant taste than other ruminants. They reject sour solutions of hydrochloric acid, acetic acid, lactic acid, or butyric acid at concentrations lower than those found in the rumen, yet the volatile fatty acids must surely be tasted when the sheep ruminates. A bitter solution of quinine (0.004 M) was rejected, but not one of urea, even at concentrations high enough to produce fatal toxicity.[832] Experience also plays a role in that sheep that initially rejected quinine-treated hay eventually accepted it even when non-bitter hay was available.[710]

Sheep are more likely to consume poisonous plants while food is restricted.[162] Lambs will more readily eat food their dam has eaten, but the influences can begin prenatally. Feeding oregano essential oil to the pregnant ewe will result in acceptance of oregano-flavored food in her lamb after weaning.[2125] Secondary compounds in plants can be harmful, but ingestion of one type, tannins, can increase the intake of another, ergotamine, and possibly buffer the toxic effects.[1146] When a fungus such as endophyte infests fescue, the sheep avoid it, apparently because they are nauseated.[25]

Defense of Body Weight

Not surprisingly, fasted sheep eat faster, taking larger bites than those who have been grazing at will, but it is interesting that their food preferences change, tending toward higher roughage feeds, such as grass, rather than the higher protein plant, clover. Within 24 hours of being fed a fiber-free diet, sheep will pseudoruminate (regurgitate without cud chewing) and ingest plastic fiber. Placing a pompom of fiber in the reflexogenic areas of the reticulorumen reduces this fiber hunger.[381]

Rumen Factors

Fiber decreases intake, and the smaller the particle size, the greater the intake of those diets in which rumen distention limits intake. There is additivity of ruminal acetate and intraportal propionate in suppressing intake of sheep, indicating that several factors acting in concert could be necessary for satiety. This is the more natural situation than an increase or decrease in a single metabolite or hormone. When given a choice, sheep do not eat the most calorically dense food but choose sufficient long fiber to optimize rumen function.

Intestinal Receptors

Factors such as CCK and propionate act additively in suppressing ruminant intake, but immunizing lambs against endogenous CCK did not result in a significant increase in intake.[2158,2290] If digesta enters the duodenum more rapidly, the sheep eats more, which suggests that abomasal fill may produce satiety.[1447] GLP1 suppresses intake in sheep, and ghrelin stimulates it.[2176]

Grazing and Selectivity

In contrast to goats, sheep are not very selective and are willing to choose a high-fiber diet. Sheep graze up to 12 h/day, and 90% of that time is spent biting.[2115,2118] A sheep takes 0.34 seconds to open and close its mouth in a prehension bite; therefore, it prehends at a rate of 60–80 bites/min.[406] Sheep masticate (chew) 60–70 times/min. Sheep prehend grass by breaking it between their lower incisors and upper dental pad. That and their narrow muzzle enable them to be more selective than cattle. They select leaves rather than stems. When the protein content of a diet is insufficient, food intake may be depressed. This may occur on poor-quality pastures. The rate of food intake depends on the plants grazed. For example, sheep can prehend and masticate clover faster than grass.[1789] Sheep expend energy moving from place to place while grazing, and they increase their food intake 20–50% over that in confinement to compensate for the extra energy expended. Sheep have peaks of grazing activity every eight hours. They graze most intensely just before sunset.

The factors affecting grazing are bite rate, bite size, time spent grazing, and species of food selected. All of the following are important: learning, especially learning from the dam's food choice; motivation to be close to another sheep; social facilitation of the beginning, but not of the end, of a grazing bout; and physiological state. Sheep forage optimally, initially eating mostly a preferred species and later, as the height of those plants decreases, switching more frequently to the less preferred but more easily obtained plants.[1845] In general, the preferences are correlated with the dry matter and carbohydrate content of the grasses. Sheep select a diet higher in protein and lower in fiber content than that obtained from clipped pasture samples, indicating the advantage to the animal of selective grazing.[960,2194,2407]

Sheep will walk 3 or 6 m to obtain clover, but are less likely to travel 20 m, the point at which the energy they would expend reaching the clover would exceed that provided by the clover.[405]

A practical consideration in pasture management is that sheep, as well as horses, avoid fecally contaminated grasses, although they seem to prefer grass subjected to urine contamination.[1466] Sheep do not select against parasite larvae; it is the feces themselves they avoid.[453]

Sheep learn to avoid diets that exacerbate the effects of secondary plant metabolites. For example, lambs' intake decreases with increasing concentration of the terpenes found in sagebrush.[614] See the "Conditioned Taste Aversion" section in Chapter 7. The effects are worse if the animal eats a high-carbohydrate, low-nitrogen diet.[162] There are interactions between the diet and the secondary compound in that lambs innately prefer grain (barley) to sugar beets, but reverse that preference if the diets also contain terpenes.[2355] Sheep will consume more shrub if a variety of shrubs, presumably with a variety of secondary compounds, are offered. Activated charcoal that adsorbs terpenoids – the common toxin in shrubs – can be fed to encourage consumption.[1950]

It is unclear what senses are involved in forage preferences. Anosmic sheep do not avoid fecally contaminated feed as normal sheep do.[2288] Anosmic sheep and sheep with impaired vision (hooded with translucent eye coverings), however, showed preferences very similar to those of intact sheep, although the visually impaired sheep tended to graze at one level rather than grazing higher or lower on the plant to select the most succulent portions.[85] Even cutting of the gustatory nerves had little influence on forage preferences.[86] In the laboratory, anosmic sheep are no different from intact sheep in their meal patterns.[155]

Both food preferences and social factors influence food choices in sheep. Sheep in larger flocks graze for longer periods than sheep in smaller flocks.[1788] The satiety state of the grazer also influences plant selection. Previously fasted sheep eat more, as compared with non-fasted sheep, because the former take larger bites and choose fewer legumes than nonlegumes.[1687]

Environmental Temperature

Sheep eat more when they are cold and less when they are hot. For example, sheared sheep eat 50% more after shearing as a result of the loss of insulation of their wool.[2244] At very low temperatures (~10 °C or 14 °F), intake may be inhibited, and the consequences of greater losses of energy as heat will be compounded by a decrease in energy intake.

Hormonal Factors

Ewes eat less during estrus. Infusion of the amount of estrogen equivalent to that which occurs at estrus also suppresses intake.[711] Food intake decreases during late pregnancy in ewes carrying more than one lamb. The decrease can be as large as 40% if the only available forage is low-quality roughage. This can result in ketosis or pregnancy toxemia of sheep. During lactation, thin sheep eat more than fat ones – a phenomenon seen in all ruminants studied thus far.

Glucose Utilization

Cross-circulation from hungry to satiated sheep stimulates intake of the satiated animal (and depresses intake of the hungry one), indicating the existence of humoral factors that influence feeding.[2084] Glucose or insulin levels may be among the humoral factors. Because virtually everything that the ruminant eats is exposed to rumen bacteria before reaching the intestine, very little dietary glucose becomes available to the animal. Instead, the ruminant depends on the volatile fatty acids for energy and produces glucose by the process of gluconeogenesis. Plasma glucose is low, approximately half that of simple-stomached animals. For these reasons, ruminants were assumed to be fairly independent of glucose utilization and not expected to eat in response to glucoprivation. However, as has been demonstrated in both sheep and goats, food intake can be markedly increased by insulin and the glucose analog 2DG.[1064]

Control of Food Intake in Goats

Meal Patterns and Grazing

Goats eat 12 meals a day (remarkably similar to cattle and sheep), eight of them during the day. Goats are more selective feeders than sheep and have a longer vertical reach than sheep of the same weight.[711] Goats select low-fiber material. Browsing behavior is a skill that must be learned. Goats learn to break twigs off the plants rather than to chew them off.[1738] Attempts to increase consumption among goats with plentiful, but not particularly palatable, foods such as sagebrush have not been successful,[1934] but goats will consume more shrubs than sheep.[1950] Goat selectivity is strongly influenced by their dam and peers and by the plants to which they were exposed in their first year of life.[251] When fed as a group, food intake and time spent eating decline when feeding space is restricted. The dominant goat shows less reduction in intake.[1161] Goats in a warm climate will eat longer and consume more when their feed is in the shade, emphasizing the importance of ambient temperature on food intake.[50]

Inexperienced kids consumed similar proportions of shrubs and grasses in their diets compared with adult goats. However, kids browsed a larger proportion of DMI (dry matter intake) from lower strata than adult goats, possibly due to their smaller height. In addition, kids consumed a smaller proportion of large bites compared with adult goats. These behavioral features are likely related to differences in mouth size between kids and adult goats.[2763]

Goats readily consume glucose and sucrose solutions at concentrations as high as 40%.[226] Goats do not prefer bitter substances but will accept quinine-adulterated water at nearly 10 times the concentration that a rat will.[226,228] Field studies confirm that goats have a high tolerance for bitter taste.[459] Castrated male angora goats are in danger of urolithiasis. It is possible to increase their water intake, and thereby decrease their risk of urethral blockage, by adding vinegar or orange flavor to the water.[454] Increasing the crude protein of concentrates fed to goats increases their food intake and their milk production.[121] Propionate and lactate suppress intake in goats, but the site of action is beyond the rumen, presumably in the liver.

Central Neural Mechanisms in Ruminants

The easiest generalization that can be made about central stimulants of intake is that factors that depress activity, such as anesthetics and opiates, increase feeding. For example, central nervous system depressants, such as calcium, barbiturates, and benzodiazepines, also stimulate intake in ruminants.[186,552,1259,1467,2083,2084]

As the number of known neurotransmitters and neuromodulators grows, the hope of gaining a complete understanding of the pharmacology of central neural controls of feeding and other behaviors grows dimmer. CCK, discussed in this chapter as a peripheral satiety factor, also exists in the brain, where it can act to produce satiety in sheep.[127]

The opioid peptides are also involved in feeding behavior. The mu and kappa receptor agonists given intracranially appear to stimulate intake in sheep; gamma agonists depress intake.[128] A mu opioid receptor ligand, syndyphalin, stimulates food intake over 48 hours.[1714]

Although sheep increase their food intake when norepinephrine is injected via the cerebral ventricles, cattle do not show the same response, nor does a clear picture emerge when adrenergic agonists or antagonists are injected.[129] Cerebrospinal fluid from hungry sheep stimulates intake by satiated sheep, indicating that humoral factors within the brain (or the ventricles) influence feeding.[1467] The serotonin antagonist cyproheptadine increases food intake in sheep.[598]

It is not yet clear whether these drugs, which stimulate intake over the short term, would, if administered chronically, produce a long-term increase in food intake or meat and milk production.[2127] The problem of the effects of barbiturates and tranquilizers on human consumers also remains unknown. The latest approach is to stimulate production with bovine growth hormone or somatotropin and rely on the animal to increase intake to match the increased production (output).

Obesity can be produced in sheep by offering a free-choice pelleted diet. The sheep will consume three to six times their maintenance requirements. After the sheep have gained weight, their intake falls and they actually eat more slowly than lean sheep. This indicates that the feedback from fat, presumably leptin (ob protein), is inhibiting intake. These sheep are more sensitive to the anorexic effects of opiate blockers.[17] See Figure 8.14 for controls of intake in ruminants.

Chickens

They forage approximately 40% of the day, peaking just after sunrise and before sunset. They prefer to forage in low stress (low risk of predators) environments.[2910] They forage by scratching at the substrate, presumably to dislodge insects, worms, etc., and then peck at the surface which they scratched. Chickens shake their heads and wipe their bills if they encounter unpalatable objects. They swallow with their eyes closed, but drink with their eyes open. When a chicken encounters a large food item she may run with it, either to prevent other chickens from obtaining the prize or to encourage others to follow and help tear the object into bite-sized pieces.

Vision is more important in birds' choice of foods than taste. They have no sweet taste preference, but have a calcium-specific hunger similar to the salt hunger of herbivores mammals. They reject acid and bitter tastes. Chickens will contra-free load. There is social facilitation of feeding in chickens.[2648,2906,2910]

Chickens can learn to choose a food that is higher in protein or some other nutrient, but only if they can taste the food. They do not form preferences for food given by tube into the crop.[2746] Chicks prefer a single, balanced food to a choice between high protein and low protein as demonstrated by Rovee-Collier et al.,[2957] who offered a choice between high- and low-protein foods during the 12 hours of daylight but a food with an adequate protein content at night.[2957] The birds adopted a nocturnal feeding pattern (although they did eat a little food during the day), showing that if necessary the chick will eat at night in order to get a single, complete food even though it is normally a diurnal feeder. Intake is controlled to meet requirements over a period of several days.[2956]

Water Intake

At least three types of stimuli elicit thirst: a dry mouth, an increase in the osmotic pressure of the blood, and a decrease in the blood volume. In addition to these internal signals, taste preferences and aversions influence water intake. For example, high concentrations of magnesium (4 g/l), but not sodium sulfate, found in some natural water sources suppress water intake.[862]

Increase in Osmotic Pressure

Hypertonic sodium chloride infused intravenously causes thirst in pigs,[1110] horses,[2203] and dogs.[2489] An increase in the osmotic pressure of the blood is believed to stimulate osmoreceptors located in the brain.[2480] Goats drink copiously when hypertonic saline solutions (2% NaCl) are injected into the brain through a cannula.[63] Similarly, a mare whose water intake is restricted to half her normal intake will exhibit thirst as a result of an increase in the osmotic pressure of her blood and consequent stimulation of osmoreceptors.[1054] Free-ranging cattle drink once a day. Under these conditions, lactating cattle drink larger amounts but drink no more frequently.[1985] Pigs weighing 30 kg drink about 6 l/day. Feeding excessive protein increases water intake. In general, if 2.5–3 g of food is consumed, a gram of water will be drunk.

Decrease in Blood Volume

Decrease in blood volume, for instance as a result of hemorrhage or peritoneal dialysis, may stimulate thirst.[428] A decrease in the blood volume would also be expected in a cow that produces 36 kg (80 lb.) of milk (95% water) per day. A lactating cow drinks 45 kg (100 lb.) more water a day than a dry cow for this reason.[879] The drug furosemide, frequently administered to racehorses shortly before they perform, causes a decrease in plasma volume and thus stimulates thirst in horses[2203] and sheep.[2520] Water is lost when animals are heat stressed, whether they cool themselves primarily by panting (dogs), saliva spreading (cats), or sweating (horses). Therefore, water intake increases with environmental temperature.

Angiotensin

Another type of drinking occurs in response to the hormone angiotensin. Angiotensinogen is acted upon by the kidney hormone renin, and then by a pulmonary-converting enzyme to form the octapeptide angiotensin II, which has several actions. It releases another hormone, aldosterone, which is involved in sodium reabsorption by the kidney. High doses of angiotensin II can increase blood pressure, and angiotensin II is the most potent dipsogen known. Angiotensin II, or procedures known to release the hormone, stimulates water intake in a wide variety of animals, including dogs,[702] cats,[448,2201] sheep,[3] goats,[64] pigs,[152] and horses.[65] The role that angiotensin release may play in normal thirst remains to be determined.

Situations in which blood supply to the kidneys is compromised stimulate renin release and, therefore, angiotensin release that could be expected to lead to thirst. Indeed, dogs in congestive heart failure show increased water intake.[1888]

Dry Mouth

A desalivate animal takes frequent small draughts of water in order to swallow dry food. This type of drinking, prandial drinking, is also seen in intact pigs that take a small quantity of water into their mouths before swallowing a mouthful of grain.[1002]

Multiple Causes of Thirst

Just as most food intake appears to occur without a major change in body energy balance, most drinking occurs without a change in body fluid balance. The osmotic and volume depletion stimuli to drinking are emergency mechanisms to restore body water under life-threatening conditions.

Most drinking in domestic animals is prandial, that is, in association with meals. For example, 75% of water intake in pigs is in association with meals. Twenty percent of the drinking occurs after feeding (within 10 minutes); 30%, as pauses in feeding; and 25% precedes meals. The drinking occurs before any changes take place in blood volume or osmolality. The animals appear to be drinking in anticipation of their needs, and the physiological mechanisms are the same as those that control the cephalic phase of gastric secretion.[1069]

Thirst produced by overnight water deprivation is a combination of osmotic thirst and hypovolemic thirst. In contrast to the osmoreceptors that stimulate vasopressin secretion, those that stimulate thirst in the dog appear to be located on the blood side of the blood–brain barrier.[2256] Water intake of thirsty dogs is reduced by 80% if water is injected intracarotidly so that the osmoreceptors of the brain are no longer stimulated. Intravenous administration of an equal volume of water has no effect. If thirsty dogs are injected with isotonic saline so that peripheral blood volume is returned to normal, their water intake is reduced by 20%. If both intravenous isotonic saline and intracarotid water are administered, water-deprived dogs do not drink.[1889] Despite this evidence that thirst is inhibited when blood volume and osmotic pressure return to normal, dogs cease drinking before these parameters return to normal.[2489] There may be signals from the gastrointestinal tract that inhibit water intake, as there appear to be signals that inhibit food intake. The stomach has been implicated,[2287] but gastric fill alone does not suppress drinking in dogs;[2146] duodenal osmoreceptors are more likely candidates for the source of inhibition.

Water intake falls with environmental temperature, and this may account for the increased incidence of impaction colic during the winter when horses eat more and drink less.[334,2639] Providing warm water with meals increases water intake by 40%.[1268] Horses drink more water from a bucket than from automatic waterers. These methods of providing water may lead to negative fluid balance.[1712] Horses prefer float-valve to push-lever drinkers.[1265]

Water intake increases from 2 l/day when horses are on pasture to 6 l/day when they are maintained in stalls and fed hay. Despite that increase in water intake, fecal output decreases when horses are stalled. These changes can explain why colic is a frequent consequence of changing the horse's environment.[2459] Figure 8.15 illustrates seasonal changes in water intake of horses.

Cattle fed silage – a somewhat wet feed – and limited amounts of concentrates drink four times a day. The drinks ranged from 1 to 13 l (1 to 14 quarts).[711] Dairy cows spend 25 seconds drinking per bout, consuming 9 l in 15 sips.[2236] There may be central sodium receptors in cattle that, when stimulated by an increase in NaCl in the cerebrospinal fluid, increase water intake. Water intake increases in the heat and decreases in the cold, but when the environmental temperature falls below 0 °C (32 °F), water intake increases with the increased food intake necessary to control body temperature. Dogs may not be as thirsty in the cold. Their threshold for osmotic stimuli is higher, and their blood volume is elevated.[2146]

If given access to water, veal calves will drink a large quantity (3–8 l/day) in addition to milk replacer and will exhibit less nonnutritive oral behavior.[845] Early-weaned (18 days) piglets may both overdrink and waste water, particularly when provided with a nipple drinker. They may associate the nipple with suckling. Provision of a push-lever drinker reduces both water intake wastage and belly nosing of pen-mates.[2281] When given a choice, pigs will drink cold water when the environmental temperature is high and warm water

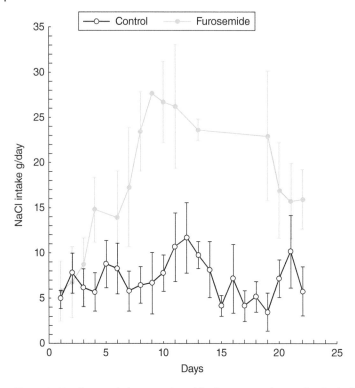

Figure 8.15   Seasonal changes of total body water and water intake in Shetland ponies measured by an isotope dilution technique. *Source:* Brinkmann *et al.* (2013).[2639]

when the environmental temperature is low, so water intake can be used for temperature regulation.[1019]

During the dry months, female African wild ass with young foals visited permanent water once a day, traveled on average 9 km and drank only at night. Nonreproductive adult females and males traveled to water every 5–10 days. In rainfall months, females with young foals drank twice a day and on average traveled 3 km to water.[3004]

Cats drink about a liter a day, and although fountains are recommended for cats, intake is not much greater from a flowing water source.[1749]

Adipsia and Hyponatremia

This syndrome is rarely encountered, but it has been found in Miniature Schnauzer dogs[466] and in cats. It is interesting because it demonstrates two principles of ingestive behavior: (1) that there are multiple controls of thirst and (2) that animals will increase their intake of a diluted diet in order to keep their caloric intake constant. These animals do not drink in response to the osmotic stimuli, so they present with hypernatremia. They will, however, respond to hypovolemia, so they drink when furosemide, a diuretic that lowers blood volume, is administered. To ensure that the animals consume enough water, they can be maintained on a slurry of canned food and water. The controls of food intake are normal, so they inadvertently ingest water while eating.

Specific Hungers and Salt Appetite

The concept of the nutritional wisdom of animals has not been validated. Animals apparently cannot innately choose a diet containing a vitamin or other nutrient in which the animal is deficient.[1987] Horses fed a diet deficient in calcium will not eat more of a calcium supplement to correct the deficiency.[2055] There is better evidence for a phosphorus-specific hunger. Cattle and other ruminants chew on bones, and some will consume phosphorus supplements. Animals, at least laboratory animals, can learn to associate a particular diet with improvement in health. Conversely, animals can learn to avoid a diet they associate with a feeling of malaise. Given proper clues, such as a distinctive flavor, most domestic animals could probably learn to choose a diet that would correct a deficiency rather than choose a deficient diet. Examples of this ability are that lambs fed a diet high in energy, but low in protein, would preferentially eat feed that was high in protein and low in energy, and lambs fed a diet high in protein but low in energy would also choose a diet that rectified their imbalances.[2068]

There is, however, one nutrient that nearly all species select innately when they are deficient: sodium.[1025] Salt hunger is a well-recognized phenomenon, especially in herbivores, whose diet tends to be low in sodium, but even dogs exhibit salt appetite when sodium deficient.[1025] In most species, removal of the adrenal glands and the consequent hyponatremia are followed by life-saving ingestion of sodium chloride. Pigs, for instance, drink sodium chloride solutions and survive, following experimental adrenalectomy.[1422] Ruminants can be made experimentally sodium deficient by creating a salivary fistula. The large loss of sodium bicarbonate in saliva produces a deficiency that sheep can correct by drinking precisely the quantity of sodium solution they need to bring their sodium levels up to normal. Treatment with a diuretic also stimulates sodium appetite in sheep.[2520]

Salt appetite is not stimulated during pregnancy and lactation in sheep despite the extra sodium demands.[1577] Sheep can be divided into those that excrete sodium predominantly in the feces (i.e., they do not absorb excess sodium) and those that excrete sodium predominantly in the urine. The fecal excretors have a greater sodium preference.[1576] Although sodium is usually in low concentrations in the herbivore diet, in some environments it may be in high concentrations that result in decreased intake and digestibility. When consuming a high-salt diet, sheep will select a supplemental diet for energy rather than protein.[2248]

Cattle will travel farther for water than for salt.[786] Sodium-deficient cattle and sheep are able to learn an operant response to obtain a sodium reward.[2,2139] Sodium status is apparently assessed in the brain, where changes in the concentration of intracellular sodium act to initiate transcription and translation processes. The protein synthesized alters the ionic or membrane characteristics or increases the neurotransmitter capacity of the neurons.[540] The hormones that mediate salt hunger are angiotensin and aldosterone acting in synchrony. Because of the hormonal involvement, there is a latency for the appearance of the salt appetite.

Salt intake varies from 19 to 143 g/day in horses.[2054] Furosemide causes a loss of sodium as well as water in the urine. Sodium appetite as well as thirst are stimulated in horses treated with furosemide.[1059] This phenomenon may be important because of the widespread use of furosemide in racehorses.

The preference for sodium is innate, but animals can learn to associate a given mineral with post-ingestive consequences. For example, phosphorus- or calcium-deficient sheep will prefer a flavor associated with a feed containing the deficient mineral or even with ruminal infusion of phosphorus.[2354,2356]

9

The Genome and the Microbiome

In this chapter, sex and breed differences in behavior, means of determining temperament, laterality and the few examples in which a gene has been identified that is responsible, at least in part, for a given behavior will be presented. The use of DNA sequencing tools to explore microbial biodiversity has allowed correlations with behavior to be made. In genomic mating the genetic information and the estimated marker effects are used to decide which genotypes should be crossed to obtain the next breeding population.[2642]

The microbiome can affect human behavior.[3079] The relative abundance of *Blautia*, *Bacteroides*, and *Odoribacter* in the microbiome is found to be decreased in humans suffering from anxiety, but there is still a lack of a causal account of how microbiota changes and interactions between competing microorganisms in the gut environment are connected to brain and behavioral states.[2733,2748] Manipulating the microbiome by diet, probiotics, or even fecal transplantation may be used to treat behavior problems.

Cats

Coat Color and Breed

The frequencies of the orange allele were high in rural habitats, which were characterized by low densities and a polygynous mating system.

Low frequencies of the orange allele were found in urban populations, which had high densities and a promiscuous mating system.[1842]

Coat color appears to be associated with temperament in cats. Sex-linked orange female (tortoiseshells, calicos, and "torbies"), black-and-white, and gray-and-white cats tend to be more frequently aggressive toward humans.[2178] See Figure 9.1.

In a survey of over 500 cat owners, differences in feline behavior were associated with breed and coat color. Red-coated cats were more likely to exhibit fear-related aggression toward unfamiliar people, whereas Tonkinese and Siamese were more likely to display separation anxiety. Agouti-colored cats are more likely to display inter-cat aggression and red cats have more prey drive, but many of differences are within breed. For instance, lilac-coated Tonkinese had significantly higher playfulness and attention-seeking scores than non-lilac-coated non-Tonkinese, but lilac-coated non-Tonkinese did not have higher playfulness and attention-seeking scores. Birmans and Persian were less playful, but Devon rexes and Tonkinese demonstrated significantly higher scores. Birmans and Persians demonstrated significantly lower scores for predatory behavior than cats not of those breeds, whereas Bengals demonstrated significantly higher scores.[3032] Norwegian Forest kittens differ from kittens of Oriental breeds in that they are more active and vocal when

Domestic Animal Behavior for Veterinarians and Animal Scientists, Seventh Edition. Katherine A. Houpt.
© 2024 John Wiley & Sons, Inc. Published 2024 by John Wiley & Sons, Inc.
Companion website: www.wiley.com/go/houpt/7e

(A)

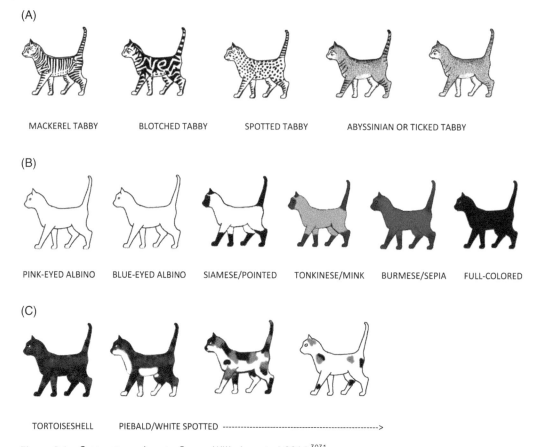

MACKEREL TABBY   BLOTCHED TABBY   SPOTTED TABBY   ABYSSINIAN OR TICKED TABBY

(B)

PINK-EYED ALBINO   BLUE-EYED ALBINO   SIAMESE/POINTED   TONKINESE/MINK   BURMESE/SEPIA   FULL-COLORED

(C)

TORTOISESHELL   PIEBALD/WHITE SPOTTED -->

Figure 9.1   Coat patterns in cats. *Source:* Wilhelmy *et al.* 2016.[3031]

exposed to a novel, mildly frightening object – a spring loaded cylinder.[2869] Not surprisingly, these differences in behavior are heritable.[2965] Microsatellite polymorphism adjacent to the oxytocin receptor gene are associated with feline personality.[2649]

A survey of 80 feline practitioners found that the most desirable cats are Ragdolls.[920] Bengals – a cross of Asian leopard cats and domestic cats – were the most aggressive. Male cats are affectionate to family members and playful but likely to urine spray. Female cats are more fearful and aggressive to other cats. Siamese and Tonkinese are most vocal, while Persians, Maine Coon, and Ragdolls are the quietest.[920] See Figures 9.2 and 9.3.

See Figures 9.2 and 9.3.

Feline Temperament Tests

Several attempts have been made to categorize feline temperament in the following ways: (1) recording behavior in the home environment, whether that is the barnyard, the living room, or the laboratory; (2) recording behavior in a structured test situation, usually while exposing the cat to a familiar and/or a strange person and a novel stimulus; (3) rating various characteristics (active, aggressive, agile, curious, excitable, playful, solitary, tense, vocal, voracious, and/or watchful), reactions to other cats (equable, hostile, fearful, or sociable), and reactions to people (equable, hostile, fearful, or sociable); or (4) accepting owner reports.[670,1559] Seventeen

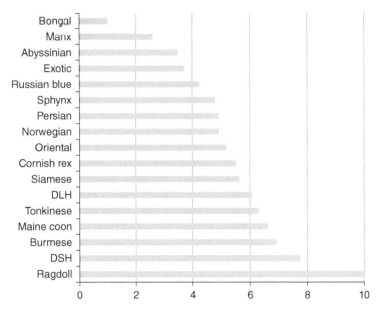

Figure 9.2 Breed differences in feline affection to human family members. Ten is a high score. *Source:* Hart and Hart (2013).[920] Reproduced with permission of Purdue University Press.

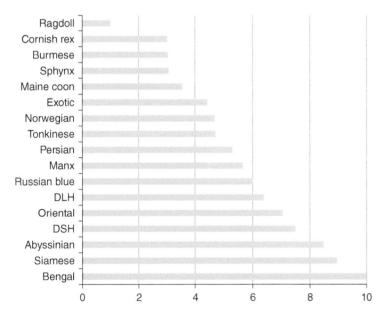

Figure 9.3 Breed differences in feline aggression to other cats. Ten is a high score. *Source:* Hart and Hart (2013).[920] Reproduced with permission of Purdue University Press.

studies of feline temperament revealed that the factors *sociable*, *dominant*, and *curious* were most valid.[798] Female spayed cats with the A form of the oxytocin receptor allele in the single nucleotide polymorphism (SNP) G738A were more likely to be dominant (aggressive).[73,2649] One study found that cats temperament varied in six dimensions: Cat Social,

Active, Human Nonsocial, Human Aggressive, and Intense.[2721] The second study found seven factors, but one was over-grooming which is a medical problem.[2887]

A laboratory test of sociability showed that as early as 10 weeks, cats differed among themselves in their reactions to strange people, to rats, and to the aggressive vocalization of adult cats.[6] The cats that demonstrated fearful behavior in those three situations were classified as defensive and represented 25% of the population. These differences in personality appear to be inherited, because a paternal effect has been noted.[6,670,1923]

Another kitten temperament test reveals that cats that are vocal as kittens are vocal as adults, that very active kittens were less likely to spend time with people as adults, and that some kittens were timid.[1181]

Dogs

Microbiome

Aggressive dog microbiomes were found to be characterized by a peculiar gut microbiome structure, with high biodiversity and enrichment in generally subdominant bacterial genera (i.e., *Catenibacterium* and *Megamonas*). On the other hand, phobic dogs were enriched in *Lactobacillus*.[3086] There are microbiome correlates to abilities of working dogs.[2701]

Sex Differences

There are sex differences in many behaviors in addition to sexual behavior itself. Males are more reactive, more confident, and more aggressive. Females are more social.[731] Females are easier to housebreak, more obedient, and more affectionate, but less active as indicated in surveys from several countries, whereas males are more aggressive, more active, more playful, and more likely to bark and be destructive.[928,1707]

Breed Differences

Breed differences reveal the influence of geographic origin, migration and hybridization on modern dog breeds.[2923,2924] When considering the influence of breed on behavior of dogs there are several ways of determining behavior: the owner's perspective exemplified by C-BARQ and that of veterinarians.[583,2780] The former found that Dachshunds were most aggressive to strangers whereas the latter found that Akitas, American Stafford terriers, and Chesapeake Bay Retrievers were more likely to exhibit territorial defense and Chihuahuas, Chows, Cocker Spaniels, and Dalmatians most likely to snap.

There are breed differences in behavioral neoteny, social signaling, prevalence of behavior problems, and so on. However, substantial within-breed differences in behavior also exist – even in the most controlled experimental studies, according to an extensive review of the literature.[1548]

Retriever breeds gazed longer at the human face than shepherds and poodles and there is significant heritability in human-directed social behavior by dogs.[1125, 2930] Breeds vary in their ability to follow a human's pointing gesture. Border collies do better than Airedales, who do better than Anatolian shepherds, probably because of the tasks for which they were selected rather than cognitive differences.[2301]

Behavioral and physical characteristics may have been simultaneously selected. Some, like pugs, have puppy-like facial features (short nose and full cheeks), whereas German shepherds are fully adult in appearance. Breeds can be ranked by developmental stages: heelers (Huskies and Corgis), headers-stalkers (collies), object players (hounds, retrievers, and poodles), and adolescents (St. Bernards, Komondors, and Great Pyrenees). The sheep-guarding dogs are classified as adolescents, and they show juvenile behavior such as play and lack of mature sexual behavior.[455]

Most impressive is the effect of breed on the response to early isolation and handling.

If puppies are completely isolated from the 3rd to the 20th week of life, they are markedly disturbed. Beagles react most fearfully, and Scottish terriers are more hyperactive and show an impaired (higher) threshold to pain.[1558] Partial isolation from 3 to 16 weeks has different effects on different breeds. Beagles become less active; terriers become more active.[754,769] The early environment of puppies had no effect on the reaction of some breeds to mild punishment (saying "No" and hitting with a newspaper). Basenjis ignored the punishment; Shetland sheepdogs were always inhibited by the punishment. Beagles and Wirehaired fox terriers were inhibited only if they had not been punished in early life.

Ten breeds of dogs were compared to wolves. Dogs of each breed lived in groups, ranging in size from four to seven. They were observed for several hours, and the number of behaviors they exhibited was compared to those of wolves. Siberian huskies were more like wolves than Labrador retrievers. The fewest behaviors were observed in the Cavalier King Charles spaniels, Norfolk terriers, and French bulldogs. The authors interpreted this as meaning that behaviors had been lost with domestication due to pedomorphosis.[841]

Veterinarians and obedience judges were surveyed as to 13 traits in 56 breeds of dog. Principle component analysis revealed three factors – reactivity, aggressiveness, and trainability – and a fourth factor that included playfulness and destructiveness. Cluster analysis of breeds with similar traits revealed seven clusters. It is interesting that snapping at children clusters with reactivity, not with aggression.[928,2780] See Table 9.1 for a comparison of canine fear and aggression measures.

Scott and Fuller studied five breeds of dog and found differences between the breeds, but there were greater differences within breeds than between breeds.[2066]

The extensive studies at Jackson indicate that care must be taken in comparing intelligence, even within a species, because breeds differ markedly in their relative performance, depending on the task to be learned.

Jack Russell terriers and Staffordshire bull terriers were found to be most impulsive, and Labradors and Poodles least.[2495] Impulsivity is a trait that may be linked to aggressiveness. Border collies were more impulsive and aggressive than Labradors, especially if they were field rather than show strains, indicating different selective pressures on the dogs depending on their purpose.[661] Nevertheless, pit bulls, Akitas, and Jack Russell terriers ranked high in inter-dog aggression among the owners surveyed. In the same survey, Dachshunds, Chihuahuas, and Jack Russell terriers were most likely to bite owners or strangers. Labradors used as show dogs were less likely to exhibit aggression than those used for field work. The opposite is true of Springer spaniels. The recent popularity of cross breeds, especially with poodles, such as Labradoodles have revealed interesting behavior problems of these dogs (see Figure 9.4).[2623,2978]

Genome wide association can be used to map Mendelian traits.[2821] There are 10 major canine genetic lineages and their behavioral correlates show that breed diversification is predominantly driven by noncoding regulatory variation.[2727] It should now be possible to use genotyping and DNA sequencing data to determine optimum matings.[2694]

Sensitivity to pointing gestures and attention to human faces during speech were estimated to have the highest heritability.[2807] In the point-following task, genetic factors accounted for 43% of variation between dogs.[3112]

Behavior Problems

There are significant neuroanatomical variation among dog breeds which can explain the differences in behavior as well as disease.[2783,2784,3044] Coat color is genetically determined, and, because the precursor molecules of pigment are also the precursor molecules for neurotransmitters, it is not surprising that behavior differs with coat color. Yellow, as

Table 9.1 Summary of canine fear and aggression GWAS results. Fear and aggression trait peaks are given for separate GWAS studies using Vaysse (marked "V"; Illumina HD) and Boyko ("B"; Affymetrix v.2) genotype datasets. Loci shared with both are green, and others are gray. Coordinates use CanFam2 assembly.

Locus (chr:Mb position)	1:65.7	3:43.4	3:44.8	5:17.2	7:5.9	10:10.8-11.1	10:43.3	11:24.8	12:3.2	15:44.2	18:23.2	26:5.9	32:8.7	34:21.6	34:29.4	X:105.2-106.1
Stranger-directed fear	V	V							B		V, B					V[c]
Dog-directed fear	V									B	V, B			B		V[c], B
Stranger-directed aggression				V							V, B					V[a]
Dog-directed aggression											V					V[b]
Touch sensitivity			B			V, B[f]			B	B	V[e], B					V[c]
Nonsocial fear				V		V		B	B		V[e], B					B
Separation anxiety						V, B[f]			B	B						V[c], B
Dog rivalry							B			B			B			
Owner-directed aggression			B		B		B			V[g], B		B	B		V	
Candidate (favored in bold)	*TRDN*	*CERS3*	*IGF1R*	*PVRL1*	*NR5A2*	*MSRB3, HMGA2*	*TMEM182*	*FSTL4*	*ARG1, MED23*	*IGF1*	*GNAT3, TMEM132C, CD36*	*TMEM132C CD36*	*RASGEF1B*	*SFRS10*	*SMC4*[h]	*ARHGAP36, IGSF1, FIRRE, STK26*[i]

[a-c] The peak SNPs chrX:105,245,495, chrX:105,770,058, chrX:105,877,339, and chrX:106,189,665 (numbered [a-c] in superscript, respectively) lie within one LD block. At least SNPs 2 and 3 are presumed to implicate the same haplotype/functional variant; candidate genes refer to these peaks.

[e] The peak SNP is 23,298,242 (vs. chr18:23,260,370 for the others).

[f] The peak SNP for Vaysse is chr10:11,169,956 and for Boyko is chr10:10,859,628.

[g] Vaysse peak SNP: chr15:44,258,017; Boyko peak SNP: chr15:44,226,659.

[h] Peak SNP is a coding variant at a generally mammalian-conserved position.

[i] *ARHGAP36, IGSF1,* and long noncoding RNA *FIRRE* are co-expressed, including in the pituitary gland and hypothalamus (see text).

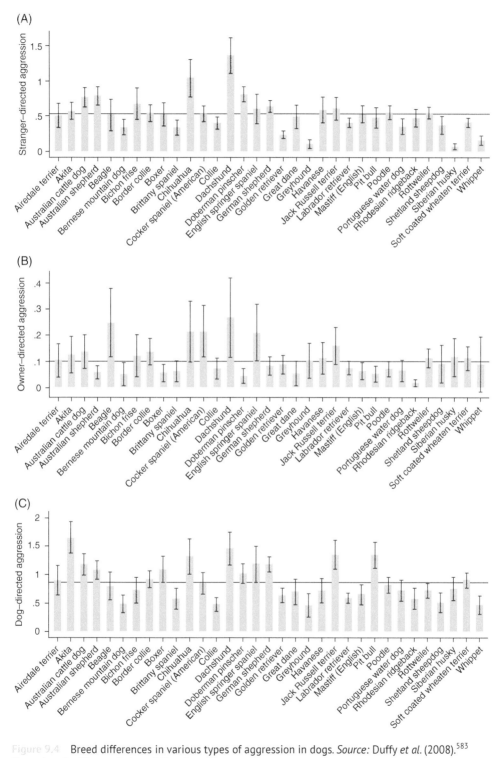

Figure 9.4   Breed differences in various types of aggression in dogs. *Source:* Duffy *et al.* (2008).[583] Reproduced with permission of Elsevier.

(D)

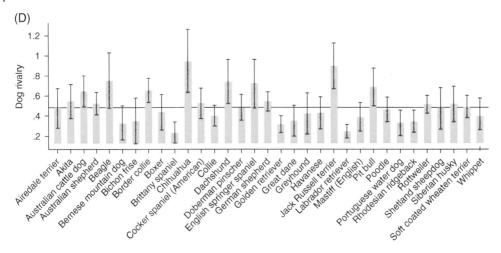

Figure 9.4 (Continued)

opposed to black or chocolate, Labradors are more likely to have backyard problems (barking, chewing, and digging)[1243] and present to a behavior clinic for aggression.[1047] Black Labradors made more errors and took longer to reach criterion (16/20) in a visual discrimination test than yellow ones.[1320]

Fears and Phobias

There are differences in fearfulness among breeds. When owners were surveyed about noise phobias in particular, Soft coated Wheaten terriers were most likely to be fearful, whereas Boxers and Great Danes were least likely.[2192]

Flank Sucking

Flank sucking, a very specific and easily recognized compulsive problem, is a behavior seen almost exclusively in Doberman pinschers. Occasionally, a blanket or another material can serve as the substrate for sucking. It is not a serious behavior problem because the irritation to the skin is mild. More owners complain about fabric sucking because the material must be replaced. The sucking behavior occurs mostly as the dog is resting prior to sleeping. Using genome-wide analysis, an association of SNPs peaking on canine chromosome 7 was found. The most significantly associated SNP

is located within the *CDH2* gene.[555] *CDH2* is widely expressed, mediating synaptic activity-regulated neuronal adhesion.

In an interesting follow-up to the genetic basis of this abnormal behavior, the brains of flank-sucking Dobermans differed from those of unaffected Dobermans. Magnetic resonance imaging revealed higher total brain and gray matter volumes and lower dorsal anterior cingulate cortex and right anterior insula gray matter densities in the affected dogs. The affected Dobermans also had higher fractional anisotropy in the splenium of the corpus callosum, the degree of which correlated with the severity of the behavioral signs.[1728]

Dogs showing multiple compulsive behaviors have a higher frequency of the risk allele than do dogs with a less severe phenotype (60 and 43%, respectively), compared with 22% in unaffected dogs. More recently, four genes, all with synaptic function, have the most obsessive-compulsive disorder (OCD) case-only variation: neuronal cadherin (CDH2), catenin alpha2 (CTNNA2), ataxin-1 (ATXN1), and plasma glutamate carboxypeptidase (PGCP). In the 2 Mb gene desert between the cadherin genes CDH2 and DSC3, two different variants, which disrupt the same highly conserved regulatory element, are found only in dogs with OCD.[2229]

Narcolepsy

Narcolepsy is a syndrome characterized by attacks of inappropriate sleep. The affected dog will collapse and fall asleep for several seconds or minutes at a time. Play or food, especially very palatable food, often elicits the behavior. Doberman pinschers are the breed most affected; Dachshunds, Labradors, as well as Poodles may also be affected. In the Doberman breed, an autosomal recessive gene coding hypocretin (also called "orexin") receptor 2 is involved.[719,2275]

Orexin was believed to be a gene stimulating feeding, hence the name, but its main action seems to be to stimulate wakefulness; therefore, it is now called the "hypocretin (orexin) receptor 2" (*Hcrt2*). Less stimulation of the receptor for hypocretin might allow rapid eye movement (REM) sleep to occur at inappropriate times. It is a single autosomal recessive trait with full penetrance. The *Hcrt2* gene encodes a G-protein-coupled receptor with high affinity for the hypocretin neuropeptides.

Sequence analysis of the reverse transcription polymerase chain reaction (RT-PCR) product in narcoleptic and control animals indicated a 116 base pair (bp) deletion. The *Hcrtr2* transcripts produced in narcoleptic animals are grossly abnormal messenger RNA (mRNA) molecules. In Doberman pinschers, the mRNA potentially encodes a protein with 38 amino acids deleted within the fifth transmembrane domain followed by a frameshift and a premature stop codon at position 932 in the encoded RNA. A SINE insertion mutation is the cause of narcolepsy in Dobermans.[1382] More recent work indicates that this mutation reduces the expression of the neuropeptide precursor molecules, tachykinin precursor 1 (*TAC1*) and proenkephalin (*PENK*), as well as that of suppressor of cytokine signaling 2 (*SOCS2*), in narcoleptic brains. The difference was particularly pronounced in the amygdala, where mRNA levels of *PENK* were 6.2-fold lower in narcoleptic dogs than in heterozygous siblings, and *TAC1* and *SOCS2* showed 4.4-fold and 2.8-fold decrease in expression, respectively.[1385]

Not all canine narcolepsy arises from the same mutation. Analysis of the intron–exon boundaries and sequencing of exon 6 revealed a G-to-A (guanine-to-adenine) transition in the 5′ splice junction consensus sequence (position 5, exon 6–intron 6) in genomic DNA of narcoleptic Labrador retrievers. The C terminus of the protein encoded by narcoleptic Labradors is also truncated and does not include a seventh transmembrane domain. These changes most likely disrupt proper membrane localization and/or cause loss of function of this strongly evolutionarily conserved protein.[1382]

Aggression

The statistics on deaths caused by dogs allow one to determine breed differences in aggression. Between 1979 and 1998, pit bulls killed the greatest number of people, followed by Rottweilers, German shepherds, Huskies, Malamutes, Dobermans, and Chows. These are all large-breed dogs, but other popular large breeds such as Labradors and Golden retrievers are not on the list. It is most interesting that Rottweilers have overtaken pit bulls and in 1998 killed more people per year. The number of Rottweilers registered had increased fivefold between 1979 and 1998, but the number of fatalities increased sevenfold.[2014,2015] The statement is often made that popularity ruins the breed, but what probably happens is that while the percentage of aggressive dogs within a breed remains the same, the total numbers increase so there are more aggressive dogs of that particular breed. Unfortunately, these statistics and the tendency of people to sue if bitten have led insurance companies to refuse policies to owners of pit bulls or Staffordshire terriers, German shepherds, Chows, and Dobermans. Breed-specific legislation has been enacted in only a few communities, but the insurance companies are essentially doing that nationwide. When pit bulls were compared to other breeds of dogs that were adopted from a shelter, there were no differences in aggression and the pit bulls were more likely to cuddle and sleep on the owner's bed.[2594]

Dog breeds can be grouped into: ancient breeds, toy, terrier, working, herding, retrieving, spaniels, and mastiffs. When owners in Japan and the United States were surveyed about behavior problems, toy dogs are the most aggressive group to strangers and household members and most afraid of strange dogs, but terriers and ancient breeds are most aggressive to them.[2274] Breeds differ in behavior and heritability of most behavior traits is 25%, but breed explains only 9% of behavioral variation.[2727] In other words, the behavior of the parents is more important than the breed of the parents. Nevertheless, there are breed differences in social cognition, inhibitory control, and spatial problem-solving ability in dogs.[3113]

Spaniel Aggression

Canine aggression is the most common problem presented to clinical animal behaviorists and results in human injuries and canine euthanasia. One goal of canine behavioral geneticists is to eliminate aggressive dogs, or dogs carrying genes for aggression, from the gene pool. Because aggression in hunting dogs such as spaniels is always undesirable and because the aggression displayed is impulsive (i.e., unpredictable and extreme), the so-called "Springer rage" syndrome has been identified and studied. A similar syndrome is present in English cocker spaniels, and in these dogs the yellow coat color is associated with aggression.[52] The heritability of their aggression is 0.20.[1795]

The types of aggression treated in an urban consultation were as follows: dominance aggression was most common in English springer spaniels (ESS), Doberman pinschers, toy Poodles, and Lhasa apsos; resource guarding was most common in Cocker spaniels and German shepherds, but fear aggression was also common in both breeds and in miniature Poodles.[287]

When comparing a private practice in Ontario, a private practice in Kansas, and a university clinic in upstate New York, ESS were most often presented to the eastern clinics but not to the Midwestern one.[1301] The geographical differences implicate genetic difference between the populations in the East and the Midwest. Two other behaviors problems, separation anxiety and thunder phobia, revealed no breed differences.

Of course, breed differences in prevalence have to be compared with the numbers of dogs of each breed in the catchment area. Historically, ESS present with aggression to owners more than would be predicted by regional breed distributions and by national breed registration statistics.[210,1301] A survey of over 200 ESS owners revealed that 65% of ESS with a history of biting (27% of total ESS) had bitten a familiar person.[2617]

The hunt for the gene involved in aggression is very difficult. For example, one may select one neurotransmitter – for example, serotonin. The difference between aggressive and nonaggressive dogs could be due to a gene controlling synthesis of the neurotransmitter, a gene controlling reuptake of the neurotransmitter, the enzymes that inactivate the neurotransmitter, or genes that control expression of any of the above genes. For example, aggressive dogs have lower serum serotonin levels than nonaggressive dogs, and aggressive English cocker spaniels have lower serum serotonin than aggressive dogs of other breeds.[51,370,1344]

Genetic and Humoral Differences and Aggression

Mean regional 5-HT2A (serotonin receptor 2A) binding index was significantly higher in impulsive dogs than in controls in all cortical regions and in the global cortex using single-photon emission tomography (SPET).[1795]

Monoamine oxidase A is an enzyme that breaks down dopamine, and a mutation that lowers the amount of that enzyme is associated with incarceration of humans, if they had a bad childhood environment.[396] There is evidence in dogs that aggressive individuals have lower cerebrospinal levels of 5-hydroxyindole acetic acid and homovanillic acid, the major metabolites of serotonin and dopamine, respectively.[1922] The DBH (dopamine beta hydroxylase) gene catalyzes the conversion of dopamine into norepinephrine. When over a hundred dogs of various breeds were tested the CC genotype was more common in aggressive (0.8) than in nonaggressive dogs (0.4).[3091]

There is high heritability of aggression – at least in Golden retrievers, with heritability estimate scores of 0.9 for aggression toward strangers, and 0.88 for aggression to owners.[2320] Heritability of aggression toward other dogs is 0.91.[1380] Investigation of genes involved in serotonin function – serotonin receptor 1A (htr1A), serotonin receptor 1B (htr1B) and serotonin receptor 2A (htr2A), and serotonin transporter gene (slc6A4) – using linkage analysis of pedigrees of Golden retrievers did not demonstrate that any of these genes were linked with aggression.[2320]

The heritability of temperament was determined using German shepherds from the Division of Biosensor Research of the US Army. The specifics of the temperament test were not mentioned, but they were all determined by one person and were composite scores used to predict future performance, and indicated the animal's ability to chase and attack a decoy. The hip dysplasia scores also were assigned by one person. There was a negative correlation between temperament and hip dysplasia.[1435]

Genes for aggression and impulsivity in specific breeds have been identified. A polymorphism of the neuronal/epithelial high-affinity glutamate transporter is associated with aggression toward strangers in Shiba Inu dogs.[2223] The neuronal/epithelium high-affinity glutamate transporter was also associated with activity in Labrador retrievers, as was a polymorphism of the catecholamine methyl transferase gene.[2222]

Police and pet German shepherd dogs diagnosed with hyperactivity and impulsivity based on questionnaires were genotyped, and the dopamine D4 receptor subtypes 2/2 were compared with 2a/3a and 3a/3a (combined because 3a/3a is rare) with the behaviors. There was no difference in the activity–impulsivity scores between dogs with the 2/2 genotype versus the 2/3a and 3a/3a combined genotype group either in the total sample or in the pet dog group. In contrast, police dogs with the 2/2 genotype showed significantly lower activity–impulsivity scores compared with police dogs with the 2/3a or 3a/3a genotype.[973]

German shepherds with the short form of the TH (tyrosine hydroxylase, the enzyme involved in dopamine formation) gene were more active and impulsive.[1280] Siberian huskies with the short form of the TH gene were more impulsive. Siberian huskies possessing at least one short dopamine D4 allele displayed greater activity–impulsivity in the behavioral tests than did those with two long alleles; dogs with the short allele also tended to receive higher ratings on the activity–impulsivity scale of the questionnaire.[2382]

By using one breed, English cocker spaniels, a breed in which aggressive behavior has been noted for the past 40 years, breed differences in the genotype can be eliminated so that any differences found should reflect differences in temperament. In a study comparing nonaggressive English cocker spaniels with English cockers that had bitten and broken skin, there were significant associations between aggression and four SNPS in the region of the dopamine D1 receptor (DRD1), two SNPS in the serotonin ID receptor (HTR1D), and five SNPS in a glutamate receptor (SLC6A1).[2312]

Most dogs are homozygous for the DAT-VNTR (dopamine transporter–variable number tandem repeat) two-tandem-repeat allele (2/2). The one-tandem-repeat allele is overrepresented in American Malinois, both as heterozygotes and as homozygotes (1/2 or 1/1). All American Malinois with reported seizures were 1/1 genotype. Those with at least one "1" allele (1/1 or ½ genotype) were more likely to display hypervigilance and exhibit episodic aggression as well as more fearful postures.[1402]

Trainability and boldness do not always segregate together between dog breed clusters.[3010] Boldness is associated with certain SNP markers on the candidate genes CNIH and PCDH9.[2575]

In a study of the association of genomics and behavior, all prick-eared and small dogs were classified as bold, whereas all drop-eared dogs were classified as non-bold, with the exception of the Bernese mountain dog.[2632]

Canine fear and aggression traits have been mapped to single haplotypes at the GNAT3–CD36 and IGSF1 loci. CD36 is widely expressed, but areas of the amygdala and hypothalamus are among the brain regions with highest enrichment (Figure 9.4).[583]

Dogs

Gut microbiota in dogs and cats consist primarily of the genus *Firmicutes*, *Bacteroides* species, and *Fusobacteria*. The canine GI tract contains large amounts of *Enterococcus* and lactic acid-producing species.

The meconium microbiota resembled bacteria from the maternal vagina in vaginally delivered puppies, the meconium microbiota of puppies born by Cesarean section indicated a relative resemblance to maternal oral and vaginal microbiota.[3043,3057] Moderate predictive power of microbiome markers were observed for motivation, sociability, and gastrointestinal issues of working dogs.[2701] *Proteobacteria* and *Fusobacteria* manifested higher relative abundance in nonaggressive pit bulls, while *Firmicutes* was relatively more abundant in aggressive pit bulls. The family *Lactobacillaceae* was more abundant in aggressive dogs, while the family *Fusobacteriaceae* was more abundant in nonaggressive dogs.[2828] There is a difference in the microbiome of aggressive and nonaggressive pit bulls all fed the same diet. Clades within *Lactobacillus*, *Dorea*, *Blautia*, *Turicibacter*, and *Bacteroides* differ between the aggressive and nonaggressive groups. Nutraceuticals that alter the microbiome may have a place in treating behavior problems.[2687]

Microbiome

The relative abundance of Blautia, Bacteroides, and Odoribacter in the microbiome are found to be decreased in patients with anxiety.[2733] Caution must be taken in examining the effect of the probiotics on the microbiome and, consequently, on behavior.[2796]

Temperament

There have been many – at least 50 – publications on evaluation of canine temperament using a variety of methods from a battery of tests, experts' opinions, and ratings of individual dogs by their owners. A review of over 50 studies of canine temperament revealed seven traits: reactivity, fearfulness, sociability, activity, responsiveness to training, submissiveness, and aggression.[1157]

Owner Evaluation
Animal personality is defined as the behavioral differences between individuals that are relatively stable in time and across contexts. There have been a number of approaches to defining canine personality. The traits fearfulness, activity, sociability, responsiveness to training, submissiveness, and aggression resulted from a meta-analysis of 31 studies.[1908] Four of the five personality traits had a significant association with dominance: while more extroverted, conscientious and open dogs scored higher on dominance, more agreeable dogs scored lower. In accordance with previous studies, older dogs tend to be more dominant.[3019] In a study of 11,000 dogs, seven personality traits emerged: Insecurity, Training focus, Aggressiveness/dominance, Energy, Human sociability, Dog sociability, and Perseverance.[2964]

The dog's personality does not seem to impact the dog–owner relationship. Only fearfulness is correlated with the relationship, but the owner's personality affects the outcome of behavior problems.[2600,2936] Fear responses to less salient noises such as television or traffic may, therefore, reflect fearful personality characteristics, while responses to very salient noises, such as gunshots and fireworks, may be learned. Early experience with thunder or gunshots increased the likelihood of fear of either of these noises as adults.[258] When a large number of owners were surveyed as to the trainability and boldness of their dogs, herding dogs were more trainable than hounds, working dogs, toy dogs, and nonsporting dogs; sporting dogs were also more trainable than nonsporting dogs. In parallel, terriers were bolder than hounds and herding dogs. There are breed differences in how often a dog looks at a human.[2831] Regarding genetic relatedness, breeds with ancient Asian or African origin (ancient breeds) were less trainable than breeds in the herding/sighthound cluster and the hunting breeds. Breeds in the mastiff/terrier cluster were bolder than the ancient breeds.[2274]

Dog breeds are typically divided according to historical usage into Working, Hunting, Herding, Hound, and Terrier groups, plus the Toy group and, in some countries, a separate Gun dog group. When the results of a temperament test involving reactions to strangers who attempt to play tug-of-war with the dog are compared to the historical use of the dog, there is little correlation, but there is a similarity in response within a breed. Most interesting is that of two of the most popular breeds: the Golden retriever is fearful, and the Labrador bold. These results suggest that the present use of a dog differs from the historical use.[2206]

The ratings of individual dogs are usually based on questionnaires filled out by owners. For example, Serpell and Hsu developed a questionnaire, C-BARQ (**C**anine **B**ehavioral **A**ssessment and **R**esearch **Q**uestionnaire), designed to provide standardized evaluations of canine temperament and behavior.[2086,2801] The current version consists of 100 questions describing the different ways in which dogs typically respond to common events, situations, and stimuli in their environment. The valid factors were stranger- or dog-directed fear/aggression, nonsocial fear, energy level, owner-directed aggression, chasing, trainability, and attachment. See Figure 9.3.

Fearfulness is not a unitary phenomenon. Dogs can be separated into those that are fearful of people and those that are afraid of other dogs. Toy and female dogs are more liable to be afraid of other dogs. Dogs that are afraid of people are more likely to have female owners, to be untrained, and to have been acquired at an older age. Unrelated to fear of people or animals is *neuroticism* – defined as excitement in strange situations or places, or a fearful reaction to sudden visual or acoustic stimuli, that is, how cautiously or nervously a dog is perceived to behave.[2630] It is important to know that all fear is not the same and should be treated differently. The Dog Mentality Assessment is a series of 33 tests of a dog's personality traits and questionnaire subscales applied to Rough collies. Approximately half (45–55%) of the Rough collies typically displayed some degree of fear-related behaviors in response to sudden or loud noises. Unfortunately, selecting for less fear results in selecting for dogs that are more prone to chase, are more prone to respond aggressively if provoked by other dogs in the household, are less afraid of unfamiliar persons, and show fewer problem behaviors when left alone.[103] There is also a test for sensory processing sensitivity.[2669]

The factors that had the biggest effect on Labrador Retriever personality were sex and neuter status. A study of Golden retrievers using C-BARQ for behavior scoring revealed that substantial genetic variance for several traits, including fetching tendency and fear of loud noises, while other traits revealed negligibly small heritabilities. Dogs that are more extraverted, conscientious and open tend to rank higher in the hierarchy, while more friendly dogs tend to rank lower. In addition, older dogs tend to dominate in multi-dog households.[3019]

Effect of Owner's Personality

Owners of dogs that are aggressive to humans scored higher on neuroticism than owners of nonaggressive dogs.[2761,2792] The human's personality also contributes to improvement of canine behavior. Owner conscientiousness, extraversion and openness, and owner–dog attachment were associated with positive treatment outcomes.[2936]

Direct Evaluation
Owned Dogs

A very extensive temperament test has been developed to evaluate dogs for aggressive tendencies.[1685] In another test, barking, separation anxiety, and aggression toward cats, joggers, or other dogs could be predicted, but aggression toward the owner – conflict aggression – was not.[2326] Temperament testers are not very reliable in that their evaluation of the dog based on the same videotape of its behavior varies over time. Those testers with the most training and experience were most reliable.[548]

Most temperament tests include response to a stranger, but the stranger must be trained because dogs give very different responses to a friendly stranger in comparison to a threatening stranger even when the stranger is the same person.[2336] The friendly stranger approaches at a normal speed while talking to the dog, whereas the threatening stranger moves slowly and haltingly and stares at the dog silently. The dogs – Belgium shepherds – were consistent in their responses even a year later, but the owner's opinions of the dog's reaction did not agree with the dog's behavioral reactions.

Laboratory Dogs

A temperament test has been developed for laboratory dogs to study the dog's response to an unfamiliar person, to a novel environment, to handling of its body on a table, while restrained in a cage, and when exposed to loud noise, all traits that are important for suitability to a research or teaching environment.[2547]

Puppy Tests

Age affects the results of a temperament test. Puppies that are exploratory at 6 weeks may not be at 12 weeks, and vice versa. The same is true of social dominance.[2495] These findings indicate that tests of puppies at seven weeks, popular as a means of predicting adult behavior, are unlikely to be valid. The tests involve scoring the puppies' reactions to handling and their willingness to approach or follow people.

The Campbell Test was conducted to assess dominant behavior in puppies.[379] The test consists of five parts and must be conducted at the age of six to eight weeks old. The test leader, not previously encountered by the puppy, should remain impassive and show no signs of emotion throughout the test. Puppies are subjected to the test individually with no other person, animal, or object present that could distract them. Activity is a better predictor of later behavior than is the puppy's response to handling at seven weeks.[204] Border collie puppies that were sociable (i.e., approached a stranger) were more apt to struggle when restrained, whereas nonsocial puppies were passive. Dogs that avoided a stare were more likely to struggle when restrained. These responses were unrelated to boldness as measured by the puppies' reaction to a moving toy.[1935]

Working Dogs

Both training and breed group determine success in problem solving by dogs.[2872] Evaluation of temperament and prediction of performance of working dogs (guide and military dogs) are especially important to reduce investment in an unsuitable dog.[2464–2466] Each dog was evaluated for its response to a stranger approaching the dog, approaching the handler, and attempting to play tug-of-war with the dog; to a paper figure and a rag doll that appeared suddenly and threatened it; to gunfire; and to a threat to its handler. Using more than a thousand dogs, the evaluators calculated four factors: mental stability, willingness to please, affability, and defense drive. Breed differences appeared between German shepherds and Labradors; the latter had little prey drive. They found that defense drive (attacks threatening people) and hardness (recovers quickly from startling stimuli) could be predicted by puppy weight. Heavier females scored better.

Dogs must pass a temperament test to be used as military dogs in Sweden. Dogs that passed that test had been rated high on the C-BARQ category "Trainability" and C-BARQ items "Hyperactive/restlessness, difficulties in settling down" and "Chasing/following shadows or light spots" by the people who raised them for 18 months. They were also on average left home alone more hours per day, a surprising result. Dogs that failed were rated as fearful.[731,732]

Retrieval of objects at eight weeks and aggression to a threatening stranger at nine months have been used to predict success in police dog training. Five important traits in working dogs have been identified – playfulness, curiosity, fear, chase proneness, and sociability – all of which could be explained as a shyness/boldness trait and aggression.[2206,2207] Another test revealed three factors: exploration, reaction to novelty, and reaction to startling stimuli.[1228] The shyness/boldness trait could be used to predict success in working dogs. Only the test for fear was valid in selecting working dogs from a shelter.[2408] There appear to be two fear factors in dogs: a *social fear factor*, defined by fear of unfamiliar humans and dogs; and a *nonsocial fear factor*, defined by fear of inanimate items (e.g., wind, thunder, traffic, and loud noises).[2723]

Livestock guarding dogs have five personality traits (Trainability, Independence, Playfulness, Sociability, and Reactivity). Those dogs assessed as playful were less successful as livestock guarding, whereas those ranked high in trainability and low in reactivity were more successful.[2877] The factors that had the biggest effect on Labrador Retriever personality were sex and neuter status. The heritability for fetching was 0.38 and for noise fear 0.30.[2806]

German shepherd police dogs may show a fearful, aggressive, or ambivalent response to the approach of a stick-wielding stranger. The fearful and ambivalent dogs are the passive coping animals that have greater activation of cortisol than the active coping ones that are aggressive.[1036]

Dogs to be used for explosive detection were tested for their reaction to a black plastic bag dropped near them, to grates falling in front of and behind them, and for their willingness to climb open riser stairs, in addition to many of the situations used in another temperament test.[2098] When Labrador retrievers were rated for obedience, aggression to other dogs, concentration, affection demand, interest in the target, and anxiety, factor analysis revealed that a combination of those traits, which could be termed "willingness to work," is the key factor in determining success as a drug detection dog.[1442]

Hunting Dogs

Hunting dogs are judged on their eagerness to hunt, speed, style, independence, seeking width, cooperation, and ability to work in the field. These traits are heritable.[324]

Results of field trials revealed that Finnish hounds were found to have the highest heritability scores for pursuit and tonguing (vocalization while in pursuit of a hare or fox).[1381]

Therapy Dogs

Dogs are used in animal-assisted therapy. These dogs must be able to interact with physically and/or mentally handicapped people, so the requirements are stricter. A test was devised using a series of challenges, the first of which measured aggression to dogs and people. A dog that displayed aggression failed. Initiative was determined by the dog's approach to a person on the other side of the fence and its willingness to approach people in its enclosure. Jumping on fences or people was scored negatively because of the danger to handicapped people. Finally, the dog's response to food-lured commands such as "Sit" and "Down," and its willingness to go up and down stairs and walk on a leash, were tested. Only 5 of 23 shelter dogs tested passed the test. Another test for animals to be used in animal-assisted therapy includes a "patient" who rocks on a chair, claps his hands, grabs the dog, and screams.[2602]

Shelter Dogs

Two studies of a temperament test based loosely on the Sternberg Test have attempted to validate its use in shelter dogs. Fifty percent of dogs that passed that temperament test lunged, growled, snapped, or, rarely, bit in their new homes. Most of the aggression was in territorial situations, but 90% were still in their adoptive home.[283,415] When the behavior problems identified by the relinquishing owner are compared to those of the adoptive owner, aggression to strange people, dogs, or veterinarians and anxiety when left alone were present in both homes, indicating that the dog does not change even when the environment does; but aggressive dogs had played with a stranger much less as juveniles.[1768,2326] No one has developed an adult canine temperament test that predicts success as a pet dog based on positive qualities.

Horses

Microbiome

The abundance of *Desulfurispora*, *Helicobacter*, *Acinetobacter*, *Ruminobacter*, *Pseudobacteroides*, *Roseburia*, and members of the yet not classified *Marinilabiliaceae* family was greater with higher occurrences of oral stereotypies, while *Streptomyces* was greater with higher incidence of locomotion stereotypies. Higher frequency of aggressiveness was positively associated with overgrowth of two other bacterial genera: *Streptococcus* and *Butyrivibrio* spp. But inversely correlated to the prevalence of *Anaeroplasma*. The manifestation of unresponsiveness to the environment was positively linked to the prevalence of *Diplorickettsia*, *Anaerorhabdus*, and *Novosphingobium*.[2861] High-starch diets alter equine fecal microbiota and increase behavioral reactivity.[2680,2681] De Fombelle *et al.*[2709] showed that the cecal and right ventral colonic microbiota was modified as early as five hours after an abrupt incorporation of barley in a fiber-based diet.[2709] When horses were fed a 57% hay and 43% barley (high grain) diet, time spent in vigilance tended to be positively correlated with cecal and colonic amylolytic bacteria concentrations during the sociability test (interaction with an unfamiliar horse) and with cecal lactate-utilizing and colonic amylolytic bacteria concentrations during neophobia tests with a novel object.[2720] Horses fed with a high-barley diet were more reactive (blowing) than those fed an all-hay diet.[2719] The weaning method affects the microbione.[2859]

Breed Differences

When the genome of the domestic horse was compared with that of horses that lived thousands of years before equine domestication, there were differences not only in a group of genes controlling musculoskeletal and cardiac function but also in a group controlling cognitive function. The former group allowed selection for athletic performance in the horse, but the latter allowed selection for tameness, tractability, and trainability.[2056] When Quarter Horses and Thoroughbreds were compared on their ability to learn a visual discrimination, the Quarter Horses did better, apparently because they were less distracted.[1439] Non-warmbloods learned more quickly than warmbloods (Thoroughbreds and Arabians).[1384] Anglo–Arabs took longer to train to accept a rider than either Thoroughbreds or Arabians.[1130] Horses bred to be jumpers are less fearful of a visual and auditory stimulus than those bred for dressage, whether or not they have been trained, indicating a selection for that characteristic.[2371]

When testing the ability to learn a simple operant conditioning task – touching a target – certain mare lines, sire lines, and mare/sire groups were found to learn more efficiently and to display fewer signs of avoidance than others.[285] When Thoroughbreds and Haflingers were observed on the same pasture, Thoroughbreds were more active, ate more hay, and drank more water, whereas the Haflingers grazed more.[3040] The heritability of reactivity (moving when they were supposed to stand still) in warmbloods

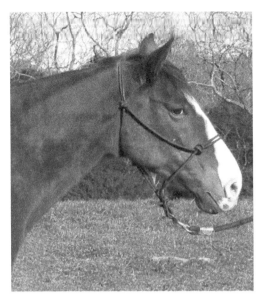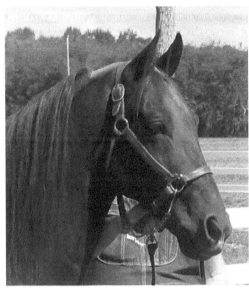

Figure 9.5 Behavioral independence in Tennessee Walker mares varies with agouti signaling protein (ASIP) loci. Black mares (aa) (on the right) are more independent (self-reliant) than bay mares (A−) (on the left). *Source:* Courtesy of Ann Staiger.

is 0.17.[1984] The heart rate of young race horses increases in anticipation of a novel event, and Thoroughbred colts exhibit a greater response than Thoroughbred fillies or Arabians of either sex.[1130] Ponies show a similar increase in epinephrine before a treadmill exercise.[160]

There are breed differences in the incidence of behavior problems.[2086] Thoroughbreds are more likely to crib, whereas Arabians are more likely to stall walk and reject their foals.[20,1419,1531] Standardbreds are less likely to crib than Thoroughbreds.[1910]

In Mongolian horses, BDNF, DBH, SLC6A4, and COMT were associated with the behavior trait of biting. In the BDNF gene, the SNPs in 222 bp (C→T) and 261 bp (G→C) were identified, and the association analysis showed that the biting behavior was significantly affected by BDNF genes as C222T and G261C.[2949]

Coat Color

Coat color influences horse behavior too. When surveyed, owners identified only resistance to having feet picked up by strangers as the only difference between bays and chestnuts, but chestnuts do seem to be bolder – more likely to approach a novel object. Likely to approach unfamiliar objects and animals than bays.[692,2743] Bay Tennessee Walker mares that carry the A− genotype of agouti signaling protein (ASIP) are more likely to exhibit separation anxiety than black (aa) mares[1122,2997] (see Figure 9.5). Silver Icelandic horses carry a missense mutation in exon 11 (Arg618Cys) in the PMEL/SILV gene that codes for the glycolprotein PMEL. Silver horses are slower to approach a novel object than horses of other coat colors, but are no more fearful of a noisy rapidly moving object.[338]

Equine Temperament Tests

Several equine temperament tests have been developed. All these tests measure reaction to stimuli that are frightening. Mackenzie's test involves leading a horse over a measured distance and then attempting to lead the horse after an umbrella had been snapped open in front of it, after a bunch of pots and pans fell from 10 feet, or when there was a piece of plastic on the ground.[1434] In another test, a balloon was burst beside a horse, a mechanical pig moved in front of the horse, or an umbrella opened. The umbrella gave the most accurate results.[2526]

Physiological responses to environmental changes vary with the type of changes. Horses are more likely to defecate when isolated, but more likely to walk when confronted with a novel object (a tricycle). Heart rate is the best physiological measure of emotionality when the horse's activity is controlled.[1495] Horses' cardiac responses to auditory (white noise) or visual (orange traffic cone) stimuli were similar, but their behavioral responses were different. They backed away from the visual stimulus.[420]

The horse's response to an umbrella lowered from the ceiling when the horse was free in an arena and the ease with which the horse could be led across a bridge were measured. The horse's heart rate was correlated with its behavior. Flightiness and sensitivity were measured by the novel object (umbrella) test, and patience and willingness to perform by the handling (bridge) tests. There was some relationship between the reactions of an individual horse at one and at two years old to novel objects and between that reaction and the horse's performance (number of jumps taken correctly) at age three, but there was no single test that consistently predicted performance.[2364] A simplified four-minute temperament test utilizing stationary and rolling balls, a wooden bridge, traffic cones, an alleyway formed of plastic sheeting, and a blue bar on the ground was applied to over a thousand horses and gave a wide range of scores for reactivity; warmbloods and Thoroughbreds were more reactive than ponies and draft breeds.[2565] The horses' response – movement and heart rate – to a large rotating weather balloon was correlated with the handlers' assessment of their temperament.[1611] The greater the number of defecations when exposed to the balloons, the more anxious the horse had been rated by

its caretakers.[1610] Shaking a red-and-white garland in the horse's home stall and, in a separate test, covering its head for an hour revealed that jumpers are no more reactive than therapeutic riding horses.[1598] Reactivity can be measured objectively by quantifying the speed with which a horse rejoins its herd mates after being startled.[1700] Even when tested six times, the horses did not seem to habituate, so riders should realize that their mount will spook at the same fallen tree during their next ride.

The most extensive equine temperament testing has been performed by Hausberger and her associates.[943] The test involved releasing the horse alone in an arena and measuring its behavior before and after a novel object – in this case, colored rails – was put in the arena. Included in the temperament tests was a learning task. The horse had to manipulate a lid with its muzzle for a food reward. Of the breeds tested, the Icelandic pony was the most successful. This breed has been genetically isolated for hundreds of years, which indicates that we have not been selecting for equine intelligence. (See Chapter 6 for more detail on early handling effects.) Most interesting was the finding that the reaction of horses of the same breed revealed differences in their temperament depending on the use to which they were put. Dressage horses were most flighty than jumpers. Exploration was significantly higher in the jumping and equine assisted therapy groups than in the eventing and dressage groups, although in another study, all horses needed a similar length of time to approach the person after the opening of the umbrella.[2885] This is an interesting finding because it means that, independent of the activity they have been trained to practice, horses will demonstrate the same response to a sudden stimulus: running away and then returning and exploring the area. In a similar test of riding school horses, the horses kept in box stalls were more reactive than those kept in paddocks.[1346]

Most temperament tests are performed only once, so it is important to know how repeatable they are. Male yearlings are more fearful of unfamiliar humans than females, but mares showed more anxiety and less affability than geldings in a training situation.[580,2498] Training horses may not influence their physiological fear reactions, but it reduces the behavioral expression of fear if the trainer is present.[1463]

Diet

Diet has an effect on temperament. Weaned foals fed a high-fat and high-fiber diet were more likely to investigate a novel object or person than those fed a high-starch, high-sugar diet.[1021] Adult horses fed a high-fat diet reacted as quickly to a startling stimulus (tiger head on a spring) than those fed a high-sugar diet, but they did not move as far or as long.[1912]

The microbiome of the domesticated horse is less diverse than that of the free ranging ones. When comparing the microbiome of Przewalski horses born in European semi-reserves and those born in Mongolia, the latter had a more diverse microbiome than the former.[2824]

Crib-biting horses showed greater abundance of Campylobacteria, Campylobacteriaceae, Campylobacteriales, Synergistales, Synergistaceae, Synergistota, Synergista, and F0B2 in feces.[3120] There are clearly stratified communities of bacteria from individuals trained for dressage and jumping differ from those used for other types of disciplines. In addition, the microbiota of horses housed in stalls on straw bedding were clustered apart from those housed in stalls on shavings and wood pellets. In general, straw bedding is considered more comfortable for horses. There is a correlation between aggressiveness and lactate-producing bacteria indicating that acidosis may be involved in the misbehavior.[2826] A broad spectrum of factors are known to affect the equine intestinal microbiome, including feed, environmental conditions (e.g., geographic location, climate, hygiene, fasting, transportation, and exercise), inflammation, and the use of external compounds, such as prebiotics, probiotics, and antibiotics. Fecal microbiome transplantation may be considered for behavior problems as well as digestive ones.

Age

Reactivity to humans, whether active or passive and whether the human was familiar or strange, was stable at least from 8 months to 2.5 years.[1307] The same group found that horses' reactions to isolation were consistent over time. The number of neighs was particularly stable. A horse's attraction to other horses was not stable over time.[1309]

There have been numerous attempts to describe horse personality. Rankin and Wickens reviewed 113 publications dealing with equine personality.[2944] Reactivity to environmental stimuli, gregariousness, reactivity to humans, sensory sensitivity, and locomotor activity are some of the most assessed traits. One study of equine personality described four components of equine personality. Component 1 included the attributes of anxious, stressed, and excitable and was defined as the equine personality scale "temperament." Component 2 contained the descriptors of affectionate, sociable, and curious and was termed "character." Component 3 included imaginative, dominant, and clever and was defined as "intelligence." Component 4 was composed of cooperative, focused, and sensible and was defined as "willingness (to work)."[3037]

In addition to an academic exercise, the personality test is supposed to help assign the correct horse to the correct user (e.g., riding for the handicapped or open jumping). A horse and its femalemale rider may have similar personality traits.[3037] Usually, the handlers are given a list of adjectives and asked to apply these to a horse. Those adjectives that are correlated with one another can be identified by factor analysis. The experimenter can then name the factors. When this method was used, there were three factors: (a) agreeableness (obedience, nonaggression, "kindness," and sociality), (b) intelligence and curiosity, and

(c) emotionality or nervousness.[1534] The easiest equine personality trait to identify is nervousness, and this can be compared to the human personality trait neuroticism.[1610,1611] Conscientiousness and extraversion also seem to be valid terms.[1404,1592,2364] Trainability and affability (aggression to people or other horses) are other important factors. In a large survey in which over a thousand people rated horses, Thoroughbreds, Arabians, and Welsh ponies were rated most anxious and excitable, but also most inquisitive.[1405] Horses used for competition were less anxious than those used for leisure.[1666] Finally, the five dimensions of temperament (fearfulness, gregariousness, reactivity to humans, level of locomotor activity, and tactile sensitivity) have been identified.[1307] When a subjective rating by caretakers for agreeableness, extraversion, and neuroticism was compared to performance in a temperament test that involved the horses' reaction to the sudden opening of an umbrella, to a large colorful toy, and to be asked to cross a plastic sheet, extraversion predicted time to cross the plastic and refusal behavior during this test. It also predicted minimum distance to the novel object. Neuroticism predicted how reactive an individual was to the opening of the umbrella.[2573] Horses that misbehaved during veterinary examinations were judged by their owners to be anxious and aggressive, and were not likely to be sociable or learn well.[1784] *Boldness* in horses is defined as a general lack of fear. Older horses were more likely to be bolder than younger horses, but horses started under saddle at a relatively older age were less bold and less independent. In Australia, boldness was positively associated with breed (Australian Stock Horses) and disciplines (breeding conformation, equitation, eventing, and working cow horse) and negatively associated with dressage and therapy horses. Independence was positively associated with breed (Australian Stock Horses, heavy horses, and ponies).[2682]

When American horse owners, most of whom were pleasure rather than competitive riders, were surveyed, three personality traits emerged: nervousness, curiosity, and threatening. Arabians, Thoroughbreds, Saddlebreds, and Walking horses were the most nervous, and Quarter Horses, Paints, Appaloosas, and Drafts were the least nervous.[2962]

Microbiome

The abundance of *Desulfurispora*, *Helicobacter*, *Acinetobacter*, *Ruminobacter*, *Pseudobacteroides*, *Roseburia*, and members of the yet not classified *Marinilabiliaceae* family was greater with higher occurrences of oral stereotypies, while *Streptomyces* was greater with higher incidence of locomotion stereotypies. Higher frequency of aggressiveness was positively associated with overgrowth of two other bacterial genera: *Streptococcus* and *Butyrivibrio* spp. But inversely correlated to the prevalence of *Anaeroplasma* The manifestation of unresponsiveness to the environment was positively linked to the prevalence of *Diplorickettsia*, *Anaerorhabdus*, and *Novosphingobium*.[2861] The microbiome of foals can predict their response to weaning. Most genera in community type 2 (i.e., *Eubacterium*, *Coprococcus*, *Clostridium* XI, and *Blautia* spp.) were negatively correlated with salivary cortisol levels.[2861]

Genetic Differences in Temperament

One basic genetic difference between horses is sex; geldings are believed to have better temperaments.[3062] There is a polymorphism in the horse – an A-to-G substitution – in the dopamine D4 receptor gene. This may code for an asparagine for aspartic acid amino acid substitution. Over 100 two-year-old Thoroughbreds were genotyped and evaluated for temperament. Those horses that carried the G allele were more curious (examined novel objects) and less vigilant than horses carrying the A allele according to their caretakers.[1610] When the temperament of yearling Thoroughbreds in training was evaluated for tractability, those carrying the A allele form of the serotonin 1A receptor gene were less tractable.[1031]

A study of Tennessee Walking Horses iden
tified loci (ECA1, ECA23, and ECA13) that
may contribute to the anxious, tractable, and
agnostic traits.[3073] There are other equine
genes orthologous to human genes related to
the Big Five personality traits, and 18
personality-related candidate genes in horses
were identified but have not been tested
behaviorally.[3042]

When the learning ability (target training to
touch) was measured among ponies significant
differences were found among sire, dam, and
full sibling lines.[2655] Thoroughbreds were
slower than other breeds in learning to back
through a corridor.[3062]

Cattle

Breed Differences

Social, Sexual, and Maternal Behavior
Dominance is clearly influenced by heredity,
for twin cattle are often of equal dominance.[651]
Also, breed differences in dominance exist
among dairy cattle. Among beef breeds, which
do not differ markedly in weight, definite differences in temperament can also be found.[2373]
Success (or failure) in dominance interactions
is genetically determined in heifers.[1876] In
northern Italy each year, dual-purpose cows of
the Valdostan breed are paired to establish
dominance. Heritability of fighting ability was
estimated to be 0.08–0.09.[2031]

Intra-individual and intra-breed differences
in sexual behavior may be noted. For example,
the Brown Swiss breed shows the least marked
estrous activity of the dairy breeds. Black cattle
exhibit stronger signs of estrus than red, roan,
or white cattle.[42] Male sexual behavior is definitely under genetic control, as indicated by
the nearly identical performance within pairs
of twin bulls but the marked difference
between twin pairs (Figure 9.6). German
(Aberdeen Angus × German) dual-purpose
cattle showed more maternal protectiveness
than Simmental when their day-old calves

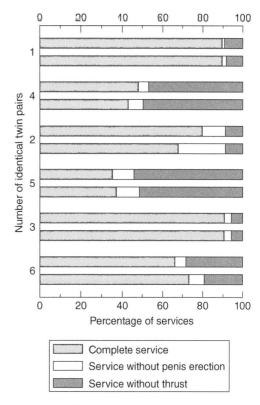

Figure 9.6   Percentage distribution of complete
copulations, mounts without penis erections, and
mounts without thrusts in pairs of twin bulls.
Source: Hafez (1975).[879] Reproduced with
permission of Elsevier.

were ear tagged.[1028] There are marked genetic
effects on maze-learning ability in cattle.[74]

Feeding Behavior
Cows sired by Piedmontese bulls were willing
to graze farther from water than those sired by
Angus.[2335] Piedmontese cattle were developed
in mountainous regions, so they may make
more uniform use of a rough-terrain environment. A high bite rate and low mastication rate
are an adaption to maximize intake. Therefore,
it is not surprising that Holsteins, a breed
selected for high food intake, have a higher
bite rate and slower mastication rate than
Norwegian reds.[1723]

When Charolais and Holstein cattle cross
breeds were tested for fearfulness (of an
approaching human and in response to

separation from pen mates), two quantitative loci for the fear test scores showed the same mode of action, with both significant additive and dominance effects. The Charolais allele was associated with less fearful animals in the fear test, and those cattle showed dominance relative to those with the Holstein allele. The two quantitative trait loci (QTLs) detected on chromosome 25 showed an additive mode of inheritance, where the Holstein allele was associated with an increased frequency of vocalization during separation. No overlapping QTLs were identified for the traits measured by the two different tests, supporting the hypothesis that different genetic factors influence behavioral responses to different situations.[873]

Bovine Temperament Tests

A tethering test at three weeks of age, a weighing test at three months of age, and a separation and restraint test at seven to eight months of age have been used to evaluate temperament in cattle. A region on BTA29 with a putative QTL in the proximal part and the candidate gene, *DRD4*, appear to be involved in a trait called "curiosity" (willingness to explore the scale).[829] Approach to a novel object and to familiar and unfamiliar humans has been used as a temperament test in cattle, as has the response to a novel environment with or without a novel object. The temperament factors identified were fearfulness, activity, exploration, and attention toward the environment. The characteristic high activity is associated with low food motivation and, consequently, poor performance on an operant task.[2403]

Individual differences in the fearfulness of cattle are measured by their response to a novel object, a different environment, feed in an unfamiliar place, or a startling stimulus.[277] One cattle temperament test consists of leading, restraining in a corner, and stroking. There were genetic effects, a heritability factor of 0.22 for docility, and environmental effects as well. Cattle kept indoors were more docile than those kept outside.[1304]

When observed in an auction ring, sensitivity or temperament was based on whether the cattle stood still or walked or slowly trotted, or tried to escape the ring. Holsteins were more sound sensitive (sudden yell or air hose) than beef cattle, but were no more sensitive to sudden movements (hand waving or children running).[1304]

The response of beef cattle in a chute is correlated with their behavior in a pen when the animals are ranked from 1 to 5 on temperament, where 1 is a calm animal and 5 is extremely agitated.[490] Speed of leaving a chute (flight speed or exit velocity) is also used as a measure of temperament and is correlated with the animal's response to social separation and attempts by a person to move it – the docility tests. The animals that freeze when separated are probably more fearful. Those who move around when isolated have high rates of weight gain.[1644] Cattle that react more negatively to human handling are more likely to be behaviorally and physiologically stressed at slaughter.[303]

QTLs (i.e., loci explaining a portion of the variation in the traits of interest) for behavioral traits have been found, especially on chromosomes 1, 8, 9, 16, and 29. A dopamine receptor gene is associated with docility in cattle. A study of temperament and meat quality in Nellore–Angus beef cattle found an association between response to social separation in a pen and a gene regulating sodium ion transport. A study in Brown Swiss cattle identified regions with high influence on temperament and aggression on chromosomes 4, 8, and 14. There have been a number of studies on QTLs for temperament, especially response to entering a chute or scale, flightiness, aggression to humans, and milking temperament.[936]

Sheep

Social Behavior

Breed differences exist in the tendency to aggregate. For example, Clun Forest sheep gather in large groups, whereas Dalesbred and

Jacob sheep are more dispersed and form smaller groups.[2105] Similarly, breed differences appear in the tendency to form separate subgroups within large flocks. Merinos rarely form subgroups, whereas Dorsets and Southdowns do. The grouping depends on the sheep's activity. Some sheep form subgroups only when grazing, whereas others form subgroups both when grazing and when camping (resting at night).[95] Leadership in sheep is negatively correlated with the tendency to join the flock. In other words, independent sheep lead; the others follow. There are breed differences, but these may be cultural in that lambs raised by Blackface ewes have shorter inter-individual distance and smaller group size than those raised by Suffolk ewes. There are breed differences in environmental preferences. Blackface sheep prefer uplands despite the poorer quality forage, whereas Suffolks prefer lowlands.

Reactivity

Sheep have been selected to be either more active and likely to approach humans or less active and less likely to approach. Although less afraid of humans, the more active sheep found dogs more aversive.[207] A calm and a nervous strain of sheep have been developed at the University of South Australia. The calm sheep were less stressed by isolation when exposed to lavender odor whereas there was no effect of the odor on the nervous sheep.[3067] This may explain why many odors and other products reduce fear in laboratory dogs, but not in phobic pets.

Sexual and Maternal Behavior

There are breed differences in the duration of estrus in sheep, even in estrogen-induced estrus in ovariectomized ewes.[2120] Great breed differences appear in the frequency of abandonment of one of a pair of twin lambs. Merino sheep are much more likely to abandon one of their twin lambs than are Dorsets or Romney.[40] The more primitive breeds of sheep such as Romanov and those kept extensively such as

Scottish Blackface show stronger maternal behavior than Merinos or Suffolks.[606] Maternal behavior is moderately heritable (0.35). The more agitated the animal when isolated and the faster the flight time when released from restraint, the higher the litter survival in its progeny.[1829]

Another example of genetic differences is that Targhee sheep do not show as strong maternal behavior as other breeds.[2145] An interesting study involved embryo transfer of lambs into ewes of another breed. This allows separation of genetic and learned components of behavior.[607] Lambs play a part in ewe–lamb proximity. Suffolk lambs stay closer to their mothers and vocalize more often than Blackface lambs. Blackface lambs also play more, and female lambs stay closer than males. Lambs born to Blackface sheep were more active, and Suffolk ewes nursed their lambs more often. Blackface lambs grazed more and Suffolk lambs raised by a Blackface ewe grazed more than Suffolk lambs raised by a Suffolk ewe – a breed and learning interaction.

Ovine Temperament Tests

One ovine temperament test consists of isolating the sheep, then measuring its approach to a novel object (usually, a red balloon dropping from the ceiling) and to a human. In some tests, the human sits in front of a partition separating the test sheep from its pen mates, so the sheep's desire to approach its flock competes with its desire to avoid a human. Sheep can be divided, according to their responses to isolation and to humans, into one group that is very active and vocal (More Active) and another that is Less Active. The more active sheep were less physiologically stressed and actually spent more time close to the human.[206] Another test involves exposure to six novel objects (bottle brush, rattle, teething rings, and boxes of herbs), and those sheep that visited four or more novel objects were considered bold and the other shy. This is consistent with cat and dog temperaments.

Shy sheep graze closer to their nearest neighbor and stayed farther from humans.[2118] Ewes are more fearful than rams, and ewes given testosterone are less fearful.[2331] Ewes that have lambed are less fearful than nulliparous ones.[2352] Sheep respond more to carnivores (stuffed, moving wolverine, lynx, and bear, and a real dog) by fleeing and flocking together than they respond to novel objects such as a moving ball. Other signs of fear are alarm vocalizations, urinating, or defecating. Lighter weight sheep are more responsive than heavy sheep. A calm and a nervous strain of sheep have been developed at the University of South Australia. Sheep breeds differ in their reactivity and selection within one breed (Romane) has resulted in reactive and nonreactive sheep. It is interesting that the reactive sheep respond more positively to brushing.[3004] There is low heritability of behaviors associated with an approach–avoidance test in which the lamb must approach a human to gain access its flock mates in an adjacent pen as measured by number of bleats, locomotion, and time near the human.[2481]

Goats

Caprine Temperament

Goats have been divided into four temperament groups: aggressive, affiliative, passive, and avoiders. The aggressive goats were the largest, but they did worse in a simple maze test; the passive goats did best.[1774] The response of goats to an arena is a repeatable and valid test. Vocalizations are the usual measure.[714] Kids can be divided into timid and bold animals on the basis of their approach to humans. The behavior of the mother and, in the case of timid kids, that of even strange goats affected the willingness of the kids to approach humans.[1429] Diet can have an effect on temperament. Goats would obtain plenty of long-chain polyunsaturated acid when grazing, but a cereal and silage diet is deficient in linoleic acid, the precursor of docosahexaenoic and arachidonic acid. Goat kids whose mother was supplemented with linoleic acid were less inhibited by a novel object.[602]

Pigs

Breed Differences

Breed differences appear in aggression, learning, sexual behavior, and maternal behavior. Yorkshires are more aggressive than Berkshires.[1487] Breed differences appear in dominance by sex; more Hampshire males are dominant over females than are Durocs.[218] Small pigs and newcomers to an established group are usually subordinate.[744] Yorkshires are easier to train to mount a dummy than Durocs, but Durocs make more correct response in an avoidance test than Hampshires (Figure 9.7).[42,1261] Poor libido is seen more frequently in Landrace than in boars of the Large white breed.[66] Play back of nursing calls decreased nursing intervals in one genotype of pigs (Meishan), but not others (Yorkshire and Landrace).[667] There are breed differences in feeding strategies. Duroc pigs are "meal and slow eaters," Landrace pigs are "meal and fast eaters," Large white pigs are "nibblers and fast eaters," and Pietrain pigs are "nibblers and slow eaters."

Minipigs are often used in biomedical research, and there are several breeds. Göettingen minipigs were developed by crossing Vietnamese minipigs (that tend to be aggressive) with Minnesota minipigs and a conventional breed (Landrace) to produce small white pigs. Heritability of Göettingen minipigs' reaction to being handled was low to moderate, with a range from 0.09 to 0.22.[1246] When two breeds of minipigs were compared, Pitman–Moore piglets systematically expressed more locomotion, vocalizations, and exploratory behavior than Vietnamese piglets. They were also more prone to initiate contact with an unknown human during an open-field test, but less easy to catch in their home pen.[2316] Minipigs and low-birth-weight conventional

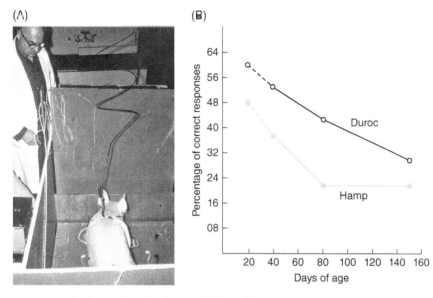

Figure 9.7 Avoidance learning in pigs. (A) To avoid shock, the pig must jump a barrier when a buzzer sounds. (B) The ability to learn to avoid shock decreases with age in Duroc and Hampshire pigs. *Source:* Kratzer (1969).[1261] Reproduced with permission of American Society of Animal Science.

pigs learned a conditioned discrimination better than normal-weight conventional pigs.[1653]

Care must be taken when breeding for specific characteristics. Sows selected for high survivability of piglets in outdoor systems were more likely to savage their piglets when indoors, whereas unselected sows were more likely to crush their piglets in both environments.[187]

Porcine Temperament Test

Restraining a pig by placing it on its back – the back test or tonic immobility test – has been used to assess active (high resistance) and passive personality (low resistance) in pigs.[715,1006] The pigs that resisted most at three days of age were more likely to approach people or venture out of their pens at two months of age, although some investigators did not find that correlation.[1128] Lean growth is higher in pigs that resisted least.[397] When strange pigs are mixed, the high-resisting pigs are more aggressive both to one another and to low resistors if they are dominant.[1999] When stressed by restraint in a cage, low-resistance pigs, but not high-resistance pigs, showed less standing alert behavior and pinned their ears back less with the pen mate present than without the pen mate present.[1917] The back test does not predict the response to novelty.[2156]

Although aggression over food appears to be a consistent characteristic of a pig, response to the back test and to novelty is not.[1999] By the time of puberty, most behavioral differences between these two groups have disappeared, but the low-resistance pigs have higher baseline cortisol and gain more weight.[811] Large white pigs are more easily immobilized in the back test than Landrace pigs.[524]

There appear to be three important temperament traits: aggression, sociability, and exploration, as measured by aggression to an intruder, social dependence, and response to novelty, respectively. Aggression as an individual personality trait can be measured by adding a smaller "intruder" to a pig's home cage. The latency to attack is stable over time.[640]

Other important traits are activity (in an open field or other novel environment) and anxiety or fear.[55] Pigs raised in an enriched environment show more diverse behaviors and are more active in response to a novel object, and vocalize more in an open-field test, but they are less tractable.[202,2420] Pigs find an unpredictable intermittent sound more aversive than a continuous one and will avoid it.[2227] Another test of fear used a ball that rose from the trough from which the pigs had become accustomed to eat. A horn behind a curtain adjacent to the trough was the auditory stimulus, and carbon dioxide in the trough the olfactory one. The pig's approach time, locomotion, and latency to eat were measured. Younger pigs were more frightened than older finishing pigs. The anxiolytic midazolam reduced fear in the younger pigs.[502] Elevated mazes in which the pig has a choice of open or closed arms and dark-versus-light tests have been used to measure fear in pigs.[715] Willingness to approach a human is another measure of temperament; pigs initially reluctant to approach people become less reluctant with repeated testing, but the relative rank is consistent across time.[957] Pigs that approach humans are more likely to be subordinate in a feed competition test. The latency to approach novel objects (traffic cones, bucket, or basketball) was not correlated with latency to approach a person; nevertheless, it was correlated with latency to leave the pen.[344] In a review of 83 papers on the subject of porcine personality, exploration, aggressiveness, reactivity to humans, and fearfulness are the most common personality traits studied in pigs.[2915]

Chickens

Personality

There are breed differences in aggressiveness; consider game cocks versus meat breed roosters. Three personality traits emerge in chickens – boldness, activity/exploration, and vigilance.[2736] There are strain differences in chickens personality. For example, tonic immobility Tetras are more social than ISA Browns and the latter showed longer tonic immobility.[2725]

A common problem of chickens, especially caged chicken is feather pecking, in which chickens pull feathers from their cage mates. The microbiome of chickens selected for low feather picking differ from that of chickens selected for high feather picking. The orders of *Clostridiales* and *Lactobacillales* had the highest relative abundance in both pools. The higher feather pickers had a higher relative abundance of *Clostridiales* and the lower feather pickers had a higher relative abundance of *Lactobacillales*.[2663]

Faecalibacterium, Oscillibacter, Butyricicoccus, and Bacteroides were enriched in line less aggressive white Leghorns strain) birds, while *Clostridiales vadin BB60, Alistipes, Mollicutes RF39 were dominant* in the more aggressive strain.[3070] From the predicted bacterial functional genes, the kynurenine pathway was upregulated suggesting a functional linkage of gut microbes with serotonin activity and stress levels.[3115]

Laterality or Handedness in Animals

Lateralization is a term used to describe the idea that external stimuli are perceived and processed differently on each side of the brain and/or that some behaviors are preferentially performed by one side of the body.

Handedness reflects which side of the brain is dominant. Therefore, differences between right- and left-handed humans and, probably most important, between ambidextrous people and the others have been related to various behavior patterns in humans. Recently, this has been extended to animals. Happy faces were associated with a right hemisphere bias in dogs.[2140,2675, 2676,2677]

Horses

Horses show laterality. Colts are more often born with their left foreleg anterior to the right and retain this left bias.[1655] Foals approach their dam to suckle on the left side.[2819,2820] Grooming was lateralized for the right side.[2704,2734] Ponies looked with their left eye at actors displaying angry expressions and with their right eye when the actors were expressing joy.[2887]

The left tendency increased with age, which may indicate a training effect.[1527] This hypothesis is strengthened by the finding that Przewalski horses exhibit laterality as foals, but not as adults.[113] There are breed differences in laterality based on which leg is forward while grazing. Thoroughbreds are significantly left lateral, Standardbred pacers slightly less so, and Quarter Horses used for cutting had no laterality. Horses loading into a trailer or stepping off a step show a left limb bias, so there may be an emotional component.[2129] The side from which the horse was handled is also important. Horses were faster at backing when handled on the right side than the left side.

Horses turn their right ear toward a familiar whinny, indicating a left-brain recognition.[179] Horses, including Przewalski horses, are more vigilant to stimuli on their left and are more likely to attack with the left eye facing the opponent.[113] Horses tend to look at a novel object (a box covered with shiny red tape) with their left eye if they are afraid of it, although there are breed differences. French saddle horses are less likely to use the left eye than the more excitable Trotters.[1311] In general, horses look at humans with their left eye, especially if the person has been interacting with them or has an angry expression.[668,2140] Horses seem to perform the task of recognizing humans cross modally with a left-brain hemispheric specialization: they correctly matched stimuli across modalities only when the visual stimulus was presented in their right visual hemifield.[1866]

Horses preferentially approached pictures of persons with the left eye in all situations, but this was expressed more strongly when the pictures showed a person with an aggressive facial expression.[2984] The same appears to be the case for auditory laterality, as horses reacted to voices of persons they matched to negative prior experiences predominantly with the left ear.[3114] When sniffing at epinephrine and estrous mare urine, horses showed a clear right-nostril bias accompanied by increasing cardiac activity and behavioral reactivity, strengthening the role of the right hemisphere in the analysis of intense emotion and sexual behavior.[2128] Bear in mind that the olfactory stimuli are ipsilateral whereas the visual ones are contralateral. Australian feral horses have been found to show left bias in sensory laterality in the form of head posture and eye preference during agonistic interactions but, interestingly, there was no significant motor laterality on population level. About 40% demonstrated a left leg preference while grazing, and about 40% a right leg preference, while about 20% were ambidextrous, with young horses being more strongly lateralized than mature horses.[37] The study was later repeated on Przewalski horses and, again, no significant population bias in motor laterality in terms of forelimb preferences was found. About 30% were left leg biased, 30% right leg biased, and 40% were bilateral.

Dog

There are several ways to test for laterality: the paw used to remove tape from the nose, to overturn a can under which a treat had been hidden, to remove a blanket placed over the dog's head, or to hold a Kong toy; the first step taken downstairs; or the paw raised when the dog is told to "Shake" or "Give paw,"[1880,2415] or the paw used to retrieve an object from underneath furniture.[1880,2415] Dogs display right- and left-paw preferences and this can reflect the owner's handedness.[2693] Male and female dogs showed paw preferences at the level of the population but in opposite directions. Female dogs had a greater preference for using their right paw on all tasks, while males were more inclined to use their left paw, although this is not seen in all studies.[2049] When dolichocephalic dogs were compared to brachycephalic breeds, there were no differences in laterality.[1528] Brain laterality influences immunity through effects on cytokines. Interleukin-2 (IL2) and (IL6) gene expression is higher in left-pawed dogs than in right-pawed and ambidextrous dogs. After rabies vaccine administration, decreasing levels of IL2 and IL6 gene expression are observed in left-pawed and right-pawed dogs, but not in ambidextrous dogs.[1880] Ambidextrous dogs are more likely to suffer from noise phobias, such as storm phobia and fear of fireworks.[320] Ambidextrous dogs were faster at solving a manipulative task (opening a container by pushing a treadle).[2596] Dogs with stronger laterality are more relaxed and confident.[183] The emotional valence hypothesis states that positive emotions are processed predominantly by the left hemisphere while negative emotions are processed predominantly by the right hemisphere.[1879,3026] When dogs are startled while eating they turn their heads left.[2981] When the left eye of an animal is covered it does not exhibit the usual signs of positive emotion when signaled that a treat is coming, whereas the animal's response to a negative stimulus is unchanged. No correlations were found between measures of paw preference and a test of dogs' predisposition to emotionality.[2980] Stranger-directed aggression, stranger-directed fear, and attention-seeking behavior were associated with right-pawedness.[3030]

Dogs inspect the left side of photographs of human faces whether the photographs are right side up or upside down.[869] When observing photographs, dogs displayed left bias toward negative expression (no significant bias toward neutral expression and a significant right bias toward positive expressions).[2942] They do not display similar laterality to dog faces unless the dog face displays aggression, in which they show a left bias.[869,2613] Dogs process meaningful sounds in their left brain, which they indicate by turning their head to the right; they turn toward the left when meaningless sounds are heard.[1904] Dogs initially show a consistent right-nostril bias when sniffing a veterinarian's sweat and a left-nostril bias when sniffing food or canine vaginal secretion.[2131]

When exposed to the odors of dogs or humans in various emotional states, the dogs consistently used their right nostril to sniff the dog odor and the left nostril to sniff the human fear stimuli.[2132]

There is also a side bias in tail wagging. Dogs wag their tails to the right when facing the owner or an unfamiliar person, although the amplitude of the wag is smaller to an unfamiliar person. Heart rates are lower when the dog wags to the right, indicating a positive emotional state. Dogs looking at moving video images of conspecifics showed higher cardiac activity and higher scores of anxious behavior when observing left- rather than right-biased tail wagging.[2613] A cat also elicits a right-sided bias, but a strange dominant dog elicits a left-sided bias.[1879]

Cats

Cats, like dogs, show definite paw preferences especially when trying to manipulate something out of a jar. Although both sexes exhibit paw preferences, more females are right pawed and more males are left pawed.[2413] There are breed differences; Bengals tend to be left pawed, Ragdolls right pawed, and Persians ambidextrous, although only the Bengal preference was significant.[3029]

Pigs

The eye with which the pig is viewing a scene influences his emotional reaction.[2761]

Ruminants

Sheep with stronger laterality in either direction were more attached to their lamb or ewe if they consistently chose one side to pass an obstacle.[166] Lambs tend to suckle from the left.[2820] It is easier for goats to learn to turn left in a maze, which may indicate a right-brain bias in the processing of visual-spatial cues.[1303] When passing an object, 40% of cattle pass to the right and 40% to the left.[1218]

Hair Whorls

There is an association between laterality and the presence and direction of hair whorls in dogs. The presence of a whorl on the left side of the head and thorax was associated with a right visual bias. In addition, right visual bias was probable if the ventricular mandibular whorl had a clockwise direction.[2269]

There is a correlation of position of hair whorls in cattle and agitation in a chute.[850,1305]

A whorl above the eyes may predict agitation.[849,850] Cattle with high whorls had higher crush scores, that is, were more agitated. Cattle with lower facial hair whorls had smaller flight distance and less interest in an unfamiliar human than those with whorls located higher on their faces.[1895] Only crush scores (pushing, head tossing, and shaking) rather than flight speed or weight gain varied with hair whorl position.[1731]

References

The uncited references are presented in bold in the reference list.

1 Abitbol, M. L., & S. R. Inglis. 1997. Role of amniotic fluid in newborn acceptance and bonding in canines. *J. Matern. Fetal. Med.* 6:49–52.

2 Abraham, I., S. R. Baker, D. A. Denton, F. Kraintz, L. Kraintz, & L. Purser. 1973. Components in the regulation of salt balance: Salt appetite studied by operant behaviour. *Aust. J. Exper. Biol. Med. Sci.* 51:5–81.

3 Abraham, S. F., R. M. Baker, E. H. Blaine, D. A. Denton, & M. J. McKinley. 1975. Water drinking induced in sheep by angiotensin – a physiological or pharmacological effect? *J. Comp. Physiol. Psychol.* 88:503–518.

4 **Adachi, I., H. Kuwahata, & K. Fujita. 2007. Dogs recall their owner's face upon hearing the owner's voice. *Anim. Cogn.* 10:17–21.**

5 Adamec, R. E. 1976. The interaction of hunger and preying in the domestic cat (*Felis catus*): An adaptive hierarchy? *Behav. Biol.* 18:263–272.

6 Adamec, R. E. 1991. Anxious personality in the cat: Its ontogeny and physiology. In B. J. Carroll & J. E. Barrett (Eds.), Psychopathology and the brain, pp. 153–168. New York, NY: Raven Press.

7 Adamec, R. E., C. Stark-Adamec, & K. E. Livingston. 1983. The expression of an early developmentally emergent defensive bias in the adult domestic cat (*Felis catus*) in non-predatory situations. *Appl. Anim. Ethol.* 10:89–108.

8 Adams, D. K. 1929. Experimental studies of adaptive behavior in cats. *Comp. Psychol. Monogr.* 6:1–168.

9 **Adams, G. J., & K. G. Johnson. 1993. Sleep-wake cycles and other night-time behaviours of the domestic dog (*Canis familiaris*). *Appl. Anim. Behav. Sci.* 36:233–248.**

10 Adams, G. J., & K. G. Johnson. 1994. Behavioural responses to barking and other auditory stimuli during night-time sleeping and waking in the domestic dog (*Canis familiaris*). *Appl. Anim. Behav. Sci.* 39:151–162.

11 Adams, G. J., & K. G. Johnson. 1994. Sleep work, and the effects of shift work in drug detector dogs *Canis familiaris*. *Appl. Anim. Behav. Sci.* 41:115–126.

12 Adams, G. J., & K. G. Johnson. 1995. Guard dogs: Sleep, work and the behavioural responses of people and other stimuli. *Appl. Anim. Behav. Sci.* 46:103–115.

13 Adams, T. 1963. Hypothalamic temperature in the cat during feeding and sleep. *Science.* 139:609–610.

14 Adkins-Regan, E., P. Orgeur, & J. P. Signoret. 1989. Sexual differentiation of reproductive behavior in pigs: Defeminizing effects of prepubertal estradiol. *Horm. Behav.* 23:290–303.

Domestic Animal Behavior for Veterinarians and Animal Scientists, Seventh Edition. Katherine A. Houpt.
© 2024 John Wiley & Sons, Inc. Published 2024 by John Wiley & Sons, Inc.
Companion website: www.wiley.com/go/houpt/7e

15 Administratin, O. S. A. H. 1972. Federal regulation 37(202), part II. Occuptional safety and health standards, pp. 102–122, 356. Washington, DC: Department of Labor.

16 Agrawal, H. C., M. W. Fox, & W. A. Himwich. 1967. Neurochemical and behavioral effects of isolation-rearing in the dog. *Life Sci.* 6:71–78.

17 Alavi, F. K., J. P. McCann, A. Mauromoustakis, & S. Sangiah. 1993. Feeding behavior and its responsiveness to naloxone differ in lean and obese sheep. *Physiol. Behav.* 53:317–323.

18 Alberghina, D., A. D. Pasquale, G. Piccione, F. Vitale, & M. Panzera. 2015. Gene expression profile of cytokines in leukocytes from stereotypic horses. *J. Vet. Behav.* 10(6):556–560.

19 Albiach-Serrano, A., J. Bräuer, T. Cacchione, N. Zickert, & F. Amici. 2012. The effect of domestication and ontogeny in swine cognition (*Sus scrofa scrofa* and *S. s. domestica*). *Appl. Anim. Behav. Sci.* 141(1–2):25–35.

20 Albright, J. D., H. O. Mohammed, C. R. Heleski, C. L. Wickens, & K. A. Houpt. 2009. Crib-biting in US horses: Breed predispositions and owner perceptions of aetiology. *Equine Vet. J.* 41:455–458.

21 Albright, J. L. 1969. Social environment and growth. In E. S. E. Hafez, & I. A. Dyer (Eds.), *Animal growth and nutrition*, pp. 106–120. Philadelphia, PA: Lea & Febiger.

22 Albright, J. L., W. P. M. Gordon, W. C. Black, J. P. Dietrich, W. W. Snyder, & C. E. Meadows. 1966. Behavioral responses of cows to auditory training. *J. Dairy Sci.* 49:104–106.

23 Aldinger, S. M., V. C. Speer, V. W. Hays, & D. V. Catron. 1959. Effect of saccharin on consumption of starter rations by baby pigs. *J. Anim. Sci.* 18:1350–1355.

24 Aldis, O. 1975. Play fighting. New York, NY: Academic Press.

25 Aldrich, C. G., M. T. Rhodes, J. L. Miner, M. S. Kerley, & J. A. Paterson. 1993. The effects of endophyte-infected tall fescue consumption and use of a dopamine antagonist on intake, digestibility, body temperature, and blood constituents in sheep. *J. Anim. Sci.* 71:158–163.

26 Alexander, B. M., J. D. Rose, J. N. Stellflug, J. A. Fitzgerald, & G. E. Moss. 2001. Low-sexually performing rams but not male-oriented rams can be discriminated by cell size in the amygdala and preoptic area: A morphometric study. *Behav. Brain Res.* 119:15–21.

27 Alexander, B. M., J. N. Stellflug, J. D. Rose, J. A. Fitzgerald, & G. E. Moss. 1999. Behavior and endocrine changes in high-performing, low-performing, and male-oriented domestic rams following exposure to rams and ewes in estrus when copulation is precluded. *J. Anim. Sci.* 77:1869–1874.

28 Alexander, G. 1977. Role of auditory and visual cues in mutual recognition between ewes and lambs in merino sheep. *Appl. Anim. Ethol.* 3:65–81.

29 Alexander, G., & D. Stevens. 1981. Recognition of washed lambs by merino ewes. *Appl. Anim. Ethol.* 7:77–86.

30 Alexander, G., & D. Stevens. 1985. Fostering in sheep III. facilitation by the use of odorants. *Appl. Anim. Behav. Sci.* 14:345–354.

31 Alexander, G., & D. Williams. 1964. Maternal facilitation of sucking drive in newborn lambs. *Science* 146:65–66.

32 Alexander, G., & D. Williams. 1966. Teat-seeking activity in lambs during the first hours of life. *Anim. Behav.* 14:166–176.

33 Alexander, G., & E. E. Shillito. 1977. Importance of visual cues from various body regions in maternal recognition of the young in merino sheep (*Ovis aries*). *Appl. Anim. Ethol.* 3:137–143.

34 Alexander, G., & E. E. Shillito. 1977. The importance of odour, apearance and voice in maternal recognition of the young in merino sheep (*Ovis aries*). *Appl. Anim. Ethol.* 3:127–135.

35 Alexander, G., & E. E. Shillito. 1978. Maternal responses in merino ewes to artificially coloured lambs. *Appl. Anim. Ethol.* 4:141–152.

36 Alexander, G., & E. E. Shillito. 1978. Visual discrimination between ewes by lambs. *Appl. Anim. Ethol.* 4:81–85.

37 Alexander, G., & L. R. Bradley. 1985. Fostering in sheep IV. use of restraint. *Appl. Anim. Behav. Sci.* 14:355–364.

38 Alexander, G., D. Stevens, & L. R. Bradley. 1983. Washing lambs and confinement as aids to fostering. *Appl. Anim. Ethol.* 10:251–261.

39 Alexander, G., D. Stevens, & L. R. Bradley. 1988. Maternal behaviour in ewes following caesarian section. *Appl. Anim. Behav. Sci.* 19:273–277.

40 Alexander, G., D. Stevens, R. Kilgour, H. de Langen, B. E. Mottershead, & J. J. Lynch. 1983. Separation of ewes from twin lambs: Incidence in several breeds. *Appl. Anim. Ethol.* 10:301–317.

41 Alexander, G., G. D. Stevens, & L. R. Bradley. 1985. Fostering in sheep I. facilitation by use of textile lamb coats. *Appl. Anim. Ethol.* 14:315–334.

42 Alexander, G., J. Signoret, & E. S. E. Hafez. 1974. Sexual and maternal behavior. In E. S. E. Hafez (Ed.), *Reproduction in farm animals*, pp. 222–254. Philadelphia, PA: Lea & Febiger.

43 Algers, B., & K. Uvnas-Moberg. 2007. Maternal behavior in pigs. *Horm. Behav.* 52:78–85.

44 Algers, B., P. Jensen, & L. Steinwall. 1990. Behaviour and weight changes at weaning and regrouping of pigs in relation to teat quality. *Appl. Anim. Behav. Sci.* 26:143–155.

45 Algers, B., S. Rojanasthien, & K. Uvnas-Moberg. 1990. The relationship between teat stimulation, oxytocin release and grunting rate in the sow during nursing. *Appl. Anim. Behav. Sci.* 26:267–276.

46 Allan, C. J., P. J. Holst, & G. N. Hinch. 1991. Behaviour of parturient Australian bush goats I. doe behaviour and kid vigour. *Appl. Anim. Behav. Sci.* 32:55–64.

47 Allin, J. T., & E. M. Banks. 1972. Functional aspects of ultrasound production by infant albino rats (rattus norvegicus). *Anim. Behav.* 20:175–185.

48 Allison, T., & D. V. Cicchetti. 1976. Sleep in mammals: Ecological and constitutional correlates. *Science* 194:732–734.

49 Altmann, M. 1941. Interrelations of the sex cycle and the behavior of the sow. *J. Comp. Psychol.* 31:481–498.

50 Alvarez, L., N. Guevara, M. Reyes, A. Sánchez, & F. Galindo. 2013. Shade effects on feeding behavior, feed intake, and daily gain of weight in female goat kids. *J. Vet. Behav.* 8(6):466–470.

51 Amat, M., S. L. Brech, T. Camps, C. Torrente, V. M. Mariotti, J. L. Ruiz, & X. Manteca. 2013. Differences in serotonin serum concentration between aggressive English cocker spaniels and aggressive dogs of other breeds. *J. Vet. Behav.* 8(1):19–25.

52 Amat, M., X. Manteca, V. M. Mariotti, J. L. Ruiz, & J. Fatjó. 2009. Aggressive behavior in the English cocker spaniel. *J. Vet. Behav.* 4(3):111–117.

53 Ames, D. R., & L. A. Arehart. 1972. Physiological response of lambs to auditory stimuli. *J. Anim. Sci.* 34:994–998.

54 Andersen, I. L., K. E. Boe, & A. L. Kristiansen. 1999. The influence of different feeding arrangements and food type on competition at feeding in pregnant sows. *Appl. Anim. Behav. Sci.* 65:91–104.

55 Andersen, I. L., K. E. Boe, G. Foerevik, A. M. Janczak, & M. Bakken. 2000. Behavioural evaluation of methods for assessing fear responses in weaned pigs. *Appl. Anim. Behav. Sci.* 69:227–240.

56 Andersen, I. L., S. Berg, & K. E. Boe. 2005. Crushing of piglets by the mother sow (*Sus scrofa*) – purely accidental or a poor mother? *Appl. Anim. Behav. Sci.* 93:229–243.

57 Anderson, D. M., & N. S. Urquhart. 1986. Using digital pedometers to monitor travel of cows grazing arid rangeland. *Appl. Anim. Behav. Sci.* 16:11–23.

58 Anderson, D. M., C. V. Hulet, J. N. Smith, W. L. Shupe, & L. W. Murray. 1987.

Heifer disposition and bonding of lambs to heifers. *Appl. Anim. Behav. Sci.* 19:27–30.

59 **Anderson, D. M., C. V. Hulet, J. N. Smith, W. L. Shupe, & L. W. Murray. 1992. An attempt to bond weaned 3-month-old beef heifers to yearling ewes. *Appl. Anim. Behav. Sci.* 34:181–188.**

60 Anderson, D. M., C. V. Hulet, S. K. Hamadeh, J. N. Smith, & L. W. Murray. 1990. Diet selection of bonded and non-bonded free-ranging sheep and cattle. *Appl. Anim. Behav. Sci.* 26:231–242.

61 **Anderson, O. D., & R. Parmenter. 1941. A long-term study of the experimental neurosis in the sheep and dog. *Psychosom. Med.* 2:1–150.**

62 **Anderson, R. S. 1974. Obesity in the dog and cat. In C. S. G. Grunsell, & F. W. G. Hill (Eds.), The veterinary annual 1973, pp. 182–186. Bristol, UK: John Wright and Sons.**

63 Andersson, B., & S. M. McCann. 1955. A further study of polydipsia evoked by hypothalamic stimulation in the goat. *Acta Physiol. Scand.* 33:333–346.

64 Andersson, B., L. Eriksson, & R. Oltner. 1970. Further evidence for angiotensin-sodium interaction in central control of fluid balance. *Life Sci.* 9:1091–1096.

65 Andersson, B., O. Augustinsson, E. Bademo, J. Junkergard, C. Kvart, G. Nyman, & M. Wiberg. 1987. Systemic and centrally mediated angiotensin II effects in the horse. *Acta Physiol. Scand.* 129:143–149.

66 Anonymous. 1975. Behaviour of boars. *Vet. Rec.* 96:221.

67 Apley, M. 1999. *Buller syndrome in feedlot steers.* 29:250.

68 Apple, J. K., & J. V. Craig. 1992. The influence of pen size on toy preference in growing pigs. *Appl. Anim. Behav. Sci.* 35:149–155.

69 Appleby, M. C., & D. G. M. Wood-Gush. 1988. Effect of earth as an additional stimulus on the behaviour of confined piglets. *Behav. Processes.* 17:83–91.

70 Appleby, M. C., E. A. Pajor, & D. Fraser. 1991. Effects of management options on creep feeding by piglets. *Anim. Prod.* 53:361–366.

71 Appleby, M. C., E. A. Pajor, & D. Fraser. 1992. Individual variation in feeding and growth of piglets: Effects of increased access to creep food. *Anim. Prod.* 55:147–152.

72 Araba, B. D., & S. L. Crowell-Davis. 1994. Dominance relationships and aggression in foals (*Equus caballus*). *Appl. Anim. Behav. Sci.* 41:1–25.

73 Arahori, M., Y. Hori, A. Saito, H. Chijiiwa, S. Takagi, Y. Ito, A. Watanabe, *et al.* 2016. The oxytocin receptor gene (OXTR) polymorphism in cats (*Felis catus*) is associated with "roughness" assessed by owners. *J. Vet. Behav.* 11:109–112.

74 Arave, C. W., R. C. Lamb, M. J. Arambel, D. Purcell, & J. L. Walter. 1992. Behavior and maze learning ability of dairy calves as influenced by housing, sex and sire. *Appl. Anim. Behav. Sci.* 33:149–163.

75 Archer D. C., C. J. Proudman, G. Pinchbeck, J. E. Smith, N. P. French, & G. B. Edwards. 2004. Entrapment of the small intestine in the epiploic foramen in horses: a retrospective analysis of 71 cases recorded between 1991 and 2001. *Vet. Rec.* 155:793–796.

76 Archer, D. C., G. K. Pinchbeck, N. P. French, & C. J. Proudman. 2008. Risk factors for epiploic foramen entrapment colic: An international study. *Equine Vet. J.* 40:224–230.

77 Archer, M. 1973. The species preferences of grazing horses. *J. Br. Grassland Soc.* 28:123–128.

78 **Archibald, J. 1974. *Canine surgery*. Santa Barbara, CA: American Veterinary Publications.**

79 Arden, R., & M. J. Adams. 2016. A general intelligence factor in dogs. *Intelligence.* 55:79–85.

80 Arendt, J., A. M. Symons, C. A. Laud, & S. J. Pryde. 1983. Melatonin can induce early onset of the breeding season in ewes. *J. Endocrinol.* 97:395–400.

81 Arey, D. S. 1999. Time course for the formation and disruption of social organisation in group-housed sows. *Appl. Anim. Behav. Sci.* 62:199–207.

82 Arey, D. S., & M. F. Franklin. 1995. Effects of straw and unfamiliarity on fighting between newly mixed growing pigs. *Appl. Anim. Behav. Sci.* 45:25–30.

83 Arey, D. S., A. M. Perchey, & V. R. Fowler. 1991. The preparturient behaviour of sows in enriched pens and the effect of pre-formed nests. *Appl. Anim. Behav. Sci.* 31:61–68.

84 Arey, D. S., A. M. Petchey, & V. R. Fowler. 1992. The peri-parturient behaviour of sows housed in pairs. *Appl. Anim. Behav. Sci.* 34:49–59.

85 Arnold, G. W. 1966. The special senses in grazing animals I. sight and dietary habits in sheep. *Aust. J. Agric. Res.* 17:521–529.

86 Arnold, G. W. 1966. The special senses in grazing animals II. smell, taste, and touch and dietary habits in sheep. *Aust. J. Agric. Res.* 17:531–542.

87 **Arnold, G. W. 1984. Comparison of the time budgets and circadian patterns of maintenance activities in sheep, cattle and horses grouped together.** *Appl. Anim. Behav. Sci.* **13:19–30.**

88 Arnold, G. W., & A. Grassia. 1982. Ethogram of agonistic behaviour for thoroughbred horses. *Appl. Anim. Ethol.* 8:5–25.

89 Arnold, G. W., & M. L. Dudzinski. 1978. Ethology of free-ranging domestic animals. Amsterdam, The Netherlands: Elsevier Scientific.

90 Arnold, G. W., & P. D. Morgan. 1975. Behaviour of the ewe and lamb at lambing and its relationship to lamb mortality. *Appl. Anim. Ethol.* 2:25–46.

91 Arnold, G. W., & P. J. Pahl. 1974. Some aspects of social behaviour in domestic sheep. *Anim. Behav.* 22:592–600.

92 Arnold, G. W., & R. A. Maller. 1974. Some aspects of competition between sheep for supplementary feed. *Anim. Prod.* 19:309–319.

93 Arnold, G. W., C. A. P. Boundy, P. D. Morgan, & G. Bartle. 1975. The roles of sight and hearing in the lamb in the location and discrimination between ewes. *Appl. Anim. Ethol.* 1:167–176.

94 Arnold, G. W., S. R. Wallace, & R. A. Maller. 1979. Some factors involved in natural weaning processes in sheep. *Appl. Anim. Ethol.* 5:43–50.

95 Arnold, G. W., S. R. Wallace, & W. A. Rea. 1981. Associations between individuals and home-range behaviour in natural flocks of three breeds of domestic sheep. *Appl. Anim. Ethol.* 7:239–257.

96 Arnold, N. A., K. T. Ng, E. C. Jongman, & P. H. Hemsworth. 2007. Responses of dairy heifers to the visual cliff formed by a herringbone milking pit: Evidence of fear of heights in cows (*Bos taurus*). *J. Comp. Psychol.* 121:440–446.

97 Arnold, N. A., K. T. Ng, E. C. Jongman, & P. H. Hemsworth. 2007. The behavioural and physiological responses of dairy heifers milking facility noise with and without a pre-treatment adaptation phase. *Appl. Anim. Behav. Sci.* 106:13–25.

98 Arnold, W., T. Ruf, & R. Kuntz. 2006. Seasonal adjustment of energy budget in a large wild mammal, the przewalski horse (*Equus ferus przewalskii*) II. energy expenditure. *J. Exp. Biol.* 209:4566–4573.

99 Arnould, C., V. Piketty, & F. Levy. 1991. Behaviour of ewes at parturition toward amniotic fluids from sheep, cows, and goats. *Appl. Anim. Behav. Sci.* 32:191–196.

100 Aronson, L. R., & M. L. Cooper. 1966. Seasonal variation in mating behavior in cats after desensitization of glans penis. *Science* 152:226–230.

101 Aronson, L. R., & M. L. Cooper. 1974. Olfactory deprivation and mating behavior in sexually experienced male cats. *Behav. Biol.* 11:459–480.

102 Aronson, L. R., & M. L. Cooper. 1977. Central versus peripheral genital desensitization and mating behavior in

male cats: Tonic and phasic effects. *Ann. N Y Acad. Sci.* 290:299–313.

103 Arvelius, P., H. Eken, W. F. Fikse, E. Strandberg, & K. Nilsson. 2014. Genetic analysis of a temperament test as a tool to select against everyday life fearfulness in Rough Collie. *J. Anim. Sci.* 92(11):4843–4855.

104 **Asa, C. S. 1999. Male reproductive success in free-ranging feral horses.** ***Behav. Ecol. Sociobiol.* 47:93.**

105 Asa, C. S., D. A. Goldfoot, & O. J. Ginther. 1979. Sociosexual behavior and the ovulatory cycle of ponies (*Equus caballus*) observed in harem groups. *Horm. Behav.* 13:46–65.

106 Asa, C. S., D. A. Goldfoot, & O. J. Ginther. 1983. Assessment of the sexual behavior of pregnant mares. *Horm. Behav.* 17:405–413.

107 Aschoff, J. 1965. Circadian clocks. *Proceedings of the Feldafing Summer School*, Amsterdam, The Netherlands.

108 Ashmead, D. H., R. K. Clifton, & E. P. Reese. 1986. Development of auditory localization in dogs: Single source and precedence effect sounds. *Dev. Psychobiol.* 19:91–103.

109 **Askew, H. R. 1996.** ***Treatment of behavior problems in dogs and cats. A guide for the small animal veterinarian.* Oxford, UK: Blackwell Science.**

110 Atkeson, F. W., A. O. Shaw, & H. W. Cave. 1942. Grazing habits of dairy cattle. *J. Dairy. Sci.* 25:779–784.

111 Auffray, P., & J. C. Marcilloux. 1983. An analysis of feeding patterns in the adult pig. *Reprod. Nutr. Dev.* 23:517–524.

112 Aust, U., F. Range, M. Steurer, & L. Huber. 2008. Inferential reasoning by exclusion in pigeons, dogs, and humans. *Anim. Cogn.* 11:587–597.

113 Austin, N. P., & L. J. Rogers. 2014. Lateralization of agonistic and vigilance responses in Przewalski horses (*Equus przewalskii*). *Appl. Anim. Behav. Sci.* 151:43–50.

114 Autier-Dérian, D., B. L. Deputte, K. Chalvet-Monfray, M. Coulon, & L. Mounier. 2013. Visual discrimination of species in dogs (*Canis familiaris*). *Anim. Cogn.* 16:637–651.

115 Averósa, X., L. Brossarda, J. Y. Dourmada, K. H. Greef, H. L. Edge, S. A. Edwards, & M. C. Meunier-Salaüna. 2010. A meta-analysis of the combined effect of housing and environmental enrichment characteristics on the behaviour and performance of pigs. *Appl. Anim. Behav. Sci.* 127(3–4):73–85.

116 Awotwi, E. K., K. Oppong-Anane, P. C. Addae, & E. O. Oddoye. 2000. Behavioural interactions between west african dwarf nanny goats and their twin-born kids during the first 48 h post-partum. *Appl. Anim. Behav. Sci.* 68:281–291.

117 Back, D. G., B. W. Pickett, J. L. Voss, & G. E. Seidel Jr. 1974. Observations on the sexual behavior of nonlactating mares. *J. Am. Vet. Med. Assoc.* 165:717–720.

118 **Backus, R. C., N. J. Cave, & D. H. Keisler. 2007. Gonadectomy and high dietary fat but not high dietary carbohydrate induce gains in body weight and fat of domestic cats.** ***Brit. J. Nutr.* 98:641–650.**

119 Bacon, W. E. 1973. Aversive conditioning in neonatal kittens. *J. Comp. Physiol. Psychol.* 83:306–313.

120 **Bacon, W. E., & W. C. Stanley. 1963. Effect of deprivation level in puppies on performance maintained by a passive person reinforcer.** ***J. Comp. Physiol. Psychol.* 56:783–785.**

121 Badamana, M. S., J. D. Sutton, J. D. Oldham, & A. Mowlem. 1990. The effect of amount of protein in the concentrates on hay intake and rate of passage, diet digestibility and milk production in british saanen goats. *Anim. Prod.* 51:333–342.

122 Bado, A., M. J. Lewin, & M. Dubrasquet. 1989. Effects of bombesin on food intake

and gastric acid secretion in cats. *Am. J. Physiol.* 256:R181–R186.

123 Bado, A., M. Rodriguez, M. J. Lewin, J. Martinez, & M. Dubrasquet. 1988. Cholecystokinin suppresses food intake in cats: Structure-activity characterization. *Pharmacol. Biochem. Behav.* 31:297–303.

124 Baer, K. L., G. D. Potter, T. H. Friend, & B. V. Beaver. 1983. Observation effect on learning in horses. *Appl. Anim. Ethol.* 11:123–129.

125 Bagshaw, C. S., S. L. Ralston, & H. Fisher. 1994. Behavioral and physiological effect of orally administered tryptophan on horses subjected to acute isolation stress. *Appl. Anim. Behav. Sci.* 40:12.

126 Baile, C. A., & J. M. Forbes. 1974. Control of feed intake and regulation of energy balance in ruminants. *Physiol. Rev.* 54:160–214.

127 Baile, C. A., C. L. McLaughlin, & M. A. Della-Fera. 1986. Role of cholecystokinin and opioid peptides in control of food intake. *Physiol. Rev.* 66:172–234.

128 Baile, C. A., C. L. McLaughlin, F. C. Buonomo, T. J. Lauterio, L. Marson, & M. A. Della-Fera. 1987. Opioid peptides and the control of feeding in sheep. *Fed. Proc.* 46:173–177.

129 Baile, C. A., C. W. Simpson, L. F. Krabill, & F. H. Martin. 1972. Adrenergic agonists and antagonists and feeding in sheep and cattle. *Life Sci. I.* 11:661–668.

130 Bailey, C. J., & L. W. Porter. 1955. Relevant cues in drive discrimination in cats. *J. Comp. Physiol. Psychol.* 48:180–182.

131 Bailey, J. D., L. H. Anderson, & K. K. Schillo. 2005. Effects of novel females and stage of the estrous cycle on sexual behavior in mature beef bulls. *J. Anim. Sci.* 83:613–624.

132 **Bain, M. J., B. L. Hart, K. D. Cliff, & W. W. Ruehl. 2001. Predicting behavioral changes associated with age-related cognitive impairment in dogs. *J. Am. Vet. Med. Assoc.* 218:1792–1795.**

133 Baker, A. E. M., & B. H. Crawford. 1986. Observational learning in horses. *Appl. Anim. Behav. Sci.* 15:7–13.

134 Baker, A. E. M., & G. E. Seidel. 1985. Why do cows mount other cows? *Appl. Anim. Behav. Sci.* 13:237–241.

135 Baker, G. J., & J. Kear-Colwell. 1974. Aerophagia (windsucking) and aversion therapy in the horse. *Proc. Am. Assoc. Eq. Pract.* 20:127–130.

136 Balch, C. C. 1955. Sleep in ruminants. *Nature* 175:940–941.

137 Baldwin, B. A. 1969. The study of behaviour in pigs. *Br. Vet. J.* 125:281–288.

138 Baldwin, B. A. 1977. Ability of goats and calves to distinguish between conspecific urine samples using olfaction. *Appl. Anim. Ethol.* 3:145–150.

139 Baldwin, B. A. 1979. Operant studies on shape discrimination in goats. *Physiol. Behav.* 23:455–459.

140 Baldwin, B. A. 1981. Shape discrimination in sheep and calves. *Anim. Behav.* 29:830–834.

141 Baldwin, B. A., & C. de la Riva. 1995. Effects of the 5-HT1A agonist 8-OH-DPAT on operant feeding in pigs. *Physiol. Behav.* 58:611–613.

142 Baldwin, B. A., & D. B. Stephens. 1970. Operant conditioning procedures for producing emotional responses in pigs. *J. Physiol.* 210:127P–128P.

143 Baldwin, B. A., & D. B. Stephens. 1973. The effects of conditioned behaviour and environmental factors on plasma corticosteroid levels in pigs. *Physiol. Behav.* 10:267–274.

144 Baldwin, B. A., & D. L. Ingram. 1968. Factors influencing behavioral thermoregulation in the pig. *Physiol. Behav.* 3:409–415.

145 Baldwin, B. A., & E. E. Shillito. 1974. The effects of ablation of the olfactory bulbs on parturition and maternal behaviour in soay sheep. *Anim. Behav.* 22:220–223.

146 Baldwin, B. A., & G. B. Meese. 1977. Sensory reinforcement and illumination

preference in the domesticated pig. *Anim. Behav.* 25:497–507.

147 Baldwin, B. A., & G. B. Meese. 1977. The ability of sheep to distinguish between conspecifics by means of olfaction. *Physiol. Behav.* 18:803–808.

148 Baldwin, B. A., & G. B. Meese. 1979. Social behaviour in pigs studied by means of operant conditioning. *Anim. Behav.* 27:947–957.

149 Baldwin, B. A., & J. O. Yates. 1977. The effects of hypothalamic temperature variation and intracarotid cooling on behavioural thermoregulation in sheep. *J. Physiol.* 265:705–720.

150 Baldwin, B. A., & R. F. Parrott. 1979. Studies on intracranial electrical self-stimulation in pigs in relation to ingestive and exploratory behaviour. *Physiol. Behav.* 22:723–730.

151 Baldwin, B. A., & R. F. Parrott. 1985. Effects of intracerebroventricular injection of naloxone on operant feeding and drinking in pigs. *Pharmacol. Biochem. Behav.* 22:37–40.

152 Baldwin, B. A., & S. N. Thornton. 1986. Operant drinking in pigs following intracerebroventricular injections of hypertonic solutions and angiotensin II. *Physiol. Behav.* 36:325–328.

153 Baldwin, B. A., & T. R. Cooper. 1979. The effects of olfactory bulbectomy on feeding behaviour in pigs. *Appl. Anim. Ethol.* 5:153–159.

154 Baldwin, B. A., C. de la Riva, & I. S. Ebenezer. 1990. Effects of intracerebroventricular injection of dynorphin, leumorphin and alpha neo-endorphin on operant feeding in pigs. *Physiol. Behav.* 48:821–824.

155 Baldwin, B. A., C. L. McLaughlin, & C. A. Baile. 1977. The effect of ablation of the olfactory bulbs on feeding behaviour in sheep. *Appl. Anim. Ethol.* 3:151–161.

156 Baldwin, B. A., D. J. Conner, & G. B. Meese. 1974. Proceedings: Sensory reinforcement in the pig. *J. Physiol.* 242:27P.

157 Baldwin, B. A., I. S. Ebenezer, & C. De La Riva. 1990. Effects of intracerebroventricular injection of muscimol or GABA on operant feeding in pigs. *Physiol. Behav.* 48:417–421.

158 Bálint, A., T. Faragó, A. Dóka, Á. Miklósi, & P. Pongrácz. 2013. 'Beware, I am big and non-dangerous!' – Playfully growling dogs are perceived larger than their actual size by their canine audience. *Appl. Anim. Behav. Sci.* 148:128–137.

159 Banks, E. M. 1964. Some aspects of sexual behavior in domestic sheep, *Ovis aries*. *Behaviour* 23:249–279.

160 Baragli, P., A. Gazzano, F. Martelli, & C. Sighieri. 2009. How do horses appraise humans' actions? A brief note over a practical way to assess stimulus perception. *Equine Vet. J.* 29(10):739–742.

161 **Baranyiova, E., A. H. M. Martinikova, A. Necas, & J. Zatloukal. 2003. Epidemiology of intraspecies bite wounds in dogs in the Czech Republic. *Acta Vet. Brno.* 72:55–62.**

162 Baraza, E., J. J. Villalba, & F. D. Provenza. 2005. Nutritional context influences preferences of lambs for foods with plant secondary metabolites. *Appl. Anim. Behav. Sci.* 92:293–305.

163 Barber, J. A., & S. L. Crowell-Davis. 1994. Maternal behavior of Belgian (*Equus caballus*) mares. *Appl. Anim. Behav. Sci.* 41:161–168.

164 Bareham, J. R. 1975. The effect of lack of vision on suckling behaviour of lambs. *Appl. Anim. Ethol.* 1:245–250.

165 Bareham, J. R. 1976. The behaviour of lambs on the first day after birth. *Br. Vet. J.* 132:152–162.

166 Barnard, S., L. Matthews, S. Messori, M. Podaliri-Vulpiani, & N. Ferri. 2016. Laterality as an indicator of emotional stress in ewes and lambs during a separation test. *Anim. Cogn.* 19:207–214.

167 Barnes, R. H., A. U. Moore, & W. G. Pond. 1970. Behavioral abnormalities in young adult pigs caused by malnutrition in early life. *J. Nutr.* 100:149–155.

168 Barnett, J. L., G. M. Cronin,
T. H. McCallum, & E. A. Newman. 1993.
Effects of 'chemical intervention'
techniques on aggression and injuries
when grouping unfamiliar adult pigs. *Appl.
Anim. Behav. Sci.* 16:249–257.

169 Barnett, J. L., G. M. Cronin,
T. H. McCallum, & E. A. Newman. 1993.
Effects of pen size/shape and design on
aggression when grouping unfamiliar adult
pigs. *Appl. Anim. Behav. Sci.* 36:111–122.

170 Barnett, J. L., G. M. Cronin, T. H. McCallum,
& E. A. Newman. 1994. Effects of food and
time of day on aggression when grouping
unfamiliar adult pigs. *Appl. Anim. Behav.
Sci.* 39:339–347.

171 Barnett, J. L., P. H. Hemsworth,
C. G. Winfield, & C. Hansen. 1986. Effects
of social environment on welfare status and
sexual behaviour of female pigs I. effects of
group size. *Appl. Anim. Behav. Sci.*
16:249–257.

172 Baron, A., C. N. Stewart, & J. M. Warren.
1957. Patterns of social interaction in cats
(*Felis domestica*). *Behaviour* 11:56–66.

173 Barrett, P., & P. Bateson. 1978. The
development of play in cats. *Behaviour*
66:106–120.

174 Barroso, F. G., C. L. Alados, & J. Boza. 2000.
Social hierarchy in the domestic goat:
Effect on food habits and production. *Appl.
Anim. Behav. Sci.* 69:35–53.

175 Barry, K. J., & S. L. Crowell-Davis. 1999.
Gender differences in the social behavior of
the neutered indoor-only domestic cat.
Appl. Anim. Behav. Sci. 64:193–211.

176 Bartos, L., J. Bartosova, & L. Starostova.
2008. Position of the head is not associated
with changes in horse vision. *Equine Vet. J.*
40:599–601.

177 Bartoš, L., J. Bartošová, J. Pluhácek, &
J. Šindelárová. 2011. Promiscuous
behaviour disrupts pregnancy block in
domestic horse mares. *Behav. Ecol
Sociobiol.* 65(8):1567–1572.

178 Bartoshuk, L. M., M. A. Harned, &
L. H. Parks. 1971. Taste of water in the

cat: Effects on sucrose preference. *Science*
171:699–701.

179 Basile, M., S. Boivin, A. Boutin, C. Blois-
Heulin, M. Hausberger, & A. Lemasson.
2009. Socially dependent auditory laterality
in domestic horses (*Equus caballus*).
Anim. Cogn. 12:611–619.

180 **Bateson, P. 1978. Sexual imprinting and
optimal outbreeding. *Nature* 273:659–660.**

181 Bateson, P. 1979. How do sensitive periods
arise and what are they for? *Anim. Behav.*
27:470–486.

182 Bateson, P., M. Mendl, & J. Feaver. 1990.
Play in the domestic cat is enhanced by
rationing of the mother during lactation.
Anim. Behav. 40:514–525.

183 Batt, L. S., M. S. Batt, J. A. Baguley, &
P. D. McGreevy. 2009. The relationships
between motor lateralization, salivary
cortisol concentrations and behavior in
dogs. *J. Vet. Behav.* 4:216–222.

184 Bauer, E. B., & B. B. Smuts. 2007.
Cooperation and competition during dyadic
play in domestic dogs, *Canis familiaris*.
Anim. Behav. 73:489–499.

185 **Bauer, E., C. Ward, & B. Smits. 2009.
Play like a puppy, play like a dog. *J. Vet.
Behav.* 4:68–69.**

186 Baumgardt, B. R., & A. D. Peterson. 1970.
Hyperphagia in sheep induced by infusion
of the ventriculo cisternal system with a
depressant. *Fed. Proc.* 29:760.

187 Baxtera, E. M., S. Jarvis, L. Sherwood,
M. Farish, R. Roehe, A. B. Lawrence, &
S. A. Edwards. 2011. Genetic and
environmental effects on piglet survival
and maternal behaviour of the farrowing
sow. *Appl. Anim. Behav. Sci.* 130:28–41.

188 Beach, F. A. 1968. Coital behavior in dogs.
III. effects of early isolation on mating in
males. *Behaviour* 30:218–238.

189 Beach, F. A. 1970. Coital behavior in dogs.
VI. long-term effects of castration upon
mating in the male. *J. Comp. Physiol.
Psychol.* 70:1–32.

190 Beach, F. A. 1970. Coital behaviour in dogs
VIII. social affinity, dominance and sexual

preference in the bitch. *Behaviour* 36:131–148.

191 Beach, F. A. 1974. Effects of gonadal hormones on urinary behavior in dogs. *Physiol. Behav.* 12:1005–1013.

192 Beach, F. A., & A. Merari. 1968. Coital behavior in dogs. IV. effects of progesterone in the bitch. *Proc. Natl. Acad. Sci. U.S.A.* 61:442–446.

193 Beach, F. A., & B. J. Leboeuf. 1967. Coital behavior in dogs. I. preferential mating in the bitch. *Anim. Behav.* 15:546–558.

194 Beach, F. A., & R. E. Kuehn. 1970. Coital behavior in dogs X. effects of androgenic stimulation during development of feminine mating responses in females and males. *Horm. Behav.* 1:347–367.

195 Beach, F. A., & R. W. Gilmore. 1949. Response of male dogs to urine from females in heat. *J. Mammal.* 30:391–392.

196 Beach, F. A., A. I. Johnson, J. J. Anisko, & I. F. Dunbar. 1977. Hormonal control of sexual attraction in pseudohermaphroditic female dogs. *J. Comp. Physiol. Psychol.* 91:711–715.

197 Beach, F. A., I. F. Dunbar, & M. G. Buehler. 1982. Sexual characteristics of female dogs during successive phases of the ovarian cycle. *Horm. Behav.* 16:414–442.

198 **Beach, F. A., M. G. Buehler, & I. F. Dunbar. 1983. Development of attraction to estrous females in male dogs. *Physiol. Behav.* 31:293–297.**

199 Beach, F. A., R. E. Kuehn, R. H. Sprague, & J. J. Anisko. 1972. Coital behavior in dogs. XI. effects of androgenic stimulation during development on masculine mating responses in females. *Horm. Behav.* 3:143–168.

200 Beamer, W., G. Bermant, & M. T. Clegg. 1969. Copulatory behaviour of the ram, *Ovis aries*. II. *Factors affecting copulatory satiation. Anim. Behav.* 17:706–711.

201 Beattie, V. E., & N. E. O. O'Connell. 2002. Relationship between rooting behaviour and foraging in growing pigs. *Anim. Welf.* 11:295–303.

202 Beattie, V. E., N. Walker, & I. A. Sneddon. 1995. Effect of rearing environment and change of environment on the behaviour of gilts. *Appl. Anim. Behav. Sci.* 46:57–65.

203 Beauchemin, K. A., S. Zelin, D. Genner, & J. G. Buchanan-Smith. 1989. An automatic system for quantification of eating and ruminating activities of dairy cattle housed in stalls. *J. Dairy. Sci.* 72:2746–2759.

204 Beaudet, R. A., A. Chalifoux, & A. Dallaire. 1994. Predictive value of activity level and behavioral evaluation on future dominance in puppies. *Appl. Anim. Behav. Sci.* 40:273–284.

205 **Beausoleil, N. J., D. Blache, K. J. Stafford, D. J. Mellor, & A. D. L. Noble. 2012. Selection for temperament in sheep: Domain-general and context-specific traits. *Appl. Anim. Behav. Sci.* 139:74–85.**

206 Beausoleil, N. J., D. Blache, K. J. Stafford, D. J. Mellor, & A. D. L. Noble. 2008. Exploring the basis of divergent selection for 'temperament' in domestic sheep. *Appl. Anim. Behav. Sci.* 109:261–274.

207 Beausoleil, N. J., K. J. Stafford, & D. J. Mellor. 2006. Does direct human eye contact function as a warning cue for domestic sheep (*Ovis aries*)? *J. Comp. Psychol.* 120:269–279.

208 Beaver, B. 1980. *Veterinary aspects of feline behavior*. St. Louis, MO: C.V. Mosby.

209 **Beaver, B. V. 1983. Clinical classification of canine aggression. *Appl. Anim. Ethol.* 10:35–43.**

210 Beaver, B. V. 1993. Profiles of dogs presented for aggression. *J. Am. Anim. Hosp. Assoc.* 29:564–569.

211 **Beaver, B. V. 1999. *Canine behavior: A guide for veterinarians*. Philadelphia, PA: W.B. Saunders.**

212 Beaver, B. V., M. Fischer, & C. E. Atkinson. 1992. Determination of favorite components of garbage by dogs. *Appl. Anim. Behav. Sci.* 34:129–136.

213 Beck, A. M. 1973. *The ecology of stray dogs. A study of free-ranging urban animals.* Baltimore, MD: York Press.

214 Becker, B. A., J. J. Ford, R. K. Christenson, R. C. Manak, G. L. Hahn, & J. A. DeShazer. 1985. Cortisol response of gilts in tether stalls. *J. Anim. Sci.* 60:264–270.

215 Becker, R. F., J. E. King, & J. E. Markee. 1962. Studies on olfactory discrimination in dogs. II. discriminatory behavior in a free environment. *J. Comp. Physiol. Psychol.* 55:773–780.

216 Beckett, S. D., R. S. Hudson, & D. F. Walker. 1978. Effect of local anesthesia of the penis and dorsal penile neurectomy on the mating ability of bulls. *J. Am. Vet. Med. Assoc.* 173:838–839.

217 **Bécuwe-Bonnet, V., M.-C. Bélanger, D. Frank, J. Parent, & P. Hélie. 2012. Gastrointestinal disorders in dogs with excessive licking of surfaces. *J. Vet. Behav.* 7(4):194–204.**

218 Beilharz, R. G., & D. F. Cox. 1967. Social dominance in swine. *Anim. Behav.* 15:117–122.

219 Beilharz, R. G., & K. Zeeb. 1982. Social dominance in dairy cattle. *Appl. Anim. Ethol.* 8:79–97.

220 Beilharz, R. G., & P. J. Mylrea. 1963. Social position and behaviour of dairy heifers in yards. *Anim. Behav.* 11:522–528.

221 Beilharz, R. G., & P. J. Mylrea. 1963. Social position and movement orders of dairy heifers. *Anim. Behav.* 11:529–533.

222 Bekoff, M. 1974. Social play and play-soliciting by infant canids. *Am. Zool.* 14:323–340.

223 Bekoff, M. 1977. Social communication in canids: Evidence for the evolution of a stereotyped mammalian display. *Science* 197:1097–1099.

224 **Bekoff, M., H. L. Hill, & J. B. Mitton. 1975. Behavioural taxonomy in canids by discriminant function analyses. *Science* 190:1223–1225.**

225 Belkin, M., U. Yinon, L. Rose, & I. Reisert. 1977. Effect of visual environment on refractive error of cats. *Doc. Ophthalmol.* 42:433–437.

226 Bell, F. R. 1959. Preference thresholds for taste discrimination in goats. *J. Agric. Sci.* 52:125–128.

227 Bell, F. R. 1960. The electoencephalogram of goats during somnolence and rumination. *Anim. Behav.* 8:39–42.

228 Bell, F. R. 1963. Alkaline taste in goats assessed by the preference test technique. *J. Comp. Physiol. Psychol.* 56:174–178.

229 Bell, F. R., & H. L. Williams. 1959. Threshold values for taste in monozygotic twin calves. *Nature* 183:345–346.

230 Bellinger, L. L., & F. E. Williams. 1990. The effect of portal infusions of epinephrine on ingestion, plasma glucose and insulin in dogs. *Physiol. Behav.* 48:479–483.

231 Bellinger, L. L., G. J. Trietley, & L. L. Bernardis. 1976. Failure of portal glucose and adrenaline infusions or liver denervation to affect food intake in dogs. *Physiol. Behav.* 16:299–304.

232 Bench, C. J., & H. W. Gonyou. 2006. Effect of environmental enrichment at two stages of development on belly nosing in piglets weaned at fourteen days. *J. Anim. Sci.* 84:3397–3403.

233 **Bennett, M., K. A. Houpt, & H. N. Erb. 1988. Effects of declawing on feline behavior. *Companion Anim. Pract.* 2:7–12.**

234 Bensky, M. K., S. D. Gosling, & D. L. Sinn. 2013. The World from a Dog's Point of View: A Review and Synthesis of Dog Cognition Research. *Adv. Stud. Behav.* 45:210–387.

235 Berentsen, A. R., S. Bender, P. Bender, D. Bergman, K. Hausig, & K. C. VerCauteren. 2014. Preference among 7 bait flavors delivered to domestic dogs in Arizona: Implications for oral rabies vaccination on the Navajo Nation. *J. Vet. Behav.* 9:169–171.

236 Berg, I. A. 1944. Development of behavior: The micturition pattern in the dog. *J. Exp. Psychol.* 34:343–368.

237 Berger, A., K. Scheibe, K. Eichhorn, A. Scheibe, & J. Streich. 1999. Diurnal and

ultradian rhythms of behaviour in a mare group of Przewalski horse (*Equus ferus przewalskii*), measured through one year under semi-reserve conditions. *Appl. Anim. Behav. Sci.* 64:1–17.

238 Berger, J. 1977. Organizational systems and dominance in feral horses in the Grand Canyon. *Behav. Ecol. Sociobiol.* 2:131–146.

239 Berger, J. 1986. *Wild horses of the Great Basin.* Chicago, IL: The University of Chicago Press.

240 Berger, J. M., S. A. Bell, B. J. Holmberg, & J. E. Madigan. 2008. Successful treatment of head shaking by use of infrared diode laser deflation and coagulation of corpora nigra cysts and behavioral modification in a horse. *J. Am. Vet. Med. Assoc.* 233:1610–1612.

241 Berggren-Thomas, B., & W. D. Hohenboken. 1986. The effects of sire-breed, forage availability and weather on the grazing behavior of crossbred ewes. *Appl. Anim. Behav. Sci.* 15:217–228.

242 Berkson, G. 1968. Maturation defects in kittens. *Am. J. Ment. Defic.* 72:757–777.

243 Berman, M., & I. Dunbar. 1983. The social behavior of free-ranging urban dogs. *Appl. Anim. Ethol.* 10:5–17.

244 Bermant, G., M. T. Clegg, & W. Beamer. 1969. Copulatory behaviour of the ram, *Ovis aries. I. A normative study. Anim. Behav.* 17:700–705.

245 Bielanski, W., & S. Wierzbowski. 1961. Depletion test in stallions. *Proceedings of the IVTh International Congress on Animal Reproduction,* 279–282.

246 Bigelow, J. A., & T. R. Houpt. 1988. Feeding and drinking patterns in young pigs. *Physiol. Behav.* 43:99–109.

247 Billing, A. E., & M. A. Vince. 1987. Teat-seeking behaviour in newborn lambs I. evidence for the influence of material skin temperature. *Appl. Anim. Behav. Sci.* 18:301–313.

248 Billings, A. E., & M. A. Vince. 1987. Teat-seeking behaviour in newborn lambs II. Evidence for the influence of the dam's

surface textures and degree of surface yield. *Appl. Anim. Behav. Sci.* 18:315–325.

249 Billings, H. J., & L. S. Katz. 1999. Facilitation of sexual behavior in French-Alpine goats treated with intravaginal progesterone-releasing devices and estradiol during the breeding and nonbreeding seasons. *J. Anim. Sci.* 77:2073–2078.

250 Binev, R. 2015. Weaving horses. Etiological, clinical and paraclinical investigation. *IJAR.* 3:629–636.

251 Biquand, S., & V. Biquand-Guyot. 1992. The influence of peers, lineage and environment on food selection of the criollo goat (*Capra hircus*). *Appl. Anim. Behav. Sci.* 34:231–245.

252 **Bitterman, M. E. 1965. Phyletic differences in learning. *Am. Psychol.* 20:396–410.**

253 Bjone, S. J., W. Y. Brown, & I. R. Price. 2009. Maternal influence on grass-eating behaviour in puppies. *J. Vet. Behav.* 4:97–98.

254 Bjork, A., N. G. Olsson, E. Christensson, K. Martinsson, & O. Olsson. 1988. Effects of amperozide on biting behavior and performance in restricted-fed pigs following regrouping. *J. Anim. Sci.* 66:669–675.

255 Blackshaw, J. K., A. J. Swain, A. W. Blackshaw, F. J. M. Thomas, & K. J. Gillies. 1997. The development of playful behaviour in piglets from birth to weaning in three farrowing environments. *Appl. Anim. Behav. Sci.* 55:37–49.

256 Blackshaw, J. K., A. W. Blackshaw, & J. J. McGlone. 1997. Buller steer syndrome review. *Appl. Anim. Behav. Sci.* 54:97–108.

257 Blackwell, E. J., A. Bodnariua, J. Tyson, J. W. S. Bradshaw, & R. A. Casey. 2010. Rapid shaping of behaviour associated with high urinary cortisol in domestic dogs. *Appl. Anim. Behav. Sci.* 124:113–120.

258 Blackwell, E. J., J. W. S. Bradshaw, & R. A. Casey. 2013. Fear responses to noises in domestic dogs: Prevalence, risk factors and co-occurrence with other fear related behaviour. *Appl. Anim. Behav. Sci.* 145:15–25.

259 Blair, R., & J. FitzSimons. 1970. A note on the voluntary feed intake and growth of pigs given diets containing an extremely bitter compound. *Anim. Prod.* 12:529–530.

260 Blakemore, C., & R. C. Van Sluyters. 1975. Innate and environmental factors in the development of the kitten's visual cortex. *J. Physiol.* 248:663–716.

261 Bland, K. P., & B. M. Jubilan. 1987. Correlation of flehmen by male sheep with female behaviour and oestrus. *Anim. Behav.* 35:735–738.

262 Blaxter, K. L. 1944. Food preferences and habits in dairy cows. *British Society of Animal Prod. Second Meeting*, 85–94.

263 Bleicher, N. 1962. Behavior of the bitch during parturition. *J. Am. Vet. Med. Assoc.* 140:1076–1082.

264 Blissitt, M. J., K. P. Bland, & D. F. Cottrell. 1990. Olfactory and vomeronasal chemoreception and the discrimination of oestrous and non-oestrus ewe urine odours by the ram. *Appl. Anim. Behav. Sci.* 27:325–335.

265 Blockey, M. A. B. 1981. Development of a serving capacity test for beef bulls. *Appl. Anim. Ethol.* 7:307–319.

266 Blockey, M. A. B. 1981. Further studies on the serving capacity test for beef bulls. *Appl. Anim. Ethol.* 7:337–350.

267 Blockey, M. A. B. 1981. Modification of a serving capacity test for beef bulls. *Appl. Anim. Ethol.* 7:336.

268 Blom, A. K., K. Halse, & K. Hove. 1976. Growth hormone, insulin and sugar in the blood plasma of bulls. interrelated diurnal variations. *Acta Endocrinol.(Copenh)* 82:758–766.

269 Boe, K. E. 1991. The process of weaning in pigs: When the sow decides. *Appl. Anim. Behav. Sci.* 30:47–59.

270 **Boe, K. E. 1993. Maternal behaviour of lactating sows in a loose-housing system. *Appl. Anim. Behav. Sci.* 35:327–338.**

271 Boe, K. E. 1994. Variation in maternal behaviour and production of sows in integrated loose housing systems in Norway. *Appl. Anim. Behav. Sci.* 41:53–62.

272 Boe, K. E., & P. Jensen. 1995. Individual differences in suckling and solid food intake by piglets. *Appl. Anim. Behav. Sci.* 42:183–192.

273 Boe, K. E., S. Berg, & I. L. Andersen. 2006. Resting behaviour and displacements in ewes – effects of reduced lying space and pen shape. *Appl. Anim. Behav. Sci.* 98:249–259.

274 Bøea, K. E., R. Ehrlenbruch, G. H. Meisfjord Jørgensen, & I. L. Andersen. 2013. Individual distance during resting and feeding in age homogeneous vs. age heterogeneous groups of goats. *Appl. Anim. Behav. Sci.* 147(1–2):112–116.

275 Bohák, Zs., F. Szabó, J.-F. Beckers, N. Melo de Sousa, O. Kutasi, K. Nagy, & O. Szenci. 2013. Monitoring the circadian rhythm of serum and salivary cortisol concentrations in the horse. *Domest. Anim. Endocrin.* 45:38–42.

276 Bohnenkamp, A.-L., C. Meyer, K. Müller, & J. Krieter. 2013. Group housing with electronically controlled crates for lactating sows. Effect on farrowing, suckling and activity behavior of sows and piglets. *Appl. Anim. Behav. Sci.* 145:37–43.

277 Boissy, A., & M. Bouissou. 1995. Assessment of individual differences in behavioural reactions of heifers exposed to various fear-eliciting situations. *Appl. Anim. Behav. Sci.* 46:17–31.

278 Boissy, A., A. Aubert, L. Désiré, L. Greiveldinger, E. Delval, & I. Veissier. 2011. Cognitive sciences to relate ear postures to emotions in sheep. *Anim. Welf.* 20:47–56.

279 Boivin, X., P. Le Neindre, & J. M. Chupin. 1992. Establishment of cattle-human relationship. *Appl. Anim. Behav. Sci.* 32:325–335.

280 Boivin, X., P. Le Neindre, J. M. Chupin, J. P. Garel, & G. Trillat. 1992. Influence of breed and early management on ease of handling and open-field behaviour of cattle. *Appl. Anim. Behav. Sci.* 32:313–323.

281 Boivin, X., R. Nowak, G. Despres, H. Tournadre, & P. Le Neindre. 1997. Discrimination between shepherds by lambs reared under artificial conditions. *J. Anim. Sci.* 75:2892–2898.

282 Bolhuis, J. E., M. Oostindjer, C. W. F. Hoeks, E. N. de Haas, A. C. Bartels, M. Ooms, & B. Kemp. 2013. Working and reference memory of pigs (*Sus scrofa domesticus*) in a holeboard spatial discrimination task: the influence of environmental enrichment. *Anim. Cogn.* 16:845–850.

283 Bollen, K. S., & J. Horowitz. 2008. Behavioral evaluation and demographic information in the assessment of aggressiveness in shelter dogs. *Appl. Anim. Behav. Sci.* 112:120–135.

284 Bonanni, R., P. Valsecchi, & E. Natoli. 2010. Pattern of individual participation and cheating in conflicts between groups of free-ranging dogs. *Anim. Behav.* 79:957–968.

285 Bonnell, M. K., & S. M. McDonnell. 2016. Evidence for sire, dam, and family influence on operant learning in horses. *Equine Vet. J.* 36:69–76.

286 Booth, W. D., & B. A. Baldwin. 1980. Lack of effect on sexual behaviour or the development of testicular function after removal of olfactory bulbs in prepubertal boars. *J. Reprod. Fertil.* 58:173–182.

287 Borchelt, P. L. 1983. Aggressive behavior of dogs kept as companion animals: Classification and influence of sex, reproductive status and breed. *Appl. Anim. Ethol.* 10:45–61.

288 **Borchelt, P. L. 1991. Cat elimination behavior problems. *Vet. Clin. North Am. Small Anim. Pract.* 21:257–264.**

289 **Borchelt, P. L., & V. L. Voith. 1981. Elimination behavior problems in cats. *Comp. Contin. Ed.* 3:730–737.**

290 Borchelt, P. L., & V. L. Voith. 1985. Aggressive behavior in dogs and cats. *Comp. Contin. Ed.* 11:949–957.

291 Borchelt, P. L., & V. L. Voith. 1985. *Punishment. Comp. Contin. Ed.* 9:780–791.

292 **Borchelt, P. L., & V. L. Voith. 1996. Aggressive behavior in cats. In V. L. Voith, & P. L. Borchelt (Eds.), *Readings in companion animal*, pp. 208–216. Trenton, NJ: Veterinary Learning Systems.**

293 Borchelt, P. L., & V. L. Voith. 1996. Dominance aggression in the dog. In V. L. Voith, & P. L. Borchelt (Eds.), *Readings in companion animal behavior*, pp. 230–246. Trenton, NJ: Veterinary Learning Systems.

294 **Borchelt, P. L., R. Lockwood, A. M. Beck, & V. L. Voith. 1983. Attacks by packs of dogs involving predation on human beings. *Public Health Rep.* 98:57–66.**

295 Bordi, A., G. DeRosa, F. Napolitano, M. Litterio, V. Marino, & R. Rubino. 1994. Postpartum development of the mother-young relationship in goats. *Appl. Anim. Behav. Sci.* 42:145–152.

296 Borg, K. E., K. L. Esbenshade, & B. H. Johnson. 1993. Effects of the peri-pubertal rearing environment on endocrine and behavioural responses in oestrous female exposure in the mature bull. *Appl. Anim. Behav. Sci.* 35:245–253.

297 Borner, S., M. Derno, S. Hacke, U. Kautzsch, C. Schaff, S. ThanThan, H. Kuwayama, *et al.* 2013. Plasma ghrelin is positively associated with body fat, liver fat and milk fat content but not with feed intake of dairy cows after parturition. *J. Endocrinol.* 216:217–229.

298 Bottoms, G. D., O. F. Roesel, F. D. Rausch, & E. L. Akins. 1972. Circadian variation in plasma cortisol and corticosterone in pigs and mares. *Am. J. Vet. Res.* 33:785–790.

299 **Bouissou, M. 1965. Observations sur la hierarchie social chez les bovins domestiques. *Ann. Biol. Anim. Biochem. Biophys.* 5:327–339.**

300 Bouissou, M. 1971. Effet de l'absence d'informations optiques et de contact

physique sur la manifestation des relations hierarchiques chez les bovine domestiques *Ann. Biol. Anim. Biochem. Biophys.* 11:191–198.

301 Bouissou, M. F. 1978. Effect of injections of testosterone propionate on dominance relationships in a group of cows. *Horm. Behav.* 11:388–400.

302 Bouissou, M. F., & V. Gaudioso. 1982. Effect of early androgen treatment on subsequent social behavior in heifers. *Horm. Behav.* 16:132–146.

303 Bourguet, C., V. Deiss, M. Gobert, D. Durand, A. Boissy, & E. M. C. Terlouw. 2010. Characterising the emotional reactivity of cows to understand and predict their stress reactions to the slaughter procedure. *Appl. Anim. Behav. Sci.* 125:9–21.

304 Bourjade, M., A. de Boyer des Roches, & M. Hausberger. 2009. Adult-young ratio, a major factor regulating social behaviour of young: A horse study. *PLoS ONE.* 4(3):e4888.

305 Bowersox, S. S., T. L. Baker, & W. C. Dement. 1984. Sleep-wakefulness patterns in the aged cat. *Electroencephalogr. Clin. Neurophysiol.* 58:240–252.

306 Bowling, A. T., & R. W. Touchberry. 1990. Parentage of great-basin feral horses. *J. Wildl. Manag.* 54:424–429.

307 Boy, V., & P. Duncan. 1979. Time budgets of Camargue horses I. developmental changes in the time budgets of foals. *Behaviour* 71:187–202.

308 Boyd, L. 1998. The 24-h time budget of a takh harem stallion (*Equus ferus przewalskii*) pre- and post-reintroduction. *Appl. Anim. Behav. Sci.* 60:291–299.

309 Boyd, L. E. 1980. *The nationality, foal suvivorship, and mare-foal behavior of feral horses in Wyoming's red desert.* Laramie, WY: University of Wyoming.

310 Boyd, L., & N. Bandi. 2002. Reintroduction of takhi, *Equus ferus przewalskii*, to Hustai national park, Mongolia: Time budget and synchrony of activity pre- and post-release. *Appl. Anim. Behav. Sci.* 78:87–102.

311 Boyland, N. K., D. T. Mlynski, R. James, L. J. N. Brent, & D. P. Croft. 2016. The social network structure of a dynamic group of dairy cows: From individual to group level patterns. *Appl. Anim. Behav. Sci.* 174:1–10.

312 Bozdechová, B., G. Illmann, I. L. Andersen, J. Haman, & R. Ehrlenbruch. 2014. Litter competition during nursings and its effect on sow response on Day 2 postpartum. *Appl. Anim. Behav. Sci.* 150:9–16.

313 Bracke, M. B. M., J. J. Zonderland, P. Lenskens, W. G. P. Schouten, H. Vermeer, H. A. M. Spoolder, H. J. M. Hendriks, & H. Hopster. 2006. Formalised review of environmental enrichment for pigs in relation to political decision making. *Appl. Anim. Behav. Sci.* 98:165–182.

314 Bradshaw, J. W. S. 1992. *The behaviour of the domestic cat.* Wallingford, UK: CAB International.

315 **Bradshaw, J. W. S., E. J. Blackwell, & R. A. Casey. 2009. Dominance in domestic dogs – useful construct or bad habit?** *J. Vet. Behav.* **4:135–144.**

316 Bradshaw, J. W. S. 2014. Sociality in cats: A comparative review. *J. Vet. Behav.* 11:113–124.

317 Bradshaw, J., & C. Cameron-Beaumont. 2000. The signaling repertoire of the domestic cat and its undomesticated relatives. In D. C. Turner, & P. Bateson (Eds.), *The domestic cat: The biology of its behavior*, pp. 68–93. Cambridge, UK: Cambridge University Press.

318 **Brajon, S., J.-P. Laforest, R. Bergeron, C. Tallet, & N. Devillers. 2015. The perception of humans by piglets: Recognition of familiar handlers and generalisation to unfamiliar humans.** *Anim. Cogn.* **18:1299–1316.**

319 Brakel, W. J., & R. A. Leis. 1976. Impact of social disorganization on behavior, milk yield, and body weight of dairy cows. *J. Dairy Sci.* 59:716–721.

320 Branson, N. J., & L. J. Rogers. 2006. Relationship between paw preference strength and noise phobia in *Canis familiaris*. *J. Comp. Psychol.* 120:176–183.

321 Bray, A. R., & M. Wodzicka-Tomaszewska. 1974. Perinatal behaviour and progesterone and corticosteroid levels in sheep. *Proc. Aust. Soc. Anim. Prod.* 10:318–321.

322 Breland, K., & M. Breland. 1966. *Animal behavior*. New York, NY: Macmillan.

323 Brendle, J., & S. Hoy. 2011. Investigation of distances covered by fattening pigs measured with VideoMotionTracker®. *Appl. Anim. Behav. Sci.* 132:27–32.

324 Brenoe, U. T., A. G. Larsgard, K. Johannessen, & S. H. Uldal. 2002. Estimates of genetic parameters for hunting performance traits in three breeds of gun hunting dogs in Norway. *Appl. Anim. Behav. Sci.* 77:209–215.

325 Bressers, H. P. M., J. H. A. Te Brake, B. Engel, & J. P. T. M. Noordhuizen. 1993. Feeding order of sows at an individual electronic feed station in a dynamic group-housing system. *Appl. Anim. Behav. Sci.* 36:123–134.

326 Brewster, V., & A. Nevel. 2013. Immunocastration with Improvac reduces aggressive and sexual behaviours in male pigs. *Appl. Anim. Behav. Sci.* 145:32–36.

327 Briefer Freymond, S., D. Bardou, E. F. Briefer, R. Bruckmaier, N. Fouché, J. Fleury, A.-L. Maigrot, *et al.* 2015. The physiological consequences of crib-biting in horses in response to an ACTH challenge test. *Physiol. Behav.* 151:121–128.

328 Briefer, E., & A. G. McElligott. 2011. Mutual mother-offspring vocal recognition in an ungulate hider species (*Capra hircus*). *Anim. Cogn.* 14:585–598.

329 **Briefer, E. F., & A. G. McElligott. 2013. Rescued goats at a sanctuary display positive mood after former neglect. *Appl. Anim. Behav. Sci.* 146:45–55.**

330 Briefer, E. F., & A. G. McElligott. 2012. Social effects on vocal ontogeny in an ungulate, the goat, *Capra hircus*. *Anim. Behav.* 83:991–1000.

331 Briefer, E. F., F. Tettamanti, & A. G. McElligott. 2015. Emotions in goats: Mapping physiological, behavioural and vocal profiles. *Anim. Behav.* 99:131–143.

332 Briefer, E. F., M. Padilla de la Torre, & A. G. McElligott. 2012. Mother goats do not forget their kids' calls. *Proc. R. Soc. B.* 279:3749–3755.

333 Brindley, E. L., D. J. Bullock, & F. Maisels. 1989. Effects of rain and fly harassment on feeding behaviour of free-ranging feral goats. *Appl. Anim. Behav. Sci.* 24:31–41.

334 Brinkmann, L., M. Gerken, C. Hambly, J. R. Speakman, & A. Riek. 2014. Saving energy during hard times: Energetic adaptations of Shetland pony mares. *J. Exp. Biol.* 217:4320–4327.

335 Brisbin, I. L., Jr, & S. N. Austad. 1991. Testing the individual odour theory of canine olfaction. *Appl. Anim. Behav. Sci.* 42:63–69.

336 Bristol, F. 1982. Breeding behaviour of a stallion at pasture with 20 mares in synchronized oestrus. *J. Reprod. Fertil. Suppl.* 32:71–77.

337 Brobeck, J. R. 1955. Neural regulation of food intake. *Ann. N Y Acad. Sci.* 63:44–55.

338 Bronson, F. H., & W. K. Whitten. 1968. Oestrus-accelerating pheromone of mice: Assay, androgen-dependency and presence in bladder urine. *J. Reprod. Fertil.* 15:131–134.

339 **Bronson, R. T. 1979. Brain weight–body wright scaling in breeds of dogs and cats. *Brain Behav. Evol.* 16:227–236.**

340 Broom, D. M., & J. D. Leaver. 1978. Effects of group-rearing or partial isolation on later social behaviour of calves. *Anim. Behav.* 26:1255–1263.

341 Broom, D. M., H. Sena, & K. L. Moynihan. 2009. Pigs learn what a mirror image represents and use it to obtain information. *Anim. Behav.* 78:1037–1041.

342 Brouns, F., & S. A. Edwards. 1994. Social rank and feeding behaviour of group-housed sows fed competitively or ad libitum. *Appl. Anim. Behav. Sci.* 39:225–235.

343 Brouns, F., S. A. Edwards, & P. R. English. 1994. Effect of dietary fibre and feeding system on activity and oral behaviour of group housed gilts. *Appl. Anim. Behav. Sci.* 39:215–223.

344 Brown, J. A., C. Dewey, C. F. M. Delange, I. B. Mandell, P. P. Purslow, J. A. Robinson, E. J. Squires, & T. M. Widowski. 2009. Reliability of temperament tests on finishing pigs in group-housing and comparison to social tests. *Appl. Anim. Behav. Sci.* 118:28–35.

345 Brown, R. F., K. A. Houpt, & H. F. Schryver. 1976. Stimulation of food intake in horses by diazepam and promazine. *Pharmacol. Biochem. Behav.* 5:495–497.

346 Brown, S. M., M. Klaffenböck, I. M. Nevison, & A. B. Lawrence. 2015. Evidence for litter differences in play behaviour in pre-weaned pigs. *Appl. Anim. Behav. Sci.* 172:17–25.

347 Brownlee, A. 1954. Play in domestic cattle in Britain: An analysis of its nature. *Br. Vet. J.* 110:48–68.

348 **Brunberg, E., S. Gille, S. Mikko, G. Lindgren, & L. J. Keeling. 2013. Icelandic horses with the Silver coat colour show altered behaviour in a fear reaction test. *Appl. Anim. Behav. Sci.* 146:72–78.**

349 Bryant, M. J. 1975. A note on the effect of rearing experience upon the development of sexual behaviour in ram lambs. *Anim. Prod.* 21:97–99.

350 Bryant, M. J., & R. Ewbank. 1972. Some effects of stocking rate and group size upon agonistic behaviour in groups of growing pigs. *Br. Vet. J.* 128:64–70.

351 Bryant, M. J., & T. Tompkins. 1973. Sexual behaviour of sheep. *Vet. Rec.* 93:253.

352 Buchenauer, V. D., & B. Fritsch. 1980. Zum farbsehvermogen von hausziegen (*Capra bircus* L.). *Z. Tierpsychol.* 53:225–230.

353 Buckner, L. J., S. A. Edwards, & J. M. Bruce. 1998. Behaviour and shelter use by outdoor sows. *Appl. Anim. Behav. Sci.* 57:69–80.

354 Budzynska, M., & D. M. Weary. 2008. Weaning distress in dairy calves: Effects of alternative weaning procedures. *Appl. Anim. Behav. Sci.* 112:33–39.

355 Burger, J. F. 1952. Sex physiology of pigs. *Onderstepoort J. Vet. Res. Suppl.* 2:1–218.

356 **Burman, O., R. McGowan, M. Mendl, Y. Norling, E. Paul, T. Rehn, & L. Keeling. 2011. Using judgement bias to measure positive affective state in dogs. *Appl. Anim. Behav. Sci.* 132:160–168.**

357 Burne, T. H., P. J. Murfitt, & C. L. Gilbert. 2000. Deprivation of straw bedding alters PGF(2alpha)-induced nesting behaviour in female pigs. *Appl. Anim. Behav. Sci.* 69:215–225.

358 Burne, T. H., P. J. Murfitt, & C. L. Gilbert. 2001. Influence of environmental temperature on PGF(2alpha)-induced nest building in female pigs. *Appl. Anim. Behav. Sci.* 71:293–304.

359 Burritt, E. A., & F. D. Provenza. 1991. Ability of lambs to learn with a delay between food ingestion and consequences given meals containing novel and familiar foods. *Appl. Anim. Behav. Sci.* 32:179–189.

360 Burritt, E. A., & F. D. Provenza. 1992. Lambs form preferences for nonnutritive flavors paired with glucose. *J. Anim. Sci.* 70:1133–1136.

361 Burritt, E. A., & F. D. Provenza. 1997. Effect of an unfamiliar location on the consumption of novel and familiar foods by sheep. *Appl. Anim. Behav. Sci.* 54:317–325.

362 Burritt, E. A., H. F. Mayland, F. D. Provenza, R. L. Miller, & J. C. Burns. 2005. Effect of added sugar on preference and intake by sheep of hay cut in the morning versus the afternoon. *Appl. Anim. Behav. Sci.* 94:245–254.

363 Buskirk, D. D., A. J. Zanella, T. M. Harrigan, J. L. Van Lente, L. M. Gnagey, & M. J. Kaercher. 2003. Large round bale feeder design affects hay utilization and beef cow behavior. *J. Anim. Sci.* 81:109–115.

364 **Busnel, R. 1963. *Acoustic behaviour of animals*. Amsterdam, The Netherlands: Elsevier.**

365 **Buttner, A. P., B. Thompson, R. Strasser, & J. Santo. 2015. Evidence for a**

synchronization of hormonal states between humans and dogs during competition. *Physiol. Behav.* **147:54–62.**

366 Byosiere, S.-E., J. Espinosa, & B. Smuts. 2016. Investigating the function of play bows in adult pet dogs (*Canis lupus familiaris*). *Behav. Processes.* 125:106–113.

367 Cafazzo, S., P. Valsecchi, R. Bonanni, & E. Natoli. 2010. Dominance in relation to age, sex, and competitive contexts in a group of free-ranging domestic dogs. *Behav. Ecol.* 21(3):443–455.

368 Cafazzoa, S., & E. Natoli. 2009. The social function of tail up in the domestic cat (*Felis silvestris catus*). *Behav. Processes.* 80:60–66.

369 Cairns, R. B., & D. L. Johnson. 1965. The development of interspecies social attachments. *Psychonom. Sci.* 2:337–338.

370 Çakiroglu, D., Y. Meral, A. A. Sancak, & G. Çifti. 2007. Relationship between the serum concentrations of serotonin and lipids and aggression in dogs. *Vet. Rec.* 161:59–61.

371 Camerlink, I., S. P. Turner, M. Farish, & G. Arnott. 2015. Aggressiveness as a component of fighting ability in pigs using a game-theoretical framework. *Anim. Behav.* 108:183–191.

372 Camerlink, I., & S. P. Turner. 2013. The pig's nose and its role in dominance relationships and harmful behaviour. *Appl. Anim. Behav. Sci.* 145:84–91.

373 Cameron, E. Z., & W. L. Linklater. 2000. Individual mares bias investment in sons and daughters in relation to their condition. *Anim. Behav.* 60:359–367.

374 Cameron, E. Z., K. J. Stafford, W. L. Linklater, & C. J. Veltman. 1999. Suckling behaviour does not measure milk intake in horses, *Equus caballus. Anim. Behav.* 57:673–678.

375 Cameron, E. Z., W. L. Linklater, K. J. Stafford, & E. O. Minot. 2008. Maternal investment results in better foal condition through increased play behaviour in horses. *Anim. Behav.* 76:1511–1518.

376 Campbell, K. J., G. S. Baxter, P. J. Murray, B. E. Coblentz, & C. J. Donlan. 2007. Development of a prolonged estrus effect for use in judas goats. *Appl. Anim. Behav. Sci.* 102:12–23.

377 Campbell, R. G. 1976. A note on the use of a feed flabour to stimulate the feed intake of weaner pigs. *Anim. Prod.* 23:417–419.

378 Campbell, S. S., & I. Tobler. 1984. Animal sleep: A review of sleep duration across phylogeny. *Neurosci. Biobehav. Rev.* 8:269–300.

379 Campbell, W. E. 1989. *Better behavior in dogs and cats.* Loveland, CO: Alpine.

380 **Campbell, W. E., & A. Campbell. 1972. A behavior test for puppy selection. *Mod. Vet. Pract.* 12:29–33.**

381 Campion, D. P., & B. F. Leek. 1997. Investigation of a "fibre appetite" in sheep fed a "long fibre-free" diet. *Appl. Anim. Behav. Sci.* 52:79–86.

382 **Campitelli, S., C. Carenzi, & M. Verga. 1982. Factors which influence parturition in the mare and development of the foal. *Appl. Anim. Ethol.* 9:7–14.**

383 Canali, E., M. Varga, M. Montagna, & A. Baldi. 1986. Social interactions and induced behavioural reactions in milk-fed female calves. *Appl. Anim. Behav. Sci.* 16:207–215.

384 Candland, D. K., & D. Milne. 1966. Species differences in approach-behaviour as a function of developmental environment. *Anim. Behav.* 14:539–545.

385 Cannas, S., D. Frank, M. Minero, M. Godbout, & C. Palestrini. 2010. Puppy behavior when left home alone: Changes during the first few months after adoption. *J. Vet. Behav.* 5:94–100.

386 Carlstead, K. 1986. Predictability of feeding: Its effect on agonistic behaviour and growth in grower pigs. *Appl. Anim. Behav. Sci.* 16:25–38.

387 Caro, T. M. 1980. Effects of the mother, object play, and adult experience on predation in cats. *Behav. Neural Biol.* 29:29–51.

388 Caro, T. M. 1980. Predatory behaviour and social play in kittens. *Behaviour* 76:1–24.

389 Caro, T. M. 1980. Predatory behaviour in domestic cat mothers. *Behaviour* 74:128–148.

390 Carreras, R., L. Arroyo, E. Mainau, R. Pena, A. Bassols, A. Dalmau, L. Faucitano, *et al.* 2016. Effect of gender and halothane genotype on cognitive bias and its relationship with fear in pigs. *Appl. Anim. Behav. Sci.* 177:12–18.

391 Carroll, J., C. J. Murphy, M. Neitz, J. N. Hoeve, & J. Neitz. 2001. Photopigment basis for dichromatic color vision in the horse. *J. Vis.* 1:80–87.

392 Carson, K., & D. G. M. Wood-Gush. 1983. Equine behaviour: I. A review of the literature on social and dam foal behaviour. *Appl. Anim. Ethol.* 10:165–178.

393 Carson, K., & D. G. Wood-Gush. 1983. Behaviour of thoroughbred foals during nursing. *Equine Vet. J.* 15:257–262.

394 Carter, M. J., T. H. Friend, J. Coverdale, S. M. Garey, A. L. Adams, & C. L. Terrill. 2012. A comparison of three conventional horse feeders with the pre-vent feeder. *Equine Vet. J.* 32:252–255.

395 Carver, D. S., & H. N. Waterhouse. 1962. The variation in the water consumption of cats. *Proc. Anim. Care Panel* 12:267–270.

396 Caspi, A., J. McClay, T. E. Moffitt, J. Mill, J. Martin, I. W. Craig, A. Taylor, & R. Poulton. 2002. Role of genotype in the cycle of violence in maltreated children. *Science* 297:851–854.

397 Cassady, J. P. 2007. Evidence of phenotypic relationships among behavioral characteristics of individual pigs and performance. *J. Anim. Sci.* 85:218–224.

398 Cassini, M. H., & H. N. Hermitte. 1962. Patterns of environmental use by cattle and consumption of supplemental food blocks. *Appl. Anim. Behav. Sci.* 32:297–312.

399 Castonguay, T. W. 1981. Dietary dilution and intake in the cat. *Physiol. Behav.* 27:547–549.

400 Castren, H., B. Algers, A. M. DePassille, J. Rushen, & K. Uvnas-Moberg. 1993. Preparturient variation in progesterone, prolactin, oxytocin and somatostatin in relation to nest building in sows. *Appl. Anim. Behav. Sci.* 38:91–102.

401 Cerny, V. A. 1977. Failure of dihydrotestosterone to elicit sexual behaviour in the female cat. *J. Endocrinol.* 75:173–174.

402 Cervantes, M., R. Ruelas, & C. Beyer. 1983. Serotonergic influences on EEG synchronization induced by milk drinking in the cat. *Pharmacol. Biochem. Behav.* 18:851–855.

403 Chakraborty, P. K., W. B. Panko, & W. S. Fletcher. 1980. Serum hormone concentrations and their relationships to sexual behavior at the first and second estrous cycles of the Labrador bitch. *Biol. Reprod.* 22:227–232.

404 Chamberlain, B., F. R. Ervin, R. O. Pihl, & S. N. Young. 1987. The effect of raising or lowering tryptophan levels on aggression in vervet monkeys. *Pharmacol. Biochem. Behav.* 28:503–510.

405 Champion, R. A., N. A. Lagstrom, & A. J. Rook. 2007. Motivation of sheep to eat clover offered in a short-term closed economy test. *Appl. Anim. Behav. Sci.* 108:263–275.

406 Champion, R. A., S. M. Rutter, P. D. Penning, & A. J. Rook. 1994. Temporal variation in grazing behavior of sheep and the reliability of sampling periods. *Appl. Anim. Behav. Sci.* 42:99–108.

407 Chan, W. Y., S. Cloutier, & R. C. Newberry. 2011. Barking pigs: Differences in acoustic morphology predict juvenile responses to alarm calls. *Anim. Behav.* 82:767–774.

408 Chase, L. E., P. J. Wangsness, & B. R. Baumgardt. 1976. Feeding behavior of steers fed a complete mixed ration. *J. Dairy Sci.* 59:1923–1928.

409 Chaya, L., E. Cowan, & B. Mcguire. 2006. A note on the relationship between time spent in turnout and behaviour

during turnout in horses (***Equus caballus***). *Appl. Anim. Behav. Sci.* **98:155–160.**

410 Chemineau, P. 1986. Sexual behavior and gonadal activity during the year in the tropical creole meat goat I. Female estrous behavior and ovarian activity. *Reprod. Nutr. Dev.* 26:441–442.

411 Chen, J., Q. Weng, J. Chao, D. Hu, & K. Taya. 2008. Reproduction and development of the released Przewalski's horses (*Equus przewalskii* in Xinjiang, China). *J. Equine Sci.* 19:1–7.

412 Chepko, B. D. 1971. A preliminary study of the effects of play deprivation on young goats. *Z. Tierpsychol.* 28:517–526.

413 Chesler, P. 1969. Maternal influence in learning by observation in kittens. *Science* 166:901–903.

414 Chijiiwa, H., H. Kuroshima, Y. Hori, J. R. Anderson, & K. Fujita. 2015. Dogs avoid people who behave negatively to their owner: Third-party affective evaluation. *Anim. Behav.* 106:123–127.

415 Christensen, E., J. Scarlett, M. Campagna, & K. A. Houpt. 2007. Aggressive behavior in adopted dogs that passed a temperament test. *Appl. Anim. Behav. Sci.* 106:85–95.

416 Christensen, H. R., G. W. Seifert, & T. B. Post. 1982. The relationship between a serving capacity test and fertility of beef bulls. *Aust. Vet. J.* 58:241–244.

417 Christensen, J. W. 2016. Early-life object exposure with a habituated mother reduces fear reactions in foals. *Anim. Cogn.* 19:171–179.

418 Christensen, J. W., & M. Rundgren. 2008. Predator odour per se does not frighten domestic horses. *Appl. Anim. Behav. Sci.* 112:136–145.

419 Christensen, J. W., J. Ladewig, E. Sondergaard, & J. Malmkvist. 2002. Effects of individual versus group stabling on social behaviour in domestic stallions. *Appl. Anim. Behav. Sci.* 75:233–248.

420 Christensen, J. W., L. J. Keeling, & B. L. Nielsen. 2005. Responses of horses to novel visual, olfactory an auditory stimuli. *Appl. Anim. Behav. Sci.* 93:53–65.

421 Christensen, J. W., L. P. Ahrendt, R. Lintrup, C. Gaillard, R. Palme, & J. Malmkvist. 2012. Does learning performance in horses relate to fearfulness, baseline stress hormone, and social rank? *Appl. Anim. Behav. Sci.* 140:44–52.

422 Christensen, J. W., T. Zharkikh, & E. Chovaux. 2011. Object recognition and generalisation during habituation in horses. *Appl. Anim. Behav. Sci.* 129:83–91.

423 Christensen, J. W., T. Zharkikh, & J. Ladwig. 2008. Do horses generalise between objects during habituation? *Appl. Anim. Behav. Sci.* 114:509–520.

424 **Christiansen, F. O., M. Bakken, & B. O. Braastad. 2001. Behavioural changes and aversive conditioning in hunting dogs by the second-year confrontation with domestic sheep. *Appl. Anim. Behav. Sci.* 72:131–143.**

425 **Christiansen, F. O., M. Bakken, & B. O. Braastad. 2001. Social facilitation of predatory, sheep-chasing behaviour in Norwegian elkhounds, grey. *Appl. Anim. Behav. Sci.* 72:105–114.**

426 Christie, D. W., & E. T. Bell. 1972. Studies on canine reproductive behaviour during the normal oestrous cycle. *Anim. Behav.* 20:621–631.

427 Church, S. C., J. A. Allen, & J. W. S. Bradshaw. 1994. Anti-apostatic food selection by the domestic cat. *Anim. Behav.* 48:747–749.

428 Cizek, L. J., R. E. Semple, K. C. Huang, & M. I. Gregersen. 1951. Effect of extracellular electrolyte depletion on water intake in dogs. *Am. J. Physiol.* 164:415–422.

429 **Clark, D. K., T. H. Friend, & G. Dellmeier. 1993. The effect of orientation during trailer transport on heart rate, cortisol and balance in horses. *Appl. Anim. Behav. Sci.* 38:179–189.**

430 Clark, J. R., R. W. Bell, L. F. Tribble, & A. M. Lennon. 1985. Effects of composition and density of the group on the performance,

behaviour and age at puberty in swine. *Appl. Anim. Behav. Sci.* 14:127–135.

431 Clarke, I. J., & R. J. Scaramuzzi. 1978. Sexual behaviour and LH secretion in spayed androgenized ewes after a single injection of testosterone or oestradiol-17beta. *J. Reprod. Fertil.* 52:313–320.

432 Clegg, H. A., P. Buckley, M. A. Friend, & P. D. McGreevy. 2008. The ethological and physiological characteristics of cribbing and weaving horses. *Appl. Anim. Behav. Sci.* 109:68–76.

433 Clegg, M. T., W. Beamer, & G. Bermant. 1969. Copulatory behaviour of the ram, *Ovis aries*. III. Effects of pre- and postpubertal castration and androgen replacement therapy. *Anim. Behav.* 17:712–717.

434 Clutton-Brock, T. H., P. J. Greenwood, & R. P. Powell. 1976. Ranks and relationships in highland ponies and highland cows. *Z. Tierpsychol.* 41:202–216.

435 Cohen-Tannoudji, J., A. Locatelli, & J. P. Signoret. 1986. Non-pheromonal stimulation by the male of LH release in the anoestrous ewe. *Physiol. Behav.* 36:921–924.

436 Cohen-Tannoudji, J., J. Einhorn, & J. P. Signoret. 1994. Ram sexual pheromone: First approach of chemical identification. *Physiol. Behav.* 56:955–961.

437 Cohn, R. 1956. A contribution to the study of color vision in cat. *J. Neurophysiol.* 19:416–423.

438 Coile, D. C., C. H. Pollitz, & J. C. Smith. 1989. Behavioral determination of critical flicker fusion in dogs. *Physiol. Behav.* 45:1087–1092.

439 Cole, D. D., & J. N. Shafer. 1966. A study of social dominance in cats. *Behaviour* 27:39–53.

440 Cole, D. J. A., J. E. Duckworth, & W. Holmes. 1967. Factors affecting voluntary feed intake in pigs I. The effect of digestible energy content of the diet on the intake of castrated male pigs housed in holding pens and in metabolism crates. *Anim. Prod.* 9:141–148.

441 Collard, R. R. 1967. Fear of strangers and play behavior in kittens with varied social experience. *Child Dev.* 38:877–891.

442 Collias, N. E. 1956. The analysis of socialization in sheep and goats. *Ecology* 37:228–239.

443 Collins, J. P., & G. H. Rose. 1975. Light-dark discrimination and reversal learning in early postnatal kittens. *Dev. Psychobiol.* 8:511–518.

444 Collis, K. A. 1976. An investigation of factors related to the dominance order of a herd of dairy cows of similar age and breed. *Appl. Anim. Ethol.* 2:167–173.

445 Collis, K. A., S. J. Kay, A. J. Grant, & A. J. Quick. 1979. The effect on social organization and milk production of minor group alterations in dairy cattle. *Appl. Anim. Ethol.* 5:103–111.

446 Colson, V., P. Orgeur, A. Foury, & P. Mormède. 2006. Consequences of weaning piglets at 21 and 28 days on growth, behaviour and hormonal responses. *Appl. Anim. Behav. Sci.* 98:70–88.

447 Concannon, P. W., W. Hansel, & W. J. Visek. 1975. The ovarian cycle of the bitch: Plasma estrogen, LH and progesterone. *Biol. Reprod.* 13:112–121.

448 Cooling, M. J., & M. D. Day. 1975. Drinking behaviour in the cat induced by renin, angiotensin I, II and isoprenaline. *J. Physiol.* 244:325–336.

449 Cooper, J. J., C. Ashton, S. Bishop, R. West, D. S. Mills, & R. J. Young. 2003. Clever hounds: Social cognition in the domestic dog (*Canis familiaris*). *Appl. Anim. Behav. Sci.* 81:229–244.

450 Cooper, J. J., L. McDonald, & D. S. Mills. 2000. The effect of increasing visual horizons on stereotypic weaving: Implications for the social housing of stabled horses. *Appl. Anim. Behav. Sci.* 69:67–83.

451 Cooper, J. J., N. Mcall, S. Johnson, & H. P. B. Davidson. 2005. The short-term

effects of increasing meal frequency on stereotypic behaviour of stabled horses. *Appl. Anim. Behav. Sci.* 90:351–364.

452 Cooper, J. J., N. Mcall, S. Johnson, & H. P. B. Davidson. 2005. The short-term effects of increasing meal frequency on stereotypic behaviour of stabled horses. *Appl. Anim. Behav. Sci.* 90:351–364.

453 Cooper, J., I. J. Gordon, & A. W. Pike. 2000. Strategies for the avoidance of faeces by grazing sheep. *Appl. Anim. Behav. Sci.* 69:15–33.

454 Cooper, R. A., S. Evans, & J. A. Kirk. 1991. Effects of water additives on water consumption, urine output and urine mineral levels in angora goats. *Anim. Prod.* 52:609.

455 Coppinger, R., & R. Schneider. 2006. Evolution of working dogs. In J. Serpell (Ed.), *The domestic dog: Its evolution, behaviour and interactions with people*, pp. 21–47. Cambridge, UK: Cambridge University Press.

456 Coppinger, R., J. Lorenz, J. Glendinning, & P. Pinardi. 1983. Attentiveness of guarding dogs for reducing predation on domestic sheep. *J. Range Manag.* 36:275–279.

457 Corbett, J. L. 1953. Grazing behaviour in New Zealand. *Br. J. Anim. Behav.* 1:67–71.

458 Corson, S. A., E. L. Corson, V. Kirilcuk, J. Kirilcuk, W. Knopp, & L. E. Arnold. 1972. Differential effects of amphetamines on several types of hyperkinetic and normal dogs and on learning disability. *Psychopharmacology* 26 (Suppl.):55.

459 Cory, V. L. 1927. Activities of livestock on the range. *Tex. Agric. Exp. Sta. Bull.* 367:5–47.

460 Coulon, M., B. L. Deputte, Y. Heyman, L. Delatouce, C. Richard, & C. Baudoin. 2007. Visual discrimination by heifers (*Bos taurus*) of their own species. *J. Comp. Psychol.* 121:198–204.

461 Coulon, M., C. Baudoin, Y. Heyman, & B. L. Deputte. 2011. Cattle discriminate between familiar and unfamiliar

conspecifics by using only head visual cues. *Anim. Cogn.* 14:279–290.

462 Cowlishaw, S. J., & F. E. Alder. 1960. The grazing preferences of cattle and sheep. *J. Agric. Sci.* (Camb.) 54:257–265.

463 **Cozzi, A., C. Sighieri, A. Gazzano, C. J. Nicol, & P. Baragli. 2010. Post-conflict friendly reunion in a permanent group of horses (*Equus caballus*). *Behav. Processes.* 85:185–190.**

464 Cracknell, N. R., D. S. Mills, & P. Kaulfuss. 2008. Can stimulus enhancement explain the apparent success of the model-rival technique in the domestic dog (*Canis familiaris*)? *Appl. Anim. Behav. Sci.* 114:461–472.

465 Craig, D. P. A., C. A. Varnon, K. L. Pollock, & C. I. Abramson. 2015. An assessment of horse (*Equus ferus caballus*) responding on fixed interval schedules of reinforcement: An individual analysis. *Behav. Processes.* 120:1–13.

466 Crawford, M. A., M. D. Kittleson, & G. D. Fink. 1984. Hypernatremia and adipsia in a dog. *J. Am. Vet. Med. Assoc.* 184:818–821.

467 Creel, S. R., & J. L. Albright. 1988. The effects of neonatal social isolation on the behavior and endocrine function of Holstein calves. *Appl. Anim. Behav. Sci.* 21:293–306.

468 **Cregier, S. W. 1982. Reducing equine hauling stress: A review. *J. Equine Vet. Sci.* 2:187–198.**

469 Cresswell, E. 1959. A cattle rangemeter. *Anim. Behav.* 7:244.

470 Cresswell, E. 1960. Ranging behaviour studies with Romney marsh and cheviot sheep in New Zealand. *Anim. Behav.* 8:32–38.

471 Cronin, G. M., & J. A. Smith. 2002. Effects of accommodation type and straw bedding around parturition and during lactation on the behaviour of primiparous sows and survival and growth of piglets to weaning. *Appl. Anim. Behav. Sci.* 33:191–208.

472 Cronin, G. M., B. N. Schirmer, T. H. McCallum, J. A. Smith, & K. L. Butler. 1993. The effects of providing sawdust to pre-parturient sows in farrowing crates on sow behaviour, the duration of parturition and the occurrence of intra-partum stillborn piglets. *Appl. Anim. Behav. Sci.* 36:301–315.

473 **Cronin, G. M., P. R. Wiepkema, & J. M. van Ree. 1986. Endorphins implicated in stereotypies of tethered sows. *Experientia* 42:198–199.**

474 Crowell-Davis, S. 2002. Social behaviour, communication and development of behaviour in the cat. In D. Horwitz, D. Mills, & S. Heath (Eds.), *BSAVA canine and feline behavioural medicine.* Quidgeley, UK: British Small Animal Veterinary Society.

475 Crowell-Davis, S. L. 1985. Nursing behaviour and maternal aggression among welsh ponies (*Equus caballus*). *Appl. Anim. Behav. Sci.* 14:11–25.

476 Crowell-Davis, S. L. 1986. Spatial relations between mares and foals of the welsh pony (*Equus caballus*). *Anim. Behav.* 34:1007–1015.

477 Crowell-Davis, S. L. 1994. Daytime rest behavior of the welsh pony (*Equus caballus*) mare and foal. *Anim. Behav.* 40:197–210.

478 Crowell-Davis, S. L. 2007. Sexual behavior of mares. *Horm. Behav.* 52:12–17.

479 Crowell-Davis, S. L., & A. B. Caudle. 1989. Coprophagy by foals: Recognition of maternal feces. *Appl. Anim. Behav. Sci.* 24:267–272.

480 Crowell-Davis, S. L., & K. A. Houpt. 1985. Coprophagy by foals: Effect of age and possible functions. *Equine Vet. J.* 17:17–19.

481 Crowell-Davis, S. L., & K. A. Houpt. 1985. The ontogeny of flehmen in horses. *Anim. Behav.* 33:739–774.

482 Crowell-Davis, S. L., K. A. Houpt, & C. M. Carini. 1986. Mutual grooming and nearest-neighbor relationships among foals of *Equus caballus*. *Appl. Anim. Behav. Sci.* 15:113–123.

483 Crowell-Davis, S. L., K. A. Houpt, & J. Carnevale. 1985. Feeding and drinking behavior of mares and foals with free access to pasture and water. *J. Anim. Sci.* 60:883–889.

484 Crowell-Davis, S. L., K. A. Houpt, & J. S. Burnham. 1985. Snapping by foals of *Equus caballus*. *Z. Tierpsychol.* 69:42–54.

485 **Crowell-Davis, S. L., K. A. Houpt, & L. Kane. 1987. Play development in welsh pony (*Equus caballus*) foal. *Appl. Anim. Behav. Sci.* 18:119–131.**

486 Crowell-Davis, S. L., K. Barry, & R. Wolfe. 1997. Social behavior and aggressive problems of cats. *Vet. Clin. North Am. Small Anim. Pract.* 27:549–568.

487 **Crowell-Davis, S. L., K. Barry, J. M. Ballam, & D. P. Laflamme. 1995. The effect of caloric restriction on the behavior of pen-housed dogs: Transition from unrestricted to restricted diet. *Appl. Anim. Behav. Sci.* 43:27–41.**

488 Cuaya, L. V., R. Hernández-Pérez, & L. Concha. 2016. Our faces in the dog's brain: Functional imaging reveals temporal cortex activation during perception of human faces. *PLoS ONE.* 11(3):e0149431.

489 **Cummings, B. J., E. Head, W. Ruehl, N. W. Milgram, & C. W. Cotman. 1996. The canine as an animal model of human aging and dementia. *Neurobiol. Aging* 17:259–268.**

490 Curley, K. O., Jr, J. C. Paschal, T. H. Welsh Jr, & R. D. Randel. 2006. Technical note: Exit velocity as a measure of cattle temperament is repeatable and associated with serum concentration of cortisol in Brahman bulls. *J. Anim. Sci.* 84:3100–3103.

491 Curtis, Q. F. 1937. Experimental neurosis in the pig. *Psychol. Bull.* 34:723.

492 **Curtis, T. M., R. J. Knowles, & S. L. Crowell-Davis. 2003. Influence of familiarity and relatedness on proximity and allogrooming in domestic cats (*Felis catus*). *Am. J. Vet. Res.* 64:1151–1154.**

493 Curtis, T. M., R. J. Knowles, & S. L. Crowell-Davis. 2003. Influence of

familiarity and relatedness on proximity and allogrooming in domestic cats (Felis *catus*). *Am. J. Vet. Res.* 64:1151–1154.

494 Custance, D., & J. Mayer. 2012. Empathic-like responding by domestic dogs (*Canis familiaris*) to distress in humans: An exploratory study. *Anim. Cogn.* 15:851–859.

495 Czarkowska, J. 1983. Changes of some postural reflexes during the first postnatal weeks in the dog. *Acta Neurobiol. Exp. (Wars)* 43:27–35.

496 Dabrowska, B., W. Harmata, Z. Lenkiewicz, Z. Schiffer, & R. J. Wojtusiak. 1981. Colour perception in cows. *Behav. Processes.* 6:1–10.

497 Daels, P. F., & J. P. Hughes. 1992. The abnormal estrous cycle. In A. O. McKinnon, & J. L. Voss (Eds.), *Equine reproduction*, pp. 144–171. Malvern, PA: Lea & Febiger.

498 Dailey, J. W., & J. J. McGlone. 1997. Oral/nasal/facial and other behaviors of sows kept individually outdoors on pasture, soil or indoors in gestation crates. *Appl. Anim. Behav. Sci.* 52:25–43.

499 Dalla Costa, E., M. Minero, D. Lebelt, D. Stucke, E. Canali, & M. C. Leach. 2014. Development of the Horse Grimace Scale (HGS) as a pain assessment tool in horses undergoing routine castration. *PLoS ONE.* 9(3):e92281.

500 Dallaire, A. R. Y. 1974. Sleep and wakefulness in the housed pony under different dietary conditions. *Can. J. Comp. Med.* 38:65–71.

501 Dallaire, A., & Y. Ruckebusch. 1974. Sleep patterns in the pony with observations on partial perceptual deprivation. *Physiol. Behav.* 12:789–796.

502 Dalmau, A., E. Fabrega, & A. Velarde. 2009. Fear assessment in pigs exposed to a novel object test. *Appl. Anim. Behav. Sci.* 117:173–180.

503 Dalton, D. C., M. E. Pearson, & M. Sheard. 1967. The behaviour of dairy bulls kept in groups. *Anim. Prod.* 9:1–5.

504 Damasceno, J., & G. Genaro. 2014. Dynamics of the access of captive domestic cats to a feed environmental enrichment item. *Appl. Anim. Behav. Sci.* 151:67–74.

505 Damm, B. I., B. Forkman, & L. J. Pedersen. 2005. Lying down and rolling behaviour in sows in relation to piglet crushing. *Appl. Anim. Behav. Sci.* 9:3–20.

506 Damm, B. I., V. Moustsen, E. Jorgensen, L. J. Pedersen, T. Heiskanen, & B. Forkman. 2006. Sow preferences for walls to lean against when lying down. *Appl. Anim. Behav. Sci.* 99:53–63.

507 Daniels, T. J. 1983. The social organization of free-ranging urban dogs I. Non-estrus social behavior. *Appl. Anim. Ethol.* 10:341–363.

508 Daniels, T. J. 1983. The social organization of free-ranging urban dogs II. Estrus groups and the mating system. *Appl. Anim. Ethol.* 10:365–373.

509 Dantzer, R. 1976. Effect of diazepam on performance of pigs in a progressive ratio schedule. *Physiol. Behav.* 17:161–163.

510 Dantzer, R. 1977. Effects of diazepam on conditioned suppression in pigs. *J. Pharmacol.* 8:405–414.

511 Dantzer, R., & B. A. Baldwin. 1974. Changes in heart rate during suppression of operant responding in pigs. *Physiol. Behav.* 12:385–391.

512 Dantzer, R., & B. A. Baldwin. 1974. Effects of chlordiazepoxide on heart rate and behavioural suppression in pigs subjected to operant conditioning procedures. *Psychopharmacologia* 37:169–177.

513 Dantzer, R., P. Mormede, & B. Favre. 1976. Fear-dependent variations in continuous avoidance behavior of pigs. II. Effects of diazepam on acquisition and performance of pavlovian fear conditioning and plasma corticosteroid levels. *Psychopharmacology (Berl)* 49:75–78.

514 Dards, J. L. 1983. The behaviour of dockyard cats: Interactions of adult males. *Appl. Anim. Behav. Sci.* 19:133–153.

515 Darke, P. G. 1978. Obesity in small animals. *Vet. Rec.* 102:545–546.

516 Davis, C. N., L. E. Davis, & T. E. Powers. 1975. Comparative body compositions of the dog and goat. *Am. J. Vet. Res.* 36:309–311.

517 Davis, J. L., & R. A. Jensen. 1976. The development of passive and active avoidance learning in the cat. *Dev. Psychobiol.* 9:175–179.

518 Dawson, W. M., & R. L. Revens. 1946. Varying susceptibility in pigs to alarm. *J. Comp. Physiol. Psychol.* 39:297–305.

519 Day, J. E. L., I. Kyriazakis, & A. B. Lawrence. 1995. The effect of food deprivation on the expression of foraging and exploratory behaviour in the growing pig. *Appl. Anim. Behav. Sci.* 42:193–206.

520 De Boer, J. 1977. The age of olfactory cues functioning in chemocommunication among male domestic cats. *Behav. Processes.* 2:209–225.

521 de Jong, I. C., I. T. Prelle, J. A. van de Burgwal, E. Lambooij, S. M. Korte, H. J. Blokhuis, & J. M. Koolhaas. 2000. Effects of environmental enrichment on behavioral responses to novelty, learning, and memory, and the circadian rhythm in cortisol in growing pigs. *Physiol. Behav.* 68:571–578.

522 de Passille, A. M., & J. Rushen. 2006. What components of milk stimulate sucking in calves? *Appl. Anim. Behav. Sci.* 101:243–252.

523 De Paula Vieira, A., V. Guesdon, A. M. de Passille, M. A. G. von Keyserlingk, & D. M. Weary. 2008. Behavioural indicators of hunger in dairy calves. *Appl. Anim. Behav. Sci.* 109:180–189.

524 de Sevilla, X. F., J. Casellas, J. Tibau, & E. Fabrega. 2009. Consistency and influence on performance of behavioural differences in large white and landrace purebred pigs. *Appl. Anim. Behav. Sci.* 117:13–19.

525 De Vuyst, A., G. Thines, L. Henriet, & M. Soffie. 1964. Influence of auditory stimulations on the sexual behavior of the bull. *Experientia* 20:648–650.

526 D'Eath, R. B. 2002. Individual aggressiveness measured in a resident intruder test predicts the persistence of aggressive behaviour and weight gain of young pigs after mixing. *Appl. Anim. Behav. Sci.* 77:267–283.

527 D'Eath, R. B. 2005. Socialising piglets before weaning improves social hierarchy formation when pigs are mixed post-weaning *Appl. Anim. Behav. Sci.* 93:199–211.

528 deJonge, F. H., M. Ooms, W. W. Kuurman, J. H. R. Maes, & B. M. Spruijt. 2008. Are pigs sensitive to variability in food rewards? *Appl. Anim. Behav. Sci.* 114:93–104.

529 Delacalle, J., D. J. Burba, J. Tetens, & R. M. Moore. 2002. Nd:YAG laser-assisted modified Forssell's procedure for treatment of cribbing (crib-biting) in horses. *Vet. Surg.* 31:111–116.

530 Delagardea, R., & P. Lamberton. 2015. Daily grazing time of dairy cows is recorded accurately using the Lifecorder Plus device. *Appl. Anim. Behav. Sci.* 165:25–32.

531 deLahunta, A. 1977. *Veterinary neuroanatomy and clinical neurology*. Philadelphia, PA: W.B. Saunders.

532 Deldalle, S., & F. Gaunet. 2014. Effects of 2 training methods on stress-related behaviors of the dog (*Canis familiaris*) and on the dog-owner relationship. *J. Vet. Behav.* 9:58–65.

533 Delgadillo, J. A., J. A. Flores, H. Hernández, P. Poindron, M. Keller, G. Fitz-Rodríguez, G. Duarte, *et al.* 2015. Sexually active males prevent the display of seasonal anestrus in female goats. *Horm. Behav.* 69:8–15.

534 Delgadillo, J. A., P. Poindron, D. Krehbiel, G. Duarte, & E. Rosales. 1997. Nursing, suckling and postpartum anoestrus of creole goats kidding in January in subtropical Mexico. *Appl. Anim. Behav. Sci.* 55:91–101.

535 Deligeorgis, S. G., K. Karalis, & G. Kanzouros. 2006. The influence of drinker location and colour on drinking behaviour and water intake of newborn pigs under hot environments. *Appl. Anim. Behav. Sci.* 96:233–244.

536 Delius, K., M. Gunderoth-Palmowski, I. Krause, & W. Engelmann. 1984. Effects of lithium salts on the behaviour and the circadian system of mesocricetus auratus W. *J. Interdiscipl. Cycle Res.* 15:299.

537 Delude, L. A. 1986. Activity patterns and behavior of sled dogs. *Appl. Anim. Behav. Sci.* 15:161–168.

538 Demontigny-Bédard, I., G. Beauchamp, M.-C. Bélanger, & D. Frank. 2015. Characterization of pica and chewing behaviors in privately owned cats: A case-control study. *J. Feline Med. Surg.* 1–6.

539 DeNapoli, J. S., N. H. Dodman, L. Shuster, W. M. Rand, & K. L. Gross. 2000. Effect of dietary protein content and tryptophan supplementation on dominance aggression, territorial aggression, and hyperactivity in dogs. *J. Am. Vet. Med. Assoc.* 217:504–508.

540 Denton, D. *The hunger for salt*. Berlin, Germany: Springer-Verlag.

541 DePassille, A. M. B., J. H. M. Metz, P. Mekking, & P. R. Wiepkema. 1992. Does drinking milk stimulate sucking in young calves? *Appl. Anim. Behav. Sci.* 34:23–36.

542 DePew, C. L., D. L. Thompson Jr, J. M. Fernandez, L. L. Southern, L. S. Sticker, & T. L. Ward. 1994. Plasma concentrations of prolactin, glucose, insulin, urea nitrogen, and total amino acids in stallions after ingestion of feed or gastric administration of feed components. *J. Anim. Sci.* 72:2345–2353.

543 Deswysen, A. G., W. C. Ellis, & K. R. Pond. 1987. Interrelationships among voluntary intake, eating and ruminating behavior and ruminal motility of heifers fed corn silage. *J. Anim. Sci.* 64:835–841.

544 Devenport, J. A., M. R. Patterson, & L. D. Devenport. 2005. Dynamic averaging and foraging decisions in horses (*Equus callabus*). *J. Comp. Psychol.* 119:352–358.

545 Devilat, J., W. G. Pond, & P. D. Miller. 1970. Dietary amino acid balance in growing-finishing pigs: Effect of diet preference and performance. *J. Anim. Sci.* 30:536–543.

546 Diakow, C. 1971. Effects of genital desensitization on mating behavior and ovulation in the female cat. *Physiol. Behav.* 7:47–54.

547 Dickson, D. P., G. R. Barr, & D. A. Wieckert. 1967. Social relationship of dairy cows in a feed lot. *Behaviour* 29:195–203.

548 Diesel, G., D. Brodbelt, & D. U. Pfeiffer. 2008. Reliability of assessment of dogs' behavioural responses by staff working at a welfare charity in the UK. *Appl. Anim. Behav. Sci.* 115:171–181.

549 Dijkhuizen, T. J., & F. J. van Eerdenburg. 1997. Behavioural signs of oestrus during pregnancy in lactating dairy cows. *Vet. Q.* 19:194–196.

550 Dilks, D. D., P. Cook, S. K. Weiller, H. P. Berns, M. Spivak, & G. S. Berns. 2015. Awake fMRI reveals a specialized region in dog temporal cortex for face processing. *PeerJ.* 3:e1115.

551 Dinger, J. E., & E. E. Noiles. 1986. Effect of controlled exercise on libido in 2-yr-old stallions. *J. Anim. Sci.* 62:1220–1223.

552 Dinius, D. A., & C. A. Baile. 1977. Beef cattle response to a feed intake stimulant given alone and in combination with a propionate enhancer and an anabolic agent. *J. Anim. Sci.* 45:147–153.

553 Distel, R. A., J. J. Villalba, & H. E. Laborde. 1994. Effects of early experience on voluntary intake of low-quality roughage by sheep. *J. Anim. Sci.* 72:1191–1195.

554 Distel, R. A., J. J. Villalba, H. E. Laborde, & M. A. Burgos. 1996. Persistence of the effects of early experience on consumption of low-quality roughage by sheep. *J. Anim. Sci.* 74:965–968.

555 Dodman, N. H., E. K. Karlsson, A. Moon-Fanelli, M. Galdzicka, M. Perloski, L. Shuster, K. Lindblad-Toh, & E. I. Ginns. 2010. A canine chromosome 7 locus confers compulsive disorder susceptibility. *Mol Psychiatr* 18:8–10.

556 **Dodman, N. H., I. Reisner, L. Shuster, W. Rand, U. A. Luescher, I. Robinson, & K. A. Houpt. 1996. Effect of dietary protein content on behavior in dogs. *J. Am. Vet. Med. Assoc.* 208:376–379.**

557 Dodman, N. H., J. A. Normile, L. Shuster, & W. Rand. 1994. Equine self-mutilation syndrome (57 cases). *J. Am. Vet. Med. Assoc.* 204:1219–1223.

558 Dodman, N. H., L. Shuster, M. H. Court, & J. Patel. 1988. Use of a narcotic antagonist (nalmefene) to suppress self-mutilative behavior in a stallion. *J. Am. Vet. Med. Assoc.* 192:1585–1586.

559 Dodman, N. H., L. Shuster, M. H. Court, & R. Dixon. 1987. Investigation into the use of narcotic antagonists in the treatment of a stereotypic behavior pattern (crib-biting) in the horse. *Am. J. Vet. Res.* 48:311–319.

560 Donaldson, L. E., & J. W. James. 1963. A connection between pregnancy and crush order in cows. *Anim. Behav.* 11:286.

561 Donovan, C. A. 1967. Some clinical observations on sexual attraction and deterrence in dogs and cattle. *Vet. Med. Small Anim. Clin.* 62:1047–1051.

562 Donovan, C. A., L. Badinga, R. J. Collier, C. J. Wilcox, & R. K. Braun. 1986. Factors influencing passive transfer in dairy calves. *J. Dairy Sci.* 69:754–759. Fiset

563 **Dorais Page, D., & C. Dumas. 2009. Decision making and visibility in cats (*Felis catus*) in a progressive elimination task. *Anim. Cogn.* 12(5):679–692.**

564 Doran, C. W. 1943. Activities and grazing habits of sheep on summer ranges. *J. Forestry* 41:253–258.

565 Dore, F. Y., S. Fiset, S. Goulet, M. Dumas, & S. Gagnon. 1996. Search behavior in cats and dogs: Interspecific differences in working memory and spatial cognition. *Anim. Learn. Behav.* 24:142–149.

566 Dorries, K. M., E. Adkins-Regan, & B. P. Halpern. 1991. Sex difference in olfactory sensitivity to the boar chemosignal, androstenone, and the domestic pig. *Anim. Behav.* 42:403–411.

567 **Dorries, K. M., E. Adkins-Regan, & B. P. Halpern. 1995. Olfactory sensitivity to the pheromone, androstenone, is sexually dimorphic in the pig. *Physiol. Behav.* 57:255–259.**

568 Doty, R. L., & I. Dunbar. 1974. Attraction of beagles to conspecific urine, vaginal and anal sac secretion odors. *Physiol. Behav.* 12:825–833.

569 Dougherty, C. T., F. W. Knapp, P. B. Burrus, D. C. Willis, & N. W. Bradley. 1993. Face flies (musca autumnalis de geer) and the behavior of grazing beef cattle. *Appl. Anim. Behav. Sci.* 35:313–326.

570 Dougherty, D. M., & P. Lewis. 1993. Generalization of a tactile stimulus in horses. *J. Exp. Anal. Behav.* 59:521–528.

571 **Douglas, C., M. Bateson, C. Walsh, A. Bédué & S. A. Edwards. Environmental enrichment induces optimistic cognitive biases in pigs. *Appl. Anim. Behav. Sci.* 139:65–73.**

572 Dourmad, J. Y. 1993. Standing and feeding behaviour of the lactating sow: Effect of feeding level during pregnancy. *Appl. Anim. Behav. Sci.* 37:311–319.

573 Dove, H. R., R. G. Beilharz, & J. L. Black. 1974. Dominance patterns and positional behaviour of sheep in yards. *Anim. Prod.* 19:157–168.

574 Doyle, R. E., A. D. Fisher, G. N. Hinch, A. Boissy, & C. Lee. 2010. Release from restraint generates a positive judgement bias in sheep. *Appl. Anim. Behav. Sci.* 122:28–34.

575 Doyle, R. E., R. Freire, A. Cowling, S. A. Knott, & C. Lee. 2014. Performance of sheep in a spatial maze is impeded by negative stimuli. *Appl. Anim. Behav. Sci.* 151:36–42.

576 **Doyle, R. E., S. Vidal, G. N. Hinch, A. D. Fisher, A. Boissy, & C. Lee. 2010. The effect of repeated testing on judgement biases in sheep. *Behav. Processes.* 83:349–352.**

577 Dreschel, N. A., & D. A. Granger. 2005. Physiological and behavioral reactivity to stress in thunderstorm-phobic dogs and their caregivers. *Appl. Anim. Behav. Sci.* 95:153–168.

578 Dresher, M., I. M. A. Heitkonig, J. G. Raats, & H. H. T. Prins. 2006. The role of grass stems as structural foraging deterrents and their effects on the foraging behaviour of cattle *Appl. Anim. Behav. Sci.* 101:10–26.

579 Drickamer, L. C., R. D. Arthur, & T. L. Rosenthal. 1999. Predictors of social dominance and aggression in gilts. *Appl. Anim. Behav. Sci.* 63:121–129.

580 Duberstein, K. J., & J. A. Gilkeson. 2010. Determination of sex differences in personality and trainability of yearling horses utilizing a handler questionnaire. *Appl. Anim. Behav. Sci.* 128:57–63.

581 Duckworth, J. E., & D. W. Shirlaw. 1958. A study of factors affecting feed intake and the eating behaviour of cattle. *Anim. Behav.* 6:147–154.

582 Dudink, S., H. Simonse, I. Marks, F. H. deJonge, & B. M. Spruijt. 2006. Announcing the arrival of enrichment increases play behaviour and reduces weaning stress-induced behaviours of piglets directly after weaning. *Appl. Anim. Behav. Sci.* 101:86–101.

583 Duffy, D. L., Y. Hsu, & J. A. Serpell. 2008. Breed differences in canine aggression. *Appl. Anim. Behav. Sci.* 114:441–460.

584 Dufty, J. H. 1971. Determination of the onset of parturition in hereford cattle. *Aust. Vet. J.* 47:77–82.

585 Dufty, J. H. 1972. Clinical studies on bovine parturition. Maternal causes of dystocia and stillbirth in an experimental herd of hereford cattle. *Aust. Vet. J.* 48:1–6.

586 Dufty, J. H. 1973. Clinical studies on bovine parturition – foetal aspects. *Aust. Vet. J.* 49:177–182.

587 Dumas, C., B. St-Louis, & L. Routhier. 2006. Decision making and interference in the domestic cat (*Felis catus*). *J. Comp. Psychol.* 120:367–377.

588 Dunbar, I. F. 1978. Olfactory preferences in dogs: The response of male and female beagles to conspecific urine. *Biol. Behav.* 3:273–286.

589 Dunbar, I. F., & M. Carmichael. 1981. The response of male dogs to urine from other males. *Behav. Neural. Biol.* 31:465–470.

590 Dunbar, I., & M. Buehler. 1980. A masking effect of urine from male dogs. *Appl. Anim. Ethol.* 6:297–301.

591 Dunbar, R. I. M., D. Buckland, & D. Miller. 1990. Mating strategies of male feral goats: A problem in optimal foraging. *Anim. Behav.* 40:653–667.

592 Duncan, A. J., & S. A. Young. 2002. Can goats learn about foods through conditioned food aversions and preferences when multiple food options are simultaneously available? *J. Anim. Sci.* 80:2091–2098.

593 Duncan, P. 1980. Time-budgets of camargue horses II. Time-budgets of adult horses and weaned sub-adults. *Behaviour* 72:26–49.

594 Duncan, P. 1985. Time-budgets of camargue horses III. Environmental influences. *Behaviour* 92:188–208.

595 Duncan, P., & P. Cowtan. 1980. An unusual choice of habitat helps camargue horses to avoid blood-sucking horse-flies. *Biol. Behav.* 5:55–60.

596 Duncan, P., P. H. Harvey, & S. M. Wells. 1984. On lactation and associated behaviour in a natural herd of horses. *Anim. Behav.* 32:255–263.

597 Düpjan, S., A. Tuchscherer, J. Langbein, P.-C. Schön, G. Manteuffel, & B. Puppe. 2011. Behavioural and cardiac responses towards conspecific distress calls in domestic pigs (Sus scrofa). *Physiol. Behav.* 103:445–452.

598 Duquette, P. F., & L. A. Muir. 1979. Monitoring the effects of selected compounds on feeding behaviour of sheep. *J. Anim. Sci.* 49:1120–1124.

599 Duranton, C., T. Bedossa, & F. Gaunet. 2016. When facing an unfamiliar person, pet dogs present social referencing based on

their owners' direction of movement alone. *Anim. Behav.* 113 147–156

600 Durr, R., & C. Smith. 1997. Individual differences and their relation to social structure in domestic cats. *J. Comp. Psychol.* 111:412–418.

601 Durrer, J. L., & J. P. Hannon. 1962. Seasonal variations in caloric intake of dogs living in an arctic environment. *Am. J. Physiol.* 202:375–378.

602 Duvaux-Ponter, C., K. Rigalma, S. Roussel-Huchette, Y. Schawlb, & A. A. Ponter. 2008. Effect of a supplement rich in linolenic acid, added to the diet of gestating and lactating goats, on the sensitivity to stress and learning ability of their offspring. *Appl. Anim. Behav. Sci.* 114:373–394.

603 Duxbury, M. M., J. A. Jackson, S. W. Line, & R. K. Anderson. 2003. Evaluation of association between retention in the home and attendance at puppy socialization classes. *J. Am. Vet. Med. Assoc.* 223:61–66.

604 Dworkin, S. 1939. Conditioning neuroses in dog and cat. *Psychosom. Med.* 1:388–396.

605 Dwyer, C. M. 2003. Behavioural development in the neonatal lamb: Effect of maternal and birth-related factors. *Theriogenology* 59:1027–1050.

606 Dwyer, C. M. 2008. Individual variation in the expression of maternal behaviour: A review of the neuroendocrine mechanisms in the sheep. *J. Neuroendocrinol.* 20:526–534.

607 Dwyer, C. M., & A. B. Lawrence. 1999. Ewe-ewe and ewe-lamb behaviour in a hill and a lowland breed of sheep: A study using embryo transfer. *Appl. Anim. Behav. Sci.* 61:319–334.

608 Dwyer, C. M., & A. B. Lawrence. 2000. Effects of maternal genotype and behaviour on the behavioural development of their offspring in sheep. *Behaviour* 137:1629–1654.

609 Dwyer, C. M., & L. A. Smith. 2008. Parity effects on maternal behaviour are not related to circulating oestradiol concentrations in two breeds of sheep. *Physiol. Behav.* 93:148–154.

610 Dwyer, C. M., K. A. McLean, L. A. Deans, J. Chirnside, S. K. Calvert, & A. B. Lawrence. 1998. Vocalisations between mother and young in sheep: Effects of breed and maternal experience. *Appl. Anim. Behav. Sci.* 58:105–119.

611 Dwyer, C. M., W. S. Dingwall, & A. B. Lawrence. 1999. Physiological correlates of maternal-offspring behaviour in sheep: A factor analysis. *Physiol. Behav.* 67:443–454.

612 Dybkjaer, L., A. P. Jacobsen, F. A. Togersen, & H. D. Poulsen. 2006. Eating and drinking activity of newly weaned piglets: Effects of individual characteristics, social mixing, and addition of extra zinc to the feed. *J. Anim. Sci.* 84:702–711.

613 Dyck, G. W., E. E. Swierstra, R. M. McKay, & K. Mount. 1987. Effect of location of the teat suckled, breed and parity on piglet growth. *Can. J. Anim. Sci.* 67:929–939.

614 Dziba, L. E., & F. D. Provenza. 2008. Dietary monoterpene concentrations influence feeding patterns of lambs. *Appl. Anim. Behav. Sci.* 109:49–57.

615 Ebenezer, I. S., R. F. Parrott, & S. V. Vellucci. 1999. Effects of the 5-HT1A receptor agonist 8-OH-DPAT on operant food intake in food-deprived pigs. *Physiol. Behav.* 67:213–217.

616 Eccles, R. 1982. Autonomic innervation of the vomeronasal organ of the cat. *Physiol. Behav.* 28:1011–1015.

617 Echeverri, A. C., H. W. Gonyou, & A. W. Ghent. 1992. Preparturient behavior of confined ewes: Time budgets, frequencies, spatial distribution and sequential analysis. *Appl. Anim. Behav. Sci.* 34:329–344.

618 Eckstein, P., & S. Zuckerman. 1956. The oestrous cycle in the mammalia. In A. S. Parkes (Ed.), *Marshall's physiology of reproduction*, pp. 226–396. London, UK: Longmans, Green.

619 Eckstein, R. A., & B. L. Hart. 2000. The organization and control of grooming in cats. *Appl. Anim. Behav. Sci.* 68:131–140.

620 Edwards, S. A. 1982. Factors affecting time to first suckling in dairy calves. *Anim. Prod.* 34:339–346.

621 Edwards, S. A., & D. M. Broom. 1982. Behavioural interactions of dairy cows with their newborn calves and the effects of parity. *Anim. Behav.* 30:525–535.

622 Ehrenlechner, S., & J. Unshelm. 1997. Whisker trimming by mother cats. *Appl. Anim. Behav. Sci.* 52:181–185.

623 Ehret, C. F., V. R. Potter, & K. W. Dobra. 1975. Chronotypic action of theophylline and of pentobarbital as circadian zeitgebers in the rat. *Science* 188:1212–1215.

624 Ekkel, E. D., B. Savenije, W. G. Schouten, V. M. Wiegant, & M. J. Tielen. 1997. The effects of mixing on behavior and circadian parameters of salivary cortisol in pigs. *Physiol. Behav.* 62:181–184.

625 Eldridge, F., & Y. Suzuki. 1976. A mare mule – dam or foster mother? *J. Hered.* 67:353–360.

626 Elgier, A. M., A. Jakovcevic, A. E. Mustaca, & M. Bentosela. 2012. Pointing following in dogs: Are simple or complex cognitive mechanisms involved? *Anim. Cogn.* 15:1111–1119.

627 Elia, J. B., H. N. Erb, & Houpt, K. 2010. Motivation for hay: Effects of a pelleted diet on behavior and physiology of horses. *Physiol. Behav.* 101:623–627.

628 Ellendorff, F., N. Parvizi, D. K. Pomerantz, A. Hartjen, A. Konig, D. Smidt, & F. Elsaesser. 1975. Plasma luteinizing hormone and testosterone in the adult male pig: 24 hour fluctuations and the effect of copulation. *J. Endocrinol.* 67:403–410.

629 Elliot, O., & J. A. King. 1960. Effect of early food deprivation upon later consummatory behavior in puppies. *Psychol. Rep.* 6:391–400.

630 Elliot, O., & J. P. Scott. 1961. The development of emotional distress reactions to separation, in puppies. *J. Genet. Psychol.* 99:3–22.

631 Elliott, J. A., M. H. Stetson, & M. Menaker. 1972. Regulation of testis function in golden hamsters: A circadian clock measures photoperiodic time. *Science* 178:771–773.

632 Ellis, A. D., S. Redgate, S. Zinchenko, H. Owen, C. Barfoot, & P. Harris. 2015. The effect of presenting forage in multi-layered haynets and at multiple sites on night time budgets of stabled horses. *Appl. Anim. Behav. Sci.* 171:108–116.

633 Ellis, S. L. H., & D. L. Wells. 2010. The influence of olfactory stimulation on the behaviour of cats housed in a rescue shelter. *Appl. Anim. Behav. Sci.* 123:56–62.

634 Ellis, S. L. H., & D. L. Wells. 2008. The influence of visual stimulation on the behaviour of cats housed in a rescue shelter. *Appl. Anim. Behav. Sci.* 113:166–174.

635 Ellis, S. L. H., H. Thompson, C. Guijarro, & H. E. Zulch. 2015. The influence of body region, handler familiarity and order of region handled on the domestic cat's response to being stroked. *Appl. Anim. Behav. Sci.* 173:60–67.

636 Elmore, M. R. P., R. N. Dilger, & R. W. Johnson. 2012. Place and direction learning in a spatial T-maze task by neonatal piglets. *Anim. Cogn.* 15:667–676.

637 Ely, F., & W. E. Petersen. 1941. Factors involved in the ejection of milk. *J. Dairy Sci.* 24:211–223.

638 England, G. J. 1954. Observations on the grazing behaviour of different breeds of sheep at pantryhuad farm, carmarthenshire. *Br. J. Anim. Behav.* 2:56–60.

639 Entsu, S., H. Dohi, & A. Yamada. 1992. Visual acuity of cattle determined by the method of discrimination learning. *Appl. Anim. Behav. Sci.* 34:1–10.

640 Erhard, H. W., & M. Mendl. 1997. Measuring aggressiveness in growing pigs in a resident-intruder situation. *Appl. Anim. Behav. Sci.* 54:123–136.

641 Erhard, H. W., D. A. Elston, & G. C. Davidson. 2006. Habituation and extinction in an approach-avoidance test: An example with sheep. *Appl. Anim. Behav. Sci.* 99:132–144.

642 Erlinger, L. L., D. R. Tolleson, & C. J. Brown. 1990. Comparison of bite size, biting rate and grazing time of beef heifers from herds distinguished by mature size and rate of maturity. *J. Anim. Sci.* 68:3578–3587.

643 Escobar, J., W. G. Van Alstine, D. H. Baker, & R. W. Johnson. 2007. Behaviour of pigs with viral and bacterial pneumonia. *Appl. Anim. Behav. Sci.* 105:42–50.

644 Escos, J., C. L. Alados, & J. Boza. 1993. Leadership in a domestic goat herd. *Appl. Anim. Behav. Sci.* 38:41–47.

645 Esselmont, R. J., R. G. Glencross, M. J. Bryant, & G. S. Pope. 1980. A quantitative study of pre-ovulatory behaviour in cattle (British Friesian heifers). *Appl. Anim. Ethol.* 6:1–17.

646 Estep, D. Q., S. L. Crowell-Davis, S. Earl-Costello, & S. A. Beatey. 1993. Changes in the social behaviour of drafthorse (*Equus caballus*) mares coincident with foaling. *Appl. Anim. Behav. Sci.* 35:199–213.

647 Evans, J. W., C. M. Winget, C. De Roshia, & D. C. Holley. 1976. Ovulation and equine body temperature and heart rate circadian rhythms. *J. Interdiscip. Cycle Res.* 7:25–37.

648 Everitt, G. C., & D. S. M. Phillips. 1971. Calf rearing by multiple suckling and the effects of lactation performance of the cow. *Proc. N.Z. Soc. Anim. Prod.* 31:22–40.

649 Ewbank, R. 1963. Predicting the time of parturition in the normal cows: A study of the precalving drop in body temperature in relation to the external signs of imminent calving. *Vet. Rec.* 75:367–370.

650 Ewbank, R. 1964. Observations on the suckling habits of twin lambs. *Anim. Behav.* 12:34–37.

651 Ewbank, R. 1967. Behavior of twin cattle. *J. Dairy Sci.* 50:1510–1512.

652 Ewbank, R. 1967. Nursing and suckling behaviour amongst clun forest ewes and lambs. *Anim. Behav.* 15:251–258.

653 Ewbank, R. 1973. Abnormal behaviour and pig nutrition. An unsuccessful attempt to induce tail biting by feeding a high energy, low fibre vegetable protein ration. *Br. Vet. J.* 129:366–369.

654 Ewbank, R., & A. C. Mason. 1967. A note on the sucking behaviour of twin lambs reared as singles. *Anim. Prod.* 9:417–420.

655 Ewbank, R., & M. J. Bryant. 1972. Aggressive behaviour amongst groups of domesticated pigs kept at various stocking rates. *Anim. Behav.* 20:21–28.

656 Ewbank, R., G. B. Meese, & J. E. Cox. 1974. Individual recognition and the dominance hierarchy in the domesticated pig. *The role of sight. Anim. Behav.* 22:473–480.

657 Ewer, R. F. 1959. Suckling behaviour in kittens. *Behaviour* 15:146–162.

658 Ewer, R. F. *The carnivores*. Ithaca, *NY: Cornell University Press.*

659 Ezeh, P. I., L. J. Myers, L. A. Hanrahan, R. J. Kemppainen, & K. A. Cummins. 1992. Effects of steroids on the olfactory function of the dog. *Physiol. Behav.* 51:1183–1187.

660 Fabre-Nys, C., & H. Gelez. 2007. Sexual behavior in ewes and other domestic ruminants. *Horm. Behav.* 52:18–25.

661 Fadel, F. R., P. Driscoll, M. Pilot, H. Wright, H. Zulch, & D. Mills. 2016. Differences in trait impulsivity indicate diversification of dog breeds into working and show lines. *Sci Rep.* 6:22162.

662 Faerevik, G., I. L. Andersen, & K. E. Boe. 2005. Preferences of sheep for different types of pen flooring. *Appl. Anim. Behav. Sci.* 90:265–276.

663 Fagen, R. M., & T. K. George. 1977. Play behavior and exercise in young ponies (*Equus caballus*). *Behav. Ecol. Sociobiol.* 2:267–269.

664 Falewee, C., E. Gaultier, C. Lafont, L. Bougrat, & P. Pageat. 2006. Effect of a synthetic equine maternal pheromone during a controlled fear-eliciting situation. *Appl. Anim. Behav. Sci.* 101:144–153.

665 Farago, T., P. Pongracz, F. Range, Z. Viranyi, & A. Miklosi. 2010. 'The bone is mine': Affective

and referential aspects of dog growls. *Appl. Anim. Behav. Sci.* 79:917–925.

666 **Farley, G. R., S. M. Barlow, R. Netsell, & J. V. Chmelka. 1992. Vocalizations in the cat: Behavioral methodology and spectrographic analysis. *Exp. Brain Res.* 89:333–340.**

667 Farmer, C., & S. Robert. 2006. Behavioural responses of sows and piglets from two genotypes to recorded nursing grunts played throughout lactation. *Appl. Anim. Behav. Sci.* 96:33–42.

668 Farmer, K., K. Krueger, & R. W. Byrne. 2010. Visual laterality in the domestic horse (*Equus caballus*) interacting with humans. *Anim. Cogn.* 13:229–238.

669 Farner, D. S. 1961. Comparative physiology: Photoperiodicity. *Annu. Rev. Physiol.* 23:71–96.

670 Feaver, J., M. Mendl, & P. Bateson. 1986. A method for rating the individual distinctiveness of domestic cats. *Anim. Behav.* 34:1016–1025.

671 Feddess, J. J. R., B. A. Young, & J. A. DeShazor. 1989. Influence of temperature and light on feeding behaviour in pigs. *Appl. Anim. Behav. Sci.* 23:215–222.

672 Feh, C. 1990. Long-term paternity data in relation to different aspects of rank for camargue stallions, *Equus caballus. Anim. Behav.* 40:995–996.

673 Feh, C. 1999. Alliances and reproductive success in camargue stallions. *Anim. Behav.* 57:705–713.

674 Feh, C., & B. Munkhtuya. 2008. Male infanticide and paternity analyses in a socially natural herd of przewalski's horses: Sexual selection? *Behav. Processes* 78:335–339.

675 Feh, C., & J. de Mazieres. 1993. Grooming at a preferred site reduces heart rate in horses. *Anim. Behav.* 46:1191–1194.

676 Feist, J. D., & D. R. McCullough. 1975. Reproduction in feral horses. *J. Reprod. Fertil. Suppl.* (23):13–18.

677 Feist, J. D., & D. R. McCullough. 1976. Behavior patterns and communication in feral horses. *Z. Tierpsychol.* 41:337–371.

678 Feldman, H. N. 1993. Maternal care and differences in the use of nests in the domestic cat. *Anim. Behav.* 45:13–23.

679 Feldman, H. N. 1994. Domestic cats and passive submission. *Anim. Behav.* 47:457–459.

680 Feldmann, B. M. 1974. The problem of urban dogs. *Science* 185:903.

681 **Feldmann, B. M., & T. H. Carding. 1973. Free-roaming urban pets. *Health Serv. Rep.* 88:956–962.**

682 Fels, M., J. Hartung, & S. Hoy. 2014. Social hierarchy formation in piglets mixed in different group compositions after weaning. *Appl. Anim. Behav. Sci.* 152:17–22.

683 Fernández, J., E. Fàbrega, J. Soler, J. Tibau, J. L. Ruiz, X. Puigvert, & X. Manteca. 2011. Feeding strategy in group-housed growing pigs of four different breeds. *Appl. Anim. Behav. Sci.* 134:109–120.

684 Ferreira, A., A. Carrau, E. Rodas, E. Rubianes, & A. Benech. 1992. Diazepam facilitates acceptance of alien lambs by postparturient ewes. *Physiol. Behav.* 51:1117–1121.

685 **Ferreira, G., A. Terrazas, P. Poindron, R. Nowak, P. Orgeur, & F. Levy. 2000. Learning of olfactory cues is not necessary for early lamb recognition by the mother. *Physiol. Behav.* 69:405–412.**

686 Ferrell, F. 1984. Preference for sugars and nonnutritive sweeteners in young beagles. *Neurosci. Biobehav. Rev.* 8:199–203.

687 Feuerbacher, E. N., & C. D. L. Wynne. 2015. Shut up and pet me! Domestic dogs (*Canis lupus familiaris*) prefer petting to vocal praise in concurrent and single-alternative choice procedures. *Behav. Processes.* 110:47–59.

688 Feuerstein, N., & J. Terkel. 2008. Interrelationships of dogs (*Canis familiaris*) and cats (*Felis catus L.*) living under the same roof. *Appl. Anim. Behav. Sci.* 113:150–165.

689 Figueroa, J., D. Solà-Oriol, X. Manteca, & J. Francisco Pérez. 2013. Social learning of feeding behaviour in pigs: Effects of neophobia and familiarity with the

demonstrator conspecific. *Appl. Anim. Behav. Sci.* 148:120–127.

690 Finger, K. H., & H. Brummer. 1969. Suckling habits of calves reared without cows. *Dtsch. Tierarztl. Wochenschr.* 76:665–667.

691 Finkler, H., & J. Terkel. 2015. The relationship between individual behavioural styles, dominance rank and cortisol levels of cats living in urban social groups. *Appl. Anim. Behav. Sci.* 173:22–28.

692 Finn, J. L., B. Haase, C. E. Willet, D. van Rooy, T. Chew, C. M. Wade, N. A. Hamilton, & B. D. Velie. 2016. The relationship between coat colour phenotype and equine behaviour: A pilot study. *Appl. Anim. Behav. Sci.* 174:66–69.

693 Firth, E. C. 1980. Bilateral ventral accessory neurectomy in windsucking horses. *Vet. Rec.* 106:30–32.

694 Fiset, S., & F. Y. Dore. 2006. Duration of cats' (*Felis catus*) working memory for disappearing objects. *Anim. Cogn.* 9:62–70.

695 Fiset, S., F. Landry, & M. Ouellette. 2006. Egocentric search for disappearing objects in domestic dogs: Evidence for a geometric hypothesis of direction. *Anim. Cogn.* 9:1–12.

696 Fiset, S., S. Gagnon, & C. Beaulieu. 2000. Spatial encoding of hidden objects in dogs (*Canis familiaris*). *J. Comp. Psychol.* 114:315–324.

697 Fisher, A. D., M. Stewart, G. A. Verkerk, C. J. Morrow, & L. R. Matthews. 2003. The effects of surface type on lying behaviour and stress responses in dairy cows during periodic weather-induced removal from pasture. *Appl. Anim. Behav. Sci.* 81:1–11.

698 Fisher, R. B., & M. L. Gardner. 1976. A diurnal rhythm in the absorption of glucose and water by isolated rat small intestine. *J. Physiol.* 254:821–825.

699 Fiske, J. C., & G. D. Potter. 1979. Discrimination reversal learning in yearling horses. *J. Anim. Sci.* 49:583–588.

700 Fitzgerald, J. A., A. Perkins, & K. Hemenway. 1993. Relationship of sex and number of siblings in utero with sexual behavior of mature rams. *Appl. Anim. Behav. Sci.* 38:283–290.

701 Fitzgerald, M. & D. C. Turner. 2000. Hunting behavior of domestic cats and their impact on prey populations. In D. C. Turner, & P. Bateson, *The domestic cat: The biology of its behaviour*, 2nd ed., pp. 151–176. Cambridge, UK: Cambridge University Press.

702 Fitzsimons, J. T., & E. Szczepanska-Sadowska. 1974. Drinking and antidiuresis elicited by isoprenaline in the dog. *J. Physiol.* 239:251–267.

703 Flannery, B. 1997. Relational discrimination learning in horses. *Appl. Anim. Behav. Sci.* 54:267–280.

704 **Flannigan, G., & N. H. Dodman. 2001. Risk factors and behaviors associated with separation anxiety in dogs. *J. Am. Vet. Med. Assoc.* 219:460–466.**

705 Fletcher, I. C., & D. R. Lindsay. 1968. Sensory involvement in the mating behaviour of domestic sheep. *Anim. Behav.* 16:410–414.

706 Fleurance, G., H. Fritz, P. Duncan, I. J. Gordon, N. Edouard, & C. Vial. 2009. Instantaneous intake rate in horses of different body sizes: Influence of sward biomass and fibrousness. *Appl. Anim. Behav. Sci.* 117:84–92.

707 Folman, Y., & R. Volcani. 1966. Copulatory behaviour of the prepubertally castrated bull. *Anim. Behav.* 14:572–573.

708 **Fonberg, E. 1976. The relation between alimentary and emotional amygdalar regulation. In D. Novin, W. Wyrwicka, & G. A. Bray (Eds.), *Hunger: Basic mechanisms and clinical implications*, pp. 61–75. New York, NY: Raven Press.**

709 Fontenot, J. P., & R. E. Blaser. 1965. Symposium on factors influencing the voluntary intake of herbage by ruminants: Selection and intake by grazing animals. *J. Anim. Sci.* 24:1202–1208.

710 Foot, J. Z., & A. J. F. Russel. 1978. Pattern of intake of three roughage diets by nonpregnant, nonlactating scottish blackface ewes over a long period and the effects of previous nutritional history on current intake. *Anim. Prod.* 26:203–215.

711 Forbes, J. M. 1995. *Voluntary food intake and diet selection in farm animals.* Wallingford, UK: CAB International.

712 Ford, J. J., & H. S. Teague. 1978. Effect of floor space restriction on age at puberty in gilts and on performance of barrows and gilts. *J. Anim. Sci.* 47:828–832.

713 Ford, J. J., & R. K. Christenson. 1981. Glucocorticoid inhibition of estrus in ovariectomized pigs: Relationship to progesterone action. *Horm. Behav.* 15:427–435.

714 Forkman, B., A. Boissy, M. C. Meunier-Salaun, E. Canali, & R. B. Jones. 2007. A critical review of fear tests used on cattle, pigs, sheep, poultry and horses. *Physiol. Behav.* 92:340–374.

715 Forkman, B., I. L. Furuhaug, & P. Jensen. 1995. Personality, coping patterns, and aggression in piglets. *Appl. Anim. Behav. Sci.* 45:31–42.

716 Forssell, G. 1926. The new surgical treatment against crib-biting. *Vet. J.* 82:538–548.

717 Foss, I., & G. Flottorp. 1974. A comparative study of the development of hearing and vision in various species commonly used in experiments. *Acta Otolaryngol.* 77:202–214.

718 Foster, J. A., M. Morrison, S. J. Dean, M. Hill, & H. Frenk. 1981. Naloxone suppresses food/water consumption in the deprived cat. *Pharmacol. Biochem. Behav.* 14:419–421.

719 Foutz, A. S., M. M. Mitler, & W. C. Dement. 1980. Narcolepsy. *Vet. Clin. North Am. Small Anim. Pract.* 10:65–80.

720 Fowler, D. G., & L. D. Jenkins. 1976. The effects of dominance and infertility of rams on reproductive performance. *Appl. Anim. Ethol.* 2:327–337.

721 Fox, M. W. 1968. *Abnormal behavior in animals.* Philadelphia, PA: W.B. Saunders.

722 Fox, M. W. 1970. Reflex development and behavioral organization. In W. A. Himwich (Ed.), *Developmental neurobiology*, pp. 553–580. Springfield, IL: Charles C. Thomas.

723 Fox, M. W. 1971. *Integrative development of brain and behavior in the dog.* Chicago, IL: University of Chicago Press.

724 Fox, M. W. 1972. *Understanding your dog.* New York, NY: Coward, McCann and Geoghegan.

725 Fox, M. W. 1975. The behaviour of cats. In E. S. E. Hafez (Ed.), *The behaviour of domestic animals*, pp. 410–436. Baltimore, MD: Williams & Wilkins.

726 Fox, M. W., & D. Stelzner. 1966. Approach/withdrawal variables in the development of social behaviour in the dog. *Anim. Behav.* 14:362–366.

727 Fox, M. W., & D. Stelzner. 1966. Behavioural effects of differential early experience in the dog. *Anim. Behav.* 14:273–281.

728 Fox, M. W., & G. Stanton. 1967. A developmental study of sleep and wakefulness in the dog. *J. Small Anim. Pract.* 8:605–611.

729 Fox, M. W., & J. W. Spencer. 1967. Development of the delayed response in the dog. *Anim. Behav.* 15:162–168.

730 Fox, M. W., & M. Bekoff. 1975. The behaviour of dogs. In E. S. E. Hafez (Ed.), *The behaviour of domestic animals*, pp. 370–409. Baltimore, MD: Williams & Wilkins.

731 Foyer, P., E. Wilsson, D. Wright, & P. Jensen. 2013. Early experiences modulate stress coping in a population of German shepherd dogs. *Appl. Anim. Behav. Sci.* 146:79–87.

732 Foyer, P., N. Bjällerhag, E. Wilsson, & P. Jensen. 2014. Behaviour and experiences of dogs during the first year of life predict the outcome in a later temperament test. *Appl. Anim. Behav. Sci.* 155:93–100.

733 Francis, D., J. Diorio, D. Liu, & M. J. Meaney. 1999. Nongenomic transmission across generations of maternal behavior and stress responses in the rat. *Science* 286:1155–1158.

734 Francis-Smith, K., & D. G. Wood-Gush. 1977. Coprophagia as seen in thoroughbred foals. *Equine Vet. J.* 9:155–157.

735 Frank, D. F., H. N. Erb, & K. A. Houpt. 1999. Urine spraying in cats: Presence of concurrent disease and effects of a

pheromone treatment. *Appl. Anim. Behav. Sci.* **61:263–272.**

736 Frank, D., G. Beauchamp, & C. Palestrini. 2010. Systematic review of the use of pheromones for treatment of undesirable behavior in cats and dogs. *Sci. Rep.* 236(12):1308–1316.

737 Frank, D., M. Minero, S. Cannas, & C. Palestrini. 2007. Puppy behaviours when left home alone: A pilot study. *Appl. Anim. Behav. Sci.* 104:61–70.

738 Frank, H., & M. G. Frank. 1983. Inhibition training in wolves and dogs. *Behav. Processes.* 8:363–377.

739 Franke Stevens, E. 1990. Instability of harems of feral horses in relation to season and presence of subordinate stallions. *Behaviour* 112:149–161.

740 Fraser, A. F. 1963. Behavior disorders in domestic animals. *Cornell Vet.* 53:213–223.

741 Fraser, A. F. 1968. *Reproductive behaviour in ungulates.* New York, NY: Academic Press.

742 Fraser, A. F. 1974. *Farm animal behaviour.* Baltimore, MD: Williams & Wilkins.

743 Fraser, D. 1973. The nursing and suckling behaviour of pigs. I. The importance of stimulation of the anterior teats. *Br. Vet. J.* 129:324–336.

744 Fraser, D. 1974. The behaviour of growing pigs during experimental social encounters. *J. Agric. Sci. (Camb.)* 82:147–163.

745 Fraser, D. 1974. The vocalizations and other behaviour of growing pigs in and "open field" test. *Appl. Anim. Behav. Sci.* 1:3–16.

746 Fraser, D. 1975. The effect of straw on the behaviour of sows in tether stalls. *Anim. Prod.* 21:59–68.

747 Fraser, D. 1975. The nursing and suckling behaviour of pigs. III. Behaviour when milk ejection is elicited by manual stimulation of the udder. *Br. Vet. J.* 131:416–426.

748 Fraser, D. 1975. The nursing and suckling behaviour of pigs. IV. The effect of interrupting the sucking stimulus. *Br. Vet. J.* 131:549–559.

749 Fraser, D. 1977. Some behavioural aspects of milk ejection failure by sows. *Br. Vet. J.* 133:126–133.

750 Fraser, D. 1987. Attraction to blood as a factor in tail-biting by pigs. *Appl. Anim. Behav. Sci.* 17:61–68.

751 Fraser, D. 1987. Mineral-deficient diets and the pig's attraction to blood: Implications of tail biting. *Can. J. Anim. Sci.* 67:909–918.

752 Fraser, D., & J. Rushen. 1993. A colostrum feeder for newborn lambs. *Appl. Anim. Behav. Sci.* 35:267–276.

753 Frazer-Sissom, D. E., D. A. Rice, & G. Peters. 1991. *How cats purr. J. Zool. (Lond.)* 223:67–78.

754 Freedman, D. G. 1958. Constitutional and environmental interactions in rearing of four breeds of dogs. *Science* 127:585–586.

755 Freedman, D. G., J. A. King, & O. Elliot. 1961. Critical period in the social development of dogs. *Science* 133:1016–1017.

756 Freeman, N. C., & J. S. Rosenblatt. 1978. Specificity of litter odors in the control of home orientation among kittens. *Dev. Psychobiol.* 11:459–468.

757 Freeman, N. C., & J. S. Rosenblatt. 1978. The interrelationship between thermal and olfactory stimulation in the development of home orientation in newborn kittens. *Dev. Psychobiol.* 11:437–457.

758 Freire, R., H. A. Clegg, P. Buckley, M. A. Friend, & P. D. McGreevy. 2009. The effects of two different amounts of dietary grain on the digestibility of the diet and behaviour of intensively managed horses. *Appl. Anim. Behav. Sci.* 117:69–73.

759 Freymond, S. B., E. F. Briefer, A. Zollinger, Y. Gindrat-von Allmen, C. Wyss, & I. Bachmann. 2014. Behaviour of horses in a judgment bias test associated with positive or negative reinforcement. *Appl. Anim. Behav. Sci.* 158:34–45.

760 Friend, D. W. 1973. Self-selection of feeds and water by unbred gilts. *J. Anim. Sci.* 37:1137–1141.

761 Friend, T. H., L. O'Connor, D. Knabe, & G. Dellmeier. 1989. Preliminary trails of a sound-activated device to reduce crushing of piglets by sows. *Appl. Anim. Behav. Sci.* 24:23–29.

762 Froberg, S., & L. Lidfors. 2009. Behaviour of diary calves suckling the dam in a barn with automatic milking or being fed milk substitute from an automatic feeder in a group pen. *Appl. Anim. Behav. Sci.* 117:150–158.

763 Froberg, S., E. Gratre, K. Svennersten-Sjaunja, I. Olsson, A. Orihuela, C. S. Galina, B. Garcia, & L. Lidfors. 2008. Effect of suckling ("restricted suckling") on dairy cows' udder health and milk let-down and their calves' weight gain, feed intake and behaviour. *Appl. Anim. Behav. Sci.* 113:1–14.

764 Fuchs, T., C. Gaillard, S. Beghardt-Henrich, S. Ruefenacht, & A. Steiger. 2005. External factors and reproducibility of the behaviour test in German shepherd dogs in Switzerland. *Appl. Anim. Behav. Sci.* 94:287–301.

765 Fujita, K., A. Morisaki, A. Takaoka, T. Maeda, & Y. Hori. 2012. Incidental memory in dogs (*Canis familiaris*): Adaptive behavioral solution at an unexpected memory test. *Anim. Cogn.* 15:1055–1063.

766 Fukuzawa, M., & N. Hayashi. 2013. Comparison of 3 different reinforcements of learning in dogs (*Canis familiaris*). *J. Vet. Behav.* 8:221–224.

767 Fuller, C. A., F. M. Sulzman, & M. C. Moore-Ede. 1978. Thermoregulation is impaired in an environment without circadian time cues. *Science* 199:794–796.

768 Fuller, J. L. 1956. Photoperiodic control of estrus in the basenji. *J. Hered.* 47:179–180.

769 Fuller, J. L. 1967. Experiential deprivation and later behavior. *Science* 158:1645–1652.

770 Fuller, J. L., C. A. Easler, & E. M. Banks. 1950. Formation of conditioned avoidance responses in young puppies. *Am. J. Physiol.* 160:462–466.

771 Funston, R. N., D. D. Kress, K. M. Havstad, & D. E. Doornbos. 1991. Grazing behavior of rangeland beef cattle differing in biological type. *J. Anim. Sci.* 69:1435–1442.

772 Fureix, C., A. Gorecka-Bruzda, E. Gautier, & M. Hausberger. 2011. Cooccurrence of yawning and stereotypic behaviour in horses (*Equus caballus*). *ISRN Zoology.* 2011:271209.

773 Fureix, C., C. Beaulieu, S. Argaud, C. Rochais, M. Quinton, S. Henry, M. Hausberger, & G. Mason. 2015. Investigating anhedonia in a non-conventional species: Do some riding horses *Equus caballus* display symptoms of depression? *Appl. Anim. Behav. Sci.* 162:26–36.

774 Fureix, C., H. Benhajali, S. Henry, A. Bruchet, A. Prunier, M. Ezzaouia, C. Coste, *et al.* 2013. Plasma cortisol and faecal cortisol metabolites concentrations in stereotypic and non-stereotypic horses: Do stereotypic horses cope better with poor environmental conditions? *BMC Vet. Res.* 9:3.

775 Fureix, C., H. Menguy, & M. Hausberger. 2010. Partners with bad temper: Reject or cure? A study of chronic pain and aggression in horses. *PLoS ONE.* 5(8):e12434.

776 Fureix, C., M. Pagès, R. Bon, J.-M. Lassalle, P. Kuntz, & G. Gonzalez. 2009. A preliminary study of the effects of handling type on horses' emotional reactivity and the human-horse relationship. *Behav. Processes.* 82:202–210.

777 Fureix, C., P. Jego, C. Sankey, & M. Hausberger. 2009. How horses (*Equus caballus*) see the world: Humans as significant "objects." *Anim. Cogn.* 12:643–654.

778 **Gabor, V., & M. Gerken. 2012. Cognitive testing in horses using a computer based apparatus. *Appl. Anim. Behav. Sci.* 139:242–250.**

779 Gabor, V., & M. Gerken. 2014. Shetland ponies (*Equus caballus*) show quantity discrimination in a matching-to-sample design. *Anim. Cogn.* 17:1233–1243.

780 Gadbury, J. C. 1975. Some preliminary field observations on the order of entry of cows into herringbone parlours. *Appl. Anim. Ethol.* 1:275–281.

781 Gaebelein, C. J., R. A. Galosy, L. Botticelli, J. L. Howard, & P. A. Obrist. 1977. Blood pressure and cardiac changes during signalled and unsignalled avoidance in dogs. *Physiol. Behav.* 19:69–74.

782 Gagnon, S., & F. Y. Dore. 1994. Cross-sectional study *of object permanence in domestic puppies (Canis familiaris).* *J. Comp. Psychol.* 108:220–232.

783 Gaillard, C., R. K. Meagher, M. A. G. von Keyserlingk, & D. M. Weary. 2014. Social housing improves dairy calves' performance in two cognitive tests. *PLoS ONE.* 9(2):e90205.

784 Galvan, M., & J. Vonk. 2016. Man's other best friend: domestic cats (F. silvestris catus) and their discrimination of human emotion cues. *Anim. Cogn.* 19:193–205.

785 Ganjam, V. K., & R. M. Kenney. 1975. Androgens and oestrogens in normal and cryptorchid stallions. *J. Reprod. Fertil. Suppl.* (23):67–73.

786 Ganskopp, D. 2001. Manipulating cattle distribution with salt and water in large arid-land pastures: A GPS/GIS assessment. *Appl. Anim. Behav. Sci.* 73:251–262.

787 Ganskopp, D., R. Cruz, & D. E. Johnson. 2000. Least-effort pathways? A GIS analysis of livestock trails in rugged terrain. *Appl. Anim. Behav. Sci.* 68:179–190.

788 Garbarg, M., C. Julien, & J. C. Schwartz. 1974. Circadian rhythm of histamine in the pineal gland. *Life Sci.* 14:539–543.

789 García y González, E., A. Cuellar, H. Hernández, E. Nandayapa, L. Álvarez, J. Tórtora, & A. Terrazas. 2015. Maternal experience in Romanov sheep impairs mother-lamb recognition during the first 24 hours postpartum. *J. Vet. Behav.* 10:66–72.

790 Garcia, J., W. G. Hankins, & K. W. Rusiniak. 1974. Behavioral regulation of the milieu interne in man and rat. *Science* 185:824–831.

791 Garcia, M. C., S. M. McDonnell, R. M. Kenney, & H. G. Osborne. 1986. Bull sexual behavior tests: Stimulus cow affects performance. *Appl. Anim. Behav. Sci.* 16:1–10.

792 Gardner, L. P. 1937. Responses of horses to the same signal in different positions. *J. Comp. Psychol.* 23:305–332.

793 Gardner, L. P. 1937. The responses of cows in a discrimination problem. *J. Comp. Psychol.* 23:35–57.

794 **Gardner, L. P. 1937. The responses of cows to the same signal in different positions. *J. Comp. Psychol.* 23:333–350.**

795 Gardner, L. P. 1937. The responses of horses in a discrimination problem. *J. Comp. Psychol.* 23:13–34.

796 Gardner, L. P. 1945. Responses of sheep in a discrimination problem with variations of the position of the signal. *J. Comp. Physiol. Psychol.* 38:343–351.

797 Garner, R. H. 1963. The palatability of herbage plants. *J. Br. Grassland Soc.* 18:79–89.

798 Gartner, M. C., & A. Weiss. 2013. Personality in felids: A review. *Appl. Anim. Behav. Sci.* 144:1–13.

799 Gary, L. A., G. W. Sherritt, & E. B. Hale. 1970. Behavior of charolais cattle on pasture. *J. Anim. Sci.* 30:203–206.

800 Gastal, M. O., E. L. Gastal, M. A. Beg, & O. J. Ginther. 2007. Elevated plasma testosterone concentrations during stallion-like sexual behavior in mares (*Equus caballus*). *Horm. Behav.* 52:205–210.

801 **Gaultier, E., L. Bonnafous, D. Vienet-Legue, C. Falewee, L. Bougrat, C. Lafont-Lecuelle, & P. Pageat. 2008. Efficacy of dog-appeasing pheromone in reducing stress associated with social isolation in newly adopted puppies. *Vet. Rec.* 163:73–80.**

802 **Gaultier, E., L. Bonnafous, L. Bougrat, C. Lafont, & P. Pageat. 2005. Comparison of the efficacy of a synthetic dog-appeasing pheromone with clomipramine for the treatment of separation-related disorders in dogs. *Vet. Rec.* 156:533–538.**

803 Gaunet, F. 2008. How do guide dogs of blind owners and pet dogs of sighted owners (*Canis familiaris*) ask their owners for food? *Anim. Cogn.* 11:475–483.

804 Gazit, I., & J. Terkel. 2003. Explosives detection by sniffer dogs following strenuous physical activity. *Appl. Anim. Behav. Sci.* 81:149–161.

805 Gazit, I., A. Goldblatt, & J. Terkel. 2005. The role of context specificity in learning: The effects of training context on explosives detection in dogs. *Anim. Cogn.* 8:143–150.

806 Geary, T. W., & J. J. Reeves. 1992. Relative importance of vision and olfaction for detection of estrus by bulls. *J. Anim. Sci.* 70:2726–2731.

807 Geist, V. 1971. Mountain sheep: A study of behavior and evolution. Chicago, IL: University of Chicago Press.

808 George, J. M., & I. A. Barger. 1974. Observations of bovine parturition. *Proc. Aust. Soc. Anim. Prod.* 10:314–317.

809 Georgsson, L., & J. Svendsen. 2002. Degree of competition at feeding differentially affects behavior and performance of group-housed growing-finishing pigs of different relative weights. *J. Anim. Sci.* 80:376–383.

810 Gerritsen, R., P. Langendijk, N. Soede, & B. Kemp. 2005. Effects of artificial boar stimuli on the expression of oestrus in sows. *Appl. Anim. Behav. Sci.* 92:37–43.

811 Geverink, N. A., W. G. P. Schouten, G. Gort, & V. M. Wiegant. 2002. Individual differences in aggression and physiology in peri-pubertal breeding gilts. *Appl. Anim. Behav. Sci.* 77:43–52.

812 Ghosh, B., D. K. Choudhuri, & B. Pal. 1984. Some aspects of the sexual behaviour of stray dogs, *Canis familiaris*. *Appl. Anim. Behav. Sci.* 13:113–127.

813 Giannetto, C., F. Fazio, D. Alberghina, A. Assenza, M. Panzera, & G. Piccione. 2015. Different daily patterns of serum cortisol and locomotor activity rhythm in horses under natural photoperiod. *J. Vet. Behav.* 10:118–121.

814 Giannetto, C., M. Bazzano, S. Marafioti, C. Bertolucci, & G. Piccione. 2015. Monitoring of total locomotor activity in mares during the prepartum and postpartum period. *J. Vet. Behav.* 10:427–432.

815 Gibbons, J. M., A. B. Lawrence, & M. J. Haskell. 2009. Consistency of aggressive feeding behaviour in dairy cows. *Appl. Anim. Behav. Sci.* 121:1–7.

816 Gibbons, J. M., A. B. Lawrence, & M. J. Haskell. 2010. Measuring sociability in dairy cows. *Appl. Anim. Behav. Sci.* 122:84–91.

817 **Gibbs, J., R. C. Young, & G. P. Smith. 1973. Cholecystokinin decreases food intake in rats.** ***J. Comp. Physiol. Psychol.*** **84:488–495.**

818 Giebel, H. 1958. Visuelles lernvermogen bei einhufern. *Zool. Jahrb.* 67:487–520.

819 Gieling, E. T., M. A. Musschenga, R. E. Nordquist, & F. J. van der Staay. 2012. Juvenile pigs use simple geometric 2D shapes but not portrait photographs of conspecifics as visual discriminative stimuli. *Appl. Anim. Behav. Sci.* 142:142–153.

820 Gieling, E. T., R. E. Nordquist, & F. J. van der Staay. 2011. Assessing learning and memory in pigs. *Anim. Cogn.* 14:151–173.

821 Gifford, A. K., S. Cloutier, & R. C. Newberry. 2007. Objects as enrichment: Effects of object exposure time and delay interval on object recognition memory of the domestic pig. *Appl. Anim. Behav. Sci.* 107:206–217.

822 Gilbert, B. J., Jr, & C. W. Arave. 1986. Ability of cattle to distinguish among different wavelengths of light. *J. Dairy Sci.* 69:825–832.

823 Gill, J., K. Skwarlo, & A. Flisinska-Bojanowska. 1974. Diurnal and seasonal changes in carbohydrate metabolism in the blood of thoroughbred horses. *J. Interdiscipl.* 5:355–361.

824 Gillham, S. B., N. H. Dodman, L. Shuster, R. Kream, & W. Rand. 1994. The effect of diet on cribbing behavior and plasma b-endorphin in horses. *Appl. Anim. Behav. Sci.* 41:147–153.

825 Ginane, C., & B. Dumont. 2011. Do sheep (*Ovis aries*) categorize plant species according to botanical family? *Anim. Cogn.* 14:369–376.

826 Gleerupa, K. B., P. H. Andersen, L. Munksgaard, & B. Forkman. 2015. Pain evaluation in dairy cattle. *Appl. Anim. Behav. Sci.* 171:25–32.

827 Gleitman, H. 1974. Getting animals to understand the experimenter's instructions. *Anim. Learn. Behav.* 2:1–5.

828 Glencross, R. G., R. J. Esselmont, M. J. Bryant, & G. S. Pope. 1981. Relationships between the incidence of pre-ovulagory behavior and the concentrations of oestradiol-17b and progesterone in bovine plasma. *Appl. Anim. Ethol.* 7:141–148.

829 Glenske, K., E.-M. Prinzenberg, H. Brandt, M. Gauly, & G. Erhardt. 2011. A chromosome-wide QTL study on BTA29 affecting temperament traits in German Angus beef cattle and mapping of DRD4. *Animal.* 5(2):195–197.

830 Glunk, E. C., M. R. Hathaway, W. J. Weber, C. C. Sheaffer, & K. L. Martinson. 2014. The effect of hay net design on rate of forage consumption when feeding adult horses. *Equine Vet. J.* 34:986–991.

831 Glunk. E. C., C. C. Sheaffer, M. R. Hathaway, & K. L. Martinson. 2014. Interaction of grazing muzzle use and grass species on forage intake of horses. *Equine Vet. J.* 34:930–933.

832 Goatcher, W. D., & D. C. Church. 1970. Taste responses in ruminants. II. Reactions of sheep to acids, quinine, urea and sodium hydroxide. *J. Anim. Sci.* 30:784–790.

833 Goatcher, W. D., & D. C. Church. 1970. Taste responses in ruminants. III. Reactions of pygmy goats, normal goats, sheep and cattle to sucrose and sodium chloride. *J. Anim. Sci.* 31:364–372.

834 **Goddard, M. E., & R. G. Beilharz. 1982. Genetics of traits which determine the suitability of dogs as guide-dogs for the blind. *Appl. Anim. Ethol.* 9:299–315.**

835 Gonyou, H. W., & J. M. Stookey. 1985. Behavior of parturient ewes in group-lambing pens with and without cubicles. *Appl. Anim. Behav. Sci.* 14:163 171.

836 Gonyou, H. W., & W. R. Stricklin. 1984. Diurnal behavior of feedlot bulls during winter and spring in northern latitudes. *J. Anim. Sci.* 58:1075–1083.

837 Gonyou, H. W., R. P. Chapple, & G. R. Frank. 1992. Productivity, time budgets and social aspects of eating in pigs penned in groups of five or individually. *Appl. Anim. Behav. Sci.* 34:291–301.

838 González, M., X. Averós, I. Beltrán de Heredia, R. Ruiz, J. Arranz, & I. Estevez. 2013. The effect of social buffering on fear responses in sheep (*Ovis aries*). *Appl. Anim. Behav. Sci.* 149:13–20.

839 Goodwin, D., H. P. B. Davidson, & P. Harris. 2005. Sensory varieties in concentrate diets for stabled horses: Effects on behaviour and selection *Appl. Anim. Behav. Sci.* 90:337–349.

840 Goodwin, D., H. P. Davidson, & P. Harris. 2002. Foraging enrichment for stabled horses: Effects on behaviour and selection. *Equine Vet. J.* 34:686–691.

841 Goodwin, D., J. W. S. Bradshaw, & S. Wickens. 1997. Paedomorphosis affects agonistic visual signals of domestic dogs. *Anim. Behav.* 53:297–304.

842 Goodwin, M., K. M. Gooding, & F. Regnier. 1979. Sex pheromone in the dog. *Science* 203:559–561.

843 **Gorecka, A., M. Golonka, M. Chruszczewski, & T. Jezierski. 2007. A note on behaviour and heart rate in horses differing in facial hair whorl. *Appl. Anim. Behav. Sci.* 105:244–248.**

844 Gorniak, S. L., J. A. Pfister, E. C. Lanzonia, & E. R. Raspantini. 2008. A note on averting goats to a toxic but palatable plant, leucaena leucocephala. *Appl. Anim. Behav. Sci.* 111:396–401.

845 Gottardo, F., S. Mattiello, G. Cozzi, E. Canali, E. Scanziani, L. Ravarotto, V. Ferrante, *et al.* 2002. The provision of drinking water to veal calves for welfare purposes. *J. Anim. Sci.* 80:2362–2372.

846 Goursaud, A. P., & R. Nowak. 1999. Colostrum mediates the development of mother preference by newborn lambs. *Physiol. Behav.* 67:49–56.

847 Grace, J., & M. Russek. 1969. The influence of previous experience on the taste behavior of dogs toward sucrose and saccharin. *Physiol. Behav.* 4:553–558.

848 Grandage, J. 1972. The erect dog penis: A paradox of flexible rigidity. *Vet. Rec.* 91:141–147.

849 Grandin, T. 1993. Behavioral agitation during handling of cattle in persistent over time. *Appl. Anim. Behav. Sci.* 36:1–9.

850 Grandin, T., M. J. Deesing, J. J. Struthers, & A. M. Swinker. 1995. Cattle with hair whorl patterns above the eyes are more behaviorally agitated during restraint. *Appl. Anim. Behav. Sci.* 46:117–123.

851 Graves, H. B. 1984. Behavior and ecology of wild and feral swine (sus scrofa). *J. Anim. Sci.* 58:482–492.

852 Green, J. S., R. A. Woodruff, & T. T. Tueller. 1984. Livestock-guarding dogs for predator control: Costs, benefits and practicality. *Wildl. Soc. Bull.* 12:44–50.

853 Greene, W. A., L. Mogil, & R. H. Foote. 1978. Behavioral characteristics of freemartins administered estradiol, estrone, testosterone, and dihydrotestosterone. *Horm. Behav.* 10:71–84.

854 **Greening, L., V. Shenton, K. Wilcockson, & J. Swanson. 2013. Investigating duration of nocturnal ingestive and sleep behaviors of horses bedded on straw versus shavings. *J. Vet. Behav.* 8:82–86.**

855 Greet, T. R. 1982. Windsucking treated by myectomy and neurectomy. *Equine Vet. J.* 14:299–301.

856 Gregory, P. C., M. McFadyen, & D. V. Rayner. 1989. Relation between gastric emptying and short-term regulation of food intake in the pig. *Physiol. Behav.* 45:677–683.

857 Grenager, N. S., T. J. Divers, H. O. Mohammed, A. L. Johnson, J. Albright, & S. M. Reuss. 2010. Epidemiological features and association with crib-biting in horses with neurological disease associated with temporohyoid osteoarthropathy (1991–2008). *Equine Vet. Educ.* 22(9):467–472.

858 **Griffith, C. A., E. S. Steigerwald, & C. A. Buffington. 2000. Effects of a synthetic facial pheromone on behavior of cats. *J. Am. Vet. Med. Assoc.* 217:1154–1156.**

859 Griffith, M. K., & J. E. Minton. 1992. Effect of light intensity on circadian profiles of melatonin, prolactin, ACTH, and cortisol in pigs. *J. Anim. Sci.* 70:492–498.

860 Grignard, L., A. Boissy, X. Boivin, J. P. Garel, & P. Le Neindre. 2000. The social environment influences the behavioural responses of beef cattle to handling. *Appl. Anim. Behav. Sci.* 68:1–11.

861 Grossman, M. I., G. M. Cummins, & A. C. Ivy. 1947. The effect of insulin on food intake after vagotomy and sympathectomy. *Am. J. Physiol.* 149:100–102.

862 Grout, A. S., D. M. Veira, D. M. Weary, M. A. von Keyserlingk, & D. Fraser. 2006. Differential effects of sodium and magnesium sulfate on water consumption by beef cattle. *J. Anim. Sci.* 84:1252–1258.

863 Grubb, P. 1974. Social organizatin of soay sheep and the behaviour of ewes and lambs. In P. A. Jewell, C. Milner, & J. M. Boyd (Eds.), Island survivors: The ecology of the Soay sheep of St. Kilda, pp. 131–159. London, UK: The Athlone Press of the University of London.

864 Grubb, P. 1974. The rut and behaviour of soay rams. In P. A. Jewell, C. Milner, & J. M. Boyd (Eds.), Island survivors: The ecology of the Soay sheep of St. Kilda, pp. 195–223. London, UK: The Athlone Press of the University of London.

865 Grzimek, B. 1949. Rangordnungsversuche mit pferden. *Z. Tierpsychol.* 6:455–464.

866 Grzimek, B. 1952. Versuche uber das farbsehen von pflanzenessern. I. das farbige sehen (und die sehscharfe) von pferden. *Z. Tierpsychol.* 9:23–39.

867 Gubernick, D. J., K. C. Jones, & P. H. Klopfer. 1979. Maternal imprinting in goats. *Anim. Behav.* 27:314–315.

868 Guillemet, R., S. Comyn, J. Dourmad, & M. Meunier-Salaun. 2007. Gestating sows prefer concentrate diets to high-fibre diet in two-choice tests. *Appl. Anim. Behav. Sci.* 108:251–262.

869 Guo, K., K. Meints, C. Hall, S. Hall, & D. Mills. 2009. Left gaze bias in humans, rhesus monkeys and domestic dogs. *Anim. Cogn.* 12:409–418.

870 Gurr, M. I., J. Kirtland, M. Phillip, & M. P. Robinson. 1977. The consequences of early overnutrition for fat cell size and number: The pig as an experimental model for human obesity. *Int. J. Obes.* 1:151–170.

871 Gustafsson, M., P. Jensen, F. H. de Jonge, & T. Schuurman. 1999. Domesticatin effects on foraging strategies in pigs (sus scrofa). *Appl. Anim. Behav. Sci.* 62:305–317.

872 Gustavson, C. R., R. J. Garcia, W. G. Hankins, & K. W. Rusiniak. 1974. Coyote predation control by aversive conditioning. *Science* 184:581–583.

873 Gutierrez-Gil, B., N. Ball, D. Burton, M. Haskell, J. L. Williams, & P. Wiener. 2008. Identification of quantitative trait loci affecting cattle temperament. *J. Hered.* 99(6):629–638.

874 **Guy, N. C., U. A. Luescher, S. E. Dohoo, E. Spangler, J. B. Miller, I. R. Dohoo, & L. A. Bate. 2001. A case series of biting dogs: Characteristics of the dogs, their behaviour, and their victims. *Appl. Anim. Behav. Sci.* 74:43–57.**

875 Gygax, L., R. Siegwart, & B. Wechsler. 2007. *Effects of space allowance on the behaviour and cleanliness of finishing bulls kept in pens with fully slatted rubber coated flooring.* 107:1–12.

876 Gyori, B., M. Gácsi, & Á. Miklósi. 2010. Friend or foe: Context dependent sensitivity to human behaviour in dogs. *Appl. Anim. Behav. Sci.* 128:69–77.

877 Haag, E. L., R. Rudman, & K. A. Houpt. 1980. Avoidance, maze learning and social dominance in ponies. *J. Anim. Sci.* 50:329–335.

878 Hafez, E. S. E. 1974. *Reproduction in farm animals.* Philadelphia, PA: Lea & Febiger.

879 Hafez, E. S. E. 1975. The behaviour of cattle. In E. S. E. Hafez (Ed.), *The behaviour of domestic animals*, pp. 203–245. Baltimore, MD: Williams & Wilkins.

880 Hafez, E. S. E. 1975. *The behaviour of domestic animals.* Baltimore, MD: Williams & Wilkins.

881 Hafez, E. S. E., & J. Signoret. 1969. The behaviour of swine. In E. S. E. Hafez (Ed.), *The behaviour of domestic animals*, pp. 349–390. Baltimore, MD: Williams & Wilkins.

882 Hafez, E. S., & J. A. Lineweaver. 1968. Suckling behaviour in natural and artificially fed neonate calves. *Z. Tierpsychol.* 25:187–198.

883 Hagen, K., & D. M. Broom. 2003. Cattle discriminate between individual familiar herd members in a learning experiment. *Appl. Anim. Behav. Sci.* 82:13–28.

884 Hale, E. B. 1966. Visual stimuli and reproductive behavior in bulls. *J. Anim. Sci.* 25 Suppl:36–48.

885 Hale, L. A., & S. E. Huggins. 1980. The electroencephalogram of normal 'grade' pony in sleep and wakefulness. *Comp. Biochem. Physiol.* 66A:251–257.

886 Haley, D. B., J. Rushen, I. J. H. Duncan, T. M. Widowski, & A. M. De passille. 1998. Butting by calves, *Bos taurus*, and rate of milk flow. *Anim. Behav.* 56:1545–1551.

887 Hall, C. A., & H. J. Cassaday. 2006. An investigation into the effect of floor colour on the behaviour of the horse. *Appl. Anim. Behav. Sci.* 99:301–314.

888 Hall, C. M., J. B. Fontaine, K. A. Bryant, & M. C. Calver. 2015. Assessing the effectiveness of the Birdsbesafe® anti-predation collar cover in reducing predation on wildlife by pet cats in Western Australia. *Appl. Anim. Behav. Sci.* 173:40–51.

889 Hall, S. J. G. 1986. Chillingham cattle: Dominance and affinities and access to supplementary food. *Ethology* 71:201–215.

890 **Hall, S. J. G. 1989. Chillingham cattle: Social and maintenance behaviour in an ungulate that breeds all year round. *Anim. Behav.* 38:215–225.**

891 Hall, S. J. G. 2002. Behaviour of cattle. In P. Jensen (Ed.), *The ethology of domestic animals: An introductory text*, pp. 131–146. Wallingford, UK: CABI.

892 **Hall, S. L., J. W. S. Bradshaw, & I. H. Robinson. 2002. Object play in adult domestic cats: The roles of habituation and disinhibition. *Appl. Anim. Behav. Sci.* 79:263–271.**

893 **Hamilton, G. V. 1911. A study of trial and error reactions in mammals. *J. Anim. Behav.* 1:33–66.**

894 Hamilton, J., & J. Vonk. 2015. Do dogs (*Canis lupus familiaris*) prefer family. *Behav. Processes.* 119:123–134.

895 Hamm, D. 1977. A new surgical procedure to control crib-biting. *Proceedings of the 23rd Annual Meeting of the American Association of Equine Practice*, 301–302.

896 Hammell, D. L., D. D. Kratzer, & W. J. Bramble. 1975. Avoidance and maze learning in pigs. *J. Anim. Sci.* 40:573–579.

897 Hancock, J. 1950. Grazing habits of dairy cows in New Zealand. *Emp. J. Exp. Agric.* 18:249–263.

898 **Hanggi, E. B., & J. F. Ingersoll. 2009. Long-term memory for categories and concepts in horses. *Anim. Cogn.* 12:451–462.**

899 Hanggi, E. B., & J. F. Ingersoll. 2009. Stimulus discrimination by horses under scotopic conditions. *Behav. Processes.* 82:45–50.

900 Hanggi, E. B., & J. F. Ingersoll. 2012. Lateral vision in horses: A behavioral investigation. *Behav. Processes.* 91:70–76.

901 Hanggi, E. B. 1999. Categorization learning in horses (*Equus caballus*). *J. Comp. Psychol.* 3:243–252.

902 Hanggi, E. B. 1999. Interocular transfer of learning in horses. *Equine Vet. J.* 19(8):518–524.

903 Hanggi, E. B. 2010. Rotated object recognition in four domestic horses. *Equine Vet. J.* 30(4):175–186.

904 Hanggi, E. B., & J. F. Ingersoll. 2009. Long-term memory for categories and concepts in horses (*Equus caballus*). *Anim. Cogn.* 12:451–462.

905 Hanninen, L., H. Hepola, S. Raussi, & H. Saloniemi. 2008. Effect of colostrum feeding method and presence of dam on the sleep, reat and sucking behaviour of newborn calves. *Appl. Anim. Behav. Sci.* 112:213–222.

906 Hansen, I., & V. Lind. 2008. Are double bunks used by indoor wintering sheep? testing a proposal for organic farming in Norway. *Appl. Anim. Behav. Sci.* 115:37–43.

907 Hansen, K. E., & S. E. Curtis. 1980. Prepartal activity of sows in stall or pen. *J. Anim. Sci.* 51:456–460.

908 **Harding, E. J., E. S. Paul, & M. Mendl. 2004. Cognitive bias and affective state. *Nature.* 427:312.**

909 **Hare, B., & M. Tomasello. 1999. Domestic dogs (canis familiaris) use human and conspecific social cues to locate hidden food. *J. Comp. Psychol.* 11:173–177.**

910 **Hare, B., J. Call, & M. Tomasello. 1998. Communication of food location between human and dog (*Canis familiaris*). *Evol. Commun.* 2:137–159.**

911 Hare, B., M. Brown, C. Williamson, & M. Tomasello. 2002. The domestication of social cognition in dogs. *Science* 298:1634–1636.

912 Harker, K. W., J. I. Taylor, & D. H. L. Rollinson. 1956. Studies in the habits of zebu cattle V. Night paddocking and its effect on the animal. *J. Agric. Sci.* 47:44–49.

913 Harlow, H. F., & P. Settlage. 1939. The effect of curarization of the fore part of the body upon the retention of conditioned responses in cats. *J. Comp. Psychol.* 27:45–48.

914 Harlow, H. F., M. K. Harlow, & E. W. Hansen. 1963. The maternal affectional system of rhesus monkeys. In H. L. Rheingold (Ed.), *Maternal behavior in mammals*, pp. 254–281. New York, NY: John Wiley & Sons.

915 Harman, A. M., S. Moore, R. Hoskins, & P. Keller. 1999. Horse vision and an explanation for the visual behaviour originally explained by the "ramp retina." *Equine Vet. J.* 31:384–390.

916 Harrington, F. H. 1986. Timber wolf howling playback studies: Discrimination of pup from adult howls. *Anim. Behav.* 34:1575–1577.

917 Harrington, F. H., & L. D. Mech. 1978. Howling at two Minnesota wolf pack summer homesites. *Can. J. Zool.* 56:2024–2028.

918 Harris C. R., & C. Prouvost. 2014. Jealousy in dogs. *PLoS ONE.* 9(7):e94597.

919 Harrison, J., & J. Buchwald. 1983. Eyeblink conditioning deficits in the old cat. *Neurobiol. Aging* 4:45–51.

920 Hart, B. L., & L. A. Hart. 2013. *Your ideal cat; insights into breed and gender differences in cat behavior*, p. 147. West Lafayette, IN: Purdue University Press.

921 Hart, B. L. 1968. Role of prior experience in the effects of castration on sexual behavior of male dogs. *J. Comp. Physiol. Psychol.* 66:719–725.

922 Hart, B. L. 1970. Mating behavior in the female dog and the effects of estrogen on sexual reflexes. *Horm. Behav.* 1:93–104.

923 Hart, B. L. 1974. Environmental and hormonal influences on urine marking behavior in the adult male dog. *Behav. Biol.* 11:167–176.

924 Hart, B. L. 1978. *Feline behavior. A practitioner monograph*. Santa Barbara, CA: Veterinary Practice Publishing Co.

925 Hart, B. L. 2001. Effect of gonadectomy on subsequent development of age-related cognitive impairment in dogs. *J. Am. Vet. Med. Assoc.* 219:51–56.

926 Hart, B. L., & C. M. Haugen. 1971. Scent marking and sexual behavior maintained in anosmic male dogs. *Commun. Behav.Biol.* 6:131–135.

927 Hart, B. L., & L. A. Hart. 1985. *Canine and feline behavioral therapy*. Philadelphia, PA: Lea & Febiger.

928 Hart, B. L., & L. A. Hart. 1988. *The perfect puppy. How to choose your dog by its behavior.* New York, NY: W.H. Freeman.

929 Hart, B. L., & M. G. Leedy. 1985. Analysis of the catnip reaction: Mediation by olfactory system, not vomeronasal organ. *Behav. Neural Biol.* 44:38–46.

930 Hart, B. L., & R. E. Barrett. 1973. Effects of castration on fighting, roaming, and urine spraying in adult male cats. *J. Am. Vet. Med. Assoc.* 163:290–292.

931 Hart, B. L., & T. O. Jones. 1975. Effects of castration on sexual behavior of tropical male goats. *Horm. Behav.* 6:247–258.

932 Hart, B. L., L. A. Hart, & M. J. Bain. 2006. *Canine and feline behavior therapy*, 2nd ed. Oxford, UK: Blackwell Publishing.

933 Hartman, B. L., & W. G. Pond. 1960. Design and use of a milking machine for sows. *J. Anim. Behav.* 19:780–785.

934 Hartmann, E., L. J. Keeling, & M. Rundgren. 2011. Comparison of 3 methods for mixing unfamiliar horses. *J. Vet. Behav.* 6:39–49.

935 Hashizume, C., M. Suzuki, K. Masuda, Y. Momozawa, T. Kikusui, Y. Takeuchi, & Y. Mori. 2003. Molecular cloning of canine monoamine oxidase subtypes A (MAOA) and B (MAOB) cDNAs and their expression in the brain. *J. Vet. Med. Sci.* 65:893–898.

936 Haskell, M. J., G. Simm, & S. P. Turner. 2014. Genetic selection for temperament traits in dairy and beef cattle. *J. Equine Vet. Sci.* 5(368):1–18.

937 Haskins, R. 1977. Effect of kitten vocalizations on maternal behavior. *J. Comp. Physiol. Psychol.* 91:830–838.

938 Hatch, R. C. 1972. Effect of drugs on catnip (*Nepeta cataria*)–induced pleasure behavior in cats. *Am. J. Vet. Res.* 33:143–155.

939 Haugse, C. N., W. E. Dinusson, D. L. Erickson, J. N. Johnson, & M. L. Buchanan. 1965. A day in the life of a pig. *N. Dak. Farm Res.* 23:18–23.

940 Haulenbeek, A. M., & L. S. Katz. 2011. Female tail wagging enhances sexual performance in male goats. *Horm. Behav.* 60:244–247.

941 Hausberger, M., & C. Muller. 2002. A brief note on some possible factors involved in the reactions of horses to humans. *Appl. Anim. Behav. Sci.* 76:339–344.

942 Hausberger, M., C. Fureix, M. Bourjade, S. Wessel-Robert, & M.-A. Richard-Yris. 2012. On the significance of adult play: What does social play tell us about adult horse welfare? *Naturwiss.* 99:291–302.

943 Hausberger, M., C. Muller, & C. Lunel. 2011. Does work affect personality? *A study in horses.* PLoS ONE. 6(2):e14659.

944 Hausberger, M., E. Gautier, C. Muller, & P. Jego. 2007. Lower learning abilities in stereotypic horses. *Appl. Anim. Behav. Sci.* 107:299–306.

945 Hausberger, M., S. Henry, C. Larose, & M. A. Richard-Yris. 2007. First suckling: A crucial event for mother-young attachment? An experimental study in horses (*Equus caballus*). *J. Comp. Psychol.* 121:109–112.

946 Hauschildt, V., & M. Gerken. 2015. Individual gregariousness predicts behavioural synchronization in a foraging herbivore, the sheep. *Behav. Processes.* 113:110–112.

947 Hauschildt, V., & M. Gerken. 2015. Temporal stability of social structure and behavioural synchronization in Shetland pony mares (*Equus caballus*) kept on pasture. *Acta Agric. Scand. A Animal Sci.* 65(1):33–41.

948 Haverbeke, A., A. De Smet, E. Depiereux, J. Giffroy, & C. Diederich. 2009. Assessing undesired aggression in military working dogs. *Appl. Anim. Behav. Sci.* 117:55–62.

949 Haverbeke, A., B. Laporte, E. Depiereux, J. Giffroy, & C. Diederich. 2008. Training methods of military dog handlers and their effects on the team's performances. *Appl. Anim. Behav. Sci.* 113:110–122.

950 Hawkes, J., M. Hedges, P. Daniluk, H. F. Hintz, & H. F. Schryver. 1985. Feed preferences of ponies. *Equine Vet. J.* 17:20–22.

951 Hawking, F. 1971. Circadian rhythms in monkeys, dogs and other animals. *J. Interdiscipl. Cycle Res.* 2:153–156.

952 Hawking, F. 1971. Circadian rhythms of parasites. *J. Interdiscipl. Cycle Res.* 2:157–160.

953 Hay, M., M. C. Meunier-Salaun, F. Brulaud, M. Monnier, & P. Mormede. 2000. Assessment of hypothalamic-pituitary-adrenal axis and sympathetic nervous system activity in pregnant sows through the measurement of glucocorticoids and catecholamines in urine. *J. Anim. Sci.* 78:420–428.

954 Hayes, K. E. N., & O. J. Ginther. 1989. Relationships between estrous behavior in pregnant mares and the presence of a female conceptus. *J. Equine Vet. Sci.* 9:316–318.

955 Hayman, R. H. 1964. Exercise of mating preference by a merino ram. *Nature* 203:160–162.

956 Hayne, S. M., & H. W. Gonyou. 2003. Effects of regrouping on the individual behavioural characteristics of pigs. *Appl. Anim. Behav. Sci.* 82:267–278.

957 Hayne, S. M., & H. W. Gonyou. 2006. Behavioural uniformity or diversity? Effects on behaviour and performance following regrouping in pigs. *Appl. Anim. Behav. Sci.* 98:28–44.

958 He, J., L. Ma, S. Kim, J. Nakai, & C. R. Yu. 2008. Encoding gender and individual information in the mouse vomeronasal organ. *Science* 320:535–538.

959 Head, E., K. Moffat, P. Das, F. Sarsoza, W. W. Poon, G. Landsberg, C. W. Cotman, & M. P. Murphy. 2005. Beta-amyloid deposition and tau phosphorylation in clinically characterized aged cats. *Neurobiol. Aging* 26:749–763.

960 Heady, H. F. 1964. Palatability of herbage and animal preference. *J. Range Manag.* 17:76–82.

961 Heath, S. E., S. Barabas, & P. G. Craze. 2007. Nutritional supplementation in cases of canine cognitive dysfunction: A clinical trial. *Appl. Anim. Behav. Sci.* 105:296.

962 Heberlein, M., & D. C. Turner. 2009. Dogs, *Canis familiaris*, find hidden food by observing and interacting with a conspecific. *Anim Behav.* 78:385–391.

963 Hecht, J., A. Miklósia, & M. Gácsi. 2012. Behavioral assessment and owner perceptions of behaviors associated with guilt in dogs. *Appl. Anim. Behav. Sci.* 139:134–142.

964 Hedlund, L., M. M. Lischko, M. D. Rollag, & G. D. Niswender. 1977. Melatonin: Daily cycle in plasma and cerebrospinal fluid of calves. *Science* 195:686–687.

965 Heffner, H. E. 1983. Hearing in large and small dogs: Absolute thresholds and size of the tympanic membrane. *Behav. Neurosci.* 97:310–318.

966 Hegsted, D. M., S. N. Gershoff, & E. Lentini. 1956. The development of palatability tests for cats. *Am. J. Vet. Res.* 17:733–737.

967 **Heidenberger, E. 1997. Housing conditions and behavioural problems of indoor cats as assessed by their owners. *Appl. Anim. Behav. Sci.* 52:345–364.**

968 Hein, A., & R. Held. 1967. Dissociation of the visual placing response into elicited and guided components. *Science* 158:390–392.

969 Heird, J. C., A. M. Lennon, & R. W. Bell. 1981. Effects of early experience on the learning ability of yearling horses. *J. Anim. Sci.* 53:1204–1209.

970 **Heird, J. C., D. D. Whitaker, R. W. Bell, C. B. Ramsey, & C. E. Lokey. 1986. The effects of handling at different ages on the subsequent learning ability of 2-year-old horses. *Appl. Anim. Behav. Sci.* 15:15–25.**

971 Heitor, F., & L. Vicente. 2008. Maternal care and foal social relationships in a herd of sorraia horses: Influence of maternal rank and experience. *Appl. Anim. Behav. Sci.* 113:189–205.

972 Heitzman, R. J. 1978. The use of hormones to regulate the utilization of nutrients in farm animals: Current farm practices. *Proc. Nutr. Soc.* 37:289–293.

973 Hejjas, K., J. Vas, J. Topal, E. Szantai, Z. Ronai, A. Szekely, E. Kubinyi, et al. 2007. Association of polymorphisms in the dopamine D4 receptor gene and the activity-impulsivity endophenotype in dogs. *Anim. Genet.* 38(6):629–633.

974 **Held, S. D. E., R. W. Byrne, S. Jones, E. Murphy, M. Friel, & M. T. Mendl. 2010. Domestic pigs, Sus scrofa, adjust their foraging behaviour to whom they are foraging with. *Anim. Behav.* 79:857–862.**

975 Held, S., G. Mason, & M. Mendl. 2006. Maternal responsiveness of outdoor sows from first to fourth parities. *Appl. Anim. Behav. Sci.* 98:216–233.

976 Held, S., J. Baumgartner, A. Kilbride, R. W. Byrne, & M. Mendl. 2005. Foraging behaviour in domestic pigs (*Sus scrofa*): Remembering and prioritizing food sites of different value. *Anim. Cogn.* 8:114–121.

977 Held, S., M. Mendl, C. Devereux, & R. W. Byrne. 2002. Foraging pigs alter their behaviour in response to exploitation. *Anim. Behav.* 64:156–166.

978 Heleski, C. R., & I. Murtazashvili. 2010. Daytime shelter-seeking behavior in domestic horses. *J. Vet. Behav.* 5(5):276–282.

979 Hellekant, G., C. Hård af Segerstad, & T. W. Roberts. 1994. Sweet taste in the calf: III. *Behavioral responses to sweeteners. Physiol. Behav.* 56:555–562.

980 Hemmann, K., M. Raekallio, K. Kanerva, L. Hänninen, M. Pastell, M. Palviainen, & O. Vainio. 2012. Circadian variation in ghrelin and certain stress hormones in crib-biting horses. *Vet. J.* 193:97–102.

981 Hemsworth, P. H., & A. J. Tilbrook. 2007. Sexual behavior of male pigs. *Horm. Behav.* 52:39–44.

982 Hemsworth, P. H., & J. L. Barnett. 1992. The effects of early contact with humans on the subsequent level of fear of humans in pigs. *Appl. Anim. Behav. Sci.* 35:83–90.

983 Hemsworth, P. H., C. G. Winfield, & P. D. Mullaney. 1976. A study of the development of the teat order in piglets. *Appl. Anim. Ethol.* 2:225–233.

984 Hemsworth, P. H., C. G. Winfield, J. L. Barnett, B. Schirmer, & C. Hansen. 1986. A comparison of the effects of two estrus detection procedures and two housing systems on the oestrus detection rate of female pigs. *Appl. Anim. Behav. Sci.* 16:345–351.

985 Hemsworth, P. H., C. G. Winfield, R. G. Beilharz, & D. B. Galloway. 1977. Influence of social conditions post-puberty on the sexual behaviour of the domestic male pig. *Anim. Prod.* 25:305–309.

986 Hemsworth, P. H., E. O. Price, & A. J. Tilbrook. 1992. Influence of the sexual motivation of the boar on the sexual partner preferences of oestrous gilts. *Appl. Anim. Behav. Sci.* 33:209–215.

987 Hemsworth, P. H., G. M. Cronin, C. Hansen, & C. G. Winfield. 1984. The effects of two oestrus detection procedures and intense boar stimulation near the time of oestrus on mating efficiency of the female pig. *Appl. Anim. Behav. Sci.* 12:339–347.

988 Hemsworth, P. H., J. K. Findlay, & R. G. Bielharz. 1978. The importance of physical contact with other pigs during rearing on the sexual behaviour of the male domestic pig. *Anim. Prod.* 27:201–207.

989 Hemsworth, P. H., J. L. Barnett, & C. Hansen. 1987. The influence of inconsistent handling by humans on the behaviour, growth and corticosteroids of young pigs. *Act. Nerv. Super. (Praha).* 17:245–252.

990 Hemsworth, P. H., J. L. Barnett, A. J. Tilbrook, & C. Hansen. 1989. The effects of handling by humans at calving and during milking on the behaviour and milk cortisol concentrations of primiparous dairy cows. *Appl. Anim. Behav. Sci.* 22:313–326.

991 Hemsworth, P. H., J. L. Barnett, C. Hansen, & C. G. Winfield. 1986. Effects of social

environment on welfare status and sexual behaviour of female pigs II. Effects of space allowance. *Appl. Anim. Behav. Sci.* 16:259–267.

992 Hemsworth, P. H., R. G. Beilharz, & D. B. Galloway. 1977. Influence of social conditions during rearing on the sexual behaviour of the domestic boar. *Anim. Prod.* 24:245–251.

993 **Hendricks, J. C., A. R. Morrison, G. L. Farnbach, S. A. Steinberg, & G. Mann. 1981. A disorder of rapid eye movement sleep in a cat. *J. Am. Vet. Med. Assoc.* 178:55–57.**

994 Hendriks, W. H., M. F. Tarttelin, & P. J. Moughan. 1995. Twenty-four-hour feline excretion patterns in entire and castrated cats. *Physiol. Behav.* 58:467–469.

995 **Hendriksen, P., K. Elmgreen, & J. Ladewig. 2011. Trailer-loading of horses: Is there a difference between positive and negative reinforcement concerning effectiveness and stress-related signs? *J. Vet. Behav.* 6:261–266.**

996 Henry, S., D. Hemery, M. Richard, & M. Hausberger. 2005. Human-mare relationships and behaviour of foals toward humans. *Appl. Anim. Behav. Sci.* 93:341–362.

997 Hepper, P. G. 1986. Sibling recognition in the domestic dog. *Anim. Behav.* 34:288–289.

998 Herbel, C. H., & A. B. Nelson. 1966. Species preference of hereford and santa gertrudis cattle on a southern new Mexico range. *J. Range Manag.* 19:177–181.

999 Herd, R. M. 1988. A technique for cross-mothering beef calves which does not affect growth. *Appl. Anim. Behav. Sci.* 19:239–244.

1000 Hernádi, A., A. Kis, O. Kanizsár, K. Tóth, B. Miklósi, & J. Topál. 2015. Intranasally administered oxytocin affects how dogs (*Canis familiaris*) react to the threatening approach of their owner and an unfamiliar experimenter. *Behav. Processes.* 119:1–5.

1001 Hernandez, L., H. Barral, G. Halffter, & S. S. Colon. 1999. A note on the behavior of feral cattle in the Chihuahuan desert of

Mexico. *Appl. Anim. Behav. Sci.* 63:259–267.

1002 Herring, S. W., & R. P. Scapino. 1973. Physiology of feeding in miniature pigs. *J. Morphol.* 141:427–460.

1003 Hersher, L., J. B. Richmond, & A. U. Moore. 1963. Maternal behavior in sheep and goats. In H. L. Rheingold (Ed.), *Maternal behavior in mammals*. New York, NY: John Wilen & Sons.

1004 Herskin, M. S., L. Munksgaard, & A. M. Kristensen. 2003. Behavioural and adrenocortical responses of dairy cows toward novel food: Effects of food deprivation, milking frequency and energy density in the daily ration. *Appl. Anim. Behav. Sci.* 82:251–265.

1005 Hessel, E. F., K. Reiners, & H. F. Van den Weghe. 2006. Socializing piglets before weaning: Effects on behavior of lactating sows, pre- and postweaning behavior, and performance of piglets. *J. Anim. Sci.* 84:2847–2855.

1006 Hessing, M. J. C., A. M. Hagels, J. A. M. van Beck, P. R. Wiepkema, G. P. Schouten, & R. Krukow. 1993. Individual behavioural characteristics in pigs. *Appl. Anim. Behav. Sci.* 37:285–295.

1007 Hessle, A., M. Rutter, & K. Wallin. 2008. Effect of breed, season and pasture moisture gradient on foraging behaviour in cattle on semi-natural grasslands. *Appl. Anim. Behav. Sci.* 111:108–119.

1008 **Hetts, S. 1999. *Pet behaviour protocols*. Lakewood, CO: AAHA Press.**

1009 Hetts, S., J. Derrell Clark, J. P. Calin, C. E. Arnold, & J. M. Mateo. 1992. Influence of housing conditions on beagle behaviour. *Appl. Anim. Behav. Sci.* 34:137–155.

1010 Hetzer, H. O., & W. R. Harvey. 1967. Selection for high and low fatness in swine. *J. Anim. Sci.* 26:1244–1251.

1011 Hill, C. T., P. D. Krawczel, H. M. Dann, C. S. Ballard, R. C. Hovey, W. A. Falls, & R. J. Grant. 2009. Effect of stocking density on the short-term behavioural responses of dairy cows. *Appl. Anim. Behav. Sci.* 117:144–149.

1012 Hill, J. O., E. J. Pavlik, G. L. Smith III, G. M. Burghardt, & P. B. Coulson. 1976. Species-characteristic responses to catnip by undomesticated felids. *J. Chem. Ecol.* 2:239–253.

1013 Hinch, G. N., J. J. Lynch, & C. J. Thwaites. 1982. Patterns and frequency of social interactions in young grazing bulls and steers. *Appl. Anim. Ethol.* 9:15–30.

1014 Hintze, S., D. Scott, S. Turner, S. L. Meddle, & R. B. D'Eath. 2013. Mounting behaviour in finishing pigs: Stable individual differences are not due to dominance or stage of sexual development. *Appl. Anim. Behav. Sci.* 147:69–80.

1015 Hirsch, E., C. Dubose, & H. L. Jacobs. 1978. Dietary control of food intake in cats. *Physiol. Behav.* 20:287–295.

1016 Hite, M., H. M. Hanson, N. R. Bohidar, P. A. Conti, & P. A. Mattis. 1977. Effect of cage size on patterns of activity and health of beagle dogs. *Lab. Anim. Sci.* 27:60–64.

1017 Hoagland, T. A., & M. A. Diekman. 1982. Influence of supplemental lighting during increasing daylength on libido and reproductive hormones in prepubertal boars. *J. Anim. Sci.* 55:1483–1489.

1018 Hockenhull, J., & E. Creighton. 2010. Unwanted oral investigative behaviour in horses: A note on the relationship between mugging behaviour, hand-feeding titbits and clicker training. *Appl. Anim. Behav. Sci.* 127:104–107.

1019 Hoeck, J., & W. Büscher. 2015. Temperature-dependent consumption of drinking water in piglet rearing. *Appl. Anim. Behav. Sci.* 170:20–25.

1020 Hoffman, R. 1985. On the development of social behavior in immature males of a feral horse population (*Equus przewalski f. caballus*). *Zeitschrift Saugetierkunde* 50:302–314.

1021 Hoffman, R. M., D. S. Kronfeld, J. L. Holland, & K. M. Greiwe-Crandell. 1995. Preweaning diet and stall weaning method influences on stress response in foals. *J. Anim. Sci.* 73:2922–2930.

1022 Holcomb, K. E., C. B. Tucker, & C. L. Stull. 2014. Preference of domestic horses for shade in a hot, sunny environment. *J. Anim. Sci.* 92:1708–1717.

1023 Holland, J. L., D. S. Kronfeld, G. A. Rich, K. A. Kline, J. P. Fontenot, T. N. Meacham, & P. A. Harris. 1998. Acceptance of fat and lecithin containing diets by horses. *Appl. Anim. Behav. Sci.* 56:91–96.

1024 Holm, L., M. B. Jensen, L. J. Pedersen, & J. Ladewig. 2008. The importance of a food feedback in rooting materials for pigs measured by double demand curves with and without a common scaling factor. *Appl. Anim. Behav. Sci.* 111:68–84.

1025 Holmes, J. H., & L. J. Cizek. 1951. Observations on sodium chloride depletion in dog. *Am. J. Physiol.* 164:407–414.

1026 Holmes, L. N., G. K. Song, & E. O. Price. 1987. Head partitions facilitate feeding by subordinate horses in the presence of dominant pan-mates. *Appl. Anim. Behav. Sci.* 19:179–182.

1027 Hopkins, S. G., T. A. Schubert, & B. L. Hart. 1976. Castration of adult male dogs: Effects on roaming, aggression, urine marking, and mounting. *J. Am. Vet. Med. Assoc.* 168:1108–1110.

1028 Hoppe, S., H. R. Brandt, G. Erhardt, & M. Gauly. 2008. Maternal protective behaviour of German Angus and Simmental beef cattle after parturition and its relation to production traits. *Appl. Anim. Behav. Sci.* 114:297–306.

1029 Hoppenbrouwers, T., & M. B. Sterman. 1975. Development of sleep state patterns in the kitten. *Exp. Neurol.* 49:822–838.

1030 Horn, L., Z. Viranyi, A. Miklosi, L. Huber, & F. Range. 2012. Domestic dogs (*Canis familiaris*) flexibly adjust their human directed behavior to the actions of their human partners in a problem situation. *Anim. Cogn.* 15:57–71.

1031 Hori, Y., T. Tozako, Y. Nambo, F. Sato, M. Ishimaru, M. Inoue-Murayama, & K. Fujita. 2015. Evidence for the effect of serotonin receptor 1A gene (HTR1A) polymorphism on tractability in Thoroughbred horse. *Anim. Gen.* 47:62–67.

1032 Horowitz, A. 2009. Attention to attention in domestic dog (*Canis familiaris*) dyadic play. *Anim. Cogn.* 12:107–118.

1033 Horrell, I., & J. Hodgson. 1992. The bases of sow-piglet identification. 2. Cues used by piglets to identify their dame and home pen. *Appl. Anim. Behav. Sci.* 33:329–343.

1034 **Horrell, I., & J. Hodgson. 1992. The bases of sow-piglet identification. I. The identification by sows of their own piglets and the presence of intruders. *Appl. Anim. Behav. Sci.* 33:319–327.**

1035 Horrell, R. I., & M. Eaton. 1984. Recognition of maternal environment in piglets: Effects of age and some discrete complex stimuli. *Q. J. Exp. Psychol. B* 36:119–130.

1036 Horvath, Z., B. Z. Igyarto, A. Magyar, & A. Miklosi. 2007. Three different coping styles in police dogs exposed to a short-term challenge. *Horm. Behav.* 52:621–630.

1037 Horwitz, D. F., & J. C. Neilson. 2007. *Blackwell's five-minute veterinary consult clinical companion: Canine and feline behavior*. Oxford, UK: Blackwell Publishing.

1038 **Horwitz, D. F., D. S. Mills, & S. Heath. 2010 BSAVMA manual of canine and feline behavioural medicine. Ames, IA: Wiley.**

1039 Hosoi, E., L. R. Rittenhouse, D. M. Swift, & R. W. Richards. 1995. Foraging strategies of cattle in a Y-maze: Influence of food availability. *Appl. Anim. Behav. Sci.* 43:189–196.

1040 Hothersall, B., E. V. Gale, P. Harris, & C. J. Nicol. 2010. Cue use by foals (Equus caballus) in a discrimination learning task. *Anim. Cogn.* 13:63–74.

1041 Hothersall, B., P. Harris, L. Sörtoft, & C. J. Nicol. 2010. Discrimination between conspecific odour samples in the horse (*Equus caballus*). *Appl. Anim. Behav. Sci.* 126:37–44.

1042 Houpt, K. A. 1977. Horse behavior: Its relevancy to the equine practitioner. *J. Eq. Med. Surg.* 1:87–94.

1043 Houpt, K. A. 1978. Palatability and canine food preferences. *Canine Pract.* 5:29–35.

1044 Houpt, K. A. 1983. Disruption of the human-companion animal bond: Aggressive behavior in dogs. In A. H. Katcher, & A. M. Beck (Eds.), *New perspective on our lives with companion animals*, pp. 197–204.

1045 Houpt, K. A., & G. Wollney. 1989. Frequency of masturbation and time budgets of dairy bulls used for semen production. *Appl. Anim. Behav. Sci.* 24:217–225.

1046 Houpt, K. A., & H. F. Hintz. 1982. Some effects of maternal deprivation and maintenance behavior, spatial relationships and responses to environmental novelty in foals. *Appl. Anim. Ethol.* 9:221–230.

1047 Houpt, K. A., & M. B. Willis. 2001. Genetics of behaviour. In A. Ruvinsky, & J. Sampson (Eds.), *The genetics of the dog*, pp. 371–394. Wallingford, UK: CABI.

1048 Houpt, K. A., & R. Kusunose. 2000. Genetics of behaviour. In T. A. Bowling, & A. Ruvinsky (Eds.), *The genetics of the horse*, pp. 281–306. Wallingford, UK: CABI.

1049 Houpt, K. A., & R. R. Keiper. 1982. The position of the stallion in the equine dominance hierarchy of feral and domestic ponies. *J. Anim. Sci.* 54:945–950.

1050 Houpt, K. A., & T. R. Houpt. 1976. Comparative aspects of the ontogeny of taste. *Chem. Senses Flavor.* 2:219–228.

1051 Houpt, K. A., & T. R. Houpt. 1988. Social and illumination preferences of mares. *J. Anim. Sci.* 66:2159–2164.

1052 Houpt, K. A., & T. R. Wolski. 1979. Equine maternal behavior and aberrations. *Equine Pract.* 1:7–20.

1053 Houpt, K. A., & T. R. Wolski. 1980. Stability of equine hierarchies and the prevention of dominance related aggression. *Equine Vet. J.* 12:15–18.

1054 Houpt, K. A., A. Eggleston, K. Kunkle, & T. R. Houpt. 2000. Effect of water restriction on equine behaviour and physiology. *Equine Vet. J.* 32:341–344.

1055 Houpt, K. A., B. Coren, H. F. Hintz, & J. E. Hilderbrant. 1979. Effect of sex and reproductive status on sucrose preference, food intake, and body weight of dogs. *J. Am. Vet. Med. Assoc.* 174:1083–1085.

1056 Houpt, K. A., H. F. Hintz, & P. Shepherd. 1978. The role of olfaction in canine food preferences. *Chem. Senses Flavor.* 3:281–290.

1057 Houpt, K. A., K. Law, & V. Martinisi. 1978. Dominance hierarchies in domestic horses. *Appl. Anim. Ethol.* 4:273–283.

1058 Houpt, K. A., M. S. Parsons, & H. F. Hintz. 1982. Learning ability of orphan foals, of normal foals and of their mothers. *J. Anim. Sci.* 55:1027–1032.

1059 Houpt, K. A., N. Northrup, T. Wheatley, & T. R. Houpt. 1991. Thirst and salt appetite in horses treated with furosemide. *J. Appl. Physiol.* 71:2380–2386.

1060 Houpt, K. A., T. R. Houpt, & W. G. Pond. 1977. Food intake controls in the suckling pig: Glucoprivation and gastrointestinal factors. *Am. J. Physiol.* 232:E510–E514.

1061 Houpt, K. A., T. R. Houpt, & W. G. Pond. 1979. The pig as a model for the study of obesity and of control of food intake: A review. *Yale J. Biol. Med.* 52:307–329.

1062 Houpt, K. A., T. R. Houpt, J. L. Johnson, H. N. Erb, & S. C. Yeon. 2001. The effect of exercise deprivation on the behaviour and physiology of straight stall confined pregnant mares. *Anim. Welf.* 10:257–267.

1063 Houpt, K. A., W. Rivera, & L. Glickstein. 1989. The flehmen response of bulls and cows. *Theriogenology* 32:343–350.

1064 Houpt, T. R. 1974. Stimulation of food intake in ruminants by 2-deoxy-D-glucose and insulin. *Am. J. Physiol.* 227:161–167.

1065 Houpt, T. R. 1984. Controls of feeding in pigs. *J. Anim. Sci.* 59:1345–1353.

1066 Houpt, T. R., & H. H. Hance. 1969. Effect of 2-deoxy-D glucose on food intake by the goat, rabbit and dog. *Fed. Proc.* 28:648.

1067 Houpt, T. R., B. A. Baldwin, & K. A. Houpt. 1983. Effects of duodenal osmotic loads on spontaneous meals in pigs. *Physiol. Behav.* 30:787–795.

1068 Houpt, T. R., K. A. Houpt, & A. A. Swan. 1983. Duodenal osmoconcentration and food intake in pigs after ingestion of hypertonic nutrients. *Am. J. Physiol.* 245:R181–R189.

1069 Houpt, T. R., L. C. Weixler, & D. W. Troy. 1986. Water drinking induced by gastric secretagogues in pigs. *Am. J. Physiol.* 251:R157–R164.

1070 Houpt, T. R., S. M. Anika, & K. A. Houpt. 1979. Preabsorptive intestinal satiety controls of food intake in pigs. *Am. J. Physiol.* 236:R328–R337.

1071 Howell, T. J., S. Toukhsati, R. Conduit, & P. Bennett. 2013. Do dogs use a mirror to find hidden food? *J. Vet. Behav.* 8:425–430.

1072 Howery, L. D., F. D. Provenza, R. E. Banner, & C. B. Scott. 1998. Social and environmental factors influence cattle distribution on rangeland. *Appl. Anim. Behav. Sci.* 55:231–244.

1073 Hoy, S., S. Schamun, & C. Weirich. 2012. Investigations on feed intake and social behaviour of fattening pigs fed at an electronic feeding station. *Appl. Anim. Behav. Sci.* 139:58–64.

1074 Hubrecht, R. C. 1993. A comparison of social and environmental enrichment methods for laboratory housed dogs. *Appl. Anim. Behav. Sci.* 37:345–361.

1075 Hubrecht, R. C., J. A. Serpell, & T. B. Poole. 1992. Correlates of pen size and housing conditions on the behaviour of kennelled dogs. *Appl. Anim. Behav. Sci.* 34:365–383.

1076 **Hudson, H. J. 2012. Genetic aspects of performance in working dogs. In E. A. Ostrander, & A. Ruvinsky (Eds.), *The genetics of the dog*, 2nd ed., pp. 477–495. Cambridge, UK: CABI International.**

1077 Hudson, R., G. Raihani, D. Gonzalez, A. Bautista, & H. Diste. 2009. Nipple preference and contests in suckling kittens of the domestic cat are unrelated to presumed nipple quality. *Dev. Psychobiol.* 51:322–332.

1078 Hudson, S. J. 1977. Multiple fostering of calves onto nurse cows at birth. *Appl. Anim. Behav. Sci.* 3:57–63.

1079 Hudson, S. J., & M. M. Mullord. 1977. Investigations of maternal bonding in dairy cattle. *Appl. Anim. Ethol.* 3:271–276.

1080 Hughes, G. P., & D. Reid. 1951. Studies on the behaviour of cattle and sheep in relation to the utilization of grass. *J. Agric. Sci.* 41:350–366.

1081 Hughes, P. E., P. H. Hemsworth, & C. Hansen. 1985. The effects of supplementary olfactory and auditory stimuli on the stimulus value and mating success of the young boar. *Appl. Anim. Behav. Sci.* 14:245–252.

1082 Hulbert, L. E., & J. J. McGlone. 2006. Evaluation of drop versus trickle-feeding systems for crated or group-penned gestating sows. *J. Anim. Sci.* 84:1004–1014.

1083 Hulet, C. V. 1966. Behavioral, social and psychological factors affecting mating time and breeding efficiency in sheep. *J. Anim. Sci.* 25 Suppl:5–20.

1084 Hulet, C. V., D. M. Anderson, J. N. Smith, & W. L. Shupe. 1989. Bonding of goats to sheep and cattle for protection from predators. *Appl. Anim. Behav. Sci.* 22:261–267.

1085 Hulet, C. V., G. Alexander, & E. S. E. Hafez. 1975. *The behaviour of sheep*. Baltimore, MD: Williams & Wilkins.

1086 Hulet, C. V., R. L. Balckwell, & S. K. Ercanbrack. 1964. Observations on sexually inhibited rams. *J. Anim. Sci.* 23 1095–1097

1087 **Hulet, C. V., R. L. Balckwell, S. K. Ercanbrack, D. A. Price, & L. O. Wilson. 1962. Mating behavior of the ewe. *J. Anim. Sci.* 21:870–874.**

1088 **Hunter, D. S., S. J. Hazel, K. L. Kind, H. Liu, D. Marini, J. A. Owens, J. B. Pitcher, & K. L. Gatford. 2015. Do I turn left or right? Effects of sex, age, experience and exit route on maze test performance in sheep. *Physiol. Behav.* 139:244–253.**

1089 Hunter, L., & K. A. Houpt. 1987. Bedding material preferences of ponies. *J. Anim. Sci.* 67:1986–1991.

1090 Hunter, W. S. 1917. The delayed reaction in a child. *Psychol.* 24:74–87.

1091 **Hunthausen, W. 1997. Effects of aggressive behavior on canine welfare. *J. Am. Vet. Med. Assoc.* 210:1134–1136.**

1092 Hunthausen, W., & G. M. Landsberg. 1993. *Providing behavior services in veterinary practices.* Denver, CO: American Animal Hospital Association.

1093 Hurnik, J. F., G. J. King, & H. A. Robertson. 1975. Estrous and related behaviour in postpartum holstein cows. *Appl. Anim. Ethol.* 2:55–68.

1094 Hutson, G. D. 1980. The effect of previous experience on sheep movement through yards. *Appl. Anim. Ethol.* 6:233–240.

1095 Hutson, G. D. 1985. The influence of barley food rewards on sheep movement through a handling system. *Appl. Anim. Behav. Sci.* 14:263–273.

1096 Hutson, G. D., & M. J. Haskell. 1990. The behaviour of farrowing sows with free and operant access to an earth floor. *Appl. Anim. Behav. Sci.* 26:363–372.

1097 Hutson, G. D., E. O. Price, & L. G. Dickenson. 1993. The effect of playback volume and duration of the response of sows to piglet distress calls. *Appl. Anim. Behav. Sci.* 37:31–37.

1098 Hutson, G. D., J. L. Wilkinson, & B. G. Luxford. 1991. The response of lactating sows to tactile, visual and auditory stimuli associated with a model piglet. *Appl. Anim. Behav. Sci.* 32:129–137.

1099 Hutson, G. D., M. F. Argent, L. G. Dickenson, & B. G. Luxford. 1992. Influence of parity and time since parturition on responsiveness of sows to a piglet distress call. *Appl. Anim. Behav. Sci.* 34:303–313.

1100 Huynh, T. T. T., A. J. A. Aarnink, W. J. J. Gerrits, M. J. H. Heetkamp, T. T. Canh, H. A. M. Spoodler, B. Kemp, & M. W. A. Verstegen. 2005. Thermal behaviour of growing pigs in response to high temperature and humidity. *Appl. Anim. Behav. Sci.* 91:1–16.

1101 Iacobucci, P., V. Colonnello, L. D'Antuono, S. Cloutier, & R. C. Newberry. 2015. Piglets call for maternal attention: Vocal behaviour in Sus scrofa domesticus is modulated by mother's proximity. *Appl. Anim. Behav. Sci.* 171:88–93.

1102 Igel, G. J., & A. D. Calvin. 1960. The development of affectional responses in infant dogs. *J. Comp. Physiol. Psychol.* 53:302–305.

1103 Illius, A. W., N. B. Haynes, & G. E. Lamming. 1976. Effects of ewe proximity on peripheral plasma testosterone levels and behaviour in the ram. *J. Reprod. Fertil.* 48:25–32.

1104 Illmann, G., & J. Madlafousek. 1995. Occurrence and characteristics of unsuccessful nursing in minipigs during the first week of life. *Appl. Anim. Behav. Sci.* 44:9–18.

1105 **Illmann, G., & M. Spinka. 1993. Maternal behaviour of dairy heifers and sucking of their newborn calves in group housing. *Appl. Anim. Behav. Sci.* 36:91–98.**

1106 Illmann, G., K. Neuhauserova, Z. Pokorna, H. Chaloupkova, & M. Simeckova. 2008. Maternal responsiveness of sows towards piglet's screams during the first 24 h postpartum. *Appl. Anim. Behav. Sci.* 112:248–259.

1107 Illmann, G., M. Spinka, & Z. Stetkova. 1999. Predictability of nursings without milk ejection in domestic pigs. *Appl. Anim. Behav. Sci.* 61:303–311.

1108 Imfeld-Mueller, S., L. Van Wezemael, M. Stauffacher, L. Gygax, & E. Hillmann. 2011. Do pigs distinguish between situations of different emotional valences during anticipation? *Appl. Anim. Behav. Sci.* 131:86–93.

1109 Ingolfsdottir, H. B., & H. Sigurjonsdottir. 2008. The benefits of high rank in the wintertime: A study of the icelandic horse. *Appl. Anim. Behav. Sci.* 114:485–491.

1110 Ingram, D. L., & D. B. Stephens. 1979. The relative importance of thermal, osmoic and hypovolaemic factors in the control of drinking in the pig. *J. Physiol.* 293:501–512.

1111 Ingram, D. L., & K. F. Legge. 1974. Effects of environmental temperature on food intake in growing pigs. *Comp. Biochem. Physiol.* 48A:573–581.

1112 Ingram, D. L., & M. J. Dauncy. 1985. Circadian rhythms in the pig. *Comp. Biochem. Physiol.* 82A:1–5.

1113 Ingram, D. L., M. J. Dauncy, & K. F. Legge. 1985. Synchronization of motor activity in young pigs to a non-circadian rhythm without affecting food intake and growth. *Comp. Biochem. Physiol.* 80A:363–368.

1114 Innes, L., & S. McBride. 2008. Negative versus positive reinforcement: An evaluation of training strategies for rehabilitated horses. *Appl. Anim. Behav. Sci.* 112:357–368.

1115 Inselman-Temkin, B. R., & J. P. Flynn. 1973. Sex-dependent effects of gonadal and gonadotropic hormones on centrally-elicited attack in cats. *Brain Res.* 60:393–410.

1116 Irwin, M. R., D. R. Melendy, M. S. Amoss, & D. P. Hutcheson. 1979. Roles of predisposing factors and gonadal hormones in the Buller syndrome of feedlot steers. *J. Am. Vet. Med. Assoc.* 174:367–370.

1117 **Ishiwata, T., K. Uetake, R. J. Kilgour, Y. Eguchi, & T. Tanaka. 2007. Oral behaviors of beef steers in pen and pasture environments. *J. Appl. Anim. Welf. Sci.* 10:185–192.**

1118 Izard, M. K., & J. G. Vandenbergh. 1982. Priming pheromones from oestrous cows increase synchronization of oestrus in dairy heifers after PGF-2 alpha injection. *J. Reprod. Fertil.* 66:189–196.

1119 Jackson, B., & A. Reed. 1969. Catnip and the alteration of consciousness. *JAMA* 207:1349–1350.

1120 Jackson, B., & D. W. Robinson. 1971. Evidence of hypothalamic a and b adrenergic receptors involved in the control of food intake of the pig. *Br. Vet. J.* 127:li–liii.

1121 Jackson, S. A., R. A. Rich, & S. L. Ralston. 1984. Feeding behavior and feed efficiency in groups of horses as a function of feeding frequency and use of alfafa hay cubes. *J. Anim. Sci.* 1:152–153.

1122 Jacobs, L. N., E. A. Staiger, J. D. Albright, & S. A. Brooks. 2016. The MC1R and ASIP coat color loci may impact behavior in the horse. *J. Hered.* 107(3):214–219.

1123 Jago, J. G., C. C. Krohn, & L. R. Matthews. 1999. The influence of feeding and handling on the development of the human-animal interactions in young cattle. *Appl. Anim. Behav. Sci.* 62:137–151.

1124 Jago, J. G., N. R. Cox, J. J. Bass, & L. R. Matthews. 1997. The effect of prepubertal immunization against gonadotropin-releasing hormone on the development of sexual and social behavior of bulls. *J. Anim. Sci.* 75:2609–2619.

1125 Jakovcevic, A., A. Mustaca, & M. Bentosela. 2012. Do more sociable dogs gaze longer to the human face than less sociable ones? *Behav. Processes.* 90:217–222.

1126 Jalowiec, J. E., J. Panksepp, H. Shabshelowitz, A. J. Zolovick, W. Stern, & P. J. Morgane. 1973. Suppression of feeding in cats following 2 deoxy D glucose. *Physiol. Behav.* 10:805–807.

1127 James, W. T., & T. F. Gilbert. 1955. The effect of social facilitation on food intake of puppies fed separately and together for the first 90 days of life. *Br. J. Anim. Behav.* 3:131–133.

1128 Janczak, A. M., L. J. Pederson, & M. Bakken. 2003. Aggression, fearfullness and coping styles in female pigs. *Appl. Anim. Behav. Sci.* 81:13–28.

1129 Janczarek, I., & W. Kedzierski. 2011. Emotional response to novelty and to expectation of novelty in young race horses. *Equine Vet. J.* 31:549–554.

1130 Janczarek, I., A. Stachurska, W. Kedzierski, & I. Wilk. 2013. Responses of horses of various breeds to a sympathetic training method. *Equine Vet. J.* 33:794–801.

1131 Jankunis, E. S., & I. Q. Whishaw. 2013. Sucrose bobs and quinine gapes: Horse (*Equus caballus*) responses to taste support phylogenetic similarity in taste reactivity. *Behav. Brain Res.* 256:284–290.

1132 Janowitz, H. D., & M. I. Grossman. 1949. Effect of variations in nutritive density on intake of food of dogs and rats. *Am. J. Physiol.* 158:184–193.

1133 Janowitz, H. D., & M. I. Grossman. 1949. Some factors affecting the food intake of normal dogs and dogs with esophagostomy and gastric fistula. *Am. J. Physiol.* 159:143–148.

1134 Jansen, J., J. E. Bolhuis, W. G. P. Schouten, B. M. Spruijt, & V. M. Wiegant. 2009. Spatial learning in pigs: Effects of environmental enrichment and individual characteristics on behaviour and performance. *Anim. Cogn.* 12:303–315.

1135 Jarvis, A. M., & M. S. Cockram. 1995. Some factors affecting resting behaviour of sheep in slaughterhouse lairages after transport from farms. *Anim. Welf.* 4:53–60.

1136 Jensen, M. B. 1999. Adaptation to tethering in yearling dairy heifers assessed by the use of lying down

behaviour. *Appl. Anim. Behav. Sci.* 62:115–123.

1137 Jensen, M. B., K. S. Vestergaard, & C. C. Krohn. 1998. Play behaviour in dairy calves kept in pens: The effect of social contact and space allowance. *Appl. Anim. Behav. Sci.* 56:97–108.

1138 Jensen, M. B., K. S. Vestergaard, C. C. Krohn, & L. Munksgaard. 1997. Effect of single versus group housing and space allowance on responses of calves during open-field tests. *Appl. Anim. Behav. Sci.* 54:109–121.

1139 Jensen, P. 1980. An ethogram of social interaction patterns in grouphoused dry sows. *Appl. Anim. Ethol.* 6:341–350.

1140 Jensen, P. 1984. Effects of confinement on social interaction patters in dry sows. *Appl. Anim. Behav. Sci.* 12:93–101.

1141 Jensen, P. 1986. Observations on the maternal behavior of freeranging domestic pigs. *Appl. Anim. Behav. Sci.* 16:131–142.

1142 Jensen, P. 1993. Nest building in domestic sows: The role of external stimuli. *Anim. Behav.* 45:351–358.

1143 Jensen, P., & J. Yngvesson. 1998. Aggression between unacquainted pigs – sequential assessment and effects of familiarity and weight. *Appl. Anim. Behav. Sci.* 58:49–61.

1144 Jensen, P., G. Stangel, & B. Algers. 1991. Nursing and suckling behaviour of semi-naturally kept pigs during the first 10 days postpartum. *Appl. Anim. Behav. Sci.* 31:195–209.

1145 Jensen, P., K. Floren, & B. Hobroh. 1987. Peri-parturient changes in behaviour in free-ranging domestic pigs. *Appl. Anim. Behav. Sci.* 17:69–76.

1146 Jensen, T. L., F. D. Provenza, & J. J. Villalba. 2013. Influence of diet sequence on intake of foods containing ergotamine D tartrate, tannins and saponins by sheep. *Appl. Anim. Behav. Sci.* 144:57–62.

1147 Jeppesen, L. E. 1982. Teat-order in groups of piglets reared on an artificial sow.

I. Formation of teat-order and influence of milk yield on teat preference. *Appl. Anim. Ethol.* 8:335–345.

1148 Jeppesen, L. E. 1982. Teat-order in groups of piglets reared on an artificial sow. II. Maintenance of teat-order with some evidence for the use of odour cues. *Appl. Anim. Ethol.* 8:347–355.

1149 Jewell, P. A., S. J. Hall, & M. M. Rosenberg. 1986. Multiple mating and siring success during natural oestrus in the ewe. *J. Reprod. Fertil.* 77:81–89.

1150 Jezierski, T., Z. Jaworski, & A. Gorecka. 1999. Effects of handling on behaviour and heart rate in konik horses: Comparison of stable and forest reared youngstock. *Appl. Anim. Behav. Sci.* 62:1–11.

1151 Jimenez-Severiano, H., J. Quintal-Franco, V. Vega-Murillo, E. Zanella, M. E. Wehrman, B. R. Lindsey, E. J. Melvin, & J. E. Kinder. 2003. Season of the year influences testosterone secretion in bulls administered luteinizing hormone. *J. Anim. Sci.* 81:1023–1029.

1152 John, E. R., P. Chesler, F. Bartlett, & I. Victor. 1968. Observation learning in cats. *Science* 159:1489–1491.

1153 Johnson, A., W. Engelmann, B. Pflug, & W. Klemke. 1980. Influence of lithium ions on human circadian rhythms. *Z. Naturforsch.* 35:503–507.

1154 Johnson, B. F., & C. Chura. 1974. Diurnal variation in the effect of tolbutamide. *Am. J. Med. Sci.* 268:93–96.

1155 Johnstone-Wallace, D. B., & K. Kennedy. 1944. Grazing management practices and their relationship to the behaviour and grazing habits of cattle. *J. Agric. Sci.* 34:190–197.

1156 Joly-Mascheroni, R. M., A. Senju, & A. J. Shepherd. 2008. Dogs catch human yawns. *Biol. Lett.* 4:446–448.

1157 Jones, A. C., & S. D. Gosling. 2005. Temperament and personality in dogs (canis familiaris): A review and evaluation of past research. *Appl. Anim. Behav. Sci.* 95:1–53.

1158 Jones, C. G., K. D. Maddever, D. L. Court, & M. Phillips. 1966. The time taken by cows to eat concentrates. *Anim. Prod.* 8:489–497.

1159 **Jones, J. B., N. L. Carmichael, C. M. Wathes, R. P. White, & R. B. Jones. 2000. The effects of acute simultaneous exposure to ammonia on the detection of buried odourized food by pigs. *Appl. Anim. Behav. Sci.* 65:305–319.**

1160 Jongman, E. C., I. Bidstrup, & P. H. Hemsworth. 2005. Behavioural and physiological measures of welfare of pregnant mares fitted with a novel urine collection device. *Appl. Anim. Behav. Sci.* 93:147–163.

1161 Jorgensen, G. H. M., I. L. Andersen, & K. E. Boe. 2007. Feed intake and social interactions in dairy goats: The effects of feeding space and type of roughage. *Appl. Anim. Behav. Sci.* 107:239–251.

1162 Jorgensen, G. H. M., I. L. Andersen, & K. E. Boe. 2009. The effect of different pen partition configurations on the behaviour of sheep. *Appl. Anim. Behav. Sci.* 119:66–70.

1163 Jorgensen, G., & K. Boe. 2007. A note on the effect of daily exercise and paddock size on the behaviour of domestic horses (*Equus caballus*). *Appl. Anim. Behav. Sci.* 107:166–173.

1164 **Juarbe-Diaz, S. V., & K. A. Houpt. 1996. Comparison of two antibarking collars for treatment of nuisance barking. *J. Am. Anim. Hosp. Assoc.* 32:231–235.**

1165 Juarbe-Diaz, S. V., K. A. Houpt, & R. Kusunose. 1998. Prevalence and characteristics of foal rejection in Arabian mares. *Equine Vet. J.* 30:424–428.

1166 Kalums, H. 1955. The discrimination by the nose of the dog of individual human odours and in particular of the odours of twins. *Br. J. Anim. Behav.* 3:25–31.

1167 Kaminski, J., J. Call, & J. Fischer. 2004. Word learning in a domestic dog: Evidence for "fast mapping." *Science* 304:1682–1683.

1168 Kaminski, J., J. Fischer, & J. Call. 2008. Prospective object search in dogs: Mixed evidence for knowledge of what and where. *Anim. Cogn.* 11:367–371.

1169 Kaminski, J., J. Riedel, J. Call, & M. Tomasello. 2005. Domestic goats, *Capra hircus*, follow gaze direction and use social cues in an object choice task. *Anim. Behav.* 69:11–18.

1170 Kaminski, J., M. Neumann, J. Bräuer, J. Call, & M. Tomasello. 2011. Dogs, *Canis familiaris*, communicate with humans to request but not to inform. *Anim. Behav.* 82:651–658.

1171 Kaminski, J., M. Nitzschner, V. Wobber, C. Tennie, J. Bräuer, J. Call, & M. Tomasello. 2011. Do dogs distinguish rational from irrational acts? *Anim. Behav.* 81:195–203.

1172 Kanarck, R. B. 1975. Availability and caloric density of the diet as determinants of meal patterns in cats. *Physiol. Behav.* 15:611–618.

1173 Kanitz, E., T. Hameister, M. Tuchscherer, A. Tuchscherer, & B. Puppe. 2014. Social support attenuates the adverse consequences of social deprivation stress in domestic piglets. *Horm. Behav.* 65:203–210.

1174 Kanno, Y. 1977. Experimental studies on body temperature rhythm in dogs. I. Application of cosinor method to body temperature rhythm in dogs (author's transl). *Nippon Juigaku Zasshi* 39:69–76.

1175 Karagiannis, C. I., O. H. P. Burman, & D. S. Mills. 2015. Dogs with separation-related problems show a "less pessimistic" cognitive bias during treatment with fluoxetine (Reconcile™) and a behaviour modification plan. *BMC Vet. Res.* 11:80.

1176 Karas, G. G., R. I. Willham, & D. F. Cox. 1962. *Avoidance learning in swine. Psychol. Rep.* 11:51–54.

1177 Kare, M. R., W. C. Pond, & J. Campbell. 1965. Observations on the taste reactions in pigs. *Anim. Behav.* 13:265–269.

1178 Karlander, S., J. Mansson, & G. Tufvesson. 1965. Buccostomy as a method of treatment for arcophagia (windsucking) in the horse. *Nordisk Vet.-Med.* 17:455–458.

1179 Karn, H. W., & H. R. Malamud. 1939. The behavior of dogs on the double alternation problem in the temporal maze. *J. Comp. Psychol.* 27:461–466.

1180 Karn, J. F., & D. C. Clanton. 1974. Electronically controlled individual cattle feeding. *J. Anim. Sci.* 39:136.

1181 Karsh, E. B., & D. C. Turner. 1988. The human-cat relationship. In D. C. Turner, & P. Bateson (Eds.), *The domestic cat*, pp. 159–177. Cambridge, UK: Cambridge University Press.

1182 Kaseda, Y., & A. M. Khalil. 1996. Harem size and reproductive success of stallions in misaki feral horses. *Appl. Anim. Behav. Sci.* 47:163–174.

1183 Kasper, M., & A. M. Beck. 1997. Effect of environmental temperature on the behavior of clydesdales during preparation time before athletic performances. *Equine Pract.* 19:25–28.

1184 Katz, L. S., E. O. Price, S. J. Wallach, & J. J. Zenchak. 1988. Sexual performance of rams reared with or without females after weaning. *J. Anim. Sci.* 66:1166–1173.

1185 Kaulfuss, P., & D. S. Mills. 2008. Neophilia in domestic dogs (*Canis familiaris*) and its implication for studies of dog cognition. *Anim. Cogn.* 11:553–556.

1186 Kay, R., & C. Hall. 2009. The use of a mirror reduces isolation stress in horses being transported by trailer. *Appl. Anim. Behav. Sci.* 116:237–243.

1187 Kedzierski, W., I. Janczarek, & A. Stachurska. 2012. Emotional response of naive purebred Arabian colts and fillies to sympathetic and traditional training methods. *Equine Vet. J.* 32:752–756.

1188 Keil, N. M., & W. Langhans. 2001. The development of intersucking in dairy calves around weaning. *Appl. Anim. Behav. Sci.* 72:295–308.

1189 Keil, N. M., S. Imfeld-Mueller, J. Aschwanden, & B. Wechsler. 2012. Are head cues necessary for goats (*Capra hircus*) in recognizing group members? *Anim. Cogn.* 15:913–921.

1190 Keiper, R. R. 1976. Social organization of feral ponies. *Proc. Penn. Acad. Sci.* 50:69–70.

1191 **Keiper, R. R. 1985. *The assateague ponies*. Centreville, MD: Tidewater Press.**

1192 Keiper, R. R., & H. H. Sambraus. 1986. The stability of equine dominance hierarchies and the effects of kinship, proximity and foaling status on hierarchy rank. *Appl. Anim. Behav. Sci.* 16:121–130.

1193 **Keiper, R. R., & H. Receveur. 1992. Social interactions of free-ranging Przewalski horses in semi-reserves in the Netherlands. *Appl. Anim. Behav. Sci.* 33:303–318.**

1194 Keiper, R. R., & J. Berger. 1982. Refuge-seeking and pest avoidance by feral horses in desert and island environments. *Appl. Anim. Ethol.* 9:111–120.

1195 Keiper, R. R., & K. A. Houpt. 1984. Reproduction in feral horses: An eight-year study. *Am. J. Vet. Res.* 45:991–995.

1196 Kendrick, K. M., & B. A. Baldwin. 1987. Cells in temporal cortex of conscious sheep can respond preferentially to the sight of faces. *Science.* 236:448.

1197 Kendrick, K. M., & E. B. Keverne. 1991. Importance of progesterone and estrogen priming for the induction of maternal behavior by vaginocervical stimulation in sheep: Effects of maternal experience. *Physiol. Behav.* 49:745–750.

1198 **Kendrick, K. M., A. P. da Costa, A. E. Leigh, M. R. Hinton, & J. W. Peirce. 2001. Sheep don't forget a face. *Nature* 414:165–166.**

1199 Kendrick, K. M., E. B. Keverne, & B. A. Baldwin. 1987. Intracerebroventricular oxytocin stimulates maternal behaviour in the sheep. *Neuroendocrinology* 46:56–61.

1200 Kendrick, K. M., E. B. Keverne, B. A. Baldwin, & D. F. Sharman. 1986. Cerebrospinal fluid levels of acetylcholinesterase, monoamines and oxytocin during labour, parturition, vaginocervical stimulation, lamb separation and suckling in sheep. *Neuroendocrinology* 44:149–156.

1201 Kendrick, K. M., K. Atkins, M. R. Hinton, K. B. Broad, C. Fabre-Nys, & E. B. Keverne. 1995. Facial and vocal discrimination in sheep. *Anim. Behav.* 49:1665–1676.

1202 Kennedy, J. M., & B. A. Baldwin. 1972. Taste preferences in pigs for nutritive and non-nutritive sweet solutions. *Anim. Behav.* 20:706–718.

1203 **Kenny, F. J., & P. V. Tarrant. 1987. The behaviour of young Friesian bulls during social re-grouping at an abattoir: Influence of an overhead electrified wire grid. *Appl. Anim. Behav. Sci.* 18:233–246.**

1204 Kent, J. P. 1984. A note on multiple fostering of calves onto nurse cows at a few days post-partum. *Appl. Anim. Behav. Sci.* 12:183–186.

1205 Kerruish, B. M. 1955. The effect of sexual stimulation prior to service on the behaviour and conception rate of bulls. *Br. J. Anim. Behav.* 3:125–130.

1206 Keverne, E. B., F. Levy, P. Poindron, & D. R. Lindsay. 1983. Vaginal stimulation: An important determinant of maternal bonding in sheep. *Science* 219:81–83.

1207 Key, C., & R. M. MacIver. 1977. Factors affecting sexual preferences in sheep. *Appl. Anim. Ethol.* 3:291.

1208 Khalil, A. M., & N. Murakami. 1999. Effect of natal dispersal on the reproductive strategies of the young misaki feral stallions. *Appl. Anim. Behav. Sci.* 62:281–291.

1209 Khalil, A. M., & Y. Kaseda. 1997. Behavioral patterns and proximate reason of young male separation in misaki feral horses. *Appl. Anim. Behav. Sci.* 54:281–289.

1210 Kiddy, C. A., D. S. Mitchell, D. J. Bolt, & H. W. Hawk. 1978. Detection of estrus-related odors in cows by trained dogs. *Biol. Reprod.* 19:389–395.

1211 Kiley, M. 1972. The vocalizations of ungulates, their causation and function. *Z. Tierpsychol.* 31:171–222.

1212 Kiley, M. 1976. Fostering and adoption in beef cattle. *Br. Cattle Breeders Club Dig.* 31:42–55.

1213 Kiley-Worthington, M. 1976. The tail movements of ungulates, canids and felids with particular reference to their causation and function as displays. *Behaviour* 56:69–115.

1214 **Kiley-Worthington, M. 1977.** ***Behavioural problems of farm animals.*** **Stocksfield, UK: Oriel Press.**

1215 Kiley-Worthington, M., & P. Savage. 1978. Learning in dairy cattle using a device for economical management of behaviour. *Appl. Anim. Ethol.* 4:119–124.

1216 Kilgour, R. 1972. Some observations on the suckling activity of calves on nurse cows. *N.Z. Soc. Anim. Prod.* 32:132–136.

1217 Kilgour, R. 1981. Use of the Hebb-Williams closed-field test to study the learning ability of Jersey cows. *Anim. Behav.* 29:850–860.

1218 Kilgour, R. J., G. J. Melville, & P. L. Greenwood. 2006. Individual differences in the reaction of beef cattle to situations involving social isolation, close proximity of humans, restraint and novelty. *Appl. Anim. Behav. Sci.* 99:21–40.

1219 Kilgour, R., & C. G. Winfield. 1977. Pen-mating of pedigree sheep. *N.Z. J. Agric.* 134:25–27.

1220 Kilgour, R., & D. N. Campin. 1973. The behaviour of entire bulls of different ages at pasture. *Proc. N.Z. Soc. Anim. Prod.* 33:125–138.

1221 Kilgour, R., & T. H. Scott. 1959. Leadership in a herd of dairy cows. *Proc. N.Z. Soc. Anim. Prod.* 19:36–43.

1222 Kilgour, R., B. H. Skarsholt, J. F. Smith, K. J. Bremmer, & M. C. L. Morrison. 1977. Observations on the behaviour and factors influencing the sexually-active group in cattle. *Proc. N.Z.Soc. Anim. Prod.* 37:128–135.

1223 Kilgour, R., C. G. Winfield, K. J. Bremmer, M. M. Mullord, H. de Langen, & S. J. Hudson. 1976. Behaviour of early-weaned calves in indoor individual cubicles and group pens. *N.Z. Vet. J.* 23:119–123.

1224 **Kim, F. B., R. E. Jackson, G. D. Gordon, & M. S. Cockram. 1994. Resting behaviour of sheep in a slaughterhouse lairage.** ***Appl. Anim. Behav. Sci.*** **40:45–54.**

1225 Kimball, B. A., F. D. Provenza, & E. A. Burritt. 2002. Importance of alternative foods on the persistence of flavor aversions: Implications for applied flavor avoidance learning. *Appl. Anim. Behav. Sci.* 76:249–258.

1226 King, J. E., B. A. Becker, & J. E. Markee. 1964. Studies on olfactory discrimination in dogs: (3) Ability to detect human odour trace. *Anim. Behav.* 12:311–315.

1227 **King, S. R. B., & J. Gurnell. 2010. Effects of fly disturbance on the behaviour of a population of reintroduced Przewalski horses (*Equus ferus Przewalskii*) in Mongolia.** ***Appl. Anim. Behav. Sci.*** **125:22–29.**

1228 King, T., P. H. Hemsworth, & G. J. Coleman. 2003. Fear of novel and startling stimuli in domestic dogs. *Appl. Anim. Behav. Sci.* 82:45–64.

1229 Kirkpatrick, J. F., R. Vail, S. Devous, S. Schwend, C. B. Baker, & L. Wiesner. 1976. Diurnal variation of plasma testosterone in wild stallions. *Biol. Reprod.* 15:98–101.

1230 Kirkwood, R. N., J. M. Forbes, & P. E. Hughes. 1981. Influence of boar contact on attainment of puberty in gilts after removal of the olfactory bulbs. *J. Reprod. Fertil.* 61:193–196.

1231 Kitchell, R. L. 1972. Dogs know what they like. *Friskies Res. Dig.* 8:1–4.

1232 Klemm, W. R., C. J. Sherry, L. M. Schake, & R. F. Sis. 1983. Homosexual behavior in feedlot steers: An aggression hypothesis. *Appl. Anim. Ethol.* 11:187–195.

1233 Kling, A., & D. Coustan. 1964. Electrical stimulation of the amygdala and hypothalamus in the kitten. *Exp. Neurol.* 10:81–89.

1234 Kling, A., J. K. Kovach, & T. J. Tucker. 1969. The behaviour of cats. In E. S. E. Hafez (Ed.), *The behaviour of domestic animals*, pp. 482–512. Baltimore, MD: Williams & Wilkins.

1235 Klingel, H. 1974. A comparison of the social behaviour of the equidae. In V. Geist, & F. Walther (Eds.), *The behaviour of ungulates and its relation to management*. Morges, Switzerland: International Union for Conservation of Nature and Natural Resources.

1236 Klopfer, F. D. 1961. Early experience and discrimination learning in swine. *Am. Zool.* 1:366.

1237 Klopfer, F. D. 1966. Visual learning in swine. In L. K. Bustad, R. O. McClellan, & M. P. Burns (Eds.), *Swine in biomedical research*. Richland, WA: Battelle Memorial Institute Pacific Northwest Laboratory.

1238 Klopfer, F. D., & J. Gamble. 1966. Maternal "imprinting" on goats: The role of chemical senses. *Z. Tierpsychol.* 23:588–592.

1239 **Knecht, C. D., J. E. Oliver, R. Redding, R. Selcer, & G. Johnson. 1973. Narcolepsy in a dog and a cat. *J. Am. Vet. Med. Assoc.* 162:1052–1053.**

1240 Knight, T. W., & P. R. Lynch. 1980. Source of ram pheromones that stimulate ovulation in the ewe. *Anim. Reprod. Sci.* 3:133–136.

1241 Knowles, R. J., T. M. Curtis, & S. L. Crowell-Davis. 2004. Correlation of dominance as determined by agonistic interactions with feeding order in cats. *Am. J. Vet. Res.* 65:1548–1556.

1242 Koba, Y., & H. Tanida. 2001. How do miniature pigs discriminate between people? Discrimination between people wearing coveralls of the same colour. *Appl. Anim. Behav. Sci.* 73:45–58.

1243 Kobelt, A. J., P. H. Hemsworth, J. L. Barnett, G. J. Coleman, & K. L. Butler. 2007. The behaviour of labrador retrievers in suburban backyards: The relationships between the backyard environment and dog behaviour. *Appl. Anim. Behav. Sci.* 106:70–84.

1244 Koepke, J. E., & K. H. Pribram. 1971. Effect of milk on the maintenance of sucking behavior in kittens from birth to six months. *J. Comp. Physiol. Psychol.* 75:363–377.

1245 Kohari, D., S. Sato, & Y. Nakai. 2009. Does the maternal grooming of cattle clean bacteria from the coat of calves? *Behav. Processes.* 80:202–204.

1246 Kohn, F., A. R. Sharifi, & H. Simianer. 2009. Genetic analysis of reactivity to humans in Goettingen minipigs. *Appl. Anim. Behav. Sci.* 120:68–75.

1247 Kolb, B., & A. J. Nonneman. 1975. The development of social responsiveness in kittens. *Anim. Behav.* 23:368–374.

1248 Kondo, S., & J. F. Hurnik. 1990. Stabilization of social hierarchy in dairy cows. *Appl. Anim. Behav. Sci.* 57:287–297.

1249 **Kondo, S., N. Kawakami, H. Kohama, & S. Nishino. 1983. Changes in activity spatial pattern and social behavior in calves after grouping. *Appl. Anim. Ethol.* 11:217–228.**

1250 Kongsted, A. G., J. E. Hermansen, & T. Kristensen. 2007. Relation between parity and feed intake, fear of humans, and social behaviour in non-lactating sows group-housed under various on-farm conditions. *Anim. Welf.* 16:263–266.

1251 Konrad, K. W., & M. Bagshaw. 1970. Effect of novel stimuli on cats reared in a restricted environment. *J. Comp. Physiol. Psychol.* 70:157–164.

1252 **Kooij, E. V. E. D., A. H. Kuijpers, J. W. Schrama, F. J. C. M. van Eerdenburg, W. G. P. Schouten, & M. J. M. Tielen. 2002. Can we predict**

behaviour in pigs? Searching for consistency in behaviour over time and across situations. *Appl. Anim. Behav. Sci.* 75:293–305.

1253 Koopmans, S. J., M. Ruis, R. Dekker, H. van Diepen, M. Korte, & Z. Mroz. 2005. Surplus dietary tryptophan reduces plasma cortisol and noradrenaline concentrations and enhances recovery after social stress in pigs. *Physiol. Behav.* 85:469–478.

1254 Korda, K. W., & M. Bagshaw. 1977. Effect of stimuli emitted by sucklings on tactile contact of the bitches with sucklings and on number of licking acts. *Acta Neurobiol.* 37:99–115.

1255 Koscinczuk, P., M. N. Alabarcez, & R. P. Cainzos. 2015. Social play traits and environmental exploration in beagle and fox terriers' puppies. *Rev. Vet.* 26:1.

1256 Kouwenberg, A., C. J. Walsh, B. E. Morgan, & G. M. Martin. 2009. Episodic-like memory in crossbred Yucatan minipigs (*Sus scrofa*). *Appl. Anim. Behav. Sci.* 117:165–172.

1257 Kovach, J. K., & A. Kling. 1967. Mechanisms of neonate sucking behaviour in the kitten. *Anim. Behav.* 15:91–101.

1258 Kovalcik, K., & M. Kovalcik. 1986. Learning ability and memory testing in cattle of different ages. *Appl. Anim. Behav. Sci.* 15:27–29.

1259 Krabill, L. F., P. J. Wangsness, & C. A. Baile. 1978. Effects of elfazepam on digestibility and feeding behavior in sheep. *J. Anim. Sci.* 46:1356–1359.

1260 **Kranendonk, G., H. Van der Mheen, M. Fillerup, & H. Hopster. 2007. Social rank of pregnant sows affects their body weight gain and behavior and performance of the offspring. *J. Anim. Sci.* 85:420–429.**

1261 Kratzer, D. D. 1969. Effects of age on avoidance learning in pigs. *J. Anim. Sci.* 28:175–179.

1262 Kratzer, D. D., W. M. Netherland, R. E. Pulse, & J. P. Baker. 1977. Maze learning in quarter horses. *J. Anim. Sci.* 45:896–902.

1263 **Kraus, C., C. van Waveren, & F. Huebner. 2014. Distractible dogs, constant cats? A test of the distraction hypothesis in two domestic species. *Anim. Behav.* 93:173–181.**

1264 Krauss, V., & S. Hoy. 2011. Dry sows in dynamic groups: An investigation of social behaviour when introducing new sows. *Appl. Anim. Behav. Sci.* 130:20–27.

1265 Krawczel, P. D., T. H. Friend, & R. Johnson. 2006. A note on the preference of naive horses for different water bowls. *Appl. Anim. Behav. Sci.* 100:309–313.

1266 **Krebs, J. R., & N. B. Davies. 1978. *Behavioural ecology: An evolutionary approach*. Sunderland, MA: Sinauer Associates.**

1267 Kristal, M. B., A. C. Thompson, S. B. Heller, & B. R. Komisaruk. 1986. Placenta ingestion enhances analgesia produced by vaginal/cervical stimulation in rats. *Physiol. Behav.* 36:1017–1020.

1268 Kristula, M. A., & S. M. McDonnell. 1994. Drinking water temperature affects consumption of water during cold weather in ponies. *Appl. Anim. Behav. Sci.* 41:155–160.

1269 Krohn, C. C., & L. Munksgaard. 1993. Behaviour of dairy cows kept in extensive (loose housing/pasture) or intensive (tie stall) environments. II. Lying and lying-down behaviour. *Appl. Anim. Behav. Sci.* 37:1–16.

1270 Krohn, C. C., J. G. Jago, & X. Boivin. 2001. The effect of early handling on the socialisation of young calves to humans. *Appl. Anim. Behav. Sci.* 74:121–133.

1271 Kronberg, S. L., R. B. Muntifering, & E. L. Ayers. 1993. Feed aversion learning in cattle with delayed negative consequences. *J. Anim. Sci.* 71:1767–1770.

1272 Krueger, K., & B. Flauger. 2011. Olfactory recognition of individual competitors by means of faeces in horse (*Equus caballus*). *Anim. Cogn.* 14:245–257.

1273 Krueger, K. 2007. Behaviour of horses in the "round pen technique." *Appl. Anim. Behav. Sci.* 104:162–170.

1274 Krueger, K., B. Flauger, K. Farmer, & C. Hemelrijk. 2014. Movement initiation in groups of feral horses. *Behav. Processes.* 103:91–101.

1275 **Krueger, K., B. Flauger, K. Farmer, & K. Maros. 2011. Horses (*Equus caballus*) use human local enhancement cues and adjust to human attention. *Anim. Cogn.* 14:187–201.**

1276 Krueger, K., G. Schneider, B. Flauger, & J. Heinze. 2015. Context-dependent third-party intervention in agonistic encounters of male Przewalski horses. *Behav. Processes.* 121:54–62.

1277 Krueger, K., K. Farmer, & J. Heinze. 2014. The effects of age, rank and neophobia on social learning in horses. *Anim. Cogn.* 17:645–655.

1278 Kry, K., & R. Casey. 2007. The effect of hiding enrichment on stress levels and behaviour of domestic cats (*Felis sylvestris catus*) in a shelter setting and the implications for adoption potential. *Anim. Welf.* 16:375–383.

1279 Krzak, W. E., H. W. Gonyou, & L. M. Lawrence. 1991. Wood chewing by stabled horses: Diurnal pattern and effects of exercise. *J. Anim. Sci.* 69:1053–1058.

1280 Kubinyi, E., J. Vas, K. Hejjas, Z. Ronai, I. Brúder, B. Turcsán, M. Sasvari-Szekely, & Á. Miklósi. 2012. Polymorphism in the tyrosine hydroxylase (TH) gene is associated with activity-impulsivity in German shepherd dogs. *PLoS ONE.* 7(1):e30271.

1281 Kuhn, G., & W. Hardegg. 1988. Effects of indoor and outdoor maintenance of dogs upon food intake, body weight, and different blood parameters. *Z. Versuchstierkd.* 31:205–214.

1282 Kuhne, F., J. C. Hößler, & R. Struwe. 2012. Effects of human-dog familiarity on dogs' behavioural responses to petting. *Appl. Anim. Behav. Sci.* 142:176–181.

1283 Kuipers, M., & T. S. Whatson. 1979. Sleep in piglets: An observational study. *Appl. Anim. Ethol.* 5:145–151.

1284 Kuntz, R., C. Kubalek, T. Ruf, F. Tataruch, & W. Arnold. 2006. Seasonal adjustment of energy budget in a large wild mammal, the przewalski horse (*Equus ferus przewalskii*) I. Energy intake. *J. Exp. Biol.* 209:4557–4565.

1285 **Kuo, Z. Y. 1930. The genesis of the cat's responses to the rat. *J. Comp. Psychol.* 11:1–35.**

1286 Kurz, J. C., & R. L. Marchinton. 1972. Radiotelemetry studies of feral hogs in south Carolina. *J. Wildl. Manag.* 36:1240–1248.

1287 Kusunose, R. 1992. Diurnal pattern of cribbing in stabled horses. *Jpn. J. Equine Sci.* 3:173–176.

1288 Kusunose, R. H., H. Hatakeyama, F. Ichikawa, H. Oki, Y. Asai, & K. Ito. 1987. Behavioral studies on yearling horses in field environments 3. Effects of the pasture shape on the behavior of horses. *Bull. Equine Res. Ins.* 24:1–5.

1289 Kusunose, R. H., H. Hatakeyama, F. Ichikawa, K. Kubo, A. Kiguchi, Y. Asai, & K. Ito. 1986. Behavioural studies on yearling horses in field environments 2. Effects of the group size on the behavior of horses. *Bull. Equine Res. Ins.* 23:1–6.

1290 Kusunose, R. H., H. Hatakeyama, K. Kubo, A. Kiguchi, Y. Asai, Y. Fujii, & K. Ito. 1985. Behavioral studies on yearling horses in field environments 1. Effects of the field size on the behavior of horses. *Bull. Equine Res. Ins.* 22:1–7.

1291 Kusunose, R., & A. Yamanobe. 2002. The effect of training schedule on learned tasks in yearling horses. *Appl. Anim. Behav. Sci.* 78:225–233.

1292 Kusunose, R., & H. Sawazaki. 1984. The behavioral development of thoroughbred foals and the relationship between dams and foals. *Jap. J. Zootech.* 55:263–271.

1293 **Kusunose, R., & K. Torikai. 1996. Behavior of untethered horses during vehicle transport. *J. Eq. Sci.* 7:21–26.**

1294 Laca, E. A., E. D. Ungar, & M. W. Demment. 1994. Mechanisms of handling time and intake rate of a large mammalian grazer. *Appl. Anim. Behav. Sci.* 39:3–19.

1295 Ladewig, J., & B. L. Hart. 1980. Flehmen and vomeronasal organ function in male goats. *Physiol. Behav.* 24:1067–1071.

1296 Lagerweij, E., P. C. Nelis, V. M. Wiegant, & J. M. van Ree. 1984. The twitch in horses: A variant of acupuncture. *Science* 225:1172–1174.

1297 Laister, S., B. Stockinger, A.-M. Regner, K. Zenger, U. Knierim, & C. Winckler. 2011. Social licking in dairy cattle: Effects on heart rate in performers and receivers. *Appl. Anim. Behav. Sci.* 130:81–90.

1298 Lammers, G. J., & A. De Lange. 1986. Pre- and post-farrowing behaviour in primiparous domesticated pigs. *Appl. Anim. Behav. Sci.* 15:31–43.

1299 Lampe, J. F., & J. Andre. 2012. Cross-modal recognition of human individuals in domestic horses (*Equus caballus*). *Anim. Cogn.* 15:623–630.

1300 Landau, S., N. Silanikove, Z. Nitsan, D. Barkai, H. Baram, F. D. Provenza, & A. Perevolotsky. 2000. Short-term changes in eating patterns explain the effects of condensed tannins on feed intake in heifers. *Appl. Anim. Behav. Sci.* 69:199–213.

1301 Landsberg, G. M. 1991. The distribution of canine behavior cases at three behavior referral practices. *Vet. Med.* 86:1011–1018.

1302 Landsberg, G. M., W. Hunthausen, & L. Ackerman. 2003. Handbook of behaviour problems of the dog and cat, 2nd ed. Philadelphia, PA: Elsevier Science.

1303 Langbein, J., K. Siebert, G. Nurnberg, & G. Manteuffel. 2007. Learning to learn during visual discrimination in group housed dwarf goats (*Capra hircus*). *J. Comp. Psychol.* 121:447–456.

1304 Lanier, J. L., T. Grandin, R. D. Green, D. Avery, & K. McGee. 2000. The relationship between reaction to sudden, intermittent movements and sounds and temperament. *J. Anim. Sci.* 78:1467–1474.

1305 Lanier, J. L., T. Grandin, R. Green, D. Avery, & K. McGee. 2001. A note on hair whorl position and cattle temperament in the auction ring. *Appl. Anim. Behav. Sci.* 73:93–101.

1306 Lansade, L., & F. Simon. 2010. Horses' learning performances are under the influence of several temperamental dimensions. *Appl. Anim. Behav. Sci.* 125(1–2):30–37.

1307 Lansade, L., & M. Bouissou. 2008. Reactivity to humans: A temperament trait of horses which is stable across time and situations. *Appl. Anim. Behav. Sci.* 114:492–508.

1308 Lansade, L., G. Pichard, & M. Leconte. 2008. Sensory sensitivities: Components of a horse's temperament dimension. *Appl. Anim. Behav. Sci.* 114:534–553.

1309 Lansade, L., M. Bouissou, & H. W. Erhard. 2008. Fearfulness in horses: A temperament trait stable across time and situations. *Appl. Anim. Behav. Sci.* 115:182–200.

1310 Lansade, L., M. Bertrand, & M. Bouissou. 2005. Effects of neonatal handling on subsequent manageability, reactivity and learning ability of foals. *Appl. Anim. Behav. Sci.* 92:143–158.

1311 Larose, C., M. A. Richard-Yris, M. Hausberger, & L. J. Rogers. 2006. Laterality of horses associated with emotionality in novel situations. *Laterality.* 11(4):355–367.

1312 Lauber, M. C. Y., P. H. Hemsworth, & J. L. Barnett. 2006. The effects of age and experience on behavioural development in dairy calves. *Appl. Anim. Behav. Sci.* 99:41–52.

1313 Launchbaugh, K. L., & F. D. Provenza. 1994. The effect of flavor concentration and toxin dose on the formation and generalization of flavor aversions in lambs. *J. Anim. Sci.* 72:10–13.

1314 Laundre, J. 1977. The daytime behavior of domestic cats in a free-roaming population. *Anim. Behav.* 25:990–998.

1315 Laut, J. E., K. A. Houpt, H. F. Hintz, & T. R. Houpt. 1985. The effects of caloric dilution on meal patterns and food intake of ponies. *Physiol. Behav.* 35:549–554.

1316 Lawrence, A. B. 1990. Mother-daughter and peer relationships of Scottish hill sheep. *Anim. Behav.* 39:481–486.

1317 Lawrence, A. B., J. C. Petherick, K. McLean, C. L. Gilbert, C. Chapman, & J. A. Russell. 1992. Naloxone prevents interruption of parturition and increases plasma oxytocin following environmental disturbance in parturient sows. *Physiol. Behav.* 52:917–923.

1318 Lawson, D. C., S. S. Shiffman, & T. N. Pappas. 1993. Short-term oral sensory deprivation: Possible cause of binge eating in sham-feeding dogs. *Physiol. Behav.* 53:1231–1234.

1319 Lay, D. C., Jr, M. F. Haussmann, H. S. Buchanan, & M. J. Daniels. 1999. Danger to pigs due to crushing can be reduced by the use of a simulated udder. *J. Anim. Sci.* 77:2060–2064.

1320 Lazarowski, L., M. L. Foster, M. E. Gruen, B. L. Sherman, B. C. Case, R. E. Fish, N. W. Milgram, & D. C. Dorman. 2014. Acquisition of a visual discrimination and reversal learning task by labrador retrievers. *Anim. Cogn.* 17(3):787–792.

1321 Lazo, A. 1994. Social segregation and the maintenance of social stability in a feral cattle population. *Anim. Behav.* 48:1133–1141.

1322 Le Boeuf, B. J. 1967. Interindividual associations in dogs. *Behaviour* 29:268–295.

1323 Le Boeuf, B. J. 1970. Copulatory and aggressive behavior in the prepuberally castrated dog. *Horm. Behav.* 1:127–136.

1324 Le Neindre, P., G. Trillat, J. Sapa, F. Menissier, J. N. Bonnet, & J. M. Chupin. 1995. Individual differences in docility in Limousin cattle. *J. Anim. Sci.* 73:2249–2253.

1325 Leal, B. B., G. E. S. Alves, R. H. Douglas, B. Bringel, R. J. Young, J. P. A. Haddad, W. S. Viana, & R. R. Faleiros. 2011. Cortisol circadian rhythm ratio: A simple method to detect stressed horses at higher risk of colic? *Equine Vet. J.* 31(4):188–190.

1326 Lecoq, L., M. Gains, L. Blond, & J. Parent. 2015. Brainstem auditory evoked responses in foals: Reference values, effect of age, rate of acoustic stimulation, and neurologic deficits. *J. Vet. Intern. Med.* 29(1):362–367.

1327 Lee, C., A. D. Fisher, I. G. Colditz, J. M. Lea, & D. M. Ferguson. 2013. Preference of beef cattle for feedlot or pasture environments. *Appl. Anim. Behav. Sci.* 145(3–4):53–59.

1328 Lee, C., A. D. Fisher, M. T. Reed, & J. M. Henshell. 2008. The effect of low energy electric shock on cortisol, *β-endorphin*, heart rate and behaviour of cattle. *Appl. Anim. Behav. Sci.* 113:32–42.

1329 Lee, C., J. M. Henshall, T. J. Wark, C. C. Crossman, M. T. Reed, H. G. Brewer, J. O'Grady, & A. D. Fisher. 2009. Associative learning by cattle to enable effective and ethical virtual fences. *Appl. Anim. Behav. Sci.* 119:15–22.

1330 Lee, C., K. C. Prayaga, A. D. Fisher, & J. M. Henshall. 2008. Behavioral aspects of electronic bull separation and mate allocation in multiple-sire mating paddocks. *J. Anim. Sci.* 86:1690–1696.

1331 Lee, C., K. Prayaga, M. Reed, & J. Henshall. 2007. Methods of training cattle to avoid a location using electrical cues. *Appl. Anim. Behav. Sci.* 108:229–238.

1332 Lee, C., S. Colegate, & A. D. Fisher. 2006. Development of a maze test and its application to assess spatial learning and memory in merino sheep. *Appl. Anim. Behav. Sci.* 96:43–51.

1333 Lee, J., K. A. Houpt, & O. Dogherty. 2001. A survey of trailering problems in horses. *J. Equine Vet. Sci.* 21:23–26.

1334 Lee, J., T. Floyd, H. Erb, & K. A. Houpt. 2011. Operant and two-choice preference applied to equine welfare. *Appl. Anim. Behav. Sci.* 130:91–100.

1335 Lees, J. L., & M. Weatherhead. 1970. A note on mating preferences of Clun forest ewes. *Anim. Prod.* 12:173–175.

1336 Lefebvre, D., C. Diederich, M. Delcourt, & J. Giffroy. 2007. The quality of the relation between handler and military dogs influences efficiency and welfare of dogs. *Appl. Anim. Behav. Sci.* 104:49–60.

1337 Lehmann, K., E. Kallweit, & F. Ellendorff. 2006. Social hierarchy in exercised and untrained group-house horses: A brief report. *Appl. Anim. Behav. Sci.* 96:343–347.

1338 Lehner, P. N., C. McCluggage, D. R. Mitchell, & D. H. Neil. 1983. Selected parameters of the Fort Collins, Colorado, dog population. *Appl. Anim. Ethol.* 10:19–25.

1339 Lemasson, A., A. Boutin, S. Boivin, C. Blois-Heulin, & M. Hausberger. 2009. Horse (*Equus caballus*) whinnies: A source of social information. *Anim. Cogn.* 12(5):693–704.

1340 Lemasson, A., K. Remeuf, M. Trabalon, F. Cuir, & M. Hausberger. 2015. Mares prefer the voices of highly fertile stallions. *PLoS ONE.* 10(2):e0118468.

1341 Lenhardt, M. L. 1977. Vocal contour cues in maternal recognition of goat kids. *Appl. Anim. Ethol.* 3:211–219.

1342 Lensink, B. J., S. Raussi, X. Boivin, M. Pyykkonen, & I. I. Veissier. 2001. Reactions of calves to handling depend on housing condition and previous experience with humans. *Appl. Anim. Behav. Sci.* 70:187–199.

1343 Lensink, J., I. Veissier, & A. Boissy. 2006. Enhancement of performances in a learning task in suckler calves after weaning and relocation: Motivational versus cognitive control? A pilot study. *Appl. Anim. Behav. Sci.* 100:171–181.

1344 León, M., B. Rosado, S. García-Belenguer, G. Chacón, A. Villegas, & J. Palacio. 2012. Assessment of serotonin in serum, plasma, and platelets of aggressive dogs. *J. Vet. Behav.* 7(6):348–352.

1345 Leonardi, R. J., S. J. Vick, & V. Dufour. 2012. Waiting for more: The performance of domestic dogs (*Canis familiaris*) on exchange tasks. *Anim. Cogn.* 15(1):107–120.

1346 Lesimple, C., C. Fureix, N. Lescolan, M.-A. Richard-Yris, & M. Hausberger. 2011. Housing conditions and breed are associated with emotionality and cognitive abilities in riding school horses. *Appl. Anim. Behav. Sci.* 129(2–4):92–99.

1347 Levine, A. S., C. E. Sievert, J. E. Morley, B. A. Gosnell, & S. E. Silvis. 1984. Peptidergic regulation of feeding in the dog (*Canis familiaris*). *Peptides* 5:675–679.

1348 Levine, E. D., D. Ramos, & D. S. Mills. 2007. A prospective study of two self-help CD based desensitization conditioning programmes with the use of dog appeasing pheromone for the treatment of firework fears in dogs (*Canis familiaris*). *Appl. Anim. Behav. Sci.* 105:311–329.

1349 Levine, E. D., H. N. Erb, B. Schoenherr, & K. A. Houpt. 2016. Owner's perception of changes in behaviors associated with dieting in fat cats. *J. Vet. Behav.* 11:37–41.

1350 Levine, E., P. Perry, J. Scarlett, & K. A. Houpt. 2005. Intercat aggression in households following the introduction of a new cat. *Appl. Anim. Behav. Sci.* 90:325–336.

1351 Levis, D. G., J. L. Barnett, P. H. Hemsworth, & E. Jongman. 1995. The effect of breeding facility and sexual stimulation on plasma cortisol in boars. *J. Anim. Sci.* 73:3705–3711.

1352 Levy, F., & P. Poindron. 1987. The importance of amniotic fluids for the establishment of maternal behaviour in experienced and inexperienced ewes. *Anim. Behav.* 35:1188–1192.

1353 Levy, F., A. Locatelli, V. Piketty, Y. Tillet, & P. Poindron. 1995. Involvement of the main but not the accessory olfactory system in maternal behavior of primiparous and multiparous ewes. *Physiol. Behav.* 57:97–104.

1354 Levy, F., P. Poindron, & P. Le Neindre. 1983. Attraction and repulsion by amniotic fluids and their olfactory control in the ewe around parturition. *Physiol. Behav.* 31:687–692.

1355 Levy, F., R. Gervais, U. Kindermann, M. Litterio, P. Poindron, & R. Porter. 1991. Effects of early post-partum separation on maintenance of maternal responsiveness and selectivity in parturient ewes. *Appl. Anim. Behav. Sci.* 31:101–110.

1356 Lewis, E., L. A. Boyle, J. V. O'Doherty, P. B. Lynch, & P. Brophy. 2006. The effect of providing shredded paper or ropes to piglets in farrowing crates on their behaviour and health and the behaviour and health of their dams. *Appl. Anim. Behav. Sci.* 96:1–17.

1357 Lewis, N. J. 1999. Frustration of goal-directed behaviour in swine. *Appl. Anim. Behav. Sci.* 64:19–29.

1358 Lewis, N. J., & J. F. Hurnik. 1985. The development of nursing behaviour in swine. *Appl. Anim. Behav. Sci.* 14:225–232.

1359 **Leyhausen, P. 1973. Addictive behavior in free-ranging animals. In L. Goldberg, & F. Hoffmeister (Eds.), *Bayer symposium IV. Psychic dependence*. Berlin, Germany: Springer-Verlag.**

1360 Leyhausen, P. 1975. *Verhaltensstudien an katzen*. Berlin, Germany: Paul Parey.

1361 Leyhausen, P. 1979. *Cat behaviour*. New York, NY: Garland STPM Press.

1362 Li, X., W. Li, H. Wang, J. Cao, K. Maehashi, L. Huang, A. A. Bachmanov, *et al.* 2005. Pseudogenization of a sweet-receptor gene accounts for cats' indifference toward sugar. *PLoS ONE.* 1(1):e3.

1363 Li, Y., & H. W. Gonyou. 2002. Analysis of belly nosing and associated behaviour among pigs weaned at 12–14 days of age. *Appl. Anim. Behav. Sci.* 77:285–294.

1364 Liberg, O. 1983. Courtship behaviour and sexual selection in the domestic cat. *Appl. Anim. Ethol.* 10:117–132.

1365 Lickliter, R. E. 1984. Mother-infant spatial relationships in domestic goats. *Appl. Anim. Behav. Sci.* 13:93–100.

1366 Lickliter, R. E. 1985. Behavior associated with parturition in the domesticated goat. *Appl. Anim. Behav. Sci.* 13:335–345.

1367 Lickliter, R. E. 1987. Activity patterns and companion preferences of dometic goat kids. *Appl. Anim. Behav. Sci.* 19:137–145.

1368 Lickliter, R. E., & J. R. Heron. 1984. Recognition of mother by newborn goats. *Appl. Anim. Behav. Sci.* 12:187–192.

1369 **Liddell, H. S. 1926. A laboratory for the study of conditioned motor reflexes. *Am. J. Psychol.* 37:418–419.**

1370 Liddell, H. S. 1926. The effect of thyroidectomy on some unconditioned responses of the sheep and goat. *Am. J. Physiol.* 75:579–590.

1371 Liddell, H. S. 1954. Conditioning and emotions. *Sci. Am.* 190:48–57.

1372 Liddell, H. S., & O. D. Anderson. 1931. A comparative study of the conditioned motor reflex in the rabbit, sheep, goat, and pig. *Am. J. Physiol.* 97:539–540.

1373 Liddell, H. S., W. T. James, & O. D. Anderson. 1934. The comparative physiology of the conditioned motor reflex based on experiments with the pig, dog, sheep, goat and rabbit. *Comp. Psychol. Monogr.* 11:1–89.

1374 **Lidffors, L. M. 1993. Cross-sucking in group-housed dairy calves before and after weaning off milk. *Appl. Anim. Behav. Sci.* 38:15–24.**

1375 **Lidfors, L. M., D. Moran, J. Jung, P. Jensen, & H. Castren. 1994. Behaviour at calving and choice of calving place in cattle kept in different environments. *Appl. Anim. Behav. Sci.* 42:11–28.**

1376 Lidfors, L. M., J. Jung, & A. M. De Passillé. 2010. Changes in suckling behaviour of dairy calves nursed by their dam during the first month post partum. *Appl. Anim. Behav. Sci.* 128(1–4):23–29.

1377 Lidfors, L., & P. Jensen. 1988. Behaviour of free-ranging beef cows and calves. *Appl. Anim. Behav. Sci.* 20:237–247.

1378 Ligout, S., M. Bouissou, & X. Boivin. 2008. Comparison of the effects of two different handling methods on the subsequent behaviour of Anglo-Arabian foals toward humans and handling. *Appl. Anim. Behav. Sci.* 113:175–188.

1379 Ligout, S., R. H. Porter, & R. Bon. 2002. Social discrimination in lambs: Persistence and scope. *Appl. Anim. Behav. Sci.* 76:239–248.

1380 Liinamo, A., L. van den Berg, P. A. J. Leegwater, M. B. H. Schilder, J. A. M. van Arendonk, & B. A. van Oost. 2007. Genetic variation in aggression-related traits in golden retriever dogs. *Appl. Anim. Behav. Sci.* 104:95–106.

1381 Liinamo, A. E., L. Karjalainen, M. Ojala, & V. Vilva. 1997. Estimates of genetic parameters and environmental effects for measures of hunting performance in Finnish hounds. *J. Anim. Sci.* 75:622–629.

1382 Lin, L., J. Faraco, R. Li, H. Kadotani, W. Rogers, X. Lin, X. Qiu, *et al.* 1999. The sleep disorder canine narcolepsy is caused by a mutation in the hypocretin (orexin) receptor 2 gene. *Cell* 98:365–376.

1383 Lindahl, I. L. 1964. Time of parturition in ewes. *Anim. Behav.* 12:231–234.

1384 Lindberg, A. C., A. Kelland, & C. J. Nicol. 1999. Effects of observational learning on acquisition of an operant response in horses. *Appl. Anim. Behav. Sci.* 61:187–199.

1385 Lindberg, J., P. Saetre, S. Nishino, E. Mignot, & E. Jazin. 2007. Reduced expression of tac1, penk and socs2 in hcrtr-2 mutated narcoleptic dog brain. *BMC Neurosci.* 8:34.

1386 **Lindell, E. M., H. N. Erb, & K. A. Houpt. 1997. Intercat aggression: A retrospective study examining types of aggression, sexes of fighting pairs, and effectiveness of treatment. *Appl. Anim. Behav. Sci.* 55:153–162.**

1387 Lindsay, D. R. 1965. The importance of olfactory stimuli in the mating behaviour of the ram. *Anim. Behav.* 13:75–78.

1388 Lindsay, D. R. 1966. Mating behaviour of ewes and its effect on mating efficiency. *Anim. Behav.* 14:419–424.

1389 Lindsay, D. R. 1966. Modification of behavioural oestrus in the ewe by social and hormonal factors. *Anim. Behav.* 14:73–83.

1390 Lindsay, D. R., & I. C. Fletcher. 1968. Sensory involvement in the recognition of lambs by their dams. *Anim. Behav.* 16:415–417.

1391 Lindsay, D. R., & I. C. Fletcher. 1972. Ram-seeking activity associated with oestrous behaviour in ewes. *Anim. Behav.* 20:452–456.

1392 Lindsay, D. R., & T. J. Robinson. 1961. Studies on the efficiency of mating in the sheep. I. The effect of paddock size and number of rams. *J. Agric. Sci.* 57:137–140.

1393 Lindsay, D. R., & T. J. Robinson. 1961. Studies on the efficiency of mating in the sheep. II. The effect of freedom of rams, paddock size, and age of ewes. *J. Agric. Sci.* 57:141–145.

1394 Line, S. W., B. L. Hart, & L. Sanders. 1985. Effect of prepubertal versus postpubertal castration on sexual and aggressive behavior in male horses. *J. Am. Vet. Med. Assoc.* 186:249–251.

1395 **Linklater, W. L. 2000. Adaptive explanation in socio-ecology: Lessons from the equidae. *Biol. Rev. Camb. Philos. Soc.* 75:1–20.**

1396 Linklater, W. L., & E. Z. Cameron. 2009. Social dispersal but with philopatry reveals incest avoidance in a polygynous ungulate. *Anim. Behav.* 77:1085–1093.

1397 Linklater, W. L., E. Z. Cameron, E. O. Minot, & K. J. Stafford. 1999. Stallion harassment and the mating system of horses. *Anim. Behav.* 58:295–306.

1398 Linklater, W. L., E. Z. Cameron, K. J. Stafford, & E. O. Minot. 2013. Removal experiments indicate that subordinate stallions are not helpers. *Behav. Processes.* 94:1–4.

1399 Linnane, M. I., A. J. Brereton, & P. S. Giller. 2001. Seasonal changes in circadian grazing patterns of kerry cows (*Bos taurus*) in semi-feral conditions in Killarney National Park, Co. Kerry, Ireland. *Appl. Anim. Behav. Sci.* 71:277–292.

1400 Liptrap, R. M., & J. I. Raeside. 1978. A relationship between plasma concentrations of testosterone and corticosteroids during sexual and aggressive behaviour in the boar. *J. Endocrinol.* 76:75–85.

1401 Lit, L., & C. A. Crawford. 2006. Effects of training paradigms on search dog performance. *Appl. Anim. Behav. Sci.* 98:277–292.

1402 Lit, L., J. M. Belanger, D. Boehm, N. Lybarger, A. Haverbeke, C. Diederich, & A. M. Oberbauer. 2013. Characterization of a dopamine transporter polymorphism and behavior in Belgian Malinois. *BMC Genet.* 14:45.

1403 Littlejohn, A., & R. Munro. 1972. Equine recumbency. *Vet. Rec.* 90:83–85.

1404 Lloyd, A. S., J. E. Martin, H. L. I. Bornett-Gauci, & R. G. Wilkinson. 2007. Evaluation of a novel method of horse personality assessment: Rater-agreement and links to behaviour *Appl. Anim. Behav. Sci.* 105:205–222.

1405 Lloyd, A. S., J. E. Martin, H. L. I. Bornett-Gauci, & R. G. Wilkinson. 2008. Horse personality: Variation between breeds. *Appl. Anim. Behav. Sci.* 112:369–383.

1406 Loberg, J. M., C. E. Hernandez, T. Thierfelder, M. B. Jensen, C. Berg, & L. Lidfors. 2007. Reaction of foster cows to prevention of suckling from and separation from four calves simultaneously or in two steps. *J. Anim. Sci.* 85:1522–1529.

1407 Loberg, J. M., C. E. Hernandez, T. Thierfelder, M. B. Jensen, C. Berg, & L. Lidfors. 2008. Weaning and separation in two steps: A way to decrease stress in dairy calves suckled by foster cows. *Appl. Anim. Behav. Sci.* 111:222–234.

1408 Loberg, J., & L. Lidfors. 2001. Effect of stage of lactation and breed on dairy cows' acceptance of foster calves. *Appl. Anim. Behav. Sci.* 74:97–108.

1409 Löckener, S., S. Reese, M. Erhard, & A.-C. Wöhr. 2016. Pasturing in herds after housing in horseboxes induces a positive cognitive bias in horses. *J. Vet. Behav.* 11:50–55.

1410 **Lockwood, R. 1987. Pit bull terriers. *Arthrozoos* 1:193–194.**

1411 Lohse, C. L. 1974. Preferences of dogs for various meats. *J. Am. Anim. Hosp. Assoc.* 10:187–192.

1412 Lorenz, K. 1952. *King Solomon's ring: New light on animal ways*. New York, NY: Thomas Y. Crowell.

1413 Lorenz, K. Z. 1957. Companionship in bird life. In C. H. Schiller, & K. S. Lashley (Eds.), *Instinctive behavior: The development of a modern concept*, pp. 82–128. New York, NY: International Universities Press.

1414 Loss, S. R., T. Will, & P. P. Marra. 2013. The impact of free-ranging domestic cats on wildlife of the United States. *Nat. Commun.* 4:1396.

1415 Lou, Z., & J. F. Hurnik. 1994. An ellipsoid farrowing crate: Its ergonomical design and effects on pig productivity. *J. Anim. Sci.* 72:2610–2616.

1416 Lowe, S. E., & J. W. Bradshaw. 2001. Ontogeny of individuality in the domestic cat in the home environment. *Anim. Behav.* 61:231–237.

1417 Lowman, B. G., M. S. Hankey, N. A. Scott, D. W. Deas, & E. A. Hunter. 1981. Influence of time of feeding on time of parturition in beef cows. *Vet. Rec.* 109:557–559.

1418 **Luescher, A. U. 1993. Hyperkinesis in dogs: Six case reports. *Can. Vet. J.* 34:368–370.**

1419 Luescher, U. A., D. B. McKeown, & H. Dean. 1998. A cross-sectional study on compulsive behaviour (stable vices) in horses. *Equine Vet. J. Suppl.* 27:14–18.

1420 Lunn, D. P., P. A. Cuddon, S. Shaftoe, & R. M. Archer. 1993. Familial occurrence of narcolepsy in miniature horses. *Equine Vet. J.* 25:483–487.

1421 Lunstra, D. D., G. W. Boyd, & L. R. Corah. 1989. Effects of natural mating stimuli on serum luteinizing hormone, testosterone and estradiol-17 beta in yearling beef bulls. *J. Anim. Sci.* 67:3277–3288.

1422 Lustgarten, C., G. D. Bottoms, & J. R. Shaskas. 1973. Experimental adrenalectomy of pigs. *Am. J. Vet. Res.* 34:279–282.

1423 Luz, M. P. F., C. M. Maia, J. C. F. Pantoja, M. C. Neto, & J. N. P. Puoli Filho. 2015. Feeding time and agonistic behavior in horses: Influence of distance, proportion, and height of troughs. *Equine Vet. J.* 35(10):843–848.e841.

1424 Lyimo, Z. C., M. Nielen, W. Ouweltjes, T. A. Kruip, & F. J. van Eerdenburg. 2000. Relationship among estradiol, cortisol and intensity of estrous behavior in dairy cattle. *Theriogenology* 53:1783–1795.

1425 Lyle, S. K., R. Durand, V. P. Taylor, E. Oostelaar, D. P. Beehan, D. P. Paccamonti, & S. M. Mcdonnell. 2014. Effect of contextually congruent stallion vocalization playback on intrauterine pressure in the mare. *Equine Vet. J.* 34(1):131.

1426 Lynch, J. J., & G. Alexander. 1976. The effect of gramineous windbreaks on behaviour and lamb mortality among shorn and unshorn merino sheep during lambing. *Appl. Anim. Ethol.* 2:305–325.

1427 Lynch, J. J., & J. F. McCarthy. 1967. The effect of petting on a classically conditioned emotional response. *Behav. Res. Ther.* 5:55–62.

1428 Lynch, J. J., G. N. Hinch, & D. B. Adams. 1992. *The behaviour of sheep. Biological principles and implications of production.* Oxon, UK: CAB International.

1429 Lyons, D. M., E. O. Price, & G. P. Moberg. 1988. Social modulation of pituitary-adrenal responsiveness and individual differences in behavior of young domestic goats. *Physiol. Behav.* 43:451–458.

1430 Maarschalkerweerd, R. J., N. Endenburg, J. Kirpensteijn, & B. W. Knol. 1997. Influence of orchiectomy on canine behaviour. *Vet. Rec.* 140:617–619.

1431 Macaulay, A. S., G. L. Hahn, D. H. Clark, & D. V. Sisson. 1995. Comparison of calf housing types and tympanic temperature rhythms in Holstein calves. *J. Dairy Sci.* 78:856–862.

1432 MacDonald, D. 1981. *The behaviour and ecology of farm cats. The ecology and control of feral cats*, pp. 23–29. Potters Bar, UK: Universities Federation for Animal Welfare.

1433 Macfarlane, J. S. 1974. The effect of two post-weaning management systems on the social and sexual behaviour of zebu bulls. *Appl. Anim. Ethol.* 1:31–34.

1434 Mackenzie, S. A., & E. Thiboutot. 1997. Stimulus reactivity tests for the domestic horse (*Equus caballus*). *Equine Pract.* 19:21.

1435 Mackenzie, S. A., E. A. B. Oltenacu, & K. A. Houpt. 1986. Canine behavioral genetics: A review. *Appl. Anim. Behav. Sci.* 15:365–393.

1436 Mackenzie, S. A., E. A. Oltenacu, & E. Leighton. 1985. Heritability estimate for temperament scores in German shepherd dogs and its genetic correlation with hip dysplasia. *Behav. Genet.* 15:475–482.

1437 Macpherson, K., & W. A. Roberts. 2006. Do dogs (*Canis familiaris*) seek help in an emergency? *J. Comp. Psychol.* 120:113–119.

1438 Macuda, T., & B. Timney. 1999. Luminance and chromatic discrimination in the horse (*Equus caballus*). *Behav. Processes.* 44:301–307.

1439 Mader, D. R., & E. O. Price. 1980. Discrimination learning in horses: Effects of breed, age and social dominance. *J. Anim. Sci.* 50:962–965.

1440 Mader, D. R., & E. O. Price. 1984. The effects of sexual stimulation on the sexual performance of Hereford bulls. *J. Anim. Sci.* 59:294–300.

1441 Madigan, J. E., & S. A. Bell. 2001. Owner survey of headshaking in horses. *J. Am. Vet. Med. Assoc.* 219:334–337.

1442 Maejima, M., M. Inoue-Murayama, K. Tonosaki, N. Matsuura, S. Kato, Y. Saito, A. Weiss, *et al.* 2007. Traits and genotypes may predict the successful training of drug detection dogs. *Appl. Anim. Behav. Sci.* 107:287–298.

1443 Mahnhardt, S., J. Brietzke, E. Kanitz, P. C. Schön, A. Tuchscherer, U. Gimsa, & G. Manteuffel. 2014. Anticipation and frequency of feeding affect heart reactions in domestic pigs. *J. Anim. Sci.* 92:4878–4887.

1444 Maier, N. R. F., & T. C. Schneirla. 1964. Principles of animal psychology. New York, NY: Dover Publications.

1445 Mal, M. E., & C. A. McCall. 1996. The influence of handling during different ages on a halter training test in foals. *Appl. Anim. Behav. Sci.* 50:115–120.

1446 Mal, M. E., C. A. McCall, K. A. Cummins, & M. C. Newland. 1994. Influence of preweaning handling methods on post-weaning learning ability and manageability of foals. *Appl. Anim. Behav. Sci.* 40:187–195.

1447 Malbert, C. H., & Y. Ruckebusch. 1989. Hyperphagia induced by pylorectomy in sheep. *Physiol. Behav.* 45:495–499.

1448 Malm, K. 1995. Regurgitation in relations to weaning in the domestic dog: A questionnaire study. *Appl. Anim. Behav. Sci.* 43:111–122.

1449 Malm, K., & P. Jensen. 1993. Regurgitation as a weaning strategy: A selective review on an old subject in a new light. *Appl. Anim. Behav. Sci.* 36:47–64.

1450 Malpass, J. P., & B. J. Weigler. 1994. A simple and effective environmental enrichment device for ponies in long-term indoor confinement. *Contemp. Top. Lab. Anim. Sci.* 33:74–76.

1451 Mangalam, M., & M. Singh. 2013. Differential foraging strategies: Motivation, perception and implementation in urban free-ranging dogs, *Canis familiaris. Anim. Behav.* 85(4):763–770.

1452 Mansmann, R. A., M. C. Currie, M. T. Correa, B. Sherman, & K. Vom Orde. 2011. Equine behavior problems-around farriery: Foot pain in 11 horses. *Equine Vet. J.* 31(1):44–48.

1453 Manson, F. J., & M. C. Appleby. 1990. Spacing of dairy cows at a food trough. *Appl. Anim. Behav. Sci.* 26:69–81.

1454 Manteuffel, G., A. Mannewitz, C. Manteuffel, A. Tuchscherer, & L. Schrader. 2010. Social hierarchy affects the adaption of pregnant sows to a call feeding learning paradigm. *Appl. Anim. Behav. Sci.* 128(1–4):30–36.

1455 **Marcella, K. L. 1983. A note on canine aggression towards veterinarians. *Appl. Anim. Ethol.* 10:155–157.**

1456 Marchant, J. N., X. Whittaker, & D. M. Broom. 2001. Vocalisations of the adult female domestic pig during a standard human approach test and their relationships with behavioural and heart rate measures. *Appl. Anim. Behav. Sci.* 72:23–39.

1457 **Marchei, P., S. Diverio, N. Falocci, J. Fatjo, J. L. Ruiz-De-La-Torre, & X. Manteca. 2011. Breed differences in behavioural response to challenging situations in kittens. *Physiol. Behav.* 102(3–4):276–284.**

1458 Marcuse, F. L., & A. U. Moore. 1944. Tantrum behavior in the pig. *J. Comp. Psychol.* 37:235–241.

1459 Marcuse, F. L., & A. U. Moore. 1946. Motor criteria of discrimination. *J. Comp. Psychol.* 39:25–27.

1460 Marinier, S. L., & A. J. Alexander. 1992. Use of field observations to measure individual grazing ability in horses. *Appl. Anim. Behav. Sci.* 33:1–10.

1461 Marinier, S. L., A. J. Alexander, & G. H. Waring. 1988. Flehmen behaviour in the domestic horse: Discrimination of conspecific odours. *Appl. Anim. Behav. Sci.* 19:227–237.

1462 Maros, K., M. Gacsi, & A. Miklosi. 2008. Comprehension of human pointing gestures in horses (*Equus caballus*). *Anim. Cogn.* 11:457–466.

1463 Marsboll, A. F., & J. W. Christensen. 2015. Effects of handling on fear reactions in young Icelandic horses. *Equine Vet. J.* 47(5):615–619.

1464 Marshall-Pescini, S., C. Passalacqua, A. Ferrario, P. Valsecchi, & E. Prato-Previde. 2011. Social eavesdropping in the domestic dog. *Anim. Behav.* 81(6):1177–1183.

1465 Marshall-Pescini, S., C. Passalacqua, S. Barnard, P. Valsecchi, & E. Prato-Previde. 2009. Agility and search and rescue training differently affects pet dogs' behaviour in socio-cognitive tasks. *Behav. Processes.* 81(3):416–422.

1466 Marten, G. C., & J. E. Donker. 1964. Selective grazing induced by animal excreta. I. Evidence of occurrence and superficial remedy. *J. Dairy Sci.* 47:773–776.

1467 Martin, F. H., J. R. Seoane, & C. A. Baile. 1973. Feeding in satiated sheep elicited by intraventricular injections of CSF from fasted sheep. *Life Sci.* 13:177–184.

1468 Martin, J. E., & S. A. Edwards. 1994. Feeding behaviour of outdoor sows: The effects of diet quantity and type. *Appl. Anim. Behav. Sci.* 41:63–74.

1469 Martin, J. T. 1975. Movement of feral pigs in North Canterbury, New Zealand. *J. Mammal.* 56:914–915.

1470 Martin, P. 1984. The time and energy costs of play behaviour in the cat. *Z. Tierpsychol.* 64:298–312.

1471 Martin, P. 1986. An experimental study of weaning in the domestic cat. *Behaviour* 99:221–249.

1472 Martin, P., & P. Bateson. 1985. The ontogeny of locomotor play behaviour in the domestic cat. *Anim. Behav.* 33:502–510.

1473 Martin, R. J., J. L. Gobble, T. H. Hartsock, H. B. Graves, & J. H. Ziegler. 1973. Characterization of an obese syndrome in the pig. *Proc. Soc. Exp. Biol. Med.* 143:198–203.

1474 Martin, T. I., T. R. Zentall, & L. Lawrence. 2006. Simple discrimination reversals in the domestic horse (*Equus caballus*): Effect of discriminative stimulus modality on learning to learn. *Appl. Anim. Behav. Sci.* 101:328–338.

1475 Martins, T. 1949. Disgorging of food to the puppies by the lactating dog. *Physiol. Zool.* 22:169–172.

1476 Martinson, K. L., M. S. Wells, & C. C. Sheaffer. 2016. Horse preference, forage yield, and species persistence of 12 perennial cool-season grass mixtures under horse grazing. *Equine Vet. J.* 36:19–25.

1477 **Mason, E. 1970. Obesity in pet dogs. *Vet. Rec.* 86:612–616.**

1478 Mateo, J. M., D. Q. Estep, & J. S. McCann. 1991. Effects of differential handling on the behaviour of domestic ewes (*Ovis aries*). *Appl. Anim. Behav. Sci.* 32:45–54.

1479 Mattner, P. E., A. W. H. Braden, & K. E. Turnbill. 1967. Studies in flock mating of sheep. I. Mating behaviour. *Aust. J. Exp. Agric. Anim. Husb.* 7:103–109.

1480 May, R., J. van Dijk, J. M. Forland, R. Andersen, & A. Landa. 2008. Behavioural patterns in ewe-lamb pairs and vulnerability to predation by wolverines. *Appl. Anim. Behav. Sci.* 112:58–67.

1481 Mayes, E., & P. Duncan. 1986. Temporal patterns of feeding in free-ranging horses. *Behaviour* 96:105–129.

1482 Mayes, E.-R. E., A. Wilkinson, T. W. Pike, & D. S. Mills. 2015. Individual differences in visual and olfactory cue preference and use by cats (*Felis catus*). *Appl. Anim. Behav. Sci.* 173:52–59.

1483 McAfee, L. M., D. S. Mills, & J. J. Cooper. 2002. The use of mirrors for the control of stereotype weaving behaviour in the stabled horse. *Appl. Anim. Behav. Sci.* 78:159–173.

1484 **McBane, S. 1987. *Behaviour problems of horses*. North Pomfret, VT: David and Charles.**

1485 McBride, G. 1963. The "teat order" and communication in young pigs. *Anim. Behav.* 11:53–56.

1486 McBride, G., J. W. James, & G. S. F. Wyeth. 1965. Social behaviour of domestic animals. VII. Variation in weaning weight in pigs. *Anim. Prod.* 7:67–74.

1487 McBride, G., J. W. James, & N. Hodgens. 1964. Social behaviour of domestic animals. *IV. Growing pigs. Anim. Prod.* 6:129–139.

1488 Mcbride, S. D., N. Perentos, & A. J. Morton. 2015. Understanding the concept of a reflective surface: Can sheep improve navigational ability through the use of a mirror? *Anim. Cogn.* 18(1):361–371.

1489 McCall, C. A. 1989. *Behavior problems of horses*. North Pomfret, VT: David and Charles.

1490 McCall, C. A. 1991. Utilizing taped stallion vocalizations as a practical aid in estrus detection in mares. *Appl. Anim. Behav. Sci.* 28:305–310.

1491 McCall, C. A., & S. E. Burgin. 2002. Equine utilization of secondary reinforcement during response extinction and acquisition. *Appl. Anim. Behav. Sci.* 78:253–262.

1492 McCall, C. A., A. M. A. Salters, & S. M. Simpson. 1993. Relationship between number of conditioning trials per training session and avoidance learning in horses. *Appl. Anim. Behav. Sci.* 36:291–299.

1493 McCall, C. A., G. D. Potter, & J. L. Kreider. 1985. Locomotor, vocal and other behavioural responses to varying methods of weaning foals. *Appl. Anim. Behav. Sci.* 14:27–35.

1494 McCall, C. A., G. D. Potter, T. H. Friend, & R. S. Ingram. 1981. Learning abilities in yearling horses using the Hebb-Williams closed field maze. *J. Anim. Sci.* 53:928–933.

1495 McCall, C. A., S. Hall, W. H. McElhenney, & K. A. Cummins. 2006. Evaluation and comparison of four methods of ranking horses based on reactivity. *Appl. Anim. Behav. Sci.* 96:115–127.

1496 McClure, S. R., M. K. Chaffin, & B. V. Beaver. 1992. Nonpharmacologic management of stereotypic self-mutilative behavior in a stallion. *J. Am. Vet. Med. Assoc.* 200:1975–1977.

1497 Mccomb, K., A. M. Taylor, C. Wilson, & B. D. Charlton. 2009. The cry embedded within the purr. *Curr. Biol.* 19(13):R507–R508.

1498 McConnell, P. B. 1990. Acoustic structure and receiver response in domestic dogs, *Canis familiaris. Anim. Behav.* 39:897–904.

1499 McConnell, P. B., & J. R. Baylis. 1985. Interspecific communication in cooperative herding: Acoustic and visual signals from human shepherds and herding dogs. *Z. Tierpsychol.* 67:302–328.

1500 McCowan, B., A. M. DiLorenzo, S. Abichandani, C. Borelli, & J. S. Cullor. 2002. Bioacoustic tools for enhancing animal management and productivity: Effects of recorded calf vocalizations on milk production in dairy cows. *Appl. Anim. Behav. Sci.* 77:13–20.

1501 Mccown, S., M. Brummer, S. Hayes, G. Olson, S. R. Smith, & L. Lawrence. 2012. Acceptability of teff hay by horses. *Equine Vet. J.* 32(6):327–331.

1502 McCune, S. 1995. The impact of paternity and early socialisation on the development of cats' behaviour to people and novel objects. *Appl. Anim. Behav. Sci.* 45:109–124.

1503 McDonald, C. L., R. G. Beilharz, & J. C. McCutchan. 1981. Training cattle to control by electric fences. *Appl. Anim. Ethol.* 7:113–121.

1504 McDonnell, S. 1986. Reproductive behavior of the stallion. *Vet. Clin. North Am. Equine Pract.* 2:535–555.

1505 McDonnell, S. 2003. *A practical field guide to horse behavior: The equid ethogram.* Lexington, KY: Eclipse Press.

1506 McDonnell, S. M. 1992. Sexual behavior dysfunction in stallion. In N. E. Robinson (Ed.), *Current therapy in equine medicine*, pp. 668–671. Philadelphia, PA: W.B. Saunders.

1507 McDonnell, S. M. 2008. Practical review of self-mutilation in horses. *Anim. Reprod. Sci.* 107:219–228.

1508 McDonnell, S. M., & A. Poulin. 2002. Equid play ethogram. *Appl. Anim. Behav. Sci.* 78:263–290.

1509 **McDonnell, S. M., & J. C. S. Haviland. 1995. Agonistic ethogram of the equid bachelor band. *Appl. Anim. Behav. Sci.* 43:147–188.**

1510 Mcdonnell, S. M., J. Miller, & W. Vaala. 2013. Calming benefit of short-term alpha-casozepine supplementation during acclimation to domestic environment and basic ground training of adult semi-feral ponies. *Equine Vet. J.* 33(2):101–106.

1511 McDonnell, S. M., N. K. Diehl, M. C. Garcia, & R. M. Kenney. 1989. Gonadotropin releasing hormone (GnRH) affects precopulatory behavior in testosterone-treated geldings. *Physiol. Behav.* 45:145–149.

1512 McDonnell, S. M., R. M. Kenney, P. E. Meckley, & M. C. Garcia. 1985. Conditioned suppression of sexual behavior in stallions and reversal with diazepam. *Physiol. Behav.* 34:951–956.

1513 McDonnell, S. M., R. M. Kenney, P. E. Meckley, & M. C. Garcia. 1986. Novel environment suppression of stallion sexual behavior and effects of diazepam. *Physiol. Behav.* 37:503–505.

1514 McDonnell, S., & S. C. Murray. 1995. Bachelor and harem stallion behavior and endocrinology. *Biol. Reprod. Mono.* 1:577–590.

1515 McDougall, K. D., & W. McDougal. 1931. Insight and foresight in various animals – monkey, raccoon, rat, and wasp. *J. Comp. Psychol.* 11:237–273.

1516 McEachron, D. L., D. F. Kripke, R. Hawkins, E. Haus, D. Pavlinac, & L. Deftos. 1982. Lithium delays biochemical circadian rhythms in rats. *Neuropsychobiology* 8:12–29.

1517 McGeer, E. G., & P. L. McGeer. 1966. Circadian rhythm in pineal tyrosine hydroxylase. *Science* 153:73–74.

1518 McGinty, D. J., M. Stevenson, T. Hoppenbrouwers, R. M. Harper, M. B. Sterman, & J. Hodgman. 1977. Polygraphic studies of kitten development: Sleep state patterns. *Dev. Psychobiol.* 10:455–469.

1519 **McGlone, J. J. 1985. A quantitative ethogram of aggressive and submissive behaviors in recently regrouped pigs. *J. Anim. Sci.* 61:559–565.**

1520 McGlone, J. J. 1985. Olfactory cues and pig agonistic behavior: Evidence for a submissive pheromone. *Physiol. Behav.* 34:195–198.

1521 McGlone, J. J. 1986. Influence of resources on pig aggression and dominance. *Behav. Processes.* 12:134–144.

1522 McGlone, J. J., & D. L. Anderson. 2002. Synthetic maternal pheromone stimulates feeding behavior and weight gain in weaned pigs. *J. Anim. Sci.* 80:3179–3183.

1523 McGlone, J. J., & J. L. Morrow. 1987. Individual differences among mature boars in T-maze preference for estrous or non-estrous sows. *Appl. Anim. Behav. Sci.* 17:77–82.

1524 McGlone, J. J., & S. E. Curtis. 1985. Behavior and performance of weanling pigs in pens equipped with hide areas. *J. Anim. Sci.* 60:20–24.

1525 **McGlone, J. J., R. I. Nicholson, J. M. Hellman, & D. N. Herzog. 1993. The development of pain in young pigs associated with castration and attempts to prevent castration-induced behavioral changes. *J. Anim. Sci.* 71:1441–1446.**

1526 **McGreevy, P. D., & A. M. Masters. 2008. Risk factors for separation-related distress and feed-related aggression in dogs: Additional findings from a survey of Australian dog owners. *Appl. Anim. Behav. Sci.* 109:320–328.**

1527 McGreevy, P. D., & P. C. Thomson. 2006. Differences in motor laterality between breeds of performance horse. *Appl. Anim. Behav. Sci.* 99:183–190.

1528 McGreevy, P. D., A. Brueckner, P. C. Thomson, & N. J. Branson. 2010. Motor laterality in 4 breeds of dog. *J. Vet. Behav.* 5(6):318–323.

1529 McGreevy, P. D., J. D. Richardson, C. J. Nicol, & J. G. Lane. 1995. Radiographic and endoscopic study of horses performing an oral based stereotypy. *Equine Vet. J.* 27:92–95.

1530 McGreevy, P. D., L. A. Hawson, T. C. Habermann, & S. R. Cattle. 2001. Geophagia in horses: A short note on 13 cases. *Appl. Anim. Behav. Sci.* 71:119–125.

1531 McGreevy, P. D., N. P. French, & C. J. Nicol. 1995. The prevalence of abnormal behaviours in dressage, eventing and endurance horses in relation to stabling. *Vet. Rec.* 137:36–37.

1532 McGreevy, P. D., P. J. Cripps, N. P. French, L. E. Green, & C. J. Nicol. 1995. Management factors associated with stereotypic and redirected behaviour in the thoroughbred horse. *Equine Vet. J.* 27:86–91.

1533 McGreevy, P., & C. Nicol. 1998. Physiological and behavioral consequences associated with short-term prevention of crib-biting in horses. *Physiol. Behav.* 65:15–23.

1534 McGrogan, C., M. D. Hutchison, & J. E. King. 2008. Dimensions of horse personality based on owner and trainer supplied personality traits. *Appl. Anim. Behav. Sci.* 113:206–214.

1535 McGuire, R. A., W. M. Rand, & R. J. Wurtman. 1973. Entrainment of the body temperature rhythm in rats: Effect of color and intensity of environmental light. *Science* 181:956–957.

1536 McKinley, J., & T. D. Sambrook. 2000. Use of human-given cues by domestic dogs (*Canis familiaris*) and horses (*Equus caballus*). *Anim. Cogn.* 3:13–22.

1537 McLaughlin, C. L., C. A. Baile, L. L. Buckholtz, & S. K. Freeman. 1983. Preferred flavors and performance of weanling pigs. *J. Anim. Sci.* 56:1287–1293.

1538 McLaughlin, C. L., L. F. Krabill, G. C. Scott, & C. A. Baile. 1976. Chemical stimulants of feeding animals. *Fed. Proc.* 35:579.

1539 McLeman, M. A., M. T. Mendl, R. B. Jones, & C. M. Wathes. 2008. Social discrimination of familiar conspecifics by juvenile pigs, sus scrofa: Development of a non-invasive method to study the transmission of unimodal and bimodal cues between live stimuli. *Appl. Anim. Behav. Sci.* 115:123–137.

1540 **McPhee, C. P., G. McBride, & J. W. James. 1964. Social behaviour of domestic animals. III. *Steers in small yards. Anim. Prod.* 6:9–15.**

1541 Meagher, R. K., R. R. Daros, J. H. Costa, M. A. Von Keyserlingk, M. J. Hotzel, & D. M. Weary. 2015. Effects of degree and timing of social housing on reversal learning and response to novel objects in dairy calves. *PLoS ONE.* 10(8):e0132828.

1542 **Mech, L. D. 1975. Hunting behavior in two similar species of social canids. In M. W. Fox (Ed.), *The wild canids. their systematics, behavioral ecology and evolution*, pp. 363–368. New York, NY: Van Nostrand Reinhold.**

1543 Meese, G. B., & B. A. Baldwin. 1975. Effects of olfactory bulb ablation and maternal behaviour in sows. *Appl. Anim. Ethol.* 1:379–386.

1544 Meese, G. B., & B. A. Baldwin. 1975. The effects of ablation of the olfactory bulbs on aggressive behaviour in pigs. *Appl. Anim. Ethol.* 1:351–362.

1545 Meese, G. B., & R. Ewbank. 1973. Exploratory behaviour and leadership in the domesticated pig. *Br. Vet. J.* 129:251–259.

1546 Meese, G. B., & R. Ewbank. 1973. The establishment of and nature of the dominance hierarchy in the domesticated pig. *Anim. Behav.* 21:326–334.

1547 Meese, G. B., D. J. Conner, & B. A. Baldwin. 1975. Ability of the pig to distinguish between conspecific urine samples using olfaction. *Physiol. Behav.* 15:121–125.

1548 Mehrkam, L. R., & C. D. L. Wynne. 2014. Behavioral differences among breeds of domestic dogs (*Canis lupus familiaris*): Current status of the science. *Appl. Anim. Behav. Sci.* 155:12–27.

1549 Meier, G. W. 1961. Infantile handling and development in siamese kittens. *J. Comp. Physiol. Psychol.* 54:284–286.

1550 Meier, G. W., & J. L. Stuart. 1959. Effects of handling on the physical and behavioral development of siamese kittens. *Psychol. Rep.* 5:497–501.

1551 Meikle, D. B., L. C. Drickamer, S. H. Vessey, T. L. Rosenthal, & K. S. Fitzgerald. 1993. Maternal dominance rank and secondary sex ratio in domestic swine. *Anim. Behav.* 46:79–85.

1552 **Melese-d'Hospital, P. 1996. Eliminating urine odors in the home. In V. L. Voith, & P. L. Borchelt (Eds.), *Companion animal behavior*, pp. 191–197. Trenton, NJ: Veterinary Learning Systems.**

1553 Melin, M., G. G. N. Hermans, G. Pettersson, & H. Wiktorsson. 2006. Cow traffic in relation to social rank and motivation of cows in an automatic milking system with control gates and an open waiting area. *Appl. Anim. Behav. Sci.* 96:201–214.

1554 Melin, M., G. Pettersson, H. Svennersten-Sjaunja, & H. Wiktorsson. 2007. The effects of restricted feed access and social rank on feeding behavior, ruminating and intake for cows managed in automated milking systems. *Appl. Anim. Behav. Sci.* 107:13–21.

1555 Melo, M. I., J. R. Sereno, M. Henry, & G. D. Cassali. 1998. Peripuberal sexual development of pantaneiro stallions. *Theriogenology.* 50:727–737.

1556 Melrose, D. R., H. C. Reed, & R. L. Patterson. 1971. Androgen steroids associated with boar odour as an aid to the detection of oestrus in pig artificial insemination. *Br. Vet. J.* 127:497–502.

1557 Melzack, R. 1962. Effects of early perceptual restriction on simple visual discrimination. *Science.* 137:978–979.

1558 Melzack, R., & T. H. Scott. 1957. The effects of early experience on the response to pain. *J. Comp. Physiol. Psychol.* 50:155–161.

1559 Mendl, M., & R. Harcourt. 1988. Individuality in the domestic cat. In D. C. Turner, & P. Bateson (Eds.), *The domestic cat: The biology of its behavior*, pp. 41–54. Cambridge, UK: Cambridge University Press.

1560 Mendl, M., A. J. Zanella, & D. M. Broom. 1992. Physiological and reproductive correlates of behavioural strategies in female domestic pigs. *Anim. Behav.* 44:1107–1121.

1561 Mendl, M., A. J. Zanella, D. M. Broom, & C. T. Whittemore. 1995. Maternal social status and birth sex ratio in domestic pigs: An analysis of mechanisms. *Anim. Behav.* 50:1361–1370.

1562 **Mendl, M., J. Brooks, C. Basse, O. Burman, E. Paul, E. Blackwell, & R. Casey. 2010. Dogs showing separation-related behaviour exhibit a 'pessimistic' cognitive bias. *Curr. Biol.* 20(19):R839–R840.**

1563 Mendl, M., K. Randle, & S. Pope. 2002. Young female pigs can discriminate individual differences in odours from conspecific urine. *Anim. Behav.* 64:97–101.

1564 Mendl, M., S. Held, & R. W. Byrne. 2010. Pig cognition. *Curr. Biol.* 20(18):R796–R798.

1565 Merola, I., E. Prato-Previde, M. Lazzaroni, & S. Marshall-Pescini. 2014. Dogs' comprehension of referential emotional expressions: Familiar people and familiar emotions are easier. *Anim. Cogn.* 17(2):373–385.

1566 Merola, I., M. Lazzaroni, S. Marshall-Pescini, & E. Prato-Previde. 2015. Social referencing and cat-human communication. *Anim. Cogn.* 18(3):639–648.

1567 Merrick, A. W., & D. W. Scharp. 1971. Electroencephalography of resting behavior in cattle, with observations on the question of sleep. *Am. J. Vet. Res.* 32:1893–1897.

1568 Mersmann, H. J., M. D. MacNeil, S. C. Seiderman, & W. G. Pond. 1987. Compensatory growth in finishing pigs after feed restriction. *J. Anim. Sci.* 64:752–764.

1569 Mertens, D. R. 1987. Predicting intake and digestibility using mathematical models of ruminal function. *J. Anim. Sci.* 64:1548–1558.

1570 Metz, J. H. M. 1985. The reaction of cows to a short-term deprivation of lying. *Appl. Anim. Behav. Sci.* 13:301–307.

1571 Metz, J. H. M., & H. W. Gonyou. 1990. Effect of age and housing conditions on the behavioural and haemolytic reaction of piglets to weaning. *Appl. Anim. Behav. Sci.* 27:299–309.

1572 Metz, J. H. M., & P. Mekking. 1984. Crowding phenomena in dairy cows as related to available idling space in a cubicle housing system. *Appl. Anim. Behav. Sci.* 12:63–78.

1573 Meyer, S., G. Nurnberg, B. Puppe, & J. Langbein. 2012. The cognitive capabilities of farm animals: Categorisation learning in dwarf

goats (*Capra hircus*). *Anim. Cogn.* 15(4):567–576.

1574 Michael, R. P. 1973. The effects of hormones on sexual behavior in female cat and rhesus monkey. In R. O. Greep, & E. B. Astwood (Eds.), *Handbook of physiology, section 7, endocrinology, volume II, female reproductive system, part 1*, pp. 187–221. Washington, DC: American Physiological Society.

1575 Michelena, P., J. Gautrais, J. Gerard, R. Bon, & J. Deneubourg. 2008. Social cohesion in groups of sheep: Effect of activity level, sex composition and group size. *Appl. Anim. Behav. Sci.* 112:81–93.

1576 Michell, A. R. 1992. Sodium preference in sheep excreting sodium predominantly in urine or faeces. *Physiol. Behav.* 52:285–286.

1577 Michell, A. R., & P. Moss. 1988. Salt appetite during pregnancy in sheep. *Physiol. Behav.* 42:491–493.

1578 Miedema, H. M., M. S. Cockram, C. M. Dwyer, & A. I. Macrae. 2011. Changes in the behaviour of dairy cows during the 24h before normal calving compared with behaviour during late pregnancy. *Appl. Anim. Behav. Sci.* 131(1–2):8–14.

1579 Miklosi, A. 2007. In A. Miklosi (Ed.), *Dog behaviour, evolution, and cognition.* New York, NY: Oxford University Press.

1580 Miklosi, A., P. Pongracz, G. Lakatos, J. Topal, & V. Csanyi. 2005. A comparative study of the use of visual communicative signals in interactions between dogs (*Canis familiaris*) and humans and cats (*Felis catus*) and humans. *J. Comp. Psychol.* 119:179–186.

1581 Miklosi, A., R. Polgardi, J. Topal, & V. Csanyi. 2000. Intentional behaviour in dog-human communication: An experimental analysis of "showing" behaviour in the dog. *Anim. Cogn.* 3:159–166.

1582 Miles, R. C. 1958. Learning in kittens with manipulatory, exploratory, and food incentives. *J. Comp. Physiol. Psychol.* 51:39–42.

1583 Milgram, N. W., B. Adams, H. Callahan, E. Head, B. Mackay, C. Thirlwell, & C. W. Cotman. 1999. Landmark discrimination learning in the dog. *Learn. Mem.* 6:54–61.

1584 **Milgram, N. W., C. T. Siwak-Tapp, J. Araujo, & E. Head. 2006. Neuroprotective effects of cognitive enrichment. *Ageing Res. Rev.* 5:354–369.**

1585 **Milgram, N. W., E. Head, E. Weiner, & E. Thomas. 1994. Cognitive functions and aging in the dog: Acquisition of nonspatial visual tasks. *Behav. Neurosci.* 108:57–68.**

1586 Miller, E. R., S. Vathana, F. F. Green, J. R. Black, D. R. Romsos, & D. E. Ullrey. 1974. Dietary caloric density and caloric intake in the pig. *J. Anim. Sci.* 39:980.

1587 Miller, H. C., K. F. Pattison, C. N. Dewall, R. Rayburn-Reeves, & T. R. Zentall. 2010. Self-control without a "self": Common self-control processes in humans and dogs. *Psychol. Sci.* 21(4):534–538.

1588 Miller, P. E., & C. J. Murphy. 1995. Vision in dogs. *J. Am. Vet. Med. Assoc.* 207:1623–1634.

1589 Miller, R. M. 1991. Imprint training of the newborn foal. Colorado Springs, CO: The Western Horseman.

1590 Miller, R. R. 1981. Male aggression, dominance, and breeding behavior in red desert feral horses. *Z. Tierpsychol.* 57:340–351.

1591 Miller, R. R., & R. H. Denniston. 1979. Interband dominance in feral horses. *Z. Tierpsychol.* 51:41–47.

1592 Mills, D. S. 1998. Personality and individual differences in the horse, their significance, use and measurement. *Equine Vet. J.* (Suppl. 27):10–13.

1593 **Mills, D. S., & J. C. White. 2000. Long-term follow up of the effect of a pheromone therapy on feline spraying behaviour. *Vet. Rec.* 147:746–747.**

1594 Mills, D. S., & K. Taylor. 2003. Field study of the efficacy of three types of nose net for the treatment of headshaking in horses. *Vet. Rec.* 152:41–44.

1595 **Mills, D. S., D. Ramos, M. G. Estelles, & C. Hargrave. 2006. A triple blind placebo-controlled investigation into the assessment of the effect of dog appeasing pheromone (DAP) on anxiety related behaviour of problem dogs in the veterinary clinic. *Appl. Anim. Behav. Sci.* 98:114–126.**

1596 Mills, D. S., R. D. Alston, V. Rogers, & N. T. Longford. 2002. Factors associated with the prevalence of stereotypic behaviour amongst thoroughbred horses passing through auctioneer sales. *Appl. Anim. Behav. Sci.* 78:115–124.

1597 Mills, D., & R. Ledger. 2001. The effects of oral selegiline hydrochloride on learning and training in the dog: A psychobiological interpretation. *Prog. Neuropsychopharmacol. Biol. Psychiatry* 25:1597–1613.

1598 Minero, M., D. Zucca, & E. Canali. 2006. A note on reaction to novel stimulus and restraint by therapeutic riding horses. *Appl. Anim. Behav. Sci.* 97:335–342.

1599 Minero, M., E. Canali, V. Ferrante, M. Verga, & F. O. Odberg. 1999. Heart rate and behavioural responses of crib-biting horses to two acute stressors. *Vet. Rec.* 145:430–433.

1600 Minero, M., M. V. Tosi, E. Canali, & F. Wemelsfelder. 2009. Quantitative and qualitative assessment of the response of foals to the presence of an unfamiliar human. *Appl. Anim. Behav. Sci.* 116:74–81.

1601 **Miquel-Kergoat, S., V. Azais-Braesco, B. Burton-Freeman, & M. M. Hetherington. 2015. Effects of chewing on appetite, food intake and gut hormones: A systematic review and meta-analysis. *Physiol. Behav.* 151:88–96.**

1602 Mirza, S. N., & F. D. Provenza. 1992. Effects of age and conditions of exposure on maternally mediated food selection by lambs. *Appl. Anim. Behav. Sci.* 33:35–42.

1603 Mirza, S. N., & F. D. Provenza. 1994. Socially induced food avoidance in lambs: Direct or indirect maternal influence? *J. Anim. Sci.* 72:899–902.

1604 Mistlberger, R. E., T. A. Houpt, & M. C. Moore-Ede. 1990. Food-anticipatory rhythms under 24-hour schedules of limited access to single macronutrients. *J. Biol. Rhythms* 5:35–46.

1605 Mitler, M. M., O. Soave, & W. C. Dement. 1976. Narcolepsy in seven dogs. *J. Am. Vet. Med. Assoc.* 168:1036–1038.

1606 Mohan, R. A. B., W. J. McCaughey, W. McLauchlan, D. J. Kilpatrick, & S. McGaughey. 1991. Behavioural response to mixing of entire bulls, vasectomised bulls and steers. *Appl. Anim. Behav. Sci.* 31:157–168.

1607 **Mohr, E., & H. Krzywanek. 1990. Variations of core-temperature rhythms in unrestrained sheep. *Physiol. Behav.* 48:467–473.**

1608 Molliver, M. E. 1963. Operant control of vocal behavior in the cat. *J. Exp. Anal. Behav.* 6:197–202.

1609 Moltz, H. 1960. Imprinting: Empirical basis and theoretical significance. *Psychol. Bull.* 57:291–314.

1610 Momozawa, Y., R. Kusunose, T. Kikusui, Y. Takeuchi, & Y. Mori. 2005. Assessment of equine temperament questionnaire by comparing factor structure between two separate surveys. *Appl. Anim. Behav. Sci.* 92:77–84.

1611 Momozawa, Y., T. Ono, F. Sato, T. Kikusui, Y. Takeuchi, Y. Mori, & R. Kusunose. 2003. Assessment of equine temperament by a questionnaire survey to caretakers and evaluation of its reliability by simultaneous behavior test. *Appl. Anim. Behav. Sci.* 84:127–138.

1612 Mondard, A., & P. Duncan. 1996. Consequences of natal dispersal in female horses. *Anim. Behav.* 52:565–579.

1613 Montgomery, G. G. 1957. Some aspects of the sociality of the domestic horse. *Trans. Kansas Acad. Sci.* 60:419–424.

1614 Moore, A. S., H. W. Gonyou, & A. W. Ghent. 1993. Integration of newly introduced and resident sows following grouping. *Appl. Anim. Behav. Sci.* 38:257–267.

1615 Moore, A. S., H. W. Gonyou, J. M. Stookey, & D. G. McLaren. 1994. Effect of group composition and pen size on behaviour, productivity and immune response of growing pigs. *Appl. Anim. Behav. Sci.* 40:13–30.

1616 Moore, A. U., & F. L. Marcuse. 1945. Salivary, cardiac and motor indices of conditioning in two sows. *J. Comp. Psychol.* 38:1–16.

1617 Moore, C. L., W. G. Whittlestone, M. Mullord, P. N. Priest, R. Kilgour, & J. L. Albright. 1975. Behavior responses of dairy cows trained to activate a feeding device. *J. Dairy Sci.* 58:1531–1535.

1618 **Moore, R. M., Jr, R. B. Zehmer, J. I. Moulthrop, & R. L. Parker. 1977. Surveillance of animal-bite cases in the United States, 1971–1972. *Arch. Environ. Health* 32:267–270.**

1619 Mooring, M. S., A. J. Gavazzi, & B. L. Hart. 1998. Effects of castration on grooming in goats. *Physiol. Behav.* 64:707–713.

1620 Morag, M. 1967. Influence of diet on the behaviour pattern of sheep. *Nature* 213:110.

1621 Moretti, L., M. Hentrup, K. Kotrschal, & F. Range. 2015. The influence of relationships on neophobia and exploration in wolves and dogs. *Anim. Behav.* 107:159–173.

1622 **Morgan, C. A., B. J. Tolkamp, G. C. Emmans, & I. Kyriazakis. 2000. The way in which the data are combined affects the interpretation of short-term feeding behavior. *Physiol. Behav.* 70:391–396.**

1623 Morgan, C. A., G. C. Emmans, B. J. Tolkamp, & I. Kyriazakis. 2000.

Analysis of the feeding behavior of pigs using different models. *Physiol. Behav.* 68:395–403.

1624 **Morgan, M., & K. A. Houpt. 1989. Feline behavior problems: The influence of declawing.** *Arthrozoos.* **3:50–53.**

1625 Morgan, P. D., & G. W. Arnold. 1974. Behavioural relationships between merino ewes and lambs during the four weeks after birth. *Anim. Prod.* 19:169–176.

1626 Morgan, P. D., C. A. P. Boundy, G. W. Arnold, & D. R. Lindsay. 1975. The roles played by the senses of the ewe in the location and recognition of lambs. *Appl. Anim. Ethol.* 1:139–150.

1627 Mormede, P., & R. Dantzer. 1977. Effects of dexamethasone on fear conditioning in pigs. *Behav.Biol.* 21:225–235.

1628 Mormede, P., & R. Dantzer. 1977. Experimental studies on avoidance behavior in pigs. *Appl. Anim. Ethol.* 3:173–185.

1629 Morrison, A. R. 1983. A window on the sleeping brain. *Sci. Am.* 248:94–102.

1630 Morrison, S. R., H. F. Hintz, & R. L. Givens. 1968. A note on effect of exercise on behaviour and performance of confined swine. *Anim. Prod.* 10:341–344.

1631 Morrow, D. A. 1976. Fat cow syndrome. *J. Dairy Sci.* 59:1625–1629.

1632 Morrow, M., J. Ottobre, A. Ottobre, P. Neville, N. St-Pierre, N. Dreschel, & J. L. Pate. 2015. Breed-dependent differences in the onset of fear-related avoidance behavior in puppies. *J. Vet. Behav.* 10(4):286–294.

1633 Morrow-Tesch, J. L., J. J. McGlone, & J. L. Salak-Johnson. 1994. Heat and social stress effects on pig immune measures. *J. Anim. Sci.* 72:2599–2609.

1634 Morrow-Tesch, J., & J. J. McGlone. 1990. Sensory systems and nipple attachment behavior in neonatal pigs. *Physiol. Behav.* 47:1–4.

1635 Morrow-Tesch, J., & J. J. McGlone. 1990. Sources of maternal odors and the development of odor preferences in baby pigs. *J. Anim. Sci.* 68:3563–3571.

1636 Moser, E., & M. Mcculloch. 2010. Canine scent detection of human cancers: A review of methods and accuracy. *J. Vet. Behav.* 5(3):145–152.

1637 Motch, S. E., H. W. Harpster, S. Ralston, N. Ostiguy, & N. K. Diehl. 2007. A note on yearling horse ingestive and agonistic behaviours in three concentrate feeding systems. *Appl. Anim. Behav. Sci.* 106:167–172.

1638 Moulton, D. G., E. H. Ashton, & J. T. Eayrs. 1960. Studies in olfactory acuity. 4. Relative detectability of n-aliphatic acids by the dog. *Anim. Behav.* 8:117–128.

1639 Mounier, L., I. Veissier, S. Andanson, E. Delval, & A. Boissy. 2006. Mixing at the beginning of fattening moderates social buffering in beef bulls. *Appl. Anim. Behav. Sci.* 96:185–200.

1640 Mount, N. C. 1979. *Adaptation to thermal environment: Man and his productive animals*. Baltimore, MD: University Park Press.

1641 Mount, N. C., & M. F. Seabrook. 1993. A study of aggression when group housed sows are mixed. *Appl. Anim. Behav. Sci.* 36:383.

1642 Moya, S. L., L. A. Boyle, P. B. Lynch, & S. Arkins. 2008. Surgical castration of pigs affects the behavioural response to a low-dose lipopolysaccharide (LPS) challenge after weaning. *Appl. Anim. Behav. Sci.* 112:40–57.

1643 Mugford, R. A. 1977. External influences on the feeding of carnivores. In M. R. Kare, & O. Maller (Eds.), *The chemical senses and nutrition*, pp. 25–50. New York, NY: Academic Press.

1644 Muller, R., & M. A. G. von Keyserlingk. 2006. Consistency of flight speed and its correlation to productivity and to personality in *Bos taurus* beef cattle. *Appl. Anim. Behav. Sci.* 99:193–204.

1645 Munkenbeck, N. 1983. *A test of color vision and a spectral sensitivity curve in the sheep (Ovis aries)*. Ithaca, NY: Cornell University.

1646 Munksgaard, L., A. M. dePassille, J. Rushen, & J. Ladewig. 1999. Dairy cows' use of colour cues to discriminate between people. *Appl. Anim. Behav. Sci.* 65:1–11.

1647 Munksgaard, L., A. M. DePassille, J. Rushen, M. S. Herskin, & A. M. Kristensen. 2001. Dairy cows' fear of people: Social learning, milk yield and behaviour at milking. *Appl. Anim. Behav. Sci.* 73:15–26.

1648 Munksgaard, L., M. B. Jensen, L. J. Pedersen, S. W. Hansen, & L. Matthews. 2005. Quantifying behavioural priorities: Effects of time constraints on behaviour of dairy cows, *Bos taurus*. *Appl. Anim. Behav. Sci.* 92:3–14.

1649 Munro, J. 1956. Observations on the sucking behaviour of young lambs. *Br. J. Anim. Behav.* 4:34–36.

1650 Murphey, R. M., C. R. Ruiz-Miranda, & F. A. de Moura Duarte. 1990. Maternal recognition in gyr (*Bos indicus*) calves. *Appl. Anim. Behav. Sci.* 27:183–191.

1651 Murphey, R. M., F. A. Duarte, W. C. Novaes, & M. C. Penedo. 1981. Age group differences in bovine investigatory behavior. *Dev. Psychobiol.* 14:117–125.

1652 Murphree, O. D., J. E. Peters, & R. A. Dykman. 1969. Behavioral comparisons of nervous, stable, and crossbred pointers at ages, 2, 3, 6, 9, and 12 months. *Cond. Reflex* 4:20–23.

1653 Murphy, E., L. Kraak, J. Van Den Broek, R. E. Nordquist, & F. J. Van Der Staay. 2015. Decision-making under risk and ambiguity in low-birth-weight pigs. *Anim. Cogn.* 18(2):561–572.

1654 Murphy, E., L. Kraak, R. E. Nordquist, & F. J. Van Der Staay. 2013. Successive and conditional discrimination learning in pigs. *Anim. Cogn.* 16(6):883–893.

1655 Murphy, J., A. Sutherland, & S. Arkins. 2005. Idiosyncratic motor laterality in the horse. *Appl. Anim. Behav. Sci.* 91:297–310.

1656 Myer, J. J., F. D. Martin, & I. L. Brisbin. 2002. Characteristics of wild pig farrowing nests and beds in the upper coastal plain of south carolina. *Appl. Anim. Behav. Sci.* 78:1–17.

1657 Myers, G. C. 1916. The importance of primacy in the learning of a pig. *J. Anim. Behav.* 6:64–69.

1658 Myers, R. D., & D. C. Mesker. 1960. Operant responding in a horse under several schedules of reinforcement. *J. Exp. Anal. Behav.* 3:161–164.

1659 Mylrea, P. J., & R. G. Beilharz. 1964. The manifestation and detection of oestrous in heifers. *Anim. Behav.* 12:25–30.

1660 Nagamachi, Y. 1972. Effect of satiety center damage on food intake, blood glucose and gastric secretion in dogs. *Am. J. Dig. Dis.* 17:139–148.

1661 Nagasawa, M., A. Yatsuzuka, K. Mogi, & T. Kikusui. 2012. A new behavioral test for detecting decline of age-related cognitive ability in dogs. *J. Vet. Behav.* 7(4):220–224.

1662 Nagasawa, M., K. Murai, K. Mogi, & T. Kikusui. 2011. Dogs can discriminate human smiling faces from blank expressions. *Anim. Cogn.* 14(4):525–533.

1663 Nagasawa, M., S. Mitsui, S. En, N. Ohtani, M. Ohta, Y. Sakuma, T. Onaka, *et al.* 2015. Oxytocin-gaze positive loop and the coevolution of human-dog bonds. *Science.* 348(6232):333–336.

1664 Nagy, K., A. Schrott, & P. Kabai. 2008. Possible influence of neighbours on stereotypic behaviour in horses. *Appl. Anim. Behav. Sci.* 111:321–328.

1665 Nagy, K., G. Bodó, G. Bárdos, A. Harnos, & P. Kabai. 2009. The effect of a feeding stress-test on the behaviour and heart rate variability of control and crib-biting horses (with or without inhibition). *Appl. Anim. Behav. Sci.* 121(2):140–147.

1666 Nagy, K., G. Bodó, G. Bárdos, N. Bánszky, & P. Kabai. 2010. Differences in temperament traits between crib-biting and control horses. *Appl. Anim. Behav. Sci.* 122(1):41–47.

1667 Nagy, P., G. Duchamp, P. Chavatte-Palmer, P. F. Daels, & D. Guillaume. 2002. Induction of lactation in mares with a dopamine antagonist needs ovarian hormones. *Theriogenology* 58:589–592.

1668 Napolitano, F., V. Marino, G. De Rosa, R. Capparelli, & A. Bordi. 1995. Influence of artificial rearing on behavioral and immune response in lambs. *Appl. Anim. Behav. Sci.* 45:245–253.

1669 Natoli, E. 1985. Spacing pattern in a colony of urban stray cats (*Felis catus* L.) in the historic centre of Rome. *Appl. Anim. Behav. Sci.* 14:289–304.

1670 Natoli, E. 1990. Mating strategies in cats: A comparison of the role and importance of infanticide in domestic cats, *Felis catus* L. and lions, *Panthera leo* L. *Anim. Behav.* 40:183–186.

1671 Natoli, E., & E. De Vito. 1991. Agonistic behavior, dominance rank and copulatory success in a large multi-male feral cat, *Felis catus* L.; colony in central Rome. *Anim. Behav.* 42:227–241.

1672 Naujeck, A., J. Hill, & M. J. Gibb. 2005. Influence of sward height on diet selection by horses. *Appl. Anim. Behav. Sci.* 9:49–63.

1673 Nawroth, C., E. Von Borell, & J. Langbein. 2014. Exclusion performance in dwarf goats (*Capra aegagrus hircus*) and sheep (*Ovis orientalis aries*). *PLoS ONE.* 9(4):e93534.

1674 **Nawroth, C., E. Von Borell, & J. Langbein. 2015. "Goats that stare at men": Dwarf goats alter their behaviour in response to human head orientation, but do not spontaneously use head direction as a cue in a food-related context. *Anim. Cogn.* 18(1):65–73.**

1675 Nawroth, C., M. Ebersbach, & E. Von Borell. 2013. Are juvenile domestic pigs (sus scrofa domestica) sensitive to the attentive states of humans? The impact of impulsivity on choice behaviour. *Behav. Processes.* 96:53–58.

1676 **Neathery, M. W. 1971. Acceptance of orphan lambs by tranquilized ewes (*Ovis aries*). *Anim. Behav.* 19:75–79.**

1677 Neave, H. W., R. R. Daros, J. H. Costa, M. A. Von Keyserlingk, & D. M. Weary. 2013. Pain and pessimism: Dairy calves exhibit negative judgement bias following hot-iron disbudding. *PLoS ONE.* 8(12):e80556.

1678 Neff, W. D., & I. T. Diamond. 1958. The neural basis of auditory discriminatin. In H. F. Harlow, & C. N. Woolsey (Eds.), Biological and biochemical bases of behavior, pp. 101–126. Madison, WI: University of Wisconsin Press.

1679 **Neilson, J. C., B. L. Hart, K. D. Cliff, & W. W. Ruehl. 2001. Prevalence of behavioral changes associated with age-related cognitive impairment in dogs. *J. Am. Vet. Med. Assoc.* 218:1787–1791.**

1680 Neilson, J. C., R. A. Eckstein, & B. L. Hart. 1997. Effects of castration on problem behaviors in male dogs with reference to age and duration of behavior. *J. Am. Vet. Med. Assoc.* 211:180–182.

1681 Neitz, J., & G. H. Jacobs. 1989. Spectral sensitivity of cones in an ungulate. *Vis. Neurosci.* 2:97–100.

1682 Neitz, J., T. Geist, & G. H. Jacobs. 1989. Color vision in the dog. *Vis. Neurosci.* 3:119–125.

1683 Nelson, R. J. 2005. *An introduction to behavioral endocrinology*, 3rd ed. Sunderland, MA: Sinauer Associates.

1684 Nelson, S. H., A. D. Evans, & R. B. Bradbury. 2005. The efficacy of collar-mounted devices in reducing the rate of predation of wildlife by domestic cats. *Appl. Anim. Behav. Sci.* 94:273–285.

1685 Netto, W. J., & D. J. U. Planta. 1997. Behavioural testing for aggression in the domestic dog. *Appl. Anim. Behav. Sci.* 52:243–263.

1686 Newberry, R. C., & D. G. M. Wood-Gush. 1986. Social relationships of piglets in a seminatural environment. *Anim. Behav.* 34:1311–1318.

1687 Newman, J. A., P. D. Penning, A. J. Parson, A. Harvey, & R. J. Orr. 1994. Fasting affects intake behaviour and diet preference in grazing sheep. *Anim. Behav.* 47:185–193.

1688 Nicastro, N. 2004. Perceptual and acoustic evidence for species-level differences in meow vocalizations by domestic cats (*Felis catus*) and African wild cats (*Felis silvestris lybica*). *J. Comp. Psychol.* 118:287–296.

1689 Nicastro, N., & M. J. Owren. 2003. Classification of domestic cat (*Felis catus*) vocalizations by naive and experienced human listeners. *J. Comp. Psychol.* 117:44–52.

1690 Nicol, C. J. 2002. Equine learning: Progress and suggestions for future research. *Appl. Anim. Behav. Sci.* 78:193–208.

1691 Nicol, C. J., A. J. Badnell-Waters, R. Bice, A. Kelland, A. D. Wilson, & P. A. Harris. 2005. The effects of diet and weaning method on the behaviour of young horses. *Appl. Anim. Behav. Sci.* 95:205–221.

1692 Nicol, C. J., H. P. Davidson, P. A. Harris, A. J. Waters, & A. D. Wilson. 2002. Study of crib-biting and gastric inflammation and ulceration in young horses. *Vet. Rec.* 151:658–662.

1693 **Nikitopoulou, G., & J. L. Crammer. 1976. Change in diurnal temperature rhythm in manic-depressive illness. *Br. Med. J.* 1:1311–1314.**

1694 **Ninomiya, S., M. Aoyama, Y. Ujiie, R. Kusunose, & A. Kuwano. 2008. Effects of bedding material on the lying behavior in stabled horses. *J. Equine Sci.* 19:53–56.**

1695 Ninomiya, S., S. Sato, & K. Sugawara. 2007. Weaving in stabled horses and its relationship to other behavioural traits. *Appl. Anim. Behav. Sci.* 106:134–143.

1696 Ninomiya, S., S. Sato, R. Kusunose, T. Mitumasu, & Y. Obara. 2007. A note on

a behavioural indicator of satisfaction in stabled horses. *Appl. Anim. Behav. Sci.* 106:184–189.

1697 Ninomiya, S., T. Mitsumasu, M. Aoyama, & R. Kusunose. 2007. A note on the effect of a palatable food reward on operant conditioning in horses. *Appl. Anim. Behav. Sci.* 108:342–347.

1698 Nitzschner, M., J. Kaminski, A. Melis, & M. Tomasello. 2014. Side matters: Potential mechanisms underlying dogs' performance in a social eavesdropping paradigm. *Anim. Behav.* 90:263–271.

1699 Noble, G. K., E. Houghton, C. J. Roberts, J. Faustino-Kemp, S. S. de Kock, B. C. Swanepoel, & M. N. Sillence. 2007. Effect of exercise, training, circadian rhythm, age, and sex on insulin-like growth factor-1 in the horse. *J. Anim. Sci.* 85:163–171.

1700 Noble, G. K., K. L. Blackshaw, A. Cowling, P. A. Harris, & M. N. Sillence. 2013. An objective measure of reactive behaviour in horses. *Appl. Anim. Behav. Sci.* 144(3–4):121–129.

1701 Noble, M., & C. K. Adams. 1963. Conditioning in pigs as a function of the interval between CS and US. *J. Comp. Physiol. Psychol.* 56:215–219.

1702 **Noda, K., & K. Chikamori. 1976. Effect of ammonia via prepyriform cortex on regulation of food intake in the rat. *Am. J. Physiol.* 231:1263–1266.**

1703 Nolte, D. L., & F. D. Provenza. 1992. Food preferences in lambs after exposure to flavors in solid foods. *Appl. Anim. Behav. Sci.* 32:337–347.

1704 Nonneman, A. J., & J. M. Warren. 1977. Two-cue learning by brain-damaged cats. *Physiol. Psychol.* 5:397–402.

1705 Norman, K., S. Pellis, L. Barrett, & S. Peter Henzi. 2015. Down but not out: Supine postures as facilitators of play in domestic dogs. *Behav. Processes.* 110:88–95.

1706 Normando, S., L. Corain, M. Salvadoretti, L. Meers, & P. Valsecchi. 2009. Effects of an enhanced human interaction program on shelter dogs' behaviour analysed using a novel nonparametric test. *Appl. Anim. Behav. Sci.* 116:211–219.

1707 Notari, L., & D. Goodwin. 2007. A survey of behavioural characteristics of pure-bred dogs in Italy. *Appl. Anim. Behav. Sci.* 103:118–130.

1708 Nowak, R. 1991. Senses involved in discrimination of merino ewes at close contact and from distance by their newborn lambs. *Anim. Behav.* 42:357–366.

1709 Nowak, R., M. Keller, D. Val-Laillet, & F. Levy. 2007. Perinatal visceral events and brain mechanisms involved in the development of mother-young bonding in sheep. *Horm. Behav.* 52:92–98.

1710 Noyes, L. 1976. A behavioural comparison of gnotobiotic with normal neonate pigs, indicating stress in the former. *Appl. Anim. Ethol.* 2:113–121.

1711 Nunez, C. M. V., J. S. Adelman, C. Mason, & D. I. Rubenstein. 2009. Immunocontraception decreases group fidelity in a feral horse population during the non-breeding season. *Appl. Anim. Behav. Sci.* 117:74–83.

1712 Nyman, S., & K. Dahlborn. 2001. Effect of water supply method and flow rate on drinking behavior and fluid balance in horses. *Physiol. Behav.* 73:1–8.

1713 Oberosler, R., C. Carenzi, & M. Vega. 1982. Dominance hierarchies of cows on alpine pastures as related to phenotype. *Appl. Anim. Ethol.* 8:67–77.

1714 Obese, F. Y., B. K. Whitlock, B. P. Steele, F. C. Buonomo, & J. L. Sartin. 2007. Long-term feed intake regulation in sheep is mediated by opioid receptors. *J. Anim. Sci.* 85:111–117.

1715 O'Brien, P. H. 1984. Feral goat home range: Influence of social class and environmental variables. *Appl. Anim. Behav. Sci.* 12:373–385.

1716 **O'Brien, P. H. 1988. Feral goat organization: A review and comparative analysis. *Appl. Anim. Behav. Sci.* 21:209–221.**

1717 Ochoa, M., C.-H. Malbert, J.-P. Lallès, F. Bobillier & D. Val-Laillet. 2014. Effects of chronic intake of starch-, glucose- and fructose-containing diets on eating behaviour in adult minipigs. *Appl. Anim. Behav. Sci.* 157:61–71.

1718 O'Connell, J. M., P. S. Giller, & W. J. Meaney. 1993. Weanling training and cubicle usage as heifers. *Appl. Anim. Behav. Sci.* 37:185–195.

1719 O'Connor, C. E., A. B. Lawrence, & D. G. M. Wood-Gush. 1992. Influence of litter size and parity on maternal behaviour at parturition in Scottish blackface sheep. *Appl. Anim. Behav. Sci.* 33:345–355.

1720 Odberg, F. O. 1973. An interpretation of pawing by the horse (*Equus caballus linnaeus*), displacement activity and original functions. *Saugetierkund. Mitteil.* 21:1–12.

1721 Odberg, F. O., & K. Francis-Smith. 1977. Studies on the formation of ungrazed eliminative areas in fields used by horses. *Appl. Anim. Ethol.* 3:34.

1722 Odde, K. G., G. H. Hiracofe, & R. R. Schalles. 1985. Suckling behavior in range beef calves. *J. Anim. Sci.* 61:307–309.

1723 O'Driscoll, K., L. Boyle, & A. Hanlon. 2009. The effect of breed and housing system on dairy cow feeding and lying behaviour. *Appl. Anim. Behav. Sci.* 116:156–162.

1724 O'Farrell, V., & E. Peachey. 1990. Behavioural effects of ovariohysterectomy in bitches. *J. Small Anim. Pract.* 31:595–598.

1725 Offord, K. P., L. D. Satter, & D. A. Weickert. 1969. Study of behavioral conditioning and feed intake in dairy heifers. *J. Dairy. Sci.* 52:918.

1726 **Ogata, N., & Y. Takeuchi. 2001. Clinical trial of a feline pheromone analogue for feline urine marking. *J. Vet. Med. Sci.* 63:157–161.**

1727 **Ogata, N., C. Hashizume, Y. Momozawa, K. Masuda, T. Kikusui, Y. Takeuchi, & Y. Mori. 2006.**

Polymorphisms in the canine glutamate transporter-1 gene: Identification and variation among five dog breeds. *J. Vet. Med. Sci.* 68:157–159.

1728 Ogata, N., T. E. Gillis, X. Liu, S. M. Cunningham, S. B. Lowen, B. L. Adams, J. Sutherland-Smith, *et al.* 2013. Brain structural abnormalities in doberman pinschers with canine compulsive disorder. *Prog. Neuropsychopharmacol. Biol. Psychiatry.* 45:1–6.

1729 O'hara, S. J., & A. V. Reeve. 2011. A test of the yawning contagion and emotional connectedness hypothesis in dogs, *Canis familiaris. Anim. Behav.* 81(1):335–340.

1730 Ohkita, M., M. Nagasawa, M. Kazutaka, & T. Kikusui. 2016. Owners' direct gazes increase dogs' attention-getting behaviors. *Behav. Processes.* 125:96–100.

1731 Olmos, G., & S. P. Turner. 2008. The relationships between temperament during routine handling tasks, weight gain and facial hair whorl position in frequently handled beef cattle. *Appl. Anim. Behav. Sci.* 115:25–36.

1732 Oostindjer, M., J. E. Bolhuis, M. Mendl, S. Held, H. Van Den Brand, & B. Kemp. 2011. Learning how to eat like a pig: Effectiveness of mechanisms for vertical social learning in piglets. *Anim. Behav.* 82(3):503–511.

1733 Ordakowski-Burk, A. L., R. W. Quinn, T. A. Shellem, & L. R. Vough. 2006. Voluntary intake and digestibility of reed canarygrass and timothy hay fed to horses. *J. Anim. Sci.* 84:3104–3109.

1734 Orgeur, P. 1995. Sexual play behavior in lambs androgenized in utero. *Physiol. Behav.* 57:185–187.

1735 Orgeur, P., P. Mimouni, & J. Signoret. 1990. The influence of rearing conditions on the social relationships of young male goats (*Capra hircus*). *Appl. Anim. Behav. Sci.* 27:105–113.

1736 Orihuela, A., & C. S. Galina. 1997. Social order measured in pasture and pen conditions and its relationship to sexual behavior in brahman (*Bos indicus*) cows. *Appl. Anim. Behav. Sci.* 52:3–11.

1737 Orr, R. J., B. A. Griffith, R. A. Champion, & J. E. Cook. 2012. Defaecation and urination behaviour in beef cattle grazing semi-natural grassland. *Appl. Anim. Behav. Sci.* 139(1–2):18–25.

1738 Ortega-Reyes, L., & F. D. Provenza. 1993. Amount of experience and age affect the development of foraging skills of goats browsing blackbrus (coleogyne ramosissima). *Appl. Anim. Behav. Sci.* 36:169–183.

1739 Osterman, S., & I. I. Redbo. 2001. Effects of milking frequency on lying down and getting up behaviour in dairy cows. *Appl. Anim. Behav. Sci.* 70:167–176.

1740 Osthaus, B., L. Proops, I. Hocking, & F. Burden. 2013. Spatial cognition and perseveration by horses, donkeys and mules in a simple a-not-b detour task. *Anim. Cogn.* 16(2):301–305.

1741 **Osthaus, B., S. E. Lea, & A. M. Slater. 2005. Dogs (*Canis lupus familiaris*) fail to show understanding of means-end connections in a string-pulling task. *Anim. Cogn.* 8:37–47.**

1742 Ostojic, L., M. Tkalcic, & N. S. Clayton. 2015. Are owners' reports of their dogs' "guilty look" influenced by the dogs' action and evidence of the misdeed? *Behav. Processes.* 111:97–100.

1743 Otten, W., B. Puppe, E. Kanitz, P. C. Schon, & B. Stabenow. 2002. Physiological and behavioral effects of different success during social confrontation in pigs with prior dominance experience. *Physiol. Behav.* 75:127–133.

1744 Over, R., J. Cohen-Tannoudji, M. Dehnhard, R. Claus, & J. P. Signoret. 1990. Effect of pheromones from male goats on LH-secretion in anoestrous ewes. *Physiol. Behav.* 48:665–668.

1745 Overall, K. L. 2013. *Clinical behavioral medicine for small animals.* St. Louis, MO: Mosby.

1746 Owen, J. B., & W. J. Ridgman. 1967. The effect of dietary energy content on the voluntary intake of pigs. *Anim. Prod.* 9:107–113.

1747 Owen, R., F. J. McKeating, & D. W. Jagger. 1980. Neurectomy in windsucking horses. *Vet. Rec.* 106:134–135.

1748 Owens, J. L., T. N. Edey, B. M. Bindon, & L. R. Piper. 1984. Parturient behaviour and calf survival in a herd selected for twinning. *Appl. Anim. Behav. Sci.* 13:321–333.

1749 Pachel, C., & J. Neilson. 2010. Comparison of feline water consumption between still and flowing water sources: A pilot study. *J. Vet. Behav.* 5(3):130–133.

1750 Packwood, J., & B. Gordon. 1975. Stereopsis in normal domestic cat, siamese cat, and cat raised with alternating monocular occlusion. *J. Neurophysiol.* 38:1485–1499.

1751 Padilla De La Torre, M., E. F. Briefer, B. M. Ochocki, A. G. Mcelligott, & T. Reader. 2016. Mother-offspring recognition via contact calls in cattle, *Bos taurus. Anim. Behav.* 114:147–154.

1752 Padilla de la Torre, M., E. F. Briefer, T. Reader, & A. G. McElligott. 2015. Acoustic analysis of cattle (*Bos taurus*) mother-offspring contact calls from a source-filter theory perspective. *Appl. Anim. Behav. Sci.* 163:58–68.

1753 Pageat, P., & E. Gaultier. 2003. Current research in canine and feline pheromones. *Vet. Clin. North Am. Small Anim. Pract.* 33:187–211.

1754 Pajor, E. A., D. Fraser, & D. L. Kramer. 1991. Consumption of solid food by suckling pigs: Individual variation and relation to weight gain. *Appl. Anim. Behav. Sci.* 32:139–155.

1755 Pajor, E. A., D. M. Weary, C. Caceres, D. Fraser, & D. L. Kramer. 2002. Alternative housing for sows and litters part 3. Effects of piglet diet quality and sow-controlled housing on performance and behaviour. *Appl. Anim. Behav. Sci.* 76:267–277.

1756 Pal, S. K. 2003. Urine marking by free-ranging dogs (*Canis familiaris*) in relation to sex, season, place and posture. *Appl. Anim. Behav. Sci.* 80:45–59.

1757 Pal, S. K. 2005. Parental care in free-ranging dogs, *Canis familiaris. Appl. Anim. Behav. Sci.* 90:31–47.

1758 Pal, S. K. 2008. Maturation and development of social behaviour during early ontogeny in free-ranging dog puppies in West Bengal, India. *Appl. Anim. Behav. Sci.* 111:95–107.

1759 Pal, S. K. 2010. Play behaviour during early ontogeny in free-ranging dogs (*Canis familiaris*). *Appl. Anim. Behav. Sci.* 126(3–4):140–153.

1760 Palacio, J., M. Leon-Artozqui, E. Pastor-Villalba, F. Carrera-Martin, & S. Garcia-Belenguer. 2007. Incidence of and risk factors for cat bites: A first step in prevention and treatment of feline aggression. *J. Feline Med. Surg.* 9:188–195.

1761 Palazzolo, D. L., & S. K. Quadri. 1987. The effects of aging on the circadian rhythm of serum cortisol in the dog. *Exp. Gerontol.* 22:379–387.

1762 Palen, G. F., & G. V. Goddard. 1966. Catnip and oestrous behaviour in the cat. *Anim. Behav.* 14:372–377.

1763 Palmer, A. C., G. F. Smith, & S. J. Turner. 1980. Cataplexy in a guernsey bull. *Vet. Rec.* 106:421.

1764 Panaman, R. 1981. Behavior and ecology of free-ranging farm cats (*Felis catus*). *Z. Tierpsychol.* 56:59–73.

1765 Pappas, T. N., R. L. Melendez, K. M. Strah, & H. T. Debas. 1985. Cholecystokinin is not a peripheral satiety signal in the dog. *Am. J. Physiol.* 249:G733–G738.

1766 Parent, J.-P., M.-C. Meunier-Salaün, E. Vasseur, & R. Bergeron. 2012. Stability of social hierarchy in growing female pigs and pregnant sows. *Appl. Anim. Behav. Sci.* 142(1–2):1–10.

1767 Parker, M., E. S. Redhead, D. Goodwin, & S. D. Mcbride. 2008. Impaired instrumental choice in crib-biting horses (*Equus caballus*). *Behav. Brain Res.* 191(1):137–140.

1768 Paroz, C., S. G. Gebhardt-Henrich, & A. Steiger. 2008. Reliability and validity of behaviour tests in hovawart dogs. *Appl. Anim. Behav. Sci.* 115:67–81.

1769 Parratt, C. A., K. J. Chapman, C. Turner, P. H. Jones, M. T. Mendl, & B. G. Miller. 2006. The fighting behaviour of piglets mixed before and after weaning in the presence or absence of a sow. *Appl. Anim. Behav. Sci.* 101:54–67.

1770 **Parrott, R. F. 1993. Peripheral and central effects of CCK receptor agonists on operant feeding in pigs. *Physiol. Behav.* 53:367–372.**

1771 Parrott, R. F., & B. A. Baldwin. 1984. Olfactory stimuli and intermale aggression in androgen-treated castrated sheep. *Aggress. Behav.* 10:115–122.

1772 Parrott, R. F., & W. D. Booth. 1984. Behavioural and morphological effects of 5 alpha-dihydrotestosterone and oestradiol-17 beta in the prepubertally castrated boar. *J. Reprod. Fertil.* 71:453–461.

1773 **Parsons, S. D., & G. L. Hunter. 1967. Effect of the ram on duration of oestrus in the ewe. *J. Reprod. Fertil.* 14:61–70.**

1774 Pascual-Alonso, M., G. A. María, W. S. Sepúlveda, M. Villarroel, L. Aguayo-Ulloa, F. Galindo, & G. C. Miranda-De La Lama. 2013. Identity profiles based on social strategies, morphology, physiology, and cognitive abilities in goats. *J. Vet. Behav.* 8(6):458–465.

1775 Passalacqua, C., S. Marshall-Pescini, I. Merola, C. Palestrini, & E. P. Previde. 2013. Different problem-solving strategies in dogs diagnosed with anxiety-related disorders and control dogs in an unsolvable task paradigm. *Appl. Anim. Behav. Sci.* 147(1–2):139–148.

1776 Passalacqua, C., S. Marshall-Pescini, S. Barnard, G. Lakatos, P. Valsecchi, & E. Prato Previde. 2011. Human-directed gazing behaviour in puppies and adult dogs, *Canis lupus familiaris. Anim. Behav.* 82(5):1043–1050.

1777 Patison, K. P., D. L. Swain, G. J. Bishop-Hurley, G. Robins, P. Pattison, & D. J. Reid. 2010. Changes in temporal and spatial associations between pairs of cattle during the process of familiarisation. *Appl. Anim. Behav. Sci.* 128(1–4):10–17.

1778 **Patison, K. P., D. L. Swain, G. J. Bishop-Hurley, P. Pattison, & G. Robins. 2010. Social companionship versus food: The effect of the presence of familiar and unfamiliar conspecifics on the distance steers travel. *Appl. Anim. Behav. Sci.* 122(1):13–20.**

1779 Pavlov, I. P. 1927. *Conditioned reflexes. An investigation of the physiological activity of the cerebral cortex.* London, UK: Oxford University Press.

1780 Pedersen, L. J. 2007. Sexual behaviour in female pigs. *Horm. Behav.* 52:64–69.

1781 Pedersen, L. J., & T. Jensen. 2008. Effects of late introduction of sows to two farrowing environments on the progress of farrowing and maternal behavior. *J. Anim. Sci.* 86:2730–2737.

1782 Pedersen, L. J., E. Jørgensen, T. Heiskanen, & B. I. Damm. 2006. Early piglet mortality in loose-housed sows related to sow and piglet behaviour and to the progress of parturition. *Appl. Anim. Behav. Sci.* 96:215–232.

1783 Pedersen, L. J., T. Rojkittikhun, S. Einarsson, & L. Edqvist. 1993. Postweaning grouped sows: Effects of aggression on hormonal patterns and oestrous behaviour. *Appl. Anim. Behav. Sci.* 38:25–39.

1784 Peeters, M., D. Verwilghen, D. Serteyn, & M. Vandenheede. 2012. Relationships between young stallions' temperament and their behavioral reactions during standardized veterinary examinations. *J. Vet. Behav.* 7(5):311–321.

1785 Pekas, J. C. 1985. Animal growth during liberation from appetite suppression. *Growth* 49:19–27.

1786 **Pekas, J. C., & W. E. Trout. 1993. Cholecystokinin octapeptide immunization: Effect on growth of barrows and gilts. *J. Anim. Sci.* 71:2499–2505.**

1787 Pell, S. M., & P. D. McGreevy. 1999. A study of cortisol and beta-endorphin levels in stereotypic and normal thoroughbreds. *Appl. Anim. Behav. Sci.* 64:81–90.

1788 Penning, P. D., A. J. Parsons, J. A. Newman, R. J. Orr, & A. Harvey. 1993. The effects of group size on grazing time in sheep. *Appl. Anim. Behav. Sci.* 37:101–109.

1789 Penning, P. D., A. J. Parsons, R. J. Orr, A. Harvey, & R. A. Champion. 1995. Intake and behaviour responses by sheep, in different physiological states, when grazing monocultures of grass or white clover. *Appl. Anim. Behav. Sci.* 45:63–78.

1790 Penning, P. D., A. J. Rook, & R. J. Orr. 1991. Patterns of ingestive behaviour of sheep continuously stocked on monocultures of ryegrass or white clover. *Appl. Anim. Behav. Sci.* 31:237–250.

1791 Penny, R. H., F. W. Hill, J. E. Field, & J. T. Plush. 1972. Tail-biting in pigs: A possible sex incidence. *Vet. Rec.* 91:482–483.

1792 Pepelko, W. E., & M. T. Clegg. 1965. Influence of season of the year upon patterns of sexual behavior in male sheep. *J. Anim. Sci.* 24:633–637.

1793 Pepelko, W. E., & M. T. Clegg. 1965. Studies of mating behaviour and some factors influencing the sexual response in the male sheep *Ovis aries*. *Anim. Behav.* 13:249–258.

1794 **Peremans, K., K. Audenaert, F. Coopman, P. Blanckaert, F. Jacobs, A. Otte, F. Verschooten, *et al.* 2003. Estimates of regional cerebral blood flow and 5-ht2a receptor density in impulsive, aggressive dogs with 99mtc-ecd and 123i-5-i-r91150. *Eur. J. Nucl. Med. Mol. Imaging.* 30(11):1538–1546.**

1795 Pérez-Guisado, J., R. Lopez-Rodríguez, & A. Muñoz-Serrano. 2006. Heritability of dominant-aggressive behaviour in English cocker spaniels. *Appl. Anim. Behav. Sci.* 100(3–4):219–227.

1796 Perez-Leon, I., A. Orihuela, L. Lidfors, & V. Aguirre. 2006. Reducing mother-young separation distress by inducing ewes into oestrus at the day of weaning. *Anim. Welf.* 15:383–389.

1797 Perkins, A., & J. A. Fitzgerald. 1994. The behavioral component of the ram effect: The influence of ram sexual behavior on the induction of estrus in anovulatory ewes. *J. Anim. Sci.* 72:51–55.

1798 Peron, F., R. Ward, & O. Burman. 2014. Horses (*Equus caballus*) discriminate body odour cues from conspecifics. *Anim. Cogn.* 17(4):1007–1011.

1799 Persson, N. 1962. Self-stimulation in the goat. *Acta Physiol. Scand.* 55:276–285.

1800 Petchey, A. M., & J. Abdulkader. 1991. Intake and behaviour of cattle at different food barriers. *Anim. Prod.* 52:576–577.

1801 Petersen, H. V., K. Vestergaard, & P. Jensen. 1989. Integration of piglets into social groups of free-ranging domestic pigs. *Appl. Anim. Behav. Sci.* 23:223–226.

1802 Petersen, V. 1994. The development of feeding and investigatory behaviour in free-ranging domestic pigs during their first 18 weeks of life. *Appl. Anim. Behav. Sci.* 42:87–98.

1803 Petersen, V., H. B. Simonsen, & L. G. Lawson. 1995. The effect of environmental stimulation on the development of behaviour in pigs. *Appl. Anim. Behav. Sci.* 45:215–224.

1804 Petit, M. 1972. Emploi du temps des troupeaux de vaches-meres et de leurs veaux sur les paturages d'altitude de l'aubrac. *Ann. Zootech.* 21:5–27.

1805 Pettijohn, T. F., T. W. Wong, P. D. Ebert, & J. P. Scott. 1977. Alleviation of separation distress in 3 breeds of young dogs. *Dev. Psychobiol.* 10:373–381.

1806 Pfaffenberger, C. J., & J. P. Scott. 1959. The relationship between delayed socialization and trainability in guide dogs. *J. Genet. Psychol.* 95:145–155.

1807 Pfister, J. A., B. L. Stegelmeier, C. D. Cheney, & D. R. Gardner. 2007. Effect of previous locoweed (astragalus and oxytropis species) intoxication on conditioned taste aversions in horses and sheep. *J. Anim. Sci.* 85:1836–1841.

1808 Pfister, J. A., B. L. Stegelmeier, C. D. Cheney, M. H. Ralphs, & D. R. Gardner. 2002. Conditioning taste aversions to locoweed (oxytropis sericea) in horses. *J. Anim. Sci.* 80:79–83.

1809 Phillips, C. 2002. *Cattle behaviour & welfare.* Oxford, UK: Blackwell Science, Ltd.

1810 Phillips, C. J. C., & L. Weiguo. 1991. Brightness discrimination abilities of calves relative to those of humans. *Appl. Anim. Behav. Sci.* 31:25–33.

1811 Phillips, C. J. C., & S. A. Schofield. 1990. The effect of environment and stage of the oestrous cycle on the behaviour of dairy cows. *Appl. Anim. Behav. Sci.* 27:21–31.

1812 Phillips, C. J. C., D. Fraser, & B. K. Thompson. 1991. Preference of sows for a partially enclosed farrowing crate. *Appl. Anim. Behav. Sci.* 32:35–43.

1813 Phillips, C. J., & C. A. Lomas. 2001. The perception of color by cattle and its influence on behavior. *J. Dairy Sci.* 84:807–813.

1814 Piccione, G., C. Bertolucci, G. Caola, & A. Foa. 2007. Effects of restricted feeding on circadian activity rhythms of sheep: A brief report. *Appl. Anim. Behav. Sci.* 107:233–238.

1815 Piccione, G., C. Giannetto, S. Marafioti, S. Casella, A. Assenza, & F. Fazio. 2011. Effect of different farming management on daily total locomotor activity in sheep. *J. Vet. Behav.* 6(4):243–247.

1816 Piccione, G., C. Giannetto, S. Marafioti, S. Casella, F. Fazio, & G. Caola. 2011. Daily rhythms of rectal temperature and total locomotor activity in trained and untrained horses. *J. Vet. Behav.* 6(2):115–120.

1817 Piccione, G., S. Marafioti, C. Giannetto, M. Panzera, & F. Fazio. 2013. Daily rhythm of total activity pattern in domestic cats (*Felis silvestris catus*) maintained in two different housing conditions. *J. Vet. Behav.* 8(4):189–194.

1818 Pick, D. F., G. Lovell, S. Brown, & D. Dail. 1994. Equine color perception *revisited*. *Appl. Anim. Behav. Sci.* 42:61–65.

1819 Pickerel, T. M., S. L. Crowell-Davis, A. B. Caudle, & D. Q. Estep. 1993. Sexual preferences of mares (*Equus caballus*) for individual stallions. *Appl. Anim. Behav. Sci.* 38:1–13.

1820 Pickett, B. W., J. L. Voss, & E. L. Squires. 1977. Impotence and abnormal sexual behavior in the stallion. *Theriogenology* 8:329–347.

1821 Pickett, B. W., L. C. Faulkner, & J. L. Voss. 1975. Effect of season on some characteristics of stallion semen. *J. Reprod. Fertil. Suppl.* (23):25–28.

1822 Pinckard, K. L., J. Stellflug, & F. Stormshak. 2000. Influence of castration and estrogen replacement on sexual behavior of female-oriented, male-oriented, and asexual rams. *J. Anim. Sci.* 78:1947–1953.

1823 Pinheiro Machado Fo, L. C. 1997. Timing of the attraction towards the placenta and amniotic fluid by the parturient cow. *Appl. Anim. Behav. Sci.* 53:183–192.

1824 Pinheiro Machado, F. L. C., J. F. Hurnik, & J. H. Burton. 1997. The effect of amniotic fluid ingestion on the nociception of cows. *Physiol. Behav.* 62:1339–1344.

1825 Pisa, P. F., & C. Agrillo. 2008. Quantity discrimination in felines: A preliminary investigation of the domestic cat (*Felis silvestris catus*). *J. Ethol.* 27(2):289–293.

1826 Pitteri, E., P. Mongillo, P. Carnier, & L. Marinelli. 2014. Hierarchical stimulus processing by dogs (*Canis familiaris*). *Anim. Cogn.* 17(4):869–877.

1827 Pitts, A. D., D. M. Weary, D. Fraser, E. A. Pajor, & D. L. Kramer. 2002. Alternative housing for sows and litters part 5. Individual differences in the maternal behaviour of sows. *Appl. Anim. Behav. Sci.* 76:291–306.

1828 Pitts, A. D., D. M. Weary, E. A. Pajor, & D. Fraser. 2000. Mixing at young ages reduces fighting in unacquainted domestic pigs. *Appl. Anim. Behav. Sci.* 68:191–197.

1829 Plush, K. J., M. L. Hebart, F. D. Brien, & P. I. Hynd. 2011. The genetics of temperament in merino sheep and relationships with lamb survival. *Appl. Anim. Behav. Sci.* 134(3–4):130–135.

1830 Podberscek, A. L., & J. A. Serpell. 1997. Aggressive behaviour in English cocker spaniels and the personality of their owners. *Vet. Rec.* 141:73–76.

1831 Podberscek, A. L., & J. A. Serpell. 1997. Environmental influences on the expression of aggressive behaviour in English cocker spaniels. *Appl. Anim. Behav. Sci.* 52:215–227.

1832 Podberscek, A. L., J. K. Blackshaw, & A. W. Beattie. 1991. The behaviour of laboratory colony cats and their reactions to a familiar and unfamiliar person. *Appl. Anim. Behav. Sci.* 31:119–130.

1833 Poindron, P., A. Terrazas, L. Montes de Oca Mde, N. Serafin, & H. Hernandez. 2007. Sensory and physiological determinants of maternal behavior in the goat (*Capra hircus*). *Horm. Behav.* 52:99–105.

1834 Pollard, J. C. 1992. Effects of litter size on the vocal behaviour of ewes. *Appl. Anim. Behav. Sci.* 34:75–84.

1835 Pollard, J. C., K. J. Shaw, & R. P. Littlejohn. 1999. A note on sheltering behaviour of ewes before and after lambing. *Appl. Anim. Behav. Sci.* 61:313–318.

1836 Pollard, J. S., M. D. Baldock, & R. F. Lewis. 1971. Learning rate and use of visual information on five animal species. *Aust. J. Psychol.* 23:29–34.

1837 Pond, R. L., M. J. Darre, P. M. Scheifele, & D. G. Browning. 2010. Characterization of equine vocalization. *J. Vet. Behav.* 5(1):7–12.

1838 Pond, W. G., & J. H. Maner. 1974. *Swine production in temperate and tropical environments*. San Francisco, CA: W.H. Freeman and Co.

1839 Pongracz, P., A. Miklosi, E. Kubinyi, K. Gurobi, J. Topal, & V. Csanyi. 2001. Social learning in dogs: The effect of a human demonstrator on the performance of dogs in a detour task. *Anim. Behav.* 62:1109–1117.

1840 Pongracz, P., A. Miklósi, V. Vida, & V. Csányi. 2005. The pet dogs ability for learning from a human demonstrator in a detour task is independent from the breed and age. *Appl. Anim. Behav. Sci.* 90:309–323.

1841 Pongracz, P., V. Vida, P. Banhegyi, & A. Miklosi. 2008. How does dominance rank status affect individual and social learning performance in the dog (*Canis familiaris*)? *Anim. Cogn.* 11:75–82.

1842 Pontier, D., N. Rioux, & A. Heizmann. 1995. Evidence of selection on the orange allele in the domestic cat *Felis catus*: The role of social structure. *Oikos.* 73(3):299–308.

1843 Porter, R. H., R. Nowak, & P. Orgeur. 1995. Influence of a conspecific agemate on distress bleating by lambs. *Appl. Anim. Behav. Sci.* 45:239–244.

1844 Porter, R. H., R. Nowak, P. Orgeur, F. Levy, & B. Schaal. 1997. Twin/non-twin discrimination by lambs: An investigation of salient stimulus characteristics. *Behaviour.* 134:463–475.

1845 Prache, S., G. Bechet, & J. C. Damasceno. 2006. Diet choice in grazing sheep: A new approach to investigate the relationships between preferences and intake-rate on a daily time scale. *Appl. Anim. Behav. Sci.* 99:253–270.

1846 Prato-Previde, E., S. Marshall-Pescini, & P. Valsecchi. 2008. Is your choice my choice? The owners' effect on pet dogs' (*Canis lupus familiaris*) performance in a food choice task. *Anim. Cogn.* 11:167–174.

1847 Pratt-Phillips, S. E., S. Stuska, H. L. Beveridge, & M. Yoder. 2011. Nutritional quality of forages consumed by feral horses: The horses of Shackleford Banks. *Equine Vet. J.* 31(11):640–644.

1848 Prescott, C. W. 1973. Reproduction patterns in the domestic cat. *Aust. Vet. J.* 49:126–129.

1849 Presicce, G. A., C. C. Brockett, T. Cheng, R. H. Foote, G. F. Rivard, & W. R. Klemm. 1993. Behavioral responses of bulls kept under artificial conditions to compounds presented for olfaction, taste or with topical nasal application. *Appl. Anim. Behav. Sci.* 37:273–284.

1850 Price, E. O., & S. J. R. Wallach. 1990. Rearing bulls with females fails to enhance sexual performance. *Appl. Anim. Behav. Sci.* 26:339–347.

1851 Price, E. O., & S. J. Wallach. 1991. Development of sexual and aggressive behaviors in Hereford bulls. *J. Anim. Sci.* 69:1019–1027.

1852 Price, E. O., & S. J. Wallach. 1991. Effects of group size and the male-to-female ratio on the sexual performance and aggressive behavior of bulls in serving capacity tests. *J. Anim. Sci.* 69:1034–1040.

1853 Price, E. O., C. L. Martinez, & B. L. Coe. 1984. The effects of twinning and mother-offspring behavior in range beef cattle. *Appl. Anim. Behav. Sci.* 13:309–320.

1854 Price, E. O., G. D. Hutson, M. I. Price, & R. Borgwardt. 1994. Fostering in swine as affected by age of offspring. *J. Anim. Sci.* 72:1697–1701.

1855 Price, E. O., H. Erhard, R. Borgwardt, & M. R. Dally. 1992. Measures of libido and their relation to serving capacity in the ram. *J. Anim. Sci.* 70:3376–3380.

1856 Price, E. O., J. K. Blackhaw, A. Blackshaw, R. Borgwardt, M. R. Dally, & R. H. Bondurant. 1994. Sexual responses of rams to ovariectomized and intact estrous ewes. *Appl. Anim. Behav. Sci.* 42:67–71.

1857 Price, E. O., J. Thos, & G. B. Anderson. 1981. Maternal responses of confined beef cattle to single versus twin calves. *J. Anim. Sci.* 53:934–939.

1858 Price, E. O., L. S. Katz, S. J. R. Wallach, & J. J. Zenchak. 1988. The relationship of male-male mounting to the sexual preferences of young rams. *Appl. Anim. Behav. Sci.* 21:347–355.

1859 Price, E. O., R. Borgwardt, & A. Orihuela. 1998. Early sexual experience fails to enhance sexual performance in male goats. *J. Anim. Sci.* 76:718–720.

1860 Price, E. O., R. Borgwardt, & M. R. Dally. 1993. Effect of ewe restraint on the libido and serving capacity of rams. *Appl. Anim. Behav. Sci.* 35:339–345.

1861 Price, E. O., R. Borgwardt, & M. R. Dally. 1999. Effect of early fenceline exposure to estrous ewes on the sexual performance of yearling rams. *Appl. Anim. Behav. Sci.* 64:241–247.

1862 Price, E. O., S. J. R. Wallach, & G. V. Silver. 1990. The effects of long-term individual vs. group housing on the sexual behavior of beef bulls. *Appl. Anim. Behav. Sci.* 27:277–285.

1863 Price, E. O., V. M. Smith, & L. S. Katz. 1984. Sexual stimulation of male dairy goats. *Appl. Anim. Behav. Sci.* 13:83–92.

1864 **Prince, J. H. 1977. The eye and vision. In M. J. Swenson (Ed.), *Duke's physiology of domestic animals.* Ithaca, NY: Cornell University Press.**

1865 Proops, L., & K. Mccomb. 2010. Attributing attention: The use of human given cues by domestic horses (*Equus caballus*). *Anim. Cogn.* 13(2):197–205.

1866 Proops, L., K. McComb, & D. Reby. 2009. Cross-modal individual recognition in domestic horses (Equus caballus). *Proc. Natl. Acad. Sci.* 106(3):947–951.

1867 Proops, L., F. Burden, & B. Osthaus. 2009. Mule cognition: A case of hybrid vigour? *Anim. Cogn.* 12:75–84.

1868 Proudfoot, K. L., D. M. Weary, & M. A. G. Von Keyserlingk. 2014. Maternal isolation behavior of holstein dairy cows kept indoors. *J. Anim. Sci.* 92:277–281.

1869 Provenza, F. D., & J. C. Malechek. 1986. A comparison of feed selection and foraging behavior in juvenile and adult goats. *Appl. Anim. Behav. Sci.* 16:49–61.

1870 Provenza, F. D., L. Ortega-Reyes, C. B. Scott, J. J. Lynch, & E. A. Burritt. 1994. Antiemetic drugs attenuate food aversions in sheep. *J. Anim. Sci.* 72:1989–1994.

1871 **Pryor, P. A., B. L. Hart, M. J. Bain, & K. D. Cliff. 2001. Causes of urine marking in cats and effects of environmental management on frequency of marking. *J. Am. Vet. Med. Assoc.* 219:1709–1713.**

1872 Pullen, A. J., R. J. Merrill, & J. W. Bradshaw. 2012. Habituation and dishabituation during object play in kennel-housed dogs. *Anim. Cogn.* 15(6):1143–1150.

1873 Pullen, A. J., R. J. N. Merrill, & J. W. S. Bradshaw. 2010. Preferences for toy types and presentations in kennel housed dogs. *Appl. Anim. Behav. Sci.* 125(3–4):151–156.

1874 Puppe, B. 1998. Effects of familiarity and relatedness on agonistic pair relationships in newly mixed domestic pigs. *Appl. Anim. Behav. Sci.* 58:233–239.

1875 Puppe, B., K. Ernst, P. C. Schön, & G. Manteuffel. 2007. Cognitive enrichment affects behavioural reactivity in domestic pigs. *Appl. Anim. Behav. Sci.* 105:75–86.

1876 Purcell, D., & C. W. Arave. 1991. Isolation vs. group rearing in monozygous twin heifer calves. *Appl. Anim. Behav. Sci.* 31:147–156.

1877 Purcell, D., C. W. Arava, & J. L. Walters. 1988. Relationship of three measures of behavior to milk production. *Appl. Anim. Behav. Sci.* 21:307–313.

1878 Putnam, P. A., & R. E. Davis. 1963. Ration effects on drylot steer feeding patterns. *J. Anim. Sci.* 22:437–443.

1879 Quaranta, A., M. Siniscalchi, & G. Vallortigara. 2007. Asymmetric tail-wagging responses by dogs to different emotive stimuli. *Curr. Biol.* 17:R199–R201.

1880 Quaranta, A., M. Siniscalchi, M. Albrizio, S. Volpe, C. Buonavoglia, & G. Vallortigara. 2008. Influence of behavioural lateralization on interleukin-2 and interleukin-6 gene expression in dogs before and after immunization with rabies vaccine. *Behav. Brain Res.* 186:256–260.

1881 Ralphs, M. H., & C. D. Cheney. 1993. Influence of cattle age, lithium chloride dose level, and food type in the retention of food aversions. *J. Anim. Sci.* 71:373–379.

1882 Ralston, S. L. 1984. Controls of feeding in horses. *J. Anim. Sci.* 59:1354–1361.

1883 Ralston, S. L., & C. A. Baile. 1983. Effects of intragastric loads of xylose, sodium chloride and corn oil on feeding behavior of ponies. *J. Anim. Sci.* 56:302–308.

1884 Ralston, S. L., D. E. Freeman, & C. A. Baile. 1983. Volatile fatty acids and the role of the large intestine in the control of feed intake in ponies. *J. Anim. Sci.* 57:815–825.

1885 Ramirez, A., A. Quiles, M. Hevia, & F. Sotillo. 1995. Behavior of Murciano-Granadina goat in the hour before parturition. *Appl. Anim. Behav. Sci.* 44:29–35.

1886 Ramirez, A., A. Quiles, M. L. Hevia, & F. Sotillo. 1998. Behaviour of the

Murciano-Granadina goat during the first hour after parturition. *Appl. Anim. Behav. Sci.* 56:223–230.

1887 Ramonet, Y., J. Bolduc, R. Bergeron, S. Robert, & M. Meunier-Salaun. 2000. Feeding motivation in pregnant sows: Effects of fibrous diets on an operant conditioning procedure. *Appl. Anim. Behav. Sci.* 66:21–29.

1888 Ramsay, D. J., B. J. Rolls, & R. J. Wood. 1975. The relationship between elevated water intake and oedema associated with congestive cardiac failure in the dog. *J. Physiol.* 244:303–312.

1889 Ramsay, D. J., B. J. Rolls, & R. J. Wood. 1977. Thirst following water deprivation in dogs. *Am. J. Physiol.* 232:R93–R100.

1890 Ramseyer, A., A. Boissy, B. Dumont, & B. Thierry. 2009. Decision making in group departures of sheep is a continuous process. *Anim. Behav.* 78(1):71–78.

1891 Randall, G. C. 1972. Observations on parturition in the sow. I. Factors associated with the delivery of the piglets and their subsequent behaviour. *Vet. Rec.* 90:178–182.

1892 Randall, R. P., W. A. Schurg, & D. C. Church. 1978. Response of horses to sweet, salty, sour and bitter solutions. *J. Anim. Sci.* 47:51–55.

1893 Randall, W., & V. Lakso. 1968. Body weight and food intake rhythms and their relationship to the behavior of cats with brain stem lesions. *Psychonom. Sci.* 11:33–34.

1894 **Randall, W., R. Swenson, V. Parsons, J. Elbin, & M. Trulson. 1975. The influence of seasonal changes in light on hormones in normal cats and in cats with lesions of the superior colliculi and pretectum. *J. Interdiscip. Cycle Res.* 6:253–266.**

1895 Randle, H. D. 1998. Facial hair whorl position and temperament in cattle. *Appl. Anim. Behav. Sci.* 56:139–147.

1896 **Range, F., L. Horn, T. Bugnyar, G. K. Gajdon, & L. Huber. 2009.**

Social attention in keas, dogs, and human children. *Anim. Cogn.* 12(1):181–192.

1897 Range, F., L. Horn, T. Bugnyar, G. K. Gajdon, & L. Huber. 2009. Social attention in keas, dogs, and human children. *Anim. Cogn.* 12:181–192.

1898 Range, F., L. Horn, Z. Viranyi, & L. Huber. 2009. The absence of reward induces inequity aversion in dogs. *Proc. Natl. Acad. Sci. U.S.A.* 106(1):340–345.

1899 Range, F., U. Aust, M. Steurer, & L. Huber. 2008. Visual categorization of natural stimuli by domestic dogs. *Anim. Cogn.* 11:339–347.

1900 Ransom, J. I., J. G. Powers, H. M. Garbe, M. W. Oehler, T. M. Nett, & D. L. Baker. 2014. Behavior of feral horses in response to culling and GNRH immunocontraception. *Appl. Anim. Behav. Sci.* 157:81–92.

1901 Rashotte, M. E., J. C. Smith, T. Austin, C. Pollitz, T. W. Castonguay, & L. Jonsson. 1984. Twenty-four-hour free-feeding patterns of dogs eating dry food. *Neurosci. Biobehav. Rev.* 8:205–210.

1902 Rasmussen, D. K., R. Weber, & B. Wechsler. 2006. Effects of animal/ feeding-place ratio on the behaviour and performance of fattening pigs fed via sensor-controlled liquid feeding. *Appl. Anim. Behav. Sci.* 98:45–53.

1903 Rasmussen, O. G., E. M. Banks, T. H. Berry, & D. E. Becker. 1962. Social dominance in gilts. *J. Anim. Sci.* 21:520–522.

1904 Ratcliffe, V. F., K. Mccomb, & D. Reby. 2014. Cross-modal discrimination of human gender by domestic dogs. *Anim. Behav.* 91:127–135.

1905 Raussi, S., A. Boissy, E. Delval, P. Pradel, J. Kaihilahti, & I. Veissier. 2005. Does repeated regrouping alter the social behaviour of heifers? *Appl. Anim. Behav. Sci.* 93:1–12.

1906 **Raussi, S., S. Niskanen, J. Siivonen, L. Hanninen, H. Hepola, L. Jauhiainen, & I. Veissier. 2010.**

The formation of preferential relationships at early age in cattle. *Behav. Processes.* 84(3):726–731.

1907 Ray, D. E., & C. B. Roubicek. 1971. Behavior of feedlot cattle during two seasons. *J. Anim. Sci.* 33:72–76.

1908 Rayment, D. J., B. De Groef, R. A. Peters, & L. C. Marston. 2015. Applied personality assessment in domestic dogs: Limitations and caveats. *Appl. Anim. Behav. Sci.* 163:1–18.

1909 Rayner, D. V., & S. Miller. 1993. Voluntary intake and gastric emptying in pigs: Effects of fat and a CCK inhibitor. *Physiol. Behav.* 54:917–922.

1910 Redbo, I., P. Redbo-Torstensson, F. O. Odberg, A. Hadendahl, & J. Holm. 1998. Factors affecting behavioural disturbances in race-horses. *Anim. Sci.* 66:475–481.

1911 Redgate, S. E., J. J. Cooper, S. Hall, P. Eady, & P. A. Harris. 2014. Dietary experience modifies horses' feeding behavior and selection patterns of three macronutrient rich diets. *J. Anim. Sci.* 92:1524–1530.

1912 Redondo, A. J., J. Carranza, & P. Trigo. 2009. Fat diet reduces stress and intensity of startle reaction in horses. *Appl. Anim. Behav. Sci.* 118:69–75.

1913 Reed, H. C., D. R. Melrose, & R. L. Patterson. 1974. Androgen steroids as an aid to the detection of oestrus in pig artificial insemination. *Br. Vet. J.* 130:61–67.

1914 Reefmann, N., B. Wechsler, & L. Gygax. 2009. Behavioural and physiological assessment of positive and negative emotion in sheep. *Anim. Behav.* 78(3):651–659.

1915 Reefmann, N., F. Bütikofer Kaszàs, B. Wechsler, & L. Gygax. 2009. Ear and tail postures as indicators of emotional valence in sheep. *Appl. Anim. Behav. Sci.* 118(3–4):199–207.

1916 Rehkamper, G., & A. Gorlach. 1998. Visual identification of small sizes by

adult dairy bulls. *J. Dairy Sci.* 81:1574–1580.

1917 Reimert, I., J. E. Bolhuis, B. Kemp, & T. B. Rodenburg. 2014. Social support in pigs with different coping styles. *Physiol. Behav.* 129:221–229.

1918 **Reimert, I., J. E. Bolhuis, B. Kemp, & T. B. Rodenburg. 2015. Emotions on the loose: Emotional contagion and the role of oxytocin in pigs. *Anim. Cogn.* 18(2):517–532.**

1919 Reinhardt, V., F. M. Mutiso, & A. Reinhardt. 1978. Resting habits of zebu cattle in a nocturnal enclosure. *Appl. Anim. Ethol.* 4:261.

1920 Reinhardt, V., F. M. Mutiso, & A. Reinhardt. 1978. Social behaviour and social relationships between female and male prepubertal bovine calves (*Bos indicus*). *Appl. Anim. Ethol.* 4:43–54.

1921 **Reisner, I. 1991. The pathophysiologic basis of behavior problems. *Vet. Clin. North Am. Small Anim. Pract.* 21:207–224.**

1922 Reisner, I. R., J. J. Mann, M. Stanley, Y. Y. Huang, & K. A. Houpt. 1996. Comparison of cerebrospinal fluid monoamine metabolite levels in dominant-aggressive and non-aggressive dogs. *Brain Res.* 714:57–64.

1923 Reisner, I. R., K. A. Houpt, H. N. Erb, & F. W. Quimby. 1994. Friendliness to humans and defensive aggression in cats: The influence of handling and paternity. *Physiol. Behav.* 55:1119–1124.

1924 **Reisner, I. R., M. L. Nance, J. S. Zeller, E. M. Houseknecht, N. Kassam-Adams, & D. J. Wiebe. 2011. Behavioural characteristics associated with dog bites to children presenting to an urban trauma centre. *Inj. Prev.* 17(5):348–353.**

1925 **Remmers, J. E., & H. Gautier. 1972. Neural and mechanical mechanisms of feline purring. *Respir. Physiol.* 16:351–361.**

1926 Renken, W. J., L. D. Howery, G. B. Ruyle, & R. M. Enns. 2008. Cattle generalise visual cues from the pen to the field to select initial feeding patches. *Appl. Anim. Behav. Sci.* 109:128–140.

1927 Rensch, B. 1956. Increase of learning capability with increase of brain-size. *Am. Nat.* 90:81–95.

1928 Reppert, S. M., H. G. Artman, S. Swaminathan, & D. A. Fisher. 1981. Vasopressin exhibits a rhythmic daily pattern in cerebrospinal fluid but not in blood. *Science* 213:1256–1257.

1929 Rheingold, H. L. 1963. Maternal behavior in the dog. In H. L. Rheingold (Ed.), Maternal behavior in mammals, pp. 169–202. New York, NY: John Wiley & Sons.

1930 Rheingold, H. L., & C. O. Eckerman. 1971. Familiar social and nonsocial stimuli and the kitten's response to a strange environment. *Dev. Psychobiol.* 4:71–89.

1931 Rhind, S. M., S. R. McMillen, E. Duff, C. E. Kyle, & S. Wright. 2000. Effect of long-term feed restriction on seasonal endocrine changes in soay sheep. *Physiol. Behav.* 71:343–351.

1932 Rhodes, R. T., M. C. Appleby, K. Chinn, L. Douglas, L. D. Firkins, K. A. Houpt, C. Irwin, *et al.* 2005. A comprehensive review of housing for pregnant sows. *Sci. Rep.* 227(10):1580–1590.

1933 Riches, J. H., & R. H. Watson. 1954. The influence of the introduction of rams on the incidence of oestrus in merino ewes. *Aust. J. Agric. Res.* 5:141–147.

1934 Richman, L. M., D. E. Johnson, & R. F. Angel. 1994. Evaluation of a positive conditioning technique for influencing big sagebrush (*Artemisia tridentata* subspp. *wyomingensis*) consumption by goats. *Appl. Anim. Behav. Sci.* 40:229–240.

1935 Riemer, S., C. Muller, Z. Viranyi, L. Huber, & F. Range. 2013. Choice of conflict resolution strategy is linked to sociability in dog puppies. *Appl. Anim. Behav. Sci.* 149(1–4):36–44.

1936 Ringo, J., M. L. Wolbarsht, H. G. Wagner, R. Crocker, & F. Amthor. 1977.

Trichromatic vision in the cat. *Science.* 198:753–755.

1937 Rioja-Lang, F. C., D. J. Roberts, S. D. Healy, A. B. Lawrence, & M. J. Haskell. 2009. Dairy cows trade-off feed quality with proximity to a dominant individual in Y-maze choice tests. *Appl. Anim. Behav. Sci.* 117:159–164.

1938 Riol, J. A., J. M. Sanchez, V. G. Eguren, & V. R. Gaudioso. 1989. Colour perception in fighting cattle. *Appl. Anim. Behav. Sci.* 23:199–206.

1939 Rivas-Munoz, R., G. Fitz-Rodriguez, P. Poindron, B. Malpaux, & J. A. Delgadillo. 2007. Stimulation of estrous behavior in grazing female goats by continuous or discontinuous exposure to males. *J. Anim. Sci.* 85:1257–1263.

1940 Rivera, E., S. Benjamin, B. Nielsen, J. Shelle, & A. J. Zanella. 2002. Behavioral and physiological responses of horses to initial training: The comparison between pastured versus stalled horses. *Appl. Anim. Behav. Sci.* 78:235–252.

1941 Robert, S. J., J. J. Matte, C. Farmer, C. L. Girard, & G. P. Martineau. 1993. High-fibre diets for sows: Effects of stereotypies and adjunctive drinking. *Appl. Anim. Behav. Sci.* 37:297–309.

1942 Roberts, S. J. 1971. *Veterinary obstetrics and genital diseases (Theriogenology).* Ithaca, NY: Stephen J. Roberts.

1943 Robinson, D. W. 1975. Food intake regulation in pigs. IV. The influence of dietary threonine imbalance on food intake, dietary choice and plasma acid patterns. *Br. Vet. J.* 131:595–600.

1944 Rochais, C., S. Henry, C. Fureix, & M. Hausberger. 2016. Investigating attentional processes in depressive-like domestic horses (*Equus caballus*). *Behav. Processes.* 124:93–96.

1945 Rochais, C., S. Henry, C. Sankey, F. Nassur, A. Goracka-Bruzda, & M. Hausberger. 2014. Visual attention, an indicator of human-animal relationships? A study of domestic horses (*Equus caballus*). *Front Psychol.* 5:108.

1946 Rodiek, A. V., & B. E. Jones. 2012. Voluntary intake of four hay types by horses. *Equine Vet. J.* 32(9):579–583.

1947 Rodríguez-Estévez, V., M. Sánchez-Rodríguez, A. G. Gómez-Castro, & S. A. Edwards. 2010. Group sizes and resting locations of free range pigs when grazing in a natural environment. *Appl. Anim. Behav. Sci.* 127(1–2):28–36.

1948 Rogers, C. W., V. Walsh, E. K. Gee, & E. C. Firth. 2012. A preliminary investigation of the use of a foal image to reduce mare stress during mare-foal separation. *J. Vet. Behav.* 7(1):49–54.

1949 Rogers, V. P., G. T. Hartke, & R. L. Kitchell. 1967. Behavioral techniques to analyze a dog's ability to discriminate flavors in commercial food products. In Y. Hayashi (Ed.), *Olfaction and taste*, pp. 353–359. Oxford, UK: Pergamon Press.

1950 Rogosic, J., J. A. Pfister, F. D. Provenza, & D. Grbesa. 2006. The effect of activated charcoal and number of species offered on intake of mediterranean shrubs by sheep and goats. *Appl. Anim. Behav. Sci.* 101:305–317.

1951 Rohde, K. A., & H. W. Gonyou. 1987. Strategies of teat-seeking behavior in neonatal pigs. *Appl. Anim. Behav. Sci.* 19:57–72.

1952 Romano, J. E., C. J. Christians, & B. G. Crabo. 2000. Continuous presence of rams hastens the onset of estrus in ewes synchronized during the breeding season. *Appl. Anim. Behav. Sci.* 66:65–70.

1953 Romeyer, A., P. Poindron, & P. Orgeur. 1994. Olfaction mediates the establishment of selective bonding in goats. *Physiol. Behav.* 56:693–700.

1954 Romeyer, A., P. Poindron, R. H. Porter, F. Levy, & P. Orgeur. 1994. Establishment of maternal bonding and its mediation by vaginocervical stimulation in goats. *Physiol. Behav.* 55:395–400.

1955 **Romeyer, A., R. H. Porter, F. Levy, R. Nowak, P. Orgeur, & P. Poindron. 1993. Maternal labelling is not necessary for the establishment of discrimination between kids by recently parturient goats. *Anim. Behav.* 46:705–712.**

1956 Romsos, D. R., & D. Ferguson. 1983. Regulation of protein intake in adult dogs. *J. Am. Vet. Med. Assoc.* 182:41–43.

1957 Rook, A. J., & C. A. Huckle. 1997. Activity bout criteria for grazing dairy cows. *Appl. Anim. Behav. Sci.* 54:89–96.

1958 Rook, A. J., & P. D. Penning. 1991. Synchronisation of eating, ruminating and idling activity by grazing sheep. *Appl. Anim. Behav. Sci.* 32:157–166.

1959 Rook, A. J., S. J. Rodway-Dyer, & J. E. Cook. 2005. Effects of resource density on spatial memory and learning by foraging sheep *Appl. Anim. Behav. Sci.* 95:143–151.

1960 Rooney, N. J., J. W. S. Bradshaw, & I. H. Robinson. 2001. Do dogs respond to play signals given by humans? *Anim. Behav.* 61:715–722.

1961 Root, M. V., S. D. Johnston, & P. N. Olson. 1996. Effect of prepuberal and postpuberal gonadectomy on heat production measured by indirect calorimetry in male and female domestic cats. *Am. J. Vet. Res.* 57:371–374.

1962 **Rørvang, M. V., L. P. Ahrendt, & J. W. Christensen. 2015. A trained demonstrator has a calming effect on naïve horses when crossing a novel surface. *Appl. Anim. Behav. Sci.* 171:117–120.**

1963 Rorvang, M. V., L. P. Ahrendt, & J. W. Christensen. 2015. Horses fail to use social learning when solving spatial detour tasks. *Anim. Cogn.* 18(4):847–854.

1964 Rosa, H. J., D. T. Juniper, & M. J. Bryant. 2000. The effect of exposure to oestrous ewes on rams' sexual behaviour, plasma testosterone concentration and ability to stimulate ovulation in seasonally anoestrous ewes. *Appl. Anim. Behav. Sci.* 67:293–305.

1965 Rose, J. E. 1968. Discussion following paper, cortical representation by E. F. evans. In A. V. S. de Reuck, & J. Knight (Eds.), *Hearing mechanisms in vertebrates: CIBA foundation symposium*, pp. 287–295. London, UK: Churchill Ltd.

1966 Roselli, C. E., & F. Stormshak. 2009. The neurobiology of sexual partner preferences in rams. *Horm. Behav.* 55:611–620.

1967 Roselli, C. E., K. Larkin, J. M. Schrunk, & F. Stormshak. 2004. Sexual partner preference, hypothalamic morphology and aromatase in rams. *Physiol. Behav.* 83:233–245.

1968 Rose-Meierhöfer, S., S. Klaer, C. Ammon, R. Brunsch, & G. Hoffmann. 2010. Activity behavior of horses housed in different open barn systems. *Equine Vet. J.* 30(11):624–634.

1969 Rosenblatt, J. S. 1965. Effects of experience on sexual behavior in male cats. In F. A. Beach (Ed.), *Sex and behavior*, pp. 416–439. New York, NY: John Wiley & Sons.

1970 **Rosenblatt, J. S. 1965. The basis of synchrony in the behavioral interaction between the mother and her offspring in the laboratory rat. In B. M. Foss (Ed.), *Determinants of infant behavior*, pp. 3–45. New York, NY: John Wiley & Sons.**

1971 Rosenblatt, J. S. 1971. Suckling and home orientation in the kitten. A comparative developmental study. In E. Tobach, L. R. Aronson, & E. Shaw (Eds.), *The biopsychology of development*, pp. 345–410. New York, NY: Academic Press.

1972 Rosenblatt, J. S., & L. R. Aronson. 1958. The decline of sexual behavior in male cats after castration with special reference to the role of prior sexual experience. *Behaviour.* 12:285–338.

1973 Rosenblatt, J. S., & L. R. Aronson. 1958. The influence of experience on the behavioural effects of androgen in prepuberally castrated male cats. *Anim. Behav.* 6:171–182.

1974 Rosenblatt, J. S., & T. C. Schneirla. 1962. The behaviour of cats. In E. S. E. Hafez (Ed.), *The behaviour of domestic animals*, pp. 453–488. Baltimore, MD: Williams and Wilkins.

1975 Ross, S. 1951. Sucking behavior in neonate dogs. *J. Abnorm. Psychol.* 46:142–149.

1976 Ross, S., & J. Berg. 1956. Stability of food dominance relationships in a flock of goats. *J. Mammal.* 37:129–131.

1977 Ross, S., & J. P. Scott. 1949. Relationship between dominance and control of movement in goats. *J. Comp. Physiol. Psychol.* 42:75–80.

1978 Ross, S., J. P. Scott, M. Cherner, & V. H. Denenberg. 1960. Effects of restraint and isolation on yelping in puppies. *Anim. Behav.* 8:1–5.

1979 Rossdale, P. D. 1967. Clinical studies on the newborn thoroughbred foal. I. perinatal behaviour. *Br. Vet. J.* 123:470–481.

1980 Rossi, A. P., & C. Ades. 2008. A dog at the keyboard: Using arbitrary signs to communicate requests. *Anim. Cogn.* 11:329–338.

1981 Rossi, R., E. Del Prete, J. Rokitzky, & E. Scharrer. 1999. Circadian drinking during ad libitum and restricted feeding in pygmy goats. *Appl. Anim. Behav. Sci.* 61:253–261.

1982 Roth, B. A., E. Hillmann, M. Stauffacher, & N. M. Keil. 2008. Improved weaning reduces cross-sucking and may improve weight gain in dairy calves. *Appl. Anim. Behav. Sci.* 111:251–261.

1984 Rothmann, J., O. F. Christensen, E. Søndergaard, & J. Ladewig. 2014. A note on the heritability of reactivity assessed at field tests for Danish warmblood horses. *Equine Vet. J.* 34(2):341–343.

1985 Rouda, R. R., D. M. Anderson, J. D. Wallace, & L. W. Murray. 1994.

Free-ranging cattle water consumption in southcentral new Mexico. *Appl. Anim. Behav. Sci.* 39:29–38.

1986 Rowell, T. E. 1991. Till death do us part: Long-lasting bonds between ewes and their daughters. *Anim. Behav.* 42:681–682.

1987 Roy, J. H. B., K. W. G. Shillam, & J. Palmer. 1955. The outdoor rearing of calves on grass with special reference to growth rate and grazing behaviour. *J. Dairy Res.* 22:252–269.

1988 **Rozin, P. 1967. Thiamin specific hunger. In C. F. Code, & W. Heidel (Eds.), *Handbook of physiology: Section 6: Alimentary canal: Volume I. control of food and water intake*, pp. 411–431. Washington, DC: American Physiological Society.**

1989 Rozkowska, E., & E. Fonberg. 1973. Salivary reactions after ventromedial hypothalamic lesions in dogs. *Acta Neurobiol. Exp. (Wars)* 33:553–562.

1990 Rubenstein, D. I., & M. A. Hack. 1992. Horse signals: The sounds and scents of fury. *Evol. Ecol.* 6:254–260.

1991 Rubin, L., C. Oppegard, & H. F. Hindz. 1980. The effect of varying the temporal distribution of conditioning trials on equine learning behavior. *J. Anim. Sci.* 50:1184–1187.

1992 Ruckebusch, Y. 1972. The relevance of drowsiness in the circadian cycle of farm animals. *Anim. Behav.* 20:637–643.

1993 Ruckebusch, Y. 1974. Sleep deprivation in cattle. *Brain Res.* 78:495–499.

1994 Ruckebusch, Y. 1975. The hypnogram as an index of adaptation of farm animals to changes in their environment. *Appl. Anim. Ethol.* 2:3–18.

1995 Ruckebusch, Y., & M. Gaujoux. 1976. Sleep patterns of the laboratory cat. *Electroencephalogr. Clin. Neurophysiol.* 41:483–490.

1996 Ruckebusch, Y., M. Gaujoux, & B. Eghbali. 1977. Sleep cycles and kinesis in the foetal lamb. *Electroencephalogr. Clin. Neurophysiol.* 42:226–237.

1997 Ruckebusch, Y., R. W. Dougherty, & H. M. Cook. 1974. Jaw movements and rumen motility as criteria for measurement of deep sleep in cattle. *Am. J. Vet. Res.* 35:1309–1312.

1998 Rudge, M. R. 1970. Mother and kid behaviour in feral goats (*Capra hircus* L.). *Z. Tierpsychol.* 27:687–692.

1999 Ruis, M. A. W., J. H. A. Te Brake, B. Engel, W. G. Buist, H. J. Blokhuis, & J. M. Koolhaas. 2002. Implications of coping characteristics and social status for welfare and production of paired growing gilts. *Appl. Anim. Behav. Sci.* 75:207–231.

2000 Ruis, M. A. W., J. H. A. Te Brake, J. A. van de Burgwal, I. C. de Jong, H. J. Blokhuis, & J. M. Koolhaas. 2000. Personalities in female domesticated pigs: Behavioural and physiological indications. *Appl. Anim. Behav. Sci.* 66:31–47.

2001 Ruiz-Miranda, C. R. 1993. Use of pelage pigmentation in the recognition of mothers in a group by 2- to 4-month-old domestic goat kids. *Appl. Anim. Behav. Sci.* 36:317–326.

2002 Rushen, J. 1984. Stereotyped behaviour, adjunctive drinking and the feeding periods of tethered sows. *Anim. Behav.* 32:1059–1067.

2003 Rushen, J., & A. M. de Passille. 1995. The motivation of non-nutritive sucking in calves, *Bos taurus*. *Anim. Behav.* 49:1503–1510.

2004 Rushen, J., A. M. De Passille, & W. Schouten. 1990. Stereotypic behavior, endogenous opioids, and postfeeding hypoalgesia in pigs. *Physiol. Behav.* 48:91–96.

2005 Rushen, J., G. Foxcroft, & A. M. De Passille. 1993. Nursing-induced changes in pain sensitivity, prolactin, and somatotropin in the pig. *Physiol. Behav.* 53:265–270.

2006 **Rushen, J., J. Ladewig, & A. M. de Passille. 1995. A novel environment inhibits milk ejection in the pig but not through HPA activity. *Appl. Anim. Behav. Sci.* 45:53–61.**

2007 Russek, M., & P. J. Morgane. 1963. Anorexic effect of intraperitoneal glucose in the hypothalamic hyperphagic cat. *Nature* 199:1004–1005.

2008 Rutberg, A. T. 1990. Inter-group transfer in Assateague pony mares. *Anim. Behav.* 40:945–952.

2009 Rutberg, A. T., & R. R. Keiper. 1993. Proximate causes of natal dispersal in feral ponies: Some sex differences. *Anim. Behav.* 46:969–975.

2010 Rutberg, A. T., & S. A. Greenbrg. 1990. Dominance, aggression frequencies and modes of aggressive competition in feral pony mares. *Anim. Behav.* 40:322–331.

2011 Rutter, S. M., V. Tainton, R. A. Champion, & P. Le Grice. 2002. The effect of a total solar eclipse on the grazing behaviour of dairy cattle. *Appl. Anim. Behav. Sci.* 79:273–283.

2012 Rybarczyk, P., Y. Koba, J. Rushen, H. Tanida, & A. M. de Passille. 2001. Can cows discriminate people by their faces? *Appl. Anim. Behav. Sci.* 74:175–189.

2013 Ryder, M. L. 1976. Seasonal changes in the coat of the cat. *Res. Vet. Sci.* 21:280–283.

2014 Sacks, J. J., L. Sinclair, J. Gilchrist, G. C. Golab, & R. Lockwood. 2000. Breeds of dogs involved in fatal human attacks in the United States between 1979 and 1998. *J. Am. Vet. Med. Assoc.* 217:836–840.

2015 Sacks, J. J., R. W. Smith, & S. E. Bonzo. 1989. Dog bit-related fatalities from 1979 to 1988. *JAMA.* 262:1489–1492.

2016 **Saito, A., & K. Shinozuka. 2013. Vocal recognition of owners by domestic cats (*Felis catus*). *Anim. Cogn.* 16(4):685–690.**

2017 Salzinger, K., & M. B. Waller. 1962. The operant control of vocalization in the dog. *J. Exp. Anal. Behav.* 5:383–389.

2018 Samarakone, T. S., & H. W. Gonyou. 2009. Domestic pigs alter their social strategy in response to social group size. *Appl. Anim. Behav. Sci.* 121(1):8–15.

2019 Sambraus, H. H., & D. Sambraus. 1975. Pragung von nutztieren auf menschen. *Z. Tierpsychol.* 38:1–17.

2020 Sandem, A., & B. O. Braastad. 2005. Effects of cow-calf separation on visible eye white and behaviour in dairy cows: A brief report. *Appl. Anim. Behav. Sci.* 95:233–239.

2021 **Sandem, A., B. O. Braastad, & M. Bakken. 2006. Behaviour and percentage eye-white in cows waiting to be fed concentrate: A brief report. *Appl. Anim. Behav. Sci.* 97:145–151.**

2022 Sandem, A. I., A. M. Janczak, R. Salte, & B. O. Braastad. 2006. The use of diazepam as a pharmacological validation of eye white as an indicator of emotional state in dairy cows. *Appl. Anim. Behav. Sci.* 96:177–183.

2023 Sandem, A. I., B. O. Braastad, & K. E. Boe. 2002. Eye white may indicate emotional state on a frustration-contentedness axis in dairy cows. *Appl. Anim. Behav. Sci.* 79:1–10.

2024 Sandler, B. E., G. A. Van Gelder, D. D. Elsberg, G. G. Karas, & W. B. Buck. 1969. Dieldrin exposure and vigilance behavior in sheep. *Psychonom. Sci.* 15:261–262.

2025 Sandler, B. E., G. A. Van Gelder, G. G. Karas, & W. B. Buck. 1971. An operant feeding device for sheep. *J. Exp. Anal. Behav.* 15:95–96.

2026 Sandler, B. E., G. A. Van Gelder, W. B. Buck, & G. G. Karas. 1968. Effect of dieldrin exposure on detour behavior in sheep. *Psychol. Rep.* 23:451–455.

2027 Sankey, C., M. A. Richard-Yris, S. Henry, C. Fureix, F. Nassur, & M. Hausberger. 2010. Reinforcement as a mediator of the perception of humans by horses (*Equus caballus*). *Anim. Cogn.* 13(5):753–764.

2028 Sapolsky, R. M. 1997. The importance of a well-groomed child. *Science* 277:1620–1621.

2029 Sappington, B. F., & L. Goldman. 1994. Discrimination learning and concept formation in the Arabian horse. *J. Anim. Sci.* 72:3080–3087.

2030 **Šárová, R., M. Špinka, I. Stihulová, F. Ceacero, M. Šimeková, & R. Kotrba. 2013. Pay respect to the elders: Age,**

more than body mass, determines dominance in female beef cattle. *Anim. Behav.* 86(6):1315–1323.

2031 Šárová, R., M. Špinka, J. L. A. Panamá, & P. Šimeek. 2010. Graded leadership by dominant animals in a herd of female beef cattle on pasture. *Anim. Behav.* 79(5):1037–1045.

2032 Sartori, C. A. R. M. 2010. Genetics of fighting ability in cattle using data from the traditional battel contest of the Valdostana breed. *J. Anim. Sci.* 88:3206–3213.

2033 Sato, S. 1982. Leadership during actual grazing in a small herd of cattle. *Appl. Anim. Ethol.* 8:53–65.

2034 Sato, S. S., & A. Maeda. 1991. Social licking patterns in cattle (*Bos taurus*): Influence of environmental and social factors. *Appl. Anim. Behav. Sci.* 32:3–12.

2035 Sato, S., K. Tarumizu, & K. Hatae. 1993. The influence of social factors on allogrooming in cows. *Appl. Anim. Behav. Sci.* 38:235–244.

2036 Say, L., & D. Pontier. 2004. Spacing pattern in a social group of stray cats: Effects on male reproductive success. *Anim. Behav.* 68:175–180.

2037 Scarlett, J. M., S. Donoghue, J. Saidla, & J. Wills. 1994. Overweight cats: Prevalence and risk factors. *Int. J. Obes. Relat. Metab. Disord.* 18 Suppl 1:S22–S28.

2038 Scarpi, D. 2011. The impact of phantom decoys on choices in cats. *Anim. Cogn.* 14(1):127–136.

2039 Schafer, M. 1975. *The language of the horse*. New York, NY: Arco Publishing Co.

2040 Schake, L. M., & J. K. Riggs. 1969. Activities of lactating beef cows in confinement. *J. Anim. Sci.* 28:568–572.

2041 Schalke, E., J. Stichnoth, S. Ott, & R. Jones-Baade. 2007. Clinical signs caused by the use of electric training collars on dogs in everyday life situations. *Appl. Anim. Behav. Sci.* 105:369–380.

2042 Scheepens, C. J. M., M. J. C. Hessing, E. Laarakker, W. G. P. Schouten, & M. J. M. Tielen. 1991. Influence of intermittent daily draught on the behaviour of weaned pigs. *Appl. Anim. Behav. Sci.* 31:69–82.

2043 Schein, M. W., & M. H. Fohrman. 1955. Social dominance relationships in a herd of dairy cattle. *Br. J. Anim. Behav.* 3:45–55.

2044 Schichowski, C., E. Moors, & M. Gauly. 2008. Effects of weaning lambs in two stages or by abrupt separation on their behavior and growth rate. *J. Anim. Sci.* 86:220–225.

2045 Schino, G. 1998. Reconciliation in domestic goats. *Behaviour.* 135:343–356.

2046 Schloeth, R. 1961. Das sozialleben des camargue-rindes. qualitative und quantitative untersuchungen uber die sozialen beziehungen-insbesondere die soziale rangordnung – des halbwilden franzosischen SP – kampfrindes. *Z. Tierpsychol.* 18:574–627.

2047 Schmidt, A., E. Mostl, C. Wehnert, J. Aurich, J. Muller, & C. Aurich. 2010. Cortisol release and heart rate variability in horses during road transport. *Horm. Behav.* 57(2):209–215.

2048 Schmidt, A., J. Aurich, E. Mostl, J. Muller, & C. Aurich. 2010. Changes in cortisol release and heart rate and heart rate variability during the initial training of 3-year-old sport horses. *Horm. Behav.* 58(4):628–636.

2049 Schneider, L. A., P. H. Delfabbro, & N. R. Burns. 2013. Temperament and lateralization in the domestic dog (*Canis familiaris*). *J. Vet. Behav.* 8(3):124–134.

2050 Schneirla, T. C., J. S. Rosenblatt, & E. Tobach. 1963. Maternal behavior in the cat. In H. L. Rheingold (Ed.), *Maternal behavior in mammals*, pp. 122–168. New York, NY: John Wiley & Sons.

2051 Schoen, A. M. S., E. M. Banks, & S. E. Curtis. 1976. Behavior of young Shetland and Welsh ponies (*Equus caballus*). *Biol. Behav.* 1:199–216.

2052 Schoen, A. M. S., S. E. Curtis, E. M. Banks, & H. W. Norton. 1974. Behavior and performance of swine subjected to preweaning handling. *J. Anim. Sci.* 39:136–137.

2053 Schofield, W. L., & J. P. Mulville. 1998. Assessment of the modified Forssell's procedure for the treatment of oral stereotypies in 10 horses. *Vet. Rec.* 142:572–575.

2054 Schryver, H. F., M. T. Parker, P. D. Daniluk, K. I. Pagan, J. Williams, L. V. Soderholm, & H. F. Hintz. 1987. Salt consumption and the effect of salt on mineral metabolism in horses. *Cornell Vet.* 77:122–131.

2055 Schryver, H. F., S. VanWie, P. Daniluk, & H. F. Hintz. 1978. The voluntary intake of calcium by horses and ponies fed a calcium deficient diet. *J. Equine Med. Surg.* 2:337–340.

2056 Schubert, M., H. Jónsson, D. Chang, C. Der Sarkissian, L. Ermini, A. Ginolhac, A. Albrechtsen, *et al.* 2014. Prehistoric genomes reveal the genetic foundation and cost of horse domestication. *PNAS Early Ed.* 111(52):E5661–E5669.

2057 **Schubert, M., H. Jonsson, D. Chang, C. Der Sarkissian, L. Ermini, A. Ginolhac, A. Albrechtsen, *et al.* 2014. Prehistoric genomes reveal the genetic foundation and cost of horse domestication. *Proc. Natl. Acad. Sci. U.S.A.* 111(52):E5661–E5669.**

2058 Schutz, K., D. Davison, & L. Matthews. 2006. Do different levels of moderate feed deprivation in dairy cows affect feeding motivation? *Appl. Anim. Behav. Sci.* 101:253–263.

2059 Scott, D. W., R. W. Kirk, & J. Bentinck-Smith. 1979. Some effects of short-term methylprednisolone therapy in normal cats. *Cornell Vet.* 69:104–115.

2060 Scott, J. P. 1945. Social behavior, organization and leadership in a small flock of domestic sheep. *Comp. Psychol. Monogr.* 18:1–29.

2061 Scott, J. P. 1946. Dominance reaction in a small flock of goats. *Anat. Rec.* 94:38–381.

2062 **Scott, J. P. 1948. Dominance and the frustration-aggression hypothesis. *Physiol. Zool.* 21:31–39.**

2063 **Scott, J. P. 1958. *Aggression.* Chicago, IL: University of Chicago Press.**

2064 Scott, J. P. 1958. *Animal behavior.* Chicago, IL: University of Chicago Press.

2065 Scott, J. P. 1962. Critical periods in behavioral development. *Science* 138:949–958.

2066 Scott, J. P., & J. L. Fuller. 1974. *Dog behavior: The genetic basis.* Chicago, IL: University of Chicago Press.

2067 Scott, J. P., & M. V. Marston. 1950. Critical periods affecting the development of normal and mal-adjustive social behavior of puppies. *J. Genet. Psychol.* 77:25–60.

2068 Scott, L. L., & F. D. Provenza. 2000. Lambs fed protein or energy imbalanced diets forage in locations and on foods that rectify imbalances. *Appl. Anim. Behav. Sci.* 68:293–305.

2069 Scott, M. D., & K. Causey. 1973. Ecology of feral dogs in alabama. *J. Wildl. Manag.* 37:253–265.

2070 **Scott, P. P. 1970. Cats. In E. S. E. Hafez (Ed.), *Reproduction and breeding techniques for laboratory animals*, pp. 192–208. Philadelphia, PA: Lea & Febiger.**

2071 **Seabrook, M. F. 1972. A study to determine the influence of the herdsman's personality on milk yield. *J. Agric. Labour Sci.* 1:45–59.**

2072 Seath, D. M., & G. D. Miller. 1946. Effect of warm weather on grazing performance of milking cows. *J. Dairy Sci.* 29:199–206.

2073 Sèbe, F., J. Duboscq, T. Aubin, S. Ligout, & P. Poindron. 2010. Early vocal recognition of mother by lambs: Contribution of low- and high-frequency vocalizations. *Anim. Behav.* 79(5):1055–1066.

2074 Sechzer, J. A., & J. L. Brown. 1964. Color discrimination in the cat. *Science* 144:427–429.

2075 Segerstad, C. H., & G. Hellekant. 1989. The sweet taste in the calf. I. chorda tympani proper nerve responses to taste stimulation of the tongue. *Physiol. Behav.* 45:633–638.

2076 Seguin, M. J., R. M. Friendship, R. N. Kirkwood, A. J. Zanella, & T. M. Widowski. 2006. Effects of boar presence on agonistic behavior, shoulder scratches, and stress response of bred sows at mixing. *J. Anim. Sci.* 84:1227–1237.

2077 Seidel, W. F., T. Roth, T. Roehrs, F. Zorick, & W. C. Dement. 1984. Treatment of a 12-hour shift of sleep schedule with benzodiazepines. *Science* 224:1262–1264.

2078 Seitz, P. F. D. 1959. Infantile experiences and adult behavior in animal subjects. II. Age of separation from the mother and adult behavior in the cat. *Psychosom. Med.* 21:353–378.

2079 Seksel, K., E. J. Mazurski, & A. Taylor. 1999. Puppy socialisation programs: Short and long term behavioural effects. *Appl. Anim. Behav. Sci.* 62:335–349.

2080 Selman, I. E., A. D. McEwan, & E. W. Fisher. 1970. Studies on natural suckling in cattle during the first eight hours post partum. I. Behavioural studies (dams). *Anim. Behav.* 18:276–283.

2081 **Selman, I. E., A. D. McEwan, & E. W. Fisher. 1970. Studies on natural suckling in cattle during the first eight hours post partum. II. Behavioural studies (calves). *Anim. Behav.* 18:284–289.**

2082 Senn, C. L., & J. D. Lewin. 1975. Barking dogs as an environmental problem. *J. Am. Vet. Med. Assoc.* 166:1065–1068.

2083 Seoane, J. R., & C. A. Baile. 1973. Feeding behavior in sheep as related to the hypnotic activities of barbiturates injected into the third ventricle. *Pharmacol. Biochem. Behav.* 1:47–53.

2084 Seoane, J. R., & C. A. Baile. 1973. Feeding elicited by injections of Ca++ and Mg++ into the third ventricle of sheep. *Experientia* 29:61–62.

2085 **Seoane, J. R., C. A. Baile, & R. H. Martin. 1972. Humoral factors modifying feeding behavior of sheep. *Physiol. Behav.* 8:993–995.**

2086 Serpell, J. A., & Y. Hsu. 2001. Development and validation of a novel method for evaluating behavior and temperament in guide dogs. *Appl. Anim. Behav. Sci.* 72:347–364.

2087 Serpell, J., & J. A. Jagoe. 1995. Early experience and the development of behaviour. In J. Serpell (Ed.), *The domestic dog: Its evolution, behaviour and interactions with people*, pp. 79–102. Cambridge, UK: Cambridge University Press.

2088 Setchell, B. P. 1978. *The mammalian testis.* Ithaca, NY: Cornell University Press.

2089 Settle, R. H., B. A. Sommerville, J. McCormick, & D. M. Broom. 1994. Human scent matching using specially trained dogs. *Anim. Behav.* 48:1443–1448.

2090 Shackleton, D. M., & C. C. Shank. 1984. A review of the social behavior of feral and wild sheep and goats. *J. Anim. Sci.* 58:500–509.

2091 Shank, C. C. 1972. Some aspects of social behaviour in a population of feral goats (*Capra hircus* L.). *Z. Tierpsychol.* 30:488–528.

2092 Share, I., E. Martyniuk, & M. I. Grossman. 1952. Effect of prolonged intragastric feeding on oral food intake in dogs. *Am. J. Physiol.* 169:229–235.

2093 **Shaw, E. B., K. A. Houpt, & D. F. Holmes. 1988. Body temperature and behaviour of mares during the last two weeks of pregnancy. *Equine Vet. J.* 20:199–202.**

2094 Shaw, E., & K. A. Houpt. 1985. Pre- and post-partum behaviour in mules impregnated by embryo transfer. *Equine Vet. J.* 17:73.

2095 Shaw, R. A. 1978. A time-controlled feeding system for cattle. *Anim. Prod.* 27:277–284.

2096 Shearer, M. K., & L. S. Katz. 2006. Female-female mounting among goats stimulates sexual performance in males. *Horm. Behav.* 50:33–37.

2097 **Sheppard, A. J., R. E. Blaser, & C. M. Kincaid. 1957. The grazing habits of beef cattle on pasture. *J. Anim. Sci.* 16:681–687.**

2098 Sheppard, G., & D. S. Mills. 2003. Evaluation of dog-appeasing pheromone as a potential treatment for dogs fearful of fireworks. *Vet. Rec.* 152:432–436.

2099 Sherman, B. L., M. E. Gruen, R. B. Meeker, B. Milgram, C. Dirivera, A. Thomson, G. Clary, & L. Hudson. 2013. The use of a t-maze to measure cognitive-motor function in cats (*Felis catus*). *J. Vet. Behav.* 8(1):32–39.

2100 Sherry, C. J., T. J. Walters, J. Rodney G.G., & P. J. Henry. 1994. Behavioral chaining in the goat (*Capra hircus*). *Appl. Anim. Behav. Sci.* 40:241–251.

2101 Shi, J., & R. I. M. Dunbar. 2006. Feeding competition within a feral goat population on the isle of rum, NW Scotland. *J. Ethol.* 24:117–124.

2102 Shi, J., R. I. M. Dunbar, D. Buckland, & D. Miller. 2003. Daytime activity budgets of feral goats (*Capra hircus*) on the Isle of Rum: Influence of season, age, and sex. *Can. J. Zool.* 81:803–815.

2103 Shillito Walser, E. E. 1986. Recognition of the sow's voice by neonatal piglets. *Behaviour.* 99:177–187.

2104 Shillito Walser, E., & P. Hague. 1980. Variations in the structure of bleats from sheep of four different breeds. *Behaviour.* 75:22–35.

2105 Shillito Walser, E., & P. Hague. 1981. Field observations on a flock of ewes and lambs made of Clun Forest, Dalesbred and Jacob sheep. *Appl. Anim. Ethol.* 7:175–178.

2106 **Shillito Walser, E., E. Walters, & P. Hague. 1981. A statistical analysis of the structure of bleats from sheep of four different breeds. *Behaviour.* 77:67–76.**

2107 Shillito Walser, E., S. Willadsen, & P. Hague. 1982. Maternal vocal recognition in lambs born to Jacob and Dalesbred ewes after embryo transplantation between breeds. *Appl. Anim. Ethol.* 8:479–486.

2108 Shillito, E. E. 1975. A comparison of the role of vision and hearing in lambs finding their own dams. *Appl. Anim. Ethol.* 1:369–377.

2109 Shillito, E. E., & V. J. Hoyland. 1971. Observations on parturition and maternal care in soay sheep. *J. Zool.* 165:509–512.

2110 **Shillito, E., & G. Alexander. 1975. Mutual recognition amongst ews and lambs of four breeds of sheep (*Ovis aries*). *Appl. Anim. Ethol.* 1:151–165.**

2111 Shipka, M. P., & L. C. Ellic. 1998. No effect of bull exposure on expression of estrous behavior in high-producing dairy cows. *Appl. Anim. Behav. Sci.* 57:1–7.

2112 Shipka, M. P., & S. P. Ford. 1991. Relationship of circulating estrogen and progesterone concentrations during late pregnancy and the onset phase of maternal behavior in the ewe. *Appl. Anim. Behav. Sci.* 31:91–99.

2113 Shreffler, C., & W. D. Hohenboken. 1974. Dominance and mating behavior in ram lambs. *J. Anim. Sci.* 39:725–731.

2114 Shuleikina, K. V. 1976. Sensory mechanisms of learning in the behaviour of newborn kittens. *Act. Nerv. Super. (Praha)* 18:48–50.

2115 Sibbald, A. M. 1997. The effect of body condition on the feeding behaviour of sheep with different times of access to food. *Anim. Sci.* 64:239–246.

2116 Sibbald, A. M., H. W. Erhard, J. E. Mcleod, & R. J. Hooper. 2009. Individual personality and the spatial distribution of groups of grazing animals: An example with sheep. *Behav. Processes.* 82(3):319–326.

2117 **Sibbald, A. M., H. W. Erhard, R. J. Hooper, B. Dumont, & A. Boissy. 2006. A test for measuring individual** variation in how far grazing animals will move away from a social group to feed. *Appl. Anim. Behav. Sci.* 98:89–99.

2118 Sibbald, A. M., L. J. Shellard, & T. S. Smart. 2000. Effects of space allowance on the grazing behaviour and spacing of sheep. *Appl. Anim. Behav. Sci.* 70:49–62.

2119 Sibbald, A. M., S. P. Oom, R. J. Hooper, & R. M. Anderson. 2008. Effects of social behaviour on the spatial distribution of sheep grazing a complex vegetation mosaic. *Appl. Anim. Behav. Sci.* 115:149–159.

2120 Signoret, J. 1967. Duree du cycle oestrien et de l'oestrus che la truie: action du benzoate d'oestradiol chez la femelle ovariectomisee. *Ann. Biol. Anim. Biochem. Biophys.* 7:407–421.

2121 Signoret, J. 1970. Sexual behaviour patterns in female domestic pigs (*Sus scrofa L.*) reared in isolation from males. *Anim. Behav.* 18:165–168.

2122 Signoret, J. 1975. Influence of the sexual receptivity of a teaser ewe on the mating preference in the ram. *Appl. Anim. Ethol.* 1:229–232.

2123 Signoret, J., & P. Mauleon. 1962. Action de l'ablatin des bulbes olfactifs sur les mecanismes de la reproductin chez la truie. *Ann. Biol. Anim. Biochem. Biophys.* 2:167–174.

2124 Signoret, J., B. A. Baldwin, D. Fraser, & E. S. E. Hafez. 1975. The behaviour of swine. In E. S. E. Hafez (Ed.), The behaviour of domestic animals, pp. 295–329. Baltimore, MD: Williams & Wilkins.

2125 Simitzis, P. E., M. A. Charismiadou, B. Kotsampasi, G. Papadomichelakis, E. P. Christopoulou, E. K. Papavlasopoulou, & S. G. Deligeorgis. 2009. Influence of maternal undernutrition on the behaviour of juvenile lambs. *Appl. Anim. Behav. Sci.* 116:191–197.

2126 Simpson, B. S. 2002. Neonatal foal handling. *Appl. Anim. Behav. Sci.* 78:303–317.

2127 Simpson, C. W., C. A. Baile, & L. F. Krabill. 1975. Neurochemical coding for feeding in sheep and steers. *J. Comp. Physiol. Psychol.* 88:176–182.

2128 Siniscalchi, M., B. Padalino, L. Aube, & A. Quaranta. 2015. Right-nostril use during sniffing at arousing stimuli produces higher cardiac activity in jumper horses. *Laterality.* 20(4):483–500.

2129 Siniscalchi, M., B. Padalino, R. Lusito, & A. Quaranta. 2014. Is the left forelimb preference indicative of a stressful situation in horses? *Behav. Processes.* 107:61–67.

2130 **Siniscalchi, M., R. Lusito, G. Vallortigara, & A. Quaranta. 2013. Seeing left- or right-asymmetric tail wagging produces different emotional responses in dogs. *Curr. Biol.* 23(22):2279–2282.**

2131 Siniscalchi, M., R. Sasso, A. M. Pepe, S. Dimatteo, G. Vallortigara & A. Quaranta. 2011. Sniffing with the right nostril: Lateralization of response to odour stimuli by dogs. *Anim. Behav.* 82(2):399–404.

2132 Siniscalchi, M., S. D'ingeo, & A. Quaranta. 2016. The dog nose "knows" fear: Asymmetric nostril use during sniffing at canine and human emotional stimuli. *Behav. Brain Res.* 304:34–41.

2133 **Sinn, D. L., S. D. Gosling, & S. Hilliard. 2010. Personality and performance in military working dogs: Reliability and predictive validity of behavioral tests. *Appl. Anim. Behav. Sci.* 127(1–2):51–65.**

2134 Sivak, J., & B. D. Allen. 1975. An evaluation of the "ramp" retina of the horse eye. *Vision Res.* 15:1353–1356.

2135 **Siwak, C. T., H. L. Murphey, B. A. Muggenburg, & N. W. Milgram. 2002. Age-dependent decline in locomotor activity in dogs is environment specific. *Physiol. Behav.* 75:65–70.**

2136 Skinner, B. F. 1938. The behavior of organisms. New York, NY: Appleton-Century.

2137 Slabbert, J. M., & J. S. J. Odendaal. 1999. Early prediction of adult police dog efficiency – a longitudinal study. *Appl. Anim. Behav. Sci.* 64:269–288.

2138 **Slabbert, J. M., & O. A. E. Rasa. 1997. Observational learning of an acquired maternal behaviour pattern by working dog pups: An alternative training method? *Appl. Anim. Behav. Sci.* 53:309–316.**

2139 Sly, J., & F. R. Bell. 1979. Experimental analysis of the seeking behaviour observed in ruminants when they are sodium deficient. *Physiol. Behav.* 22:499–505.

2140 Smith, A. V., L. Proops, K. Grounds, J. Wathan, & K. Mccomb. 2016. Functionally relevant responses to human facial expressions of emotion in the domestic horse (*Equus caballus*). *Biol. Lett.* 12(2):20150907.

2141 **Smith, B. L., J. H. Jones, G. P. Carlson, & J. R. Pascoe. 1994. Body position and direction preferences in horses during road transport. *Equine Vet. J.* 26:374–377.**

2142 Smith, F. V. 1965. Instinct and learning in the attachment of lamb and ewe. *Anim. Behav.* 13:84–86.

2143 **Smith, F. V., C. Van-Toller, & T. Boyes. 1966. The "critical period" in the attachment of lambs and ewes. *Anim. Behav.* 14:120–125.**

2144 Smith, S., & L. Goldman. 1999. Color discrimination in horses. *Appl. Anim. Behav. Sci.* 62:13–25.

2145 Snowder, G. D., & A. D. Knight. 1995. Breed effects of foster lamb and foster dam on lamb viability and growth. *J. Anim. Sci.* 73:1559–1566.

2146 Sobocinska, J. 1978. Gastric distention and thirst: Relevance to the osmotic thirst threshold and metering of water intake. *Physiol. Behav.* 20:497–501.

2147 Soffie, M., G. Thines, & G. De Marneffe. 1976. Relation between milking order and dominance value in a group of dairy cows. *Appl. Anim. Behav. Sci.* 2:271–276.

2148 Solà-Oriol, D., E. Roura, & D. Torrallardona. 2014. Feed preference in pigs: Relationship between cereal preference and nutrient composition and digestibility. *J. Anim. Sci.* 92:220–228.

2149 **Solomon, R. L., & L. C. Wynne. 1953. Traumatic avoidance learning: Acquisition in normal dogs. *Psychol. Monogr.* 67:1–19.**

2150 Soltysik, S., & B. A. Baldwin. 1972. The performance of goats in triple choice delayed response tasks. *Acta Neurobiol. Exp. (Wars)* 32:73–86.

2151 Somerville, S. H., & B. G. Lowman. 1979. Observations on the nursing behaviour of beef cows suckling Charolais cross calves. *Appl. Anim. Ethol.* 5:369–373.

2152 Sommer, V., A. Lowe, & T. Dietrich. 2015. Not eating like a pig: European wild boar wash their food. *Anim. Cogn.* 19(1):245–249.

2153 Sorrells, A. D., S. D. Eicher, K. A. Scott, M. J. Harris, E. A. Pajor, D. C. Lay Jr, & B. T. Richert. 2006. Postnatal behavioral and physiological responses of piglets from gilts housed individually or in groups during gestation. *J. Anim. Sci.* 84:757–766.

2154 **Souza, A. S., & A. J. Zanella. 2008. Social isolation elicits deficits in the ability of newly weaned female piglets to recognise conspecifics. *Appl. Anim. Behav. Sci.* 110:182–188.**

2155 Spain, C. V., J. M. Scarlett, & K. A. Houpt. 2004. Long-term risks and benefits of early-age gonadectomy in cats. *J. Am. Vet. Med. Assoc.* 224:372–379.

2156 Spake, J. R., K. A. Gray, & J. P. Cassady. 2012. Relationship between backtest and coping styles in pigs. *Appl. Anim. Behav. Sci.* 140(3–4):146–153.

2157 Spangenberg, E. M. F., L. Björklund, & K. Dahlborn. 2006. Outdoor housing of laboratory dogs: Effects on activity, behaviour and physiology. *Appl. Anim. Behav. Sci.* 98:260–276.

2158 Spencer, G. S. 1992. Immunization against cholecystokinin decreases appetite in lambs. *J. Anim. Sci.* 70:3820–3824.

2159 Spinka, M., & B. Algers. 1995. Functional view on udder massage after milk let-down in pigs. *Appl. Anim. Behav. Sci.* 43:197–212.

2160 **Spinka, M., G. Illmann, F. de Jonge, M. Andersson, T. Schuurman, & P. Jensen. 2000. Dimensions of maternal behaviour characteristics in domestic and wild × domestic crossbred sows. *Appl. Anim. Behav. Sci.* 70:99–114.**

2161 Spinka, M., I. J. H. Duncan, & T. M. Widowski. 1998. Do domestic pigs prefer short-term to medium-term confinement? *Appl. Anim. Behav. Sci.* 58:221–232.

2162 Sprague, R. H., & J. J. Anisko. 1973. Elimination patterns in the laboratory beagle. *Behaviour.* 47:257–267.

2163 Sprott, R. L. 1967. Barometric pressure fluctuations: Effects on the activity of laboratory mice. *Science.* 157:1206–1207.

2164 Squires, V. R., & G. T. Daws. 1975. Leadership and dominance relationships in Merino and Border Leicester sheep. *Appl. Anim. Ethol.* 1:263–274.

2165 St. Hoy, & J. Bauer. 2005. Dominance relationships between sows dependent on the time interval between separation and reunion. *Appl. Anim. Behav. Sci.* 90:21–30.

2166 **Stachurska, A., I. Janczarek, I. Wilk, & W. Kidzierski. 2015. Does music influence emotional state in race horses? *Equine Vet. J.* 35(8):650–656.**

2167 Stahlbaum, C. C., & K. A. Houpt. 1989. The role of the flehmen response in the behavioral repertoire of the stallion. *Physiol. Behav.* 45:1207–1214.

2168 Stangel, G., & P. Jensen. 1991. Behaviour of semi-naturally kept sows and piglets (except suckling) during 10 days postpartum. *Appl. Anim. Behav. Sci.* 31:211–227.

2169 Stanley, C. R., & R. I. M. Dunbar. 2013. Consistent social structure and optimal clique size revealed by social network analysis of feral goats, *Capra hircus.* *Anim. Behav.* 85(4):771–779.

2170 Stanley, W. C., & O. Elliot. 1962. Differential human handling as reinforcing events and as treatments influencing later social behavior in basenji puppies. *Psychol. Rep.* 10:775–788.

2171 Stanley, W. C., J. E. Barrett, & W. E. Bacon. 1974. Conditioning and extinction of avoidance and escape behavior in neonatal dogs. *J. Comp. Physiol. Psychol.* 87:163–172.

2172 Stanley, W. C., W. E. Bacon, & C. Fehr. 1970. Discriminated instrumental learning in neonatal dogs. *J. Comp. Physiol. Psychol.* 70:335–343.

2173 Starling, M. J., N. Branson, D. Cody, T. R. Starling, & P. D. McGreevy. 2014. Canine sense and sensibility: Tipping points and response latency variability as an optimism index in a canine judgement bias assessment. *PLoS ONE.* 9(9):e107794.

2174 Statham, P., L. Green, M. Bichard, & M. Mendl. 2009. Predicting tail-biting from behaviour of pigs prior to outbreaks. *Appl. Anim. Behav. Sci.* 121:157–164.

2175 Steigerwald, E. S., M. Sarter, P. March, & M. Podell. 1999. Effects of feline immunodeficiency virus on cognition and behavioral function in cats. *J. Acquir. Immune Defic. Syndr. Hum. Retrovirol.* 20:411–419.

2176 Steinert, R. E., C. Feinle-Bisset, N. Geary, & C. Beglinger. 2013. Digestive physiology of the pig symposium: Secretion of gastrointestinal hormones and eating control. *J. Anim. Sci.* 91:1963–1973.

2177 Stellflug, J. N., N. E. Cockett, & G. S. Lewis. 1989. Relationship between sexual behavior classifications of rams and lambs sired in a competitive breeding environment. *Horm. Behav.* 23:290–303.

2178 Stelow, E. A., M. J. Bain, & P. H. Kass. 2016. The relationship between coat color and aggressive behaviors in the domestic cat. *J. Appl. Anim. Welf. Sci.* 19(1):1–15.

2179 **Stephen, J., & R. Ledger. 2007. Relinquishing dog owners' ability to**

predict behavioural problems in shelter dogs post adoption. *Appl. Anim. Behav. Sci.* 107:88–99.

2180 **Stephens, D. B. 1974. Studies on the effect of social environment on the behaviour and growth rates of artificially reared British Friesian male calves. *Anim. Prod.* 18:23–24.**

2181 Stephens, D. B. 1975. Effects of gastric loading on the sucking response and voluntary milk intake in neonatal piglets. *J. Comp. Physiol. Psychol.* 88:796–805.

2182 Stephens, D. B. 1980. The effects of 2-deoxy-D-glucose given via the jugular or hepatic-portal vein on food intake and plasma glucose levels in pigs. *Physiol. Behav.* 25:691–697.

2183 Stephens, D. B., & B. A. Baldwin. 1971. Observations on the behaviour of groups of artificially reared lambs. *Res. Vet. Sci.* 12:219–224.

2184 Stephens, D. B., & J. L. Linzell. 1974. The development of sucking behaviour in the newborn goat. *Anim. Behav.* 22:628–633.

2185 Stephens, D. B., D. L. Ingram, & D. F. Sharman. 1983. An investigation into some cerebral mechanisms involved in schedule-induced drinking in the pig. *Q. J. Exp. Physiol.* 68:653–660.

2186 Sterman, M. B., T. Knauss, D. Lehmann, & C. D. Clemente. 1965. Circadian sleep and waking patterns in the laboratory cat. *Electroencephalogr. Clin. Neurophysiol.* 19:509–517.

2187 Stevens, B., G. M. Karlen, R. Morrison, H. W. Gonyou, K. L. Butler, K. J. Kerswell, & P. H. Hemsworth. 2015. Effects of stage of gestation at mixing on aggression, injuries and stress in sows. *Appl. Anim. Behav. Sci.* 165:40–46.

2188 Stewart, J. C., & J. P. Scott. 1947. Lack of correlation between leadership and dominance relationships in a herd of goats. *J. Comp. Physiol. Psychol.* 40:255–264.

2189 Stone, C. C., M. S. Brown, & G. H. Waring. 1974. An ethological means to improve swine production. *J. Anim. Sci.* 39:137.

2190 Stookey, J. M., & H. W. Gonyou. 1994. The effects of regrouping on behavioral and production parameters in finishing swine. *J. Anim. Sci.* 72:2804–2811.

2191 **Stookey, J. M., & H. W. Gonyou. 1998. Recognition in swine: Recognition through familiarity or genetic relatedness? *Appl. Anim. Behav. Sci.* 55:291–305.**

2192 Storengen, L. M., & F. Lingaas. 2015. Noise sensitivity in 17 dog breeds: Prevalence, breed risk and correlation with fear in other situations. *Appl. Anim. Behav. Sci.* 171:152–160.

2193 **Strain, G. M., B. M. Olcott, R. M. Archer, & B. K. McClintock. 1984. Narcolepsy in a Brahman bull. *J. Am. Vet. Med. Assoc.* 185:538–541.**

2194 Strasia, C. A., M. Thorn, R. W. Rice, & D. R. Smith. 1970. Grazing habits, diet and performance of sheep on alpine ranges. *J. Range Manag.* 23:201–208.

2195 Stricklin, W. R., & H. W. Gonyou. 1981. Dominance and eating behavior of beef cattle fed from a single stall. *Appl. Anim. Behav. Sci.* 7:135–140.

2196 Stricklin, W. R., C. C. Kautz-Scanavy, & D. L. Greger. 1985. Determination of dominance-subordinance relationships among beef heifers in a dominance tube. *Appl. Anim. Behav. Sci.* 14:111–116.

2197 Stroup, W. W., M. K. Nielsen, & J. A. Gosey. 1987. Cyclic variation in cattle feed intake data: Characterization and implications for experimental design. *J. Anim. Sci.* 64:1638–1647.

2198 Studnitz, M., & K. H. Jensen. 2002. Expression of rooting motivation in gilts following different lengths of deprivation. *Appl. Anim. Behav. Sci.* 76:203–213.

2199 **Studnitz, M., M. K. Jensen, & L. J. Pedersen. 2007. Why do pigs root and in what will they root?: A review on the exploratory behaviour of pigs in relation to environmental enrichment *Appl. Anim. Behav. Sci.* 107:183–197.**

2200 Stukenborg, A., I. Traulsen, B. Puppe, U. Presuhn, & J. Krieter. 2011. Agonistic behaviour after mixing in pigs under commercial farm conditions. *Appl. Anim. Behav. Sci.* 129(1):28–35.

2201 Sturgeon, R. D., P. D. Brophy, & R. A. Levitt. 1973. Drinking elicited by intracranial microinjection of angiotensin in the cat. *Pharmacol. Biochem. Behav.* 1:353–355.

2202 Sueda, K. L. C., B. L. Hart, & K. D. Cliff. 2008. Characterisation of plant eating in dogs. *Appl. Anim. Behav. Sci.* 111:120–132.

2203 Sufit, E., K. A. Houpt, & M. Sweeting. 1985. Physiological stimuli of thirst and drinking patterns in ponies. *Equine Vet. J.* 17:12–16.

2204 Sung, W., & S. L. Crowell-Davis. 2006. Elimination behavior patterns of domestic cats (*Felis catus*) with and without elimination behavior problems. *Am. J. Vet. Res.* 67:1500–1504.

2205 **Sutherland, G. F. 1939. Salivary conditioned reflexes in swine. *Am. J. Physiol.* 126:P640–P641.**

2206 Svartberg, K. 2002. Shyness-boldness predicts performance in working dogs. *Appl. Anim. Behav. Sci.* 79:157–174.

2207 Svartberg, K. 2006. Breed-typical behaviour in dogs: Historical remnants or recent constructs? *Appl. Anim. Behav. Sci.* 96:293–313.

2208 **Svartberg, K., & B. Forkman. 2002. Personality traits in the domestic dog (*Canis familiaris*). *Appl. Anim. Behav. Sci.* 79:133–155.**

2209 **Svobodova, I., P. Vapenik, L. Pinc, & L. Bartos. 2008. Testing German shepherd puppies to assess their chances of certification. *Appl. Anim. Behav. Sci.* 113:139–149.**

2210 Sweeting, M. P., C. E. Houpt, & K. A. Houpt. 1985. Social facilitation of feeding and time budgets in stabled ponies. *J. Anim. Sci.* 60:369–374.

2211 **Sweetwood, H. L., D. F. Kripke, I. Grant, J. Yager, & M. S. Gerst. 1976. Sleep disorder and psychobiological symptomatology in male psychiatric outpatients and male nonpatients. *Psychosom. Med.* 38:373–378.**

2212 **Swenson, R. M., & W. Randall. 1977. Grooming behavior in cats with pontile lesions and cats with tectal lesions. *J. Comp. Physiol. Psychol.* 91:313–326.**

2213 Syme, G. J., L. A. Syme, & T. P. Jefferson. 1974. A note on variations in the level of aggression within a herd of goats. *Anim. Prod.* 18:309–312.

2214 Syme, L. A., G. J. Syme, T. G. Waite, & A. J. Pearson. 1975. Spatial distribution and social status in a small herd of dairy cows. *Anim. Behav.* 23:609–614.

2215 Symoens, J., & M. Van Den Brande. 1969. Prevention and cure of aggressiveness in pigs using the sedative azaperone. *Vet. Rec.* 85:64–67.

2216 Szabó, D., N. R. Gee, & Á. Miklósi. 2016. Natural or pathologic? Discrepancies in the study of behavioral and cognitive signs in aging family dogs. *J. Vet. Behav.* 11:86–98.

2217 **Szenczi, P., O. Banszegi, A. Urrutia, T. Farago, & R. Hudson. 2016. Mother-offspring recognition in the domestic cat: Kittens recognize their own mother's call. *Dev. Psychobiol.* 58(5):568–577.**

2218 Takagi, S., H. Chijiiwa, M. Arahori, M. Tsuzuki, A. Hyuga, & K. Fujita. 2015. Do cats (*Felis catus*) predict the presence of an invisible object from sound? *J. Vet. Behav.* 10(5):407–412.

2219 Takaoka, A., T. Maeda, Y. Hori, & K. Fujita. 2015. Do dogs follow behavioral cues from an unreliable human? *Anim. Cogn.* 18(2):475–483.

2220 Takeda, K., S. Sato, & K. Sugawara. 2000. The number of farm mates influences social and maintenance behaviours of Japanese black cows in a communal pasture. *Appl. Anim. Behav. Sci.* 67:181–192.

2221 Takeuchi, Y., C. Hashizume, E. M. Chon, Y. Momozawa, K. Masuda, T. Kikusui, & Y. Mori. 2005. Canine tyrosine hydroxylase (TH) gene and dopamine beta-hydroxylase (DBH) gene: Their sequences, genetic polymorphisms, and diversities among five different dog breeds. *J. Vet. Med. Sci.* 67:861–867.

2222 Takeuchi, Y., C. Hashizume, S. Arata, M. Inoue-Murayama, T. Maki, B. L. Hart, & Y. Mori. 2009. An approach to canine behavioural genetics employing guide dogs for the blind. *Anim. Genet.* 40:217–224.

2223 Takeuchi, Y., F. Kaneko, C. Hashizume, K. Masuda, N. Ogata, T. Maki, M. Inoue-Murayama, *et al.* 2009. Association analysis between canine behavioural traits and genetic polymorphisms in the Shiba Inu breed. *Anim. Genet.* 40(5):616–622.

2224 Takeuchi, Y., K. A. Houpt, & J. M. Scarlett. 2000. Evaluation of treatments for separation anxiety in dogs. *J. Am. Vet. Med. Assoc.* 217:342–345.

2225 Tallet, C., I. Veissier, & X. Boivin. 2006. A note on the consistency and specificity of lambs' responses to a stockperson and to their photograph in an arena test. *Appl. Anim. Behav. Sci.* 98:308–314.

2226 **Tallet, C., I. Veissier, & X. Boivin. 2009. How does the method used to feed lambs modulate their affinity to their human caregiver?** *Appl. Anim. Behav. Sci.* **119:56–65.**

2227 Talling, J. C., N. K. Waran, C. M. Wathes, & J. A. Lines. 1998. Sound avoidance by domestic pigs depends upon characteristics of the signal. *Appl. Anim. Behav. Sci.* 58:255–266.

2228 Tan, S. S. L., & D. M. Shackleton. 1990. Effects of mixing unfamiliar individuals and of azapaerone on the social behaviour of finishing pigs. *Appl. Anim. Behav. Sci.* 26:157–168.

2229 Tang, R., H. J. Noh, D. Wang, S. Sigurdsson, R. Swofford, M. Perloski, M. Duxbury, *et al.* 2004. Candidate genes and functional noncoding variants identified in a canine model of obsessive-compulsive disorder. *Genome Biol.* 15:R25.

2230 Tanida, H., A. Miura, T. Tanaka, & T. Yoshimoto. 1995. Behavioral response to humans to individually handled weanling pigs. *Appl. Anim. Behav. Sci.* 42:249–259.

2231 Tanida, H., N. Miyazaki, T. Tanaka, & T. Yoshimoto. 1991. Selection of mating partners in boars and sows under multi-sire mating. *Appl. Anim. Behav. Sci.* 32:13–21.

2232 Tapki, I., A. Sahin, & A. G. Onal. 2006. Effect of space allowance on behaviour of newborn milk-fed dairy calves. *Appl. Anim. Behav. Sci.* 99:12–20.

2233 **Taylor, A. A., & D. M. Weary. 2000. Vocal responses of piglets to castration: Identifying procedural sources of pain.** *Appl. Anim. Behav. Sci.* **70:17–26.**

2234 **Taylor, K., & D. S. Mills. 2007. A placebo-controlled study to investigate the effect of dog appeasing pheromone and other environmental and management factors on the reports of disturbance and house soiling during the night in recently adopted puppies.** *Appl. Anim. Behav. Sci.* **105:358–368.**

2235 Taylor, N., N. Prescott, G. Perry, M. Potter, C. Le Sueur, & C. Wathes. 2006. Preference of growing pigs for illuminance. *Appl. Anim. Behav. Sci.* 96:19–31.

2236 Teixeira, D. L., M. J. Hötzel, & L. C. P. M. Filho. 2006. Designing better water troughs: 2. Surface area and height, but not depth, influence dairy cows' preference. *Appl. Anim. Behav. Sci.* 96:169–175.

2237 Telezhenko, E., & C. Bergsten. 2005. Influence of floor type on the locomotion of dairy cows. *Appl. Anim. Behav. Sci.* 93:183–197.

2238 Tellington-Jones, L., & U. Bruns. 1988. *An introduction to the Tellington Jones equine awareness method.* Millwood, NY: Breakthrough.

2239 Tennessen, T., M. A. Price, & R. T. Berg. 1985. The social interactions of young bulls and steers after regrouping. *Appl. Anim. Behav. Sci.* 14:37–47.

2240 **Tennie, C., E. Glabsch, S. Tempelmann, J. Bräuer, J. Kaminski, & J. Call. 2009. Dogs, *Canis familiaris*, fail to copy intransitive actions in third-party contextual imitation tasks. *Anim. Behav.* 77(6):1491–1499.**

2241 **Terlouw, E. M. C., A. Wiersma, A. B. Lawrence, & H. A. MacLeod. 1993. Ingestion of food facilitates the performance of stereotypies in sows. *Anim. Behav.* 46:939–950.**

2242 Terlouw, E. M., C. A. B. Lawrence, & A. W. Illius. 1991. Influences of feeding level and physical restriction on development of stereotypies in sows. *Anim. Behav.* 42:981–991.

2243 Ternman, E., M. Pastell, S. Agenäs, C. Strasser, C. Winckler, P. P. Nielsen, & L. Hänninen. 2014. Agreement between different sleep states and behaviour indicators in dairy cows. *Appl. Anim. Behav. Sci.* 160:12–18.

2244 Ternouth, J. H., & A. W. Beattie. 1970. A note on the voluntary food consumption and the sodium-potassium ratio of sheep after shearing. *Anim. Prod.* 12:343–346.

2245 **Schaffer, C. B., & Phillips, J. (Directors). 1993. *The Tuskegee behaviour test for selecting therapy dogs.* Video/DVD. Tuskegee, AL: Tuskegee University School of Veterinary Medicine.**

2246 Thiery, J. A., & J. Signoret. 1978. Effect of changing the teaser ewe on the sexual activity of the ram. *Appl. Anim. Ethol.* 4:87–90.

2247 Thinus-Blanc, C., B. Poucet, & N. Chapuis. 1982. Object permanence in cats: Analysis in locomotor space. *Behav. Processes.* 7:81–86.

2248 Thomas, D. T., A. J. Rintoul, & D. G. Masters. 2007. Sheep select combinations of high and low sodium chloride, energy and crude protein feed that improve their diet. *Appl. Anim. Behav. Sci.* 105:140–153.

2249 Thompson, L. H., & J. S. Savage. 1978. Age at puberty and ovulation rate in gilts in confinement as influenced by exposure to a boar. *J. Anim. Sci.* 47:1141–1144.

2250 Thompson, W. R., & W. Heron. 1954. The effects of early restriction on activity in dogs. *J. Comp. Physiol. Psychol.* 47:77–82.

2251 Thompson, W. R., & W. Heron. 1954. The effects of restricting early experience on the problem-solving capacity of dogs. *Can. J. Psychol.* 8:17–31.

2252 Thomsen, L. R., B. L. Nielsen, & O. N. Larsen. 2010. Implications of food patch distribution on social foraging in domestic pigs (*Sus scrofa*). *Appl. Anim. Behav. Sci.* 122(2–4):111–118.

2253 Thorhallsdotir, A. G., F. D. Provenza, & D. F. Balph. 1990. The role of the mother in the intake of harmful foods by lambs. *Appl. Anim. Behav. Sci.* 25:35–44.

2254 Thorndike, E. L. 1911. *Animal intelligence: Experimental studies.* New York, NY: Macmillan.

2255 Thorpe, W. H. 1963. *Learning and instinct in animals.* Cambridge, MA: Harvard University Press.

2256 Thrasher, T. N., C. J. Brown, L. C. Keil, & D. J. Ramsay. 1980. Thirst and vasopressin release in the dog: An osmoreceptor or sodium receptor mechanism? *Am. J. Physiol.* 238:R333–R339.

2257 Tilbrook, A. J. 1987. Physical and behavioural factors affecting the sexual "attractiveness" of the ewe. *Appl. Anim. Behav. Sci.* 17:109–115.

2258 **Tilbrook, A. J., P. H. Hemsworth, J. S. Topp, & A. W. N. Cameron. 1990. Parallel changes in the proceptive and** receptive behaviour of the ewe. *Appl. Anim. Behav. Sci.* 27:73–92.

2259 Timney, B., & K. Keil. 1992. Visual acuity in the horse. *Vision Res.* 32:2289–2293.

2260 Tischner, M. 1982. Patterns of stallion sexual behaviour in the absence of mares. *J. Reprod. Fertil. Suppl.* 32:65–70.

2261 Tischner, M., K. Kosiniak, & W. Bielanski. 1974. Analysis of the pattern of ejaculation in stallions. *J. Reprod. Fertil.* 41:329–335.

2262 Titterington, R. W., & D. Fraser. 1975. The lying behaviour of sows and piglets during early lactation in relation to the position of the creep heater. *Appl. Anim. Ethol.* 2:47–53.

2263 Tobach, E., L. R. Aronson, & E. Shaw. 1971. *The biopsychology of development.* New York, NY: Academic Press.

2264 Tod, E., D. Brander, & N. Waran. 2005. Efficacy of dog appeasing pheromone in reducing stress and fear related behaviour in shelter dogs. *Appl. Anim. Behav. Sci.* 93:295–308.

2265 Todd, N. B. 1963. *The catnip response.* Cambridge, MA: Harvard University.

2266 Toerien, C. A., T. Sahlu, & W. W. Wong. 1999. Energy expenditure of angora bucks in peak breeding season estimated with the doubly-labeled water technique. *J. Anim. Sci.* 77:3096–3105.

2267 Tolkamp, B. J., M. J. Haskell, F. M. Langford, D. J. Roberts, & C. A. Morgan. 2010. Are cows more likely to lie down the longer they stand. *Appl. Anim. Behav. Sci.* 124(1–2):1–10.

2268 Tolu, C., & T. Savas. 2007. A brief report on intra-species aggressive biting in a goat herd. *Appl. Anim. Behav. Sci.* 102:124–129.

2269 Tomkins, L. M., K. A. Williams, P. C. Thomson, & P. D. Mcgreevy. 2012. Lateralization in the domestic dog (*Canis familiaris*): Relationships between structural, motor, and sensory laterality. *J. Vet. Behav.* 7(2):70–79.

2270 Tomkins, L. M., P. C. Thomson, & P. D. McGreevy. 2010. First-stepping

test as a measure of motor laterality in dogs (*Canis familiaris*). *J. Vet. Behav.* 5(5):247–255.**

2271 Tomkins, T., & M. J. Bryant. 1974. Oestrous behaviour of the ewe and the influence of treatment with progestagen. *J. Reprod. Fert.* 41:121–132.

2272 Tomlinson, K. A., E. O. Price, & D. T. Torell. 1982. Responses of tranquilized post-partum ewes to alien lambs. *Appl. Anim. Ethol.* 8:109–117.

2273 Tomonaga, M., K. Kumazaki, F. Camus, S. Nicod, C. Pereira, & T. Matsuzawa. 2015. A horse's eye view: Size and shape discrimination compared with other mammals. *Biol. Lett.* 11:20150701.

2274 Tonoike, A., M. Nagasawa, K. Mogi, J. A. Serpell, H. Ohtsuki, & T. Kikusui. 2015. Comparison of owner-reported behavioral characteristics among genetically clustered breeds of dog (*Canis familiaris*). *Sci. Rep.* 5:17710.

2275 Tonokura, M., K. Fujita, M. Morozumi, Y. Yoshida, T. Kanbayashi, & S. Nishino. 2003. Narcolepsy in a hypocretin/orexin-deficient chihuahua. *Vet. Rec.* 152:776–779.

2276 Topal, J., A. Miklosi, & V. Csanyi. 1997. Dog-human relationship affects problem solving behavior in the dog. *Anthrozoos* 10:214.

2277 Topel, D. G., G. M. Weiss, D. G. Siers, & J. H. Magilton. 1973. Comparison of blood source and diurnal variation on blood hydrocortisone, growth hormone, lactate, glucose and electrolytes in swine. *J. Anim. Sci.* 36:531–534.

2278 Tornqvist, H., S. Somppi, A. Koskela, C. M. Krause, O. Vainio, & M. V. Kujala. 2015. Comparison of dogs and humans in visual scanning of social interaction. *R. Soc. Open Sci.* 2(9):150341.

2279 Torrey, S., & T. M. Widowski. 2006. Is belly nosing redirected suckling behaviour? *Appl. Anim. Behav. Sci.* 101:288–304.

2280 Torrey, S., & T. M. Widowski. 2007. Relationship between growth and non-nutritive massage in suckling pigs. *Appl. Anim. Behav. Sci.* **107**:32–44.

2281 Torrey, S., E. L. Toth Tamminga, & T. M. Widowski. 2008. Effect of drinker type on water intake and waste in newly weaned piglets. *J. Anim. Sci.* 86:1439–1445.

2282 Tortora, D. F. 1980. **Animal behavior therapy: The behavioral diagnosis and treatment of dominance-motivated aggression in canines: Part I.** *Canine Pract.* **7:10–19.**

2283 Tortora, D. F. 1980. **Animal behavior therapy: The behavioral diagnosis and treatment of dominance-motivated aggression in canines: Part II.** *Canine Pract.* **8:13–28.**

2284 Toscano, M. J., & D. C. Lay Jr. 2005. Parsing the characteristics of a simulated udder to determine relative attractiveness to piglets in the 72 h following parturition. *Appl. Anim. Behav. Sci.* 92:283–291.

2285 Toth, L., M. Gacsi, J. Topal, & A. Miklosi. 2008. Playing styles and possible causative factors in dogs' behaviour when playing with humans. *Appl. Anim. Behav. Sci.* 114:473–484.

2286 Toutain, P. L., C. Toutain, A. J. Webster, & J. D. McDonald. 1977. Sleep and activity, age and fatness, and the energy expenditure of confined sheep. *Br. J. Nutr.* 38:445–454.

2287 Towbin, E. J. 1949. Gastric distention as a factor in the satiation of thirst in esophagostomized dogs. *Am. J. Physiol.* 159:533–541.

2288 Tribe, D. E. 1949. The importance of sense of smell to the grazing sheep. *J. Agric. Sci. (Camb.)* 39:309–312.

2289 Trivers, R. L. 1974. Parent offspring conflict. *Am. Zool.* 14:249–264.

2290 Trout, W. E., J. C. Pekas, & B. D. Schanbacher. 1989. Immune, growth and carcass responses of ram lambs to active immunization against desulfated cholecystokinin (CCK-8). *J. Anim. Sci.* 67:2709–2714.

2291 Trumler, E. 1959. Das "rossigkeitgesicht" und ahnliches ausdrucks verhalten bei einhufern. *Z. Tierpsychol.* 16:478–488.

2292 Tuchscherer, M., B. Puppe, A. Tuchscherer, & E. Kanitz. 1998. Effects of social status after mixing on immune, metabolic, and endocrine responses in pigs. *Physiol. Behav.* 64:353–360.

2293 Tuchscherer, M., E. Kanitz, B. Puppe, & A. Tuchscherer. 2006. **Early social isolation alters behavioral and physiological responses to an endotoxin challenge in piglets.** *Horm. Behav.* **50(5):753–761.**

2294 Tucker, C. B., A. R. Rogers, G. A. Verkerk, P. E. Kendall, J. R. Webster, & L. R. Matthews. 2007. Effects of shelter and body condition on the behaviour and physiology of dairy cattle in winter. *Appl. Anim. Behav. Sci.* 105:1–13.

2295 Turcsán, B., E. Kubinyi, & Á. Miklósi. 2011. **Trainability and boldness traits differ between dog breed clusters based on conventional breed categories and genetic relatedness.** *Appl. Anim. Behav. Sci.* **132(1–2):61–70.**

2296 Turek, F. W., & S. Losee-Olson. 1986. A benzodiazepine used in the treatment of insomnia phase-shifts the mammalian circadian clock. *Nature.* 321:167–168.

2297 Turner, A. S., N. White 2nd, & J. Ismay. 1984. Modified Forssell's operation for crib biting in the horse. *J. Am. Vet. Med. Assoc.* 184:309–312.

2298 Turner, D. C., & P. Bateson. 1988. *The domestic cat: The biology of its behaviour.* New York, NY: Cambridge University Press.

2299 Turner, D. C., J. Feaver, M. Mendl, & P. Bateson. 1986. **Variation in domestic cat behaviour towards humans: A paternal effect.** *Anim. Behav.* **34:1890–1892.**

2300 Tyler, S. J. 1972. The behaviour and social organization of the new forest ponies. *Anim. Behav. Monogr.* 5:85–196.

2301 Udell, M. A. R., M. Ewald, N. R. Dorey, & C. D. L. Wynne. 2014. Exploring breed differences in dogs (*Canis familiaris*): Does exaggeration or inhibition of predatory response predict performance on human-guided tasks? *Anim. Behav.* 89:99–105.

2302 Uller, C., & J. Lewis. 2009. Horses (*Equus caballus*) select the greater of two quantities in small numerical contrasts. *Anim. Cogn.* 12(5):733–738.

2303 Ungerfeld, R. 2012. Sexual behavior of medium-ranked rams toward non-estrual ewes is stimulated by the presence of low-ranked rams. *J. Vet. Behav.* 7(2):84–87.

2304 Ungerfeld, R., & L. Silva. 2005. The presence of normal vaginal flora is necessary for normal sexual attractiveness of estrous ewes. *Appl. Anim. Behav. Sci.* 93:245–250.

2305 Ungerfeld, R., J. Giriboni, A. Freitas-De-Melo, & L. Lacuesta. 2014. Homosexual behavior in male goats is more frequent during breeding season and in bucks isolated from females. *Horm. Behav.* 65(5):516–520.

2306 **Ungerfeld, R., L. Lacuesta, J. P. Damián, & J. Giriboni. 2013. Does heterosexual experience matter for bucks' homosexual mating behavior? *J. Vet. Behav.* 8(6):471–474.**

2307 Ungerfeld, R., M. A. Ramos, & R. Möller. 2006. Role of the vomeronasal organ on ram's courtship and mating behaviour, and on mate choice among oestrous ewes. *Appl. Anim. Behav. Sci.* 99:248–252.

2308 Ursin, R. 1968. The two stages of slow wave sleep in the cat and their relation to REM sleep. *Brain Res.* 11:347–356.

2309 Ursin, R. 1970. Sleep stage relations within the sleep cycles of the cat. *Brain Res.* 20:91–97.

2310 **Ursin, R., H. Cohen, S. Henriksen, G. Mitchell, & W. Dement. 1976.** Effects of sleep of restricted sleep. A cat case study. *Electroencephalogr. Clin. Neurophysiol.* 41:96–101.

2311 Vaarst, M., M. B. Jensen, & A. Sandager. 2001. Behaviour of calves at introduction to nurse cows after the colostrum period. *Appl. Anim. Behav. Sci.* 73:27–33.

2312 Vage, J., T. B. Bønsdorff, E. Arnet, A. Tverdal, & F. Lingaas. 2010. Differential gene expression in brain tissues of aggressive and non-aggressive dogs. *BMC Vet. Res.* 6:34.

2313 Vailes, L. D., & J. H. Britt. 1990. Influence of footing surface on mounting and other sexual behaviors of estrual holstein cows. *J. Anim. Sci.* 68:2333–2339.

2314 Valenchon, M., F. Levy, A. Gorecka-Bruzda, L. Calandreau, & L. Lansade. 2013. Characterization of long-term memory, resistance to extinction, and influence of temperament during two instrumental tasks in horses. *Anim. Cogn.* 16(6):1001–1006.

2315 **Valenchon, M., F. Lévy, M. Fortin, C. Leterrier, & L. Lansade. 2013. Stress and temperament affect working memory performance for disappearing food in horses, *Equus caballus*. *Anim. Behav.* 86(6):1233–1240.**

2316 Val-Laillet, D., C. Tallet, C. Guérin, & M.-C. Meunier-Salaün. 2013. Behavioural reactivity, social and cognitive abilities of Vietnamese and Pitman-Moore weaned piglets. *Appl. Anim. Behav. Sci.* 148(1–2):108–119.

2317 Val-Laillet, D., V. Guesdon, M. A. G. von Keyserlingk, A. M. De Passille, & J. Rushen. 2009. Allogrooming in cattle: Relationships between social preferences, feeding displacements and social dominance. *Appl. Anim. Behav. Sci.* 116:141–149.

2318 Valros, A. E., M. Rundgren, M. Spinka, H. Saloniemi, L. Rydhmer, & B. Algers. 2002. Nursing behaviour of sows during 5 weeks lactation and effects on piglet growth. *Appl. Anim. Behav. Sci.* 76:93–104.

2319 Van Beirendonck, S., J. Van Thielen, G. Verbeke, & B. Driessen. 2014. **The association between sow and piglet behavior.** *J. Vet. Behav.* **9(3):107–113.**

2320 van den Berg, L., M. B. Schilder, H. de Vries, P. A. Leegwater, & B. A. van Oost. 2006. Phenotyping of aggressive behavior in golden retriever dogs with a questionnaire. *Behav. Genet.* 36:882–902.

2321 **van den Berg, L., M. Vos-Loohuis, M. B. H. Schilder, B. A. van Oost, H. A. W. Hazewinkel, C. M. Wade, E. K. Karlsson, *et al*. 2008. Evaluation of the serotonergic genes htr1A, htr1B, htr2A, and slc6A4 in aggressive behavior of Golden Retriever dogs.** *Behav. Genet.* **38(1):55–66.**

2322 Van den Berg, M., W. Y. Brown, C. Lee, & G. N. Hinch. 2015. Browse-related behaviors of pastured horses in Australia: A survey. *J. Vet. Behav.* 10(1):48–53.

2323 Van den Bos, R. 1998. Post-conflict stress-response in confined group-living cats (*Felis silvestris catus*). *Appl. Anim. Behav. Sci.* 59:323–330.

2324 **Van den Bos, R., M. K. Meijer, & B. M. Spruijt. 2000. Taste reactivity patterns in domestic cats (*Felis silvestris catus*).** *Appl. Anim. Behav. Sci.* **69:149–168.**

2325 Van der Borg, J. A. M., M. B. H. Schilder, C. M. Vinke, & H. de Vries. 2015. Dominance in domestic dogs: A quantitative analysis of its behavioural measures. *PLoS ONE.* 10(8):e0133978.

2326 van der Borg, J. A. M., W. J. Netto, & D. J. U. Planta. 1991. Behavioural testing of dogs in animal shelters to predict problem behaviour. *Appl. Anim. Behav. Sci.* 32:237–251.

2327 van der Staay, F. J., J. de Groot, T. Schuurman, & S. M. Korte. 2008. Repeated social defeat in female pigs does not induce neuroendocrine symptoms of depression, but behavioral adaptation. *Physiol. Behav.* 93,433–460.

2328 van Miert, A. S., F. Kaya, & C. T. van Duin. 1992. Changes in food intake and forestomach motility of dwarf goats by recombinant bovine cytokines (IL-1 beta, IL-2) and IFN-gamma. *Physiol. Behav.* 52:859–864.

2329 van Putten, G. 1969. An investigation into tail-biting among fattening pigs. *Br. Vet. J.* 125:511–517.

2330 Van Putten, G., & J. Dammers. 1976. A comparative study of the well-being of piglets reared conventionally and in cages. *Appl. Anim. Ethol.* 2:339–356.

2331 Van Putten, G., & R. G. Bure. 1997. Preparing gilts for group housing by increasing their social skills. *Appl. Anim. Behav. Sci.* 54:173–183.

2332 **Vandenheede, M., & M. Bouissou. 1993. Sex differences in fear reactions in sheep.** *Appl. Anim. Behav. Sci.* **37:39–55.**

2333 Van Dierendonck, M. C., H. de Vries, B. H. Schilder, B. Colenbrander, A. G. Porhallsdottir, & H. Sigurjonsdottir. 2009. Interventions in social behaviour in a herd of mares and geldings. *Appl. Anim. Behav. Sci.* 116:67–73.

2334 Van-Laillet, D., & R. Nowak. 2006. Socio-spatial criteria are important for the establishment of maternal preference in lambs. *Appl. Anim. Behav. Sci.* 96:269–280.

2335 VanWagoner, H. C., D. W. Bailey, D. D. Kress, D. C. Anderson, & K. C. Davis. 2006. Differences among beef sire breeds and relationships between terrain use and performance when daughters graze foothill rangelands as cows. *Appl. Anim. Behav. Sci.* 97:105–121.

2336 Vas, J., J. Topal, B. Gyori, & A. Miklosi. 2008. Consistency of dogs' reactions to threatening cues of an unfamiliar person. *Appl. Anim. Behav. Sci.* 112:331–344.

2337 Vas, J., R. Chojnacki, M. F. Kjøren, C. Lyngwa, & I. L. Andersen. 2013.

Social interactions, cortisol and reproductive success of domestic goats (*Capra hircus*) subjected to different animal densities during pregnancy. *Appl. Anim. Behav. Sci.* 147(1–2):117–126.

2338 **Vasdal, G., I. Møgedal, K. E. Bøe, R. Kirkden, & I. L. Andersen. 2010. Piglet preference for infrared temperature and flooring. *Appl. Anim. Behav. Sci.* 122(2–4):92–97.**

2339 Vázquez, R., A. Orihuela, F. I. Flores-Pérez, & V. Aguirre. 2015. Reducing early maternal licking of male lambs (*Ovis aries*) does not impair their sexual behavior in adulthood. *J. Vet. Behav.* 10(1):78–82.

2340 Vecchiotti, G. G., & R. Galanti. 1987. Evidence of heredity of cribbing, weaving and stall walking. *Livestock Prod. Sci.* 14:91–95.

2341 Veeckman, J., & F. O. Odberg. 1978. Preliminary studies on the behavioural detection of oestrus in Belgian "warm-blood" mares with acoustic and tactile stimuli. *Appl. Anim. Ethol.* 4:109–118.

2342 Veissier, I. 1993. Observational learning in cattle. *Appl. Anim. Behav. Sci.* 33:235–243.

2343 Veissier, I., & P. Le Neindre. 1989. Weaning of calves: Its effect on social organization. 24:43–54.

2344 Veissier, I., A. M. de Passille, G. Despres, J. Rushen, I. Charpentier, A. R. Ramirez de la Fe, & P. Pradel. 2002. Does nutritive and non-nutritive sucking reduce other oral behaviors and stimulate rest in calves? *J. Anim. Sci.* 80:2574–2587.

2345 Veissier, I., D. Lamy, & P. Le Neindre. 1990. Social behaviour in domestic beef cattle when yearling calves are left with the cows for the next calving. *Appl. Anim. Behav. Sci.* 27:193–200.

2346 Veissier, I., S. Andanson, H. Dubroeucq, & D. Pomies. 2008. The motivation of cows to walk as thwarted by tethering. *J. Anim. Sci.* 86:2723–2729.

2347 Venable, E. B., S. Bland, V. Braner, N. Gulson, & M. Halpin. 2016. Effect of

grazing muzzles on the rate of pelleted feed intake in horses. *J. Vet. Behav.* 11:56–59.

2348 Verberne, G., & J. de Boer. 1976. Chemocommunication among domestic cats, mediated by the olfactory and vomeronasal senses. *I. Chemocommunication. Z. Tierpsychol.* 42:86–109.

2349 Vercauteren, K. C., M. J. Lavelle, T. M. Gehring, & J.-M. Landry. 2012. Cow dogs: Use of livestock protection dogs for reducing predation and transmission of pathogens from wildlife to cattle. *Appl. Anim. Behav. Sci.* 140(3–4):128–136.

2350 Vervaecke, H., J. M. G. Stevens, H. Vandemoortele, H. Sigurjonsdottir, & H. De Vries. 2007. Aggression and dominance in matched groups of subadult Icelandic horses (*Equus caballus*). *J. Ethol.* 25:239–248.

2351 Vichova, J., & L. Bartos. 2005. Allosuckling in cattle: Gain or compensation? *Appl. Anim. Behav. Sci.* 94:223–235.

2352 Vierin, M., & M. Bouissou. 2002. Influence of maternal experience on fear reactions in ewes. *Appl. Anim. Behav. Sci.* 75:307–315.

2353 Villablanca, J. R., & C. E. Olmstead. 1979. Neurological development of kittens. *Dev. Psychobiol.* 12:101–127.

2354 Villalba, J. J., F. D. Provenza, & J. O. Hall. 2008. Learned appetites for calcium, phosphorus, and sodium in sheep. *J. Anim. Sci.* 86:738–747.

2355 Villalba, J. J., F. D. Provenza, & K. C. Olson. 2006. Terpenes and carbohydrate source influence rumen fermentation, digestibility, intake, and preference in sheep. *J. Anim. Sci.* 84:2463–2473.

2356 Villalba, J. J., F. D. Provenza, J. O. Hall, & C. Peterson. 2006. Phosphorus appetite in sheep: Dissociating taste from postingestive effects. *J. Anim. Sci.* 84:2213–2223.

2357 Vince, M. A. 1984. Teat seeking and presucking behaviour in newly born lambs: Possible effects of maternal skin temperatures. *Anim. Behav.* 32:249–254.

2358 Vince, M. A., & M. W. Stanier. 1991. The effect of food intake on young soay and Clun forest lambs' response to touch on the face. *Appl. Anim. Behav. Sci.* 30:37–96.

2359 Vince, M. A., & T. M. Ward. 1984. The responses of newly born Clun forest lambs to odour sources in the ewe. *Behaviour.* 89:117–121.

2360 Vince, M. A., T. M. Ward, & M. Reader. 1984. Tactile stimulation and teat seeking behaviour in newly born lambs. *Anim. Behav.* 32:1179–1184.

2361 Viranyi, Z., J. Topal, M. Gacsi, A. Miklosi, & V. Csanyi. 2004. Dogs respond appropriately to cues of humans' attentional focus. *Behav. Processes* 66:161–172.

2362 Virga, V., K. A. Houpt, & J. M. Scarlett. 2001. Efficacy of amitriptyline as a pharmacological adjunct to behavioral modification in the management of aggressive behaviors in dogs. *J. Am. Anim. Hosp. Assoc.* 37:325–330.

2363 Visser, E. K., A. D. Ellis, & C. G. Van Reenen. 2008. The effect of two different housing conditions on the welfare of young horses stabled for the first time. *Appl. Anim. Behav. Sci.* 114:521–533.

2364 Visser, E. K., C. G. van Reenen, M. B. H. Schilder, A. Barneveld, & H. J. Blokhuis. 2003. Learning performances in young horses using two different learning tests. *Appl. Anim. Behav. Sci.* 80:311–326.

2365 Visser, E. K., C. G. Van Reenen, M. Rundgren, M. Zetterqvist, K. Morgan, & H. J. Blokhuis. 2003. Responses of horses in behavioural tests correlate with temperament assessed by riders. *Equine Vet. J.* 35:176–183.

2366 Vitale Shreve, K. R., & M. A. R. Udell. 2015. What's inside your cat's head? A review of cat (*Felis silvestris catus*)

cognition research past, present and future. *Anim. Cogn.* 18(6):1195–1206.

2367 Vitale Shreve, K. R., & M. A. Udell. 2015. What's inside your cat's head? A review of cat (*Felis silvestris catus*) cognition research past, present and future. *Anim. Cogn.* 18(6):1195–1206.

2368 Vitale, A. F., M. Tenucci, M. Papini, & S. Lovari. 1986. Social behaviour of the calves of semi-wild Maremma cattle, *Bos primigenius taurus*. *Appl. Anim. Behav. Sci.* 16:217–231.

2369 Vogel, H. H., J. P. Scott, & M. Marston. 1950. Social facilitation and allelomimetic behavior in dogs I. Social facilitation in a non-competitive situation. *Behaviour.* 2:121–134.

2370 **Voith, V. L., & P. L. Borchelt. 1985. Elimination behavior and related problems in dogs. *Comp. Contin. Ed.* 7:537–546.**

2371 Von Borstel, U. U. K., I. J. H. Duncan, M. C. Lundin, & L. J. Keeling. 2010. Fear reactions in trained and untrained horses from dressage and show-jumping breeding lines. *Appl. Anim. Behav. Sci.* 125(3–4):124–131.

2372 von Borstel, U. U., I. J. H. Duncan, A. K. Shoveller, K. Merkies, L. J. Keeling, & S. T. Millman. 2009. Impact of riding in a coercively obtained rollkur posture on welfare and fear of performance horses. *Appl. Anim. Behav. Sci.* 116:228–236.

2373 von Keyserlingk, M. A., & D. M. Weary. 2007. Maternal behavior in cattle. *Horm. Behav.* 52:106–113.

2374 **Wagnon, K. A., R. G. Loy, W. C. Rollins, & F. D. Carroll. 1966. Social dominance in a herd of angus, Hereford, and shorthorn cows. *Anim. Behav.* 14:474–479.**

2375 Walker, D. B., J. C. Walker, P. J. Cavnar, J. L. Taylor, D. H. Pickel, S. B. Hall, & J. C. Suarez. 2006. Naturalistic quantification of canine olfactory sensitivity. *Appl. Anim. Behav. Sci.* 97:241–254.

2376 Walker, D. E. 1962. Suckling and grazing behaviour of beef heifers and calves. *N.Z. J. Agric. Res.* 5:331–338.

2377 Walker, S. L., R. F. Smith, D. N. Jones, J. E. Routly, & H. Dobson. 2008. Chronic stress, hormone profiles and estrus intensity in dairy cattle. *Horm. Behav.* 53:493–501.

2378 Wallace, L. R. 1949. Observations of lambing behaviour in ewes. *Proc. N.Z. Soc. Anim. Prod.* 9:85–96.

2379 Wallenbeck, A., & L. J. Keeling. 2013. Using data from electronic feeders on visit frequency and feed consumption to indicate tail biting outbreaks in commercial pig production. *J. Anim. Sci.* 91:2879–2884.

2380 Waller, G. R., G. H. Price, & E. D. Mitchell. 1969. Feline attractant, cis, trans-nepetalactone: Metabolism in the domestic cat. *Science* 164:1281–1282.

2381 Waltl, B., M. C. Appleby, & J. Solkner. 1995. Effects of relatedness on the suckling behaviour of calves in a herd of beef cattle rearing twins. *Appl. Anim. Behav. Sci.* 45:1–9.

2382 Wan, M., K. Hejjas, Z. Ronai, Z. Elek, M. Sasvari-Szekely, F. A. Champagne, A. Miklosi, & E. Kubinyi. 2013. DRD4 and TH gene polymorphisms are associated with activity, impulsivity and inattention in Siberian husky dogs. *Anim. Genet.* 44(6):717–727.

2383 Wangsness, P. J., L. E. Chase, A. D. Peterson, T. G. Hartsock, D. J. Kellmel, & B. R. Baumgardt. 1976. System of monitoring feeding behavior of sheep. *J. Anim. Sci.* 42:1544–1549.

2384 **Waran, N. K., & D. Cuddeford. 1995. Effects of loading and transport on the heart rate and behaviour of horses. *Appl. Anim. Behav. Sci.* 43:71–81.**

2385 Ward, C., & B. B. Smuts. 2007. Quantity-based judgments in the domestic dog (*Canis lupus familiaris*). *Anim. Cogn.* 10:71–80.

2386 Waring, G. H. 1982. Onset of behavior patterns in the newborn foal. *Equine Pract.* 4:28–34.

2387 Waring, G. H. 1983. *Horse behavior: The behavioral traits and adaptations of domestic and wild horses, including ponies.* Park Ridge, NJ: Noyes.

2388 **Waring, G. H., S. Wierzbowski, & E. S. E. Hafez. 1975. The behaviour of horses. In E. S. E. Hafez (Ed.), *The behaviour of domestic animals*, pp. 330–369. Baltimore, MD: Williams & Wilkins.**

2389 Warren, J. M., & A. Baron. 1956. The formation of learning sets by cats. *J. Comp. Physiol. Psychol.* 49:227–231.

2390 Warren, J. T., & I. Mysterud. 1993. Extensive ranging by sheep released onto an unfamiliar range. *Appl. Anim. Behav. Sci.* 38:67–73.

2391 Waters, A. J., C. J. Nicol, & N. P. French. 2002. Factors influencing the development of stereotypic and redirected behaviours in young horses: Findings of a four year prospective epidemiological study. *Equine Vet. J.* 34:572–579.

2392 Wathan, J., & K. Mccomb. 2014. The eyes and ears are visual indicators of attention in domestic horses. *Curr. Biol.* 24(15):677–679.

2393 Wathan, J., A. M. Burrows, B. M. Waller, & K. Mccomb. 2015. Equifacs: The equine facial action coding system. *PLoS ONE.* 10(8):e0131738.

2394 Wattanakul, W., C. A. Bulman, H. L. Edge, & S. A. Edwards. 2005. The effect of creep feed presentation method on feeding behaviour, intake and performance of suckling piglets. *Appl. Anim. Behav. Sci.* 92:27–36.

2395 Weary, D. M., & B. Chua. 2000. Effects of early separation on the dairy cow and calf. 1. Separation at 6 h, 1 day and 4 days after birth. *Appl. Anim. Behav. Sci.* 69:177–188.

2396 Weary, D. M., & D. Fraser. 1995. Calling by domestic piglets: Reliable signals of need? *Anim. Behav.* 50:1047–1055.

2397 Weary, D. M., E. A. Pajor, M. Bonenfant, D. Fraser, & D. L. Kramer. 2002. Alternative housing of sows and litters part 4. Effects of sow-controlled housing combined with a communal piglet area on pre- and post-weaning behaviour and performance. *Appl. Anim. Behav. Sci.* 76:279–290.

2398 Weary, D. M., E. A. Pajor, M. Bonenfant, S. K. Ross, D. Fraser, & D. L. Kramer. 1999. Alternative housing for sows and litters part 2. Effects of communal piglet area on pre- and post-weaning behaviour and performance. *Appl. Anim. Behav. Sci.* 65:123–135.

2399 Weary, D. M., J. M. Huzzey, & M. A. G. von Keyserlingk. 2009. Board-invited review: Using behavior to predict and identify ill health in animals. *J. Anim. Sci.* 87(2):770–777.

2400 Weary, D. M., M. C. Appleby, & D. Fraser. 1999. Responses of piglets to early separation from the sow. *Appl. Anim. Behav. Sci.* 63:289–300.

2401 Weaver, S. A., F. X. Aherne, M. J. Meaney, A. L. Schaefer, & W. T. Dixon. 2000. Neonatal handling permanently alters hypothalamic-pituitary-adrenal axis function, behaviour, and body weight in boars. *J. Endocrinol.* 164:349–359.

2402 Webb, F. M., V. N. Colenbrander, T. H. Blosser, & D. E. Waldern. 1963. Eating habits of dairy cows under drylot conditions. *J. Dairy Sci.* 46:1433–1435.

2403 Webb, L. E., C. G. Van Reenen, M. B. Jensen, O. Schmitt, & E. A. M. Bokkers. 2015. Does temperament affect learning in calves? *Appl. Anim. Behav. Sci.* 165:33–39.

2404 Weeks, J. W., S. L. Crowell-Davis, A. B. Caudle, & G. L. Heusner. 2000. Aggression and social spacing in light horse (*Equus caballus*) mares and foals. *Appl. Anim. Behav. Sci.* 68:319–337.

2405 Wehrend, A., E. Hofmann, K. Failing, & H. Bostedt. 2006. Behaviour during the first stage of labour in cattle: Influence of parity and dystocia. *Appl. Anim. Behav. Sci.* 100:164–170.

2406 Weiguo, L., & C. J. C. Phillips. 1991. The effects of supplementary light on the behaviour and performance of calves. *Appl. Anim. Behav. Sci.* 30:27–34.

2407 Weir, W. C., & D. T. Torell. 1959. Selective grazing by sheep as shown by a comparison of the chemical composition of range and pasture forage obtained by hand clipping and that collected by esophageal-fistulated sheep. *J. Anim. Sci.* 18:641–649.

2408 Weiss, E., & G. Greenberg. 1997. Service dog selection tests: Effectiveness of dogs from animal shelters. *Appl. Anim. Behav. Sci.* 53:297–308.

2409 Welch, A. R., & M. R. Baxter. 1986. Responses of newborn piglets to thermal and tactile properties of their environment. *Appl. Anim. Behav. Sci.* 15:203–215.

2410 Welch, R. A. S., & R. Kilgour. 1970. Mis-mothering among Romneys. *N.Z. J. Agric.* 121:26–27.

2411 Weldon, W. C., A. J. Lewis, G. F. Louis, J. L. Kovar, M. A. Giesemann, & P. S. Miller. 1994. Postpartum hypophagia in primiparous sows: I. Effects of gestation feeding level on feed intake, feeding behavior, and plasma metabolite concentrations during lactation. *J. Anim. Sci.* 72:387–394.

2412 Weller, R. F., & R. H. Phipps. 1985. The effect of silage preference on the performance of dairy cows. *Anim. Prod.* 42:435.

2413 Wells, D. L., & S. Millsopp. 2009. Lateralized behaviour in the domestic cat, *Felis silvestris catus. Anim. Behav.* 78(2):537–541.

2414 Wells, D. L. 2001. The effectiveness of a citronella spray collar in reducing certain forms of barking in dogs. *Appl. Anim. Behav. Sci.* 73:299–309.

2415 Wells, D. L. 2003. Lateralised behaviour in the domestic dog, *Canis familiaris.* *Behav. Processes* 61:27–35.

2416 Wells, D. L. 2006. Aromatherapy for travel-induced excitement in dogs. *J. Am. Vet. Med. Assoc.* 229:964–967.

2417 Wells, D. L., & P. G. Hepper. 1998. A note on the influence of visual conspecific contact on the behaviour of sheltered dogs. *Appl. Anim. Behav. Sci.* 60:83–88.

2418 **Wells, D. L., L. Graham, & P. G. Hepper. 2002. The influence of auditory stimulation on the behaviour of dogs housed in a rescue shelter. *Anim. Welf.* 11:385–393.**

2419 Wells, S. M., & B. von Goldschmidt-Rothschild. 1979. Social behaviour and relationships in a herd of camargue horses. *Z. Tierpsychol.* 49:363–380.

2420 Wemelsfelder, F., M. Haskell, M. T. Mendl, S. Calvert, & A. B. Lawrence. 2000. Diversity of behaviour during novel object tests is reduced in pigs housed in substrate-impoverished conditions. *Anim. Behav.* 60:385–394.

2421 Werhahn, H., E. F. Hessel, & H. F. A. Van Den Weghe. 2012. Competition horses housed in single stalls (ii): Effects of free exercise on the behavior in the stable, the behavior during training, and the degree of stress. *Equine Vet. J.* 32(1):22–31.

2422 **Werhahn, H., E. F. Hessel, H. Schulze, & H. F. A. Van Den Weghe. 2011. Temporary turnout for free exercise in groups: Effects on the behavior of competition horses housed in single stalls. *Equine Vet. J.* 31(7):417–425.**

2423 Werhahn, H., E. F. Hessel, I. Bachhausen, & H. F. A. Van Den Weghe. 2010. Effects of different bedding materials on the behavior of horses housed in single stalls. *Equine Vet. J.* 30(8):425–431.

2424 Wesley, F., & F. D. Klopfer. 1962. Visual discrimination learning in swine. *Z. Tierpsychol.* 19:93–104.

2425 Wesley, R. L., A. F. Cibils, J. T. Mulliniks, E. R. Pollak, M. K. Petersen, & E. L. Fredrickson. 2012. An assessment of behavioural syndromes in rangeland-raised beef cattle. *Appl. Anim. Behav. Sci.* 139(3–4):183–194.

2426 West, M. 1974. Social play in the domestic cat. *Am. Zool.* 14:427–436.

2427 **West, M. J. 1977. Exploration and play with objects in domestic kittens. *Dev. Psychobiol.* 10:53–57.**

2428 West, R. E., & R. J. Young. 2002. Do domestic dogs show any evidence of being able to count? *Anim. Cogn.* 5:183–186.

2429 **Westgarth, C., R. M. Christley, G. L. Pinchbeck, R. M. Gaskell, S. Dawson, & J. W. S. Bradshaw. 2010. Dog behaviour on walks and the effect of use of the leash. *Appl. Anim. Behav. Sci.* 125(1–2):38–46.**

2430 Whalen, R. E. 1963. The initiation of mating in naive female cats. *Anim. Behav.* 11:463.

2431 Whatson, T. S. 1985. Development of eliminative behaviour in piglets. *Appl. Anim. Behav. Sci.* 14:365–377.

2432 Whipp, S. C., R. L. Wood, & N. C. Lyon. 1970. Diurnal variation in concentrations of hydrocortisone in plasma of swine. *Am. J. Vet. Res.* 31:2105–2107.

2433 Whistance, L. K., D. R. Arney, L. A. Sinclair, & C. J. C. Phillips. 2007. Defaecation behaviour of dairy cows housed in straw yards or cubicle systems. *Appl. Anim. Behav. Sci.* 105:14–25.

2434 Whistance, L. K., L. A. Sinclair, D. R. Arney, & C. J. C. Phillips. 2011. Eliminative behaviour of dairy cows at pasture. *Appl. Anim. Behav. Sci.* 130(3–4):73–80.

2435 Whistance, L. K., L. A. Sinclair, D. R. Arney, & C. J. C. Phillips. 2009. Trainability of eliminative behaviour in dairy heifers using a secondary reinforcer. *Appl. Anim. Behav. Sci.* 117:128–136.

2436 **White, W., G. J. Schwartz, & T. H. Moran. 1999. Meal-synchronized**

CEA in rats: Effects of meal size, intragastric feeding, and subdiaphragmatic vagotomy. *Am. J. Physiol.* **276:R1276–R1288.**

2437 Whittlestone, W. G., & L. R. Cate. 1973. An animal activated feeding device for cattle. *J. Dairy Sci.* 56:1352–1353.

2438 Whittlestone, W. G., M. M. Mullord, R. Kilgour, & L. R. Cate. 1975. Electric shocks during machine milking. *N.Z. Vet. J.* 23:105–108.

2439 **Whittlestone, W. G., R. Kilgour, H. de Langen, & G. Duirs. 1970. Behavioral stress and the cell count of bovine milk.** *J. Milk Food Technol.* **33:217–220.**

2440 Wickens, C. L., & C. R. Heleski. 2010. Crib-biting behavior in horses: A review. *Appl. Anim. Behav. Sci.* 128(1–4):1–9.

2441 **Wickens, C. L., C. A. Mccall, S. Bursian, R. Hanson, C. R. Heleski, J. S. Liesman, W. H. Mcelhenney, & N. L. Trottier. 2013. Assessment of gastric ulceration and gastrin response in horses with history of crib-biting.** *Equine Vet. J.* **33(9):739–745.**

2442 Widdowson, E. M. 1971. Food intake and growth in the newly-born. *Proc. Nutr. Soc.* 30:127–135.

2443 Widowski, T. M., & S. W. Curtis. 1990. The influence of straw, cloth tassel, or both on the prepartum behavior of sows. *Appl. Anim. Behav. Sci.* 27:53–71.

2444 Wieckert, D. A. 1971. Social behavior in farm animals. *J. Anim. Sci.* 32:1274–1277.

2445 Wieckert, D. A., & G. R. Barr. 1966. Studies on learning ability in young pigs. *J. Anim. Sci.* 25:1280.

2446 Wieckert, D. A., L. P. Johnson, K. P. Offord, & G. R. Barr. 1966. Measuring learning ability in dairy cows. *J. Dairy Sci.* 49:729.

2447 **Wiepkema, P. R., K. K. Van Hellemond, P. Roessingh, & H. Romberg. 1987. Behaviour and abomasal damage in individual veal calves.** *Appl. Anim. Behav. Sci.* **18:257–268.**

2448 Wierbowski, S. 1959. Odruchy plciowe ogierow. *Roczn. Nauk Rolnicz.* 73:753–788.

2449 Wierbowski, S. 1978. The sexual behaviour of experimentally underfed bulls. *Appl. Anim. Ethol.* 4:55–60.

2450 Wierenga, H. K. 1990. Social dominance in dairy cattle and the influences of housing and management. *Appl. Anim. Behav. Sci.* 27:201–229.

2451 Wikmar, G., & J. M. Warren. 1972. Delayed response learning by cage-reared normal and prefrontal cats. *Psychonom. Sci.* 26:243–245.

2452 **Wilcox, S., K. Dusza, & K. A. Houpt. 1991. The relationship between recumbent rest and masturbation in stallions.** *Equine Vet. Sci.* **11:23–26.**

2453 Wilhelmy, J., J. Serpell, D. Brown, & C. Siracusa. 2016. Behavioral associations with breed, coat type, and eye color in single-breed cats. *J. Vet. Behav.* 13:80–87.

2454 Willham, R. L., D. F. Cox, & G. G. Karas. 1963. Genetic variation in a measure of avoidance learning in swine. *J. Comp. Physiol. Psychol.* 56:294–297.

2455 Willham, R. L., G. G. Karas, & D. C. Henderson. 1964. Partial acquisition and extinction of an avoidance response in two breeds of swine. *J. Comp. Physiol. Psychol.* 57:117–122.

2456 **Williams, J. L., T. H. Friend, C. H. Nevill, & G. Archer. 2004. The efficacy of a secondary reinforcer (clicker) during acquisition and extinction of an operant task in horses.** *Appl. Anim. Behav. Sci.* **88:331–341.**

2457 Williams, J. L., T. H. Friend, M. J. Toscano, M. N. Collins, A. Sisto-Burt, & C. H. Nevill. 2002. The effects of early training sessions on the reactions of foals at 1, 2, and 3 months of age. *Appl. Anim. Behav. Sci.* 77:105–114.

2458 Williams, M., & J. M. Johnston. 2002. Training and maintaining the performance of dogs (*Canis familiaris*) on an increasing number of odor discriminations in a controlled setting. *Appl. Anim. Behav. Sci.* 78:55–65.

2459 Williams, S., J. Horner, E. Orton, M. Green, S. Mcmullen, A. Mobasheri, & S. L. Freeman. 2015. Water intake, faecal output and intestinal motility in horses moved from pasture to a stabled management regime with controlled exercise. *Equine Vet. J.* 47(1):96–100.

2460 Williamson, N. B., R. S. Morris, D. C. Blood, & C. M. Cannon. 1972. A study of oestrous behaviour and oestrus detection methods in a large commercial dairy herd. I. The relative efficiency of methods of oestrus detection. *Vet. Rec.* 91:50–58.

2461 **Wilson, E. O. 1975.** *Sociobiology: The new synthesis.* **Cambridge, MA: The Belknap Press of Harvard University Press.**

2462 Wilson, M., J. M. Warren, & L. Abbott. 1965. Infantile stimulation, activity, and learning by cats. *Child Dev.* 36:843–853.

2463 Wilson, S. C., F. M. Mitlohner, J. Morrow-Tesch, J. W. Dailey, & J. J. McGlone. 2002. An assessment of several potential enrichment devices for feedlot cattle. *Appl. Anim. Behav. Sci.* 76:259–265.

2464 Wilsson, E. 1984. The social interaction between mother and offspring during weaning in German shepherd dogs: Individual differences between mothers and their effects on offspring. *Appl. Anim. Behav. Sci.* 13:101–112.

2465 **Wilsson, E., & P. Sundgren. 1997. The use of a behaviour test for the selection of dogs for service and breeding, I: Method of testing and evaluating test results in the adult dog, demands on different kinds of service dogs, sex and breed differences.** *Appl. Anim. Behav. Sci.* **53:279–295.**

2466 Wilsson, E., & P. Sundgren. 1997. The use of a behaviour test for the selection of dogs for service and breeding. II. Heritability for tested parameters and

effect of selection based on service dog characteristics. *Appl. Anim. Behav. Sci.* 54:235–241.

2467 **Wilsson, E., & P. Sundgren. 1998. Effects of weight, litter size and parity of mother on the behaviour of the puppy and the adult dog.** *Appl. Anim. Behav. Sci.* **56:245–254.**

2468 Winchester, C. F. 1943. The energy cost of standing in horses. *Science* 97:24.

2469 Winfield, C. G., & A. W. Makin. 1978. A note on the effect of continuous contact with ewes showing regular oestrus and post-weaning growth rate on the sexual activity of corriedale rams. *Anim. Prod.* 27:361–364.

2470 Winfield, C. G., & P. D. Mullaney. 1973. A note on the social behaviour of a flock of merino and wiltshire horn sheep. *Anim. Prod.* 17:93–95.

2471 Winfield, C. G., & R. Kilgour. 1976. A study of following behaviour in young lambs. *Appl. Anim. Ethol.* 2:235–243.

2472 **Winfield, C. G., G. J. Syme, & A. J. Pearson. 1981. Effect of familiarity with each and breed on the spatial behaviour of sheep in an open field.** *Appl. Anim. Ethol.* **7:67–75.**

2473 Winfield, C. G., P. H. Hemsworth, M. R. Taverner, & P. D. Mullaney. 1974. Observations on the sucking behaviour of piglets in litters of varying size. *Proc. Aust. Soc. Anim. Prod.* 10:307–310.

2474 **Winkler, W. G. 1977. Human deaths induced by dog bites, United States, 1974–75.** *Public Health Rep.* **92:425–429.**

2475 Winskill, L. C., N. K. Waran, & R. J. Young. 1996. The effect of a foraging device (a modified "Edinburgh foodball") on the behaviour of a stabled horse. *Appl. Anim. Behav. Sci.* 48:25–35.

2476 Winslow, C. N. 1944. The social behavior of cats. II. Competitive, aggressive, and food-sharing behavior when both competitors have access to the goal. *J. Comp. Psychol.* 37:315–326.

2477 Winter, A., & J. E. Hillerton. 1995. Behaviour associated with feeding and milking of early lactation cows housed in an experimental automatic milking system. *Appl. Anim. Behav. Sci.* 46:1–15.

2478 Wirant, S. C., K. T. Halvorsen, & B. McGuire. 2007. Preliminary observations on the urinary behaviour of female jack russell terriers in relation to stage of the oestrous cycle, location, and age. *Appl. Anim. Behav. Sci.* 106:161–166.

2479 **Wise, R. A., & V. Dawson. 1974. Diazepam-induced eating and lever pressing for food in sated rats. *J. Comp. Physiol. Psychol.* 86:930–941.**

2480 Wolf, A. V. 1950. Osmometric analysis of thirst in man and dog. *Am. J. Physiol.* 161:75–86.

2481 Wolf, B. T., S. D. McBride, R. M. Lewis, M. H. Davies, & W. Haresign. 2008. Estimates of the genetic parameters and repeatability of behavioural traits of sheep in an arena test. *Appl. Anim. Behav. Sci.* 112:68–80.

2482 **Wolff, A., & M. Hausberger. 1996. Learning and memorisation of two different tasks in horses: The effects of age, sex and sire. *Appl. Anim. Behav. Sci.* 46:137–143.**

2483 Wolski, T. R. 1982. Social behavior of the cat. *Vet. Clin. North Am. Small Anim. Pract.* 12:693–706.

2484 Wolski, T. R., K. A. Houpt, & R. Aronson. 1980. The role of the senses in mare-foal recognition. *Appl. Anim. Ethol.* 6:121–138.

2485 Wong, D. M., C. J. Alcott, J. L. Davis, K. L. Hepworth, L. Wulf, & J. H. Coetzee. 2015. Use of alprazolam to facilitate mare-foal bonding in an aggressive postparturient mare. *J. Vet. Intern. Med.* 29(1):414–416.

2486 Wood, M. T. 1977. Social grooming patterns in two herds of monozygotic twin dairy cows. *Anim. Behav.* 25:635–642.

2487 Wood, P. A., J. De Bie, & J. A. Clarke. 2014. Behavioural and physiological responses of domestic dogs (*Canis familiaris*) to agonistic growls from conspecifics. *Appl. Anim. Behav. Sci.* 161:105–112.

2488 **Wood, P. D., G. F. Smith, & M. F. Lisle. 1967. A survey of intersucking in dairy herds in England and Wales. *Vet. Rec.* 81:396–398.**

2489 Wood, R. J., B. J. Rolls, & D. J. Ramsay. 1977. Drinking following intracarotid infusions of hypertonic solutions in dogs. *Am. J. Physiol.* 232:R88–R92.

2490 **Wood, T., S. Stanley, & T. Tobin. 1989. Operant conditioning and its applications in equine pharmacology. *J. Equine Vet. Sci.* 9:124–130.**

2491 Wood-Gush, D. G. M. 1983. *Elements of ethology*. London, UK: Chapman and Hall.

2492 Wood-Gush, D. G. M., & K. Vestergaard. 1991. The seeking of novelty and its relation to play. *Anim. Behav.* 42:599–606.

2493 Woods, G. L., & K. A. Houpt. 1986. An abnormal facial gesture in an estrous mare. *Appl. Anim. Behav. Sci.* 16:199–202.

2494 Worobec, E. K., I. J. H. Dundan, & T. M. Widowski. 1999. The effects of weaning at 7, 14, and 28 days on piglet behaviour. *Appl. Anim. Behav. Sci.* 62:173–182.

2495 Wright, H. F., D. S. Mills, & P. M. J. Pollux. 2011. Development and validation of a psychometric tool for assessing impulsivity in the domestic dog (*Canis familiaris*). *Int. J. Comp. Psychol.* 24:210–225.

2496 **Wright, J. C. 1980. Early development of exploratory and dominance in three litters of German shepherds. *Early experiences and early behavior*, pp. 181–206. New York, NY: Academic Press.**

2497 **Wright, J. C., & M. S. Nesselrote. 1987. Classification of behavior problems in dogs: Distributions of age, breed, sex and reproductive status. *Appl. Anim. Behav. Sci.* 19:169–178.**

2498 Wulf, M., J. Aurich, A.-C. May, & C. Aurich. 2013. Sex differences in the response of yearling horses to handling by unfamiliar humans. *J. Vet. Behav.* 8(4):238–244.

2499 Xiao, H., T. Ajide, L. Zhang, G. Lu, G. Shi, & H. Li. 2015. Effect of weaning age on stress-related behavior in foals (*Equus caballus*) by abrupt – group weaning method. *J. Phylogen Evol. Biol.* 3(2):151.

2500 Yamane, A., J. Emoto, & N. Ota. 1996. Factors affecting feeding order and social tolerance to kittens in the group-living feral cat (*Felis catus*). *Appl. Anim. Behav. Sci.* 52:119–127.

2501 Yang, T. S., B. Howard, & W. V. Macfarlane. 1981. Effects of food on drinking behaviour of growing pigs. *Appl. Anim. Ethol.* 7:259–270.

2502 Yang, T. S., M. A. Price, & F. X. Aherne. 1984. The effect of level of feeding on water turnover in growing pigs. *Appl. Anim. Behav. Sci.* 12:103–109.

2503 Yaniz, J., P. Santolaria, & F. Lopez-Gatius. 2003. Relationship between fertility and the walking activity of cows at oestrus. *Vet. Rec.* 152:239–240.

2504 Yarney, T. A., G. W. Rahnefeld, R. J. Parker, & W. M. Palmer. 1982. Hourly distribution of time of parturition in beef cows. *Can. J. Anim. Sci.* 62:597–605.

2505 Yeon, S. C., G. Golden, W. Sung, H. N. Erb, A. J. Reynolds, & K. A. Houpt. 2001. A comparison of tethering and pen confinement of dogs. *J. Appl. Anim. Welf. Sci.* 4:257–260.

2506 **Yerkes, R. M. 1916. The mental life of monkeys and apes: A study of ideational behavior. *Behav. Monogr.* 3:145.**

2507 Yerkes, R. M., & C. A. Coburn. 1915. A study of the behavior of the pig (sus scrofa) by the multiple choice method. *J. Anim. Behav.* 5:185–225.

2508 Young, C. A. 1991. Verbal commands as discriminative stimuli in domestic dogs (*Canis familiaris*). *Appl. Anim. Behav. Sci.* 32:75–89.

2509 Young, R. J., J. Carruthers, & A. B. Lawrence. 1994. The effect of a foraging device (the "Edinburgh foodball") on the behaviour of pigs. *Appl. Anim. Behav. Sci.* 39:237–247.

2510 Zablocka, T. 1975. Go-no go differentiation to visual stimuli in cats with different early visual experiences. *Acta Neurobiol. Exp. (Wars)* 35:399–402.

2511 Zablocka, T., J. Konorski, & B. Zernicki. 1975. Visual discrimination learning in cats with different early visual experiences. *Acta Neurobiol. Exp. (Wars)* 35:389–398.

2512 Zahorik, D. M., & K. A. Houpt. 1977. The concept of nutritional wisdom: Applicability of laboratory learning models to large herbivores. In L. M. Barker, M. R. Best, & M. Domjan (Eds.), Learning mechanisms in food selection, pp. 45–67. Waco, TX: Baylor University Press.

2513 Zahorik, D. M., & K. A. Houpt. 1981. Species differences in feed strategies, food hazards, and the ability to learn food aversions. In A. C. Kamil, & T. D. Sargent (Eds.), Foraging behavior, pp. 289–310. New York, NY: Garland STPM Press.

2514 **Zahorik, D. M., K. A. Houpt, & J. Swartzman-Ander. 1990. Taste-aversion learning in three species of ruminants. *Appl. Anim. Behav. Sci.* 26:27–39.**

2515 Zanghi, B. M., W. Kerr, J. Gierer, C. De Rivera, J. A. Araujo, & N. W. Milgram. 2013. Characterizing behavioral sleep using actigraphy in adult dogs of various ages fed once or twice daily. *J. Vet. Behav.* 8(4):195–203.

2516 **Zapelin, H. 1989. Mammalian sleep. In K. H. Kryger, T. Roth, & W. C. Dement (Eds.), *Principles and practice of sleep medication*, pp. 30–49. Philadelphia, PA: W.B. Saunders.**

2517 Zenchak, J. J., & G. C. Anderson. 1973. Discrimination learning in sheep. *J. Anim. Sci.* 37:227.

2518 Zenchak, J. J., & G. C. Anderson. 1980. Sexual performance levels of rams (*Ovis aries*) as affected by social experiences during rearing. *J. Anim. Sci.* 50:167–174.

2519 Zicker, S. C., D. E. Jewell, R. M. Yamka, & N. W. Milgram. 2012. Evaluation of cognitive learning, memory, psychomotor, immunologic, and retinal functions in healthy puppies fed foods fortified with docosahexaenoic acid-rich fish oil from 8 to 52 weeks of age. *Sci. Rep.* 241(5):583–594.

2520 Zimmerman, M. B., E. M. Stricker, & E. H. Blaine. 1978. Water and NaCl intake after furosemide treatment in sheep (*Ovis aries*). *J. Comp. Physiol. Psychol.* 92:501–510.

2521 Zonderland, J. J., J. W. Van Riel, M. B. M. Bracke, B. Kemp, L. A. Den Hartog, & H. A. M. Spoolder. 2009. Tail posture predicts tail damage among weaned piglets. *Appl. Anim. Behav. Sci.* 121(3–4):165–170.

2522 **Zonderland, J. J., L. Cornelissen, M. Wolthuis-Fillerup, & H. A. M. Spoolder. 2008. Visual acuity of pigs at different light intensities. *Appl. Anim. Behav. Sci.* 111:28–37.**

2523 **Zupan, M., A. M. Janczak, T. Framstad, & A. J. Zanella. 2012. The effect of biting tails and having tails bitten in pigs. *Physiol. Behav.* 106(5):638–644.**

2524 Albright, J. D., T. H. Witte, B. W. Rohrbach, A. Reed, & K. A. Houpt. 2015. Efficacy and effects of various anti-crib devices on behaviour and physiology of crib-biting horses. *Eq. Vet. J.* 48: 727–737.

2525 **Alexander, G., & D. Williams. 1964. Maternal facilitation of sucking drive in newborn lambs. *Science* 146:65–66.**

2526 Anderson, M. K., T. H. Friend, J. W. Evans, & D. M. Bushong. 1999. Behavioral assessment of horses in therapeutic riding programs. *Appl. Anim. Behav. Sci.* 63.11–24.

2527 **Anderson, D. M., & N. S. Urguhart. 1986. Using digital pedometers to monitor travel of cows grazing arid rangeland. *Appl. Anim. Behav. Sci.* 16:11–23.**

2528 **Aronson, L. R., & M. L. Cooper. 1974. Olfactory deprivation and mating behavior in sexually experienced male cats. *Behav. Biol.* 11:459–480.**

2529 **Araba, B. D., & S. L. Crowell-Davis. 1994. Dominance relationships and aggression in foals (*Equus caballus*). *Appl. Anim. Behav. Sci.* 41:1–25.**

2530 **Bailey, P. J., A. H. Bishop, & C. T. Boord. 1974. Grazing behaviour of steers. *Proc. Aust. Soc. Anim. Prod.* 10:303–306.**

2531 **Beach, F. A. 1968. Coital behavior in dogs. III. Effects of early isolation on mating in males. *Behaviour* 30:218–238.**

2532 **Beach, F. A. 1974. Effects of gonadal hormones on urinary behavior in dogs. *Physiol. Behav.* 12:1005–1013.**

2533 **Beach, F. A. 1970. Coital behaviour in dogs VIII. Social affinity, dominance and sexual preference in the bitch. *Behaviour* 36:131–148.**

2534 **Beauchemin, K. A., S. Zelin, D. Genner, & J. G. Buchanan-Smith. 1989. An automatic system for quantification of eating and ruminating activities of dairy cattle housed in stalls. *J. Dairy. Sci.* 72:2746–2759.**

2535 **Bell, F. R. 1960. The electoencophalogram of goats during somnolence and rumination. *Anim. Behav.* 8:39–42.**

2536 Bertolucci, C., C. Giannetto, F. Fazio, & G. Piccione. 2008. Seasonal variations in daily rhythms of activity in athletic horses. *Animal.* 2:1055–1060.

2537 Bhadra, A., D. Bhattacharjee, M. Paul, A. Singh, P. R. Gade, P. Shrestha, & A. Bhadra. 2015. The meat of the matter: A rule of thumb for scavenging dogs? *Ethol. Ecol. Evol.* 1–14. DOI:10.1080/03949370.2015.107652

2538 Bjone, S. J., W. Y. Brown, & I. R. Price. 2009. Maternal influence on grass-eating behaviour in puppies. *J. Vet. Behav.* 4:97–98.

2539 Boe, K. E., S. Berg, & I. L. Andersen. 2006. Resting behaviour and displacements in ewes—Effects of reduced lying space and pen shape. *Appl. Anim. Behav. Sci.* 98:249–259.

2540 Boyd, L. E., D. A. Carbonaro, & K. A. Houpt. 1988. The 24-hour time budget of Przewalski horses. *Appl. Anim. Behav. Sci.* 21:5–17.

2541 Boyd, L. E. 1988. Time budgets of adult Przewalski horses: Effects of sex, reproductive status and enclosure. *Appl. Anim. Behav. Sci.* 21:19–39.

2542 Bräuer, J., M. Keckeisen, A. Pitsch, J. Kaminski, J. Call, & M. Tomasello. 2013. Domestic dogs conceal auditory but not visual information from others. *Anim. Cogn.* 16:351–359.

2543 Butler, C. L., & K. A. Houpt. 2014. Pawing by Standardbred racehorses: Frequency and patterns. *J. Equine. Sci.* 25:57–59.

2544 Castle, M. E., & R. J. Halley. 1953. The grazing behaviour of dairy cattle at the national institute of research in dairying. *Br. J. Anim. Behav.* 1:139–143.

2545 Cohn, R. 1956. A contribution to the study of color vision in cat. *J. Neurophysiol.* 19:416–423.

2546 Culley, M. J. 1938. Grazing habits of range cattle. *J. Forestry.* 36:715–717.

2547 Döring, D., B. E. Haberland, A. Ossig, H. Küchenhoff, B. Dobenecker, R. Hack, J. Schmidt, & M. H. Erhard. 2014. Behavior of laboratory beagles towards humans: Assessment in an encounter test and a simulation of experimental situations. *J. Vet. Behav.* 9: 295–303.

2548 Duffy, D. L., Y. Hsu, & J. A. Serpell. 2008. Breed differences in canine aggression. *Appl. Anim. Behav. Sci.* 114: 441–460.

2549 Eccles, R. 1982. Autonomic innervation of the vomeronasal organ of the cat. *Physiol. Behav.* 28:1011–1015.

2550 Elgier, A. M., A. Jakovcevic, A. E. Mustaca, & M. Bentosela. 2012. Pointing following in dogs: are simple or complex cognitive mechanisms involved? *Anim. Cogn.* 15:1111–1119.

2551 Feh, C., & de Mazieres, J. (1993). Grooming at a preferred site reduces heart rate in horses. *Anim. Behav.* 46:1191–1194.

2552 Feh, C., & B. Munkhtuya. 2008. Male infantacide and paternity analyses in a socially natural herd of Przewalski's horses: Sexual selection? *Behav. Proc.* 78: 335–339.

2553 Ferrell, F. 1984. Preference for sugars and nonnutritive sweeteners in young beagles. *Neurosci. Biobehav. Rev.* 8:199–203.

2554 Flannigan, G., & J. M. Stookey. 2001. Day-time time budgets of pregnant mares housed in tie stalls: A comparison of draft versus light mares. *Appl. Anim. Behav. Sci.* 78:125–144.

2555 Fraser, D. 1977. Some behavioural aspects of milk ejection failure by sows. *Br. Vet. J.* 133:126–133.

2556 Freire, R., H. A. Clegg, P. Buckley, M. A. Friend, & P. D. McGreevy. 2009. The effects of two different amounts of dietary grain on the digestibility of the diet and behaviour of intensively managed horses. *Appl. Anim. Behav. Sci.* 117:69–73.

2557 Friend, T. H., & C. E. Polan. 1974. Social rank, feeding behavior, and free stall utilization by dairy cattle. *J. Dairy Sci.* 57:1214–1220.

2558 Fujita, K., A. Morisaki, A. Takaoka, T. Maeda, & Y. Hori. 2012. Incidental memory in dogs (*Canis familiaris*): Adaptive behavioral solution at an unexpected memory test. *Anim. Cogn.* 15:1055–1063.

2559 Fukuzawa, M., & N. Hayashi. Comparison of 3 different reinforcements of learning in dogs (*Canis familiaris*). *J. Vet. Behav.* 8:221–224.

2560 Fuller, J. L. 1956. Photoperiodic control of estrus in the basenji. *J. Hered.* 47:179–180.

2561 Garcia, M. C., S. M. McDonnell, R. M. Kenney, & H. G. Osborne. 1986. Bull sexual behavior tests: Stimulus cow affects performance. *Appl. Anim. Behav. Sci.* 16:1–10.

2562 Gill, J. C., & W. Thomson. 1956. Observations on the behaviour of suckling pigs. *Br. J. Anim. Behav.* 4:46–51.

2563 Gleitman, H. 1974. Getting animals to understand the experimenter's instructions. *Anim. Learn. Behav.* 2:1–5.

2564 Gorecka, A., & T. Jezierski. 2007. Protective behaviour of Konik horses in response to insect harassment. *Anim. Welf.* 16:281–283.

2565 Graf, P., U. K. von Borstel, & M. Gauly. 2014. Practical considerations regarding the implementation of a temperament test into horse performance tests: Results of a large-scale test run. *J. Vet. Behav.* 9: 329–340.

2566 Hardison, W. A., H. L. Fisher, G. G. Graf, & N. R. Thompson. 1956. Some observations on the behavior of grazing lactating cows. *J. Dairy Sci.* 39:1735–1741.

2567 Hausberger, M., E. Gautier, V. Biquand, C. Lunel, & P. Jégo. (2009) Could work be a source of behavioural disorders? *A study in horses. PLoS ONE.* 4(10): e7625.

2568 Harlow, H. F., & P. Settlage. 1939. The effect of curarization of the fore part of the body upon the retention of conditioned responses in cats. *J. Comp. Psychol.* 27:45–48.

2569 Hein, M. A. 1935. Grazing time of beef steers on permanent pastures. *J. Am. Soc. Agron.* 27:675–679.

2570 Holder, J. M. 1960. Observations on the grazing behaviour of lactating dairy cattle in a subtropical environment. *J. Agric. Sci.* 55:261–267.

2571 Houpt, K., T. R. Houpt, J. L. Johnson, H. N. Erb, & S. C. Yeon. 2001. The effect of exercise deprivation on the behaviour and physiology of straight stall confined pregnant mares. *Anim. Welf.* 10:257–267.

2572 Hradecká, L., Bartoš, I., Svobodová, & J. Sales. 2015. Heritability of behavioural traits in domestic dogs: A meta-analysis. *Appl. Anim. Behav. Sci.* 170:1–13.

2573 Ijichi, C., L. M. Collins, E. Creighton, & R. W. Elwood. 2013. Harnessing the power of personality assessment: Subjective assessment predicts behaviour in horses. *Behav. Processes* 96:47–52.

2574 Jensen, M. B. 2012. Behaviour around the time of calving in dairy cows. *Appl. Anim. Behav. Sci.* 139:195–202.

2575 Jones, P., K. Chase, A. Martin, P. Davern, E. A. Ostrander, & K. G. Lark. 2008. Single-nucleotide-polymorphism-based association mapping of dog stereotypes. *Genetics* 179:1033–1044.

2576 Keiper, R. R., & M. A. Keenan. 1980. Nocturnal activity patterns of feral horses. *J. Mammal.* 61:116–118.

2577 Kimball, B. A., F. D. Provenza, & E. A. Burritt. 2002. Importance of alternative foods on the persistence of flavor aversions: Implications for applied flavor avoidance learning. *Appl. Anim. Behav. Sci.* 76:249–258.

2578 Kropp, J. R., J. W. Holloway, D. F. Stephens, L. Knori, R. D. Morrison, & R. Totusek. 1973. Range behavior of Hereford, Hereford X Holstein and Holstein non-lactating heifers. *J. Anim. Sci.* 36(4):797–802.

2579 Kusunose, R., & A. Yamanobe. 2002. The effect of training schedule on learned tasks in yearling horses. *Appl. Anim. Behav. Sci.* 78:225–233.

2580 Lampkin, G. H., J. Quarterman, & M. Kidner. 1958. Observations on the grazing habits of grade and zebu steers in a high altitude temperature climate. *J. Agric. Sci.* 50:211–218.

2581 Langbein, J. 2012. Investigations on training, recall and reversal learning of a Y-maze by dwarf goats (*Capra hircus*): The impact of lateralization. *Behav. Processes* 89:304–310.

2582 Larsen, H. J. 1963. Feeding habits of grazing and green feeding cows. *J. Anim. Sci.* 22:1134.

2583 Lazarowski, L., & D. C. Dorman. 2014. Explosives detection by military working dogs: Olfactory generalization from components to mixtures. *Appl. Anim. Behav. Sci.* 151:84–93.

2584 Lewis, R. C., & J. D. Johnson. 1954. Observations of dairy cow activities in loose-housing. *J. Dairy Sci.* 37:269–275.

2585 Li, Y., & H. W. Gonyou. 2002. Analysis of belly nosing and associated behaviour among pigs weaned at 12–14 days of age. *Appl. Anim. Behav. Sci.* 77:285–294.

2586 Littlejohn, A., & R. Munro. 1972. Equine recumbency. *Vet. Rec.* 90:83–85.

2587 Lofgreen, G. P., J. H. Meyer, & J. L. Hull. 1957. Behavior patterns of sheep and cattle being fed pasture of Silage. *J. Anim. Sci.* 16:773–780.

2588 Longpre, K. M., & L. S. Katz. 2011. Estrous female goats use testosterone-dependent cues to assess mates. *Horm. Behav.* 59:98–104.

2589 Loyd, K. A. T., S. M. Hernandez, J. P. Carroll, K. J. Abernathy, & G. J. Marshall. 2013. Quantifying free-roaming domestic cat predation using animal-borne video cameras. *Biol. Conserv.* 160: 183–189.

2590 Luescher, U. A., D. B. McKeown, & H. Dean. 1998. A cross-sectional study on compulsive behaviour (stable vices) in horses. *Equine Vet. J. Suppl.* 27:14–18.

2591 Luz, M. P. F., C. M. Maia, J. C. F. Pantoja, M. C. Neto, & J. N. P. P. Filho. 2015. Feeding time and agonistic behavior in horses: Influence of distance, proportion, and height of troughs. *J. Equine Vet. Sci.* 35:843–848.

2592 Lynch, J. J., & G. Alexander. 1976. The effect of gramineous windbreaks on behaviour and lamb mortality among shorn and unshorn merino sheep during lambing. *Appl. Anim. Ethol.* 2:305–325.

2593 Lynch, J. J., & G. Alexander. 1976. The effect of gramineous windbreaks on behaviour and lamb mortality among shorn and unshorn merino sheep during lambing. *Appl. Anim. Ethol.* 2:305–325.

2594 MacNeil-Allcock, A., N. M. Clarke, R. A. Ledger, & D. Fraser. 2011. Aggression, behaviour, and animal care among pit bulls and other dogs adopted from an animal shelter. *Anim. Welf.* 20:463–468.

2595 Maldonado, A., A. Orihuela, V. Aguirre, R. Vázquez, & I. Flores-Pérez. 2015. Changes in mother-offspring relationships with the increasing age of the lamb in hair sheep (*Ovis aries*). *J. Vet. Behav.* 10:166–170.

2596 Marshall-Pescini, S., S. Barnard, N. J. Branson, & P. Valsecchi. 2013. The effect of preferential paw usage on dogs' (*Canis familiaris*) performance in a manipulative problem-solving task. *Behav. Processes* 100:40–43.

2597 Matsui, K., A. M. Khalil, & K. Takeda. 2009. Do horses prefer certain substrates for rolling in grazing pasture? *J. Equine Vet. Sci.* 29:590–594.

2598 Mattner, P. E., A. W. H. Braden, & K. E. Turnbill. 1967. Studies in flock mating of sheep. I. Mating behaviour. *Aust. J. Exp. Agric. Anim. Husb.* 7:103–109.

2599 McDonnell, S. M., D. A. Freeman, N. F. Cymbaluk, H. C. Schott 2nd, K. Hinchcliff, & B. Kyle. 1999. Behavior of stabled horses provided continuous or intermittent access to drinking water. *Am. J. Vet. Res.* 60(11):1451–1456.

2600 Meyer, I., & B. Forkman. 2014. Dog and owner characteristics affecting the dog–owner relationship. *J. Vet. Behav.* 9:143–150.

2601 Mills, D. S., & K. Taylor. 2003. Field study of the efficacy of three types of nose net for the treatment of headshaking in horses. *Vet. Rec.* 152:41–44.

2602 Mongillo, P., E. Pitteri, S. Adamelli, S. Bonichini, L. Farina, & L. Marinelli. 2015. Validation of a selection protocol of dogs involved in animal-assisted intervention. *J. Vet. Behav.* 10:103–110.

2603 Morello, G., R. Imperatore, L. Palomba, C. Finelli, G. Labruna, F. Pasanisi, L. Sacchetti, *et al.* 2016. Orexin-A represses satiety-inducing POMC neurons and contributes to obesity via stimulation of endocannabinoid signaling. *PNAS.* 113:4759–4764.

2604 Moorefield, J. G., & H. H. Hopkins. 1951. Grazing habits of cattle in a mixed-prairie pasture. *J. Range Manag.* 4:151–157.

2605 Murphy, J., Waldmann, T., & Arkins, S. 2004. Sex differences in equine learning skills and visuo-spatial ability. *Appl. Anim. Behav. Sci.* 87:119–130.

2606 O'Donnell, T. G., & G. A. Walton. 1969. Some observations on the behaviour and hill-pasture utilization of Irish cattle. *J. Br. Grassland Soc.* 24:128–133.

2607 Ogilvie-Graham, T. S. 1994. *Time budget studies in stalled horses.* Edinburgh, Scotland: The University of Edinburgh.

2608 Perez, O., N. Jimenez de Perez, P. Poindron, P. Le Neindre, & J. P. Ravault. 1985. Influence of management conditions after calving on mother-young relationships and PRL response to mammary stimulation in the cow. *Reprod. Nutr. Develop.* 25:605–618.

2609 Pilley, J. W., & A. K. Reid. 2011.Border collie comprehends object names as verbal referents. *Behav. Processes* 86:184–195.

2610 Poletto, R., R. L. Meisel, B. T. Richert, H. Cheng, & J. N. Marchant-Forde. 2010. Aggression in replacement grower and finisher gilts fed a short-term high-tryptophan diet and the effect of long-term human–animal interaction. *Appl. Anim. Behav. Sci.* 122:98–110.

2611 Pond, W. G., & J. H. Maner. 1974. *Swine production in temperate and tropical environments.* San Francisco, CA: W.H. Freeman.

2612 Quimby, J. M., & K. F. Lunn. 2013. Mirtazapine as an appetite stimulant and anti-emetic in cats with chronic kidney disease: A masked placebo-controlled crossover clinical trial. *Vet. J.* 197:651–655.

2613 Racca, A., E. Amadei, S. Ligout, K. Guo, K. Meints, & D. Mills. 2010. Discrimination of human and dog faces and inversion responses in domestic dogs (*Canis familiaris*). *Anim. Cogn.* 13:525–533.

2614 Redbo, I., P. Redbo-Torstensson, F. O. Odberg, A. Hadendahl, & J. Holm. 1998. Factors affecting behavioural disturbances in race-horses. *Anim. Sci.* 66:475–481.

2615 Raihani, G., D. González, L. Arteaga, & R. Hudson. 2009. Olfactory guidance of nipple attachment and suckling in kittens of the domestic cat: Inborn and learned responses. *Dev. Psychobiol.* 51:662–671.

2616 Ralston, S. L., G. Van den Broek, & C. A. Baile. 1979. Feed intake patterns and associated blood glucose, free fatty acid and insulin changes in ponies. *J. Anim. Sci.* 49:838–845.

2617 Reisner, I. R., K. A. Houpt, & F. S. Shofer. 2005. National survey of owner-directed aggression in English springer spaniels. *JAVMA* 227:1594–1603.

2618 Rubenstein, D. I. 1981. Behavioural ecology of island feral horses. *Equine Vet. J.* 13:27–34.

2619 Salter, R.E., & R. J. Hudson. 1979. Feeding ecology of feral horse in western Alberta. *J. Range Manag.* 2:221–225.

2620 Sato, S. S., & A. Maeda. 1991. Social licking patterns in cattle (*Bos taurus*): Influence of environmental and social factors. *Appl. Anim. Behav. Sci.* 32:3–12.

2621 Schmisseur, W. E., J. L. Albright, W. M. Dillon, E. W. Kehrberg, & W. H. Morris. 1966. Animal behavior responses to loose and free stall housing. *J. Dairy Sci.* 49(1):102–104.

2622 Sechzer, J. A., & J. L. Brown. 1964. Color discrimination in the cat. *Science* 144:427–429.

2623 Segerstad, C. H., & G. Hellekant. 1989. The sweet taste in the calf. I. Chorda tympani proper nerve responses to taste stimulation of the tongue. *Physiol. Behav.* 45:633–638.

2624 Sneva, F. A. 1970. Behavior of yearling cattle on eastern Oregon range. *J. Range Manag.* 23:155–158.

2625 Søndergaard, E., & U. Halekoh. 2003.Young horses' reactions to humans in relation to handling and social environment. *Appl. Anim. Behav. Sci.* 84:265–280.

2626 Spier, S. J., J. B. Pusterla, A. Villarroel, & N. Pusterla. 2004 Outcome of tactile conditioning of neonates, or "imprint training" on selected handling measures in foals. *Vet. J.* 168:252–258.

2627 Squires, V. R. 1974. Grazing distribution and activity patterns of Merino sheep on a saltbush community in south-east Australia. *Appl. Anim. Behav. Sci.* 1:17–30.

2628 Stella, J., C. Croney, & T. Buffington. 2013. Effects of stressors on the behavior and physiology of domestic cats. *Appl. Anim. Behav. Sci.* 143: 157–163.

2629 Sugnasseelan, S., N. Prescott, D. Broom, C. Wathes, & C. J. C. Phillips. 2013. Visual discrimination learning and spatial acuity in sheep. *Appl. Anim. Behav. Sci* 147:104–111

2630 Temesi, A., B. Turcsán, & Á. Miklósi. 2014. Measuring fear in dogs by questionnaires: An exploratory study toward a standardized inventory. *Appl. Anim. Behav. Sci.* 161:121–130.

2631 Turner, R. R. 1961. Silage self-feeding. *Vet. Rec.* 73:1432–1436.

2632 Vaysse, A., A. Ratnakumar, T. Derrien, E. Axelsson, G. R. Pielberg, S. Sigurdsson, T. Fall, *et al.* 2011. Identification of genomic regions associated with phenotypic variation between dog breeds using selection mapping. *PLoS Genet.* 7(10):e1002316.

2633 Wardrop, J. C. 1953. Studies in the behaviour of dairy cows at pasture. *Br. J. Anim. Behav.* 1:23–31.

2634 Wertz-Lutz, A. E., T. J. Knight, R. H. Pritchard, J. A. Daniel, J. A. Clapper, A. J. Smart, A. Trenkle, & D. C. Beitz. 2006. Circulating ghrelin concentrations fluctuate relative to nutritional status and influence feeding behavior in cattle. *J. Anim. Sci.* 84: 3285–3300.

2635 Whisher, L., M. Raum, L. Pina, L. Pérez, H. Erb, C. Houpt, & K. Houpt. 2011. Effects of environmental factors on cribbing activity by horses. *Appl. Anim. Behav. Sci.* 135:63–69.

2636 Willard, J. G., J. C. Willard, S. A. Wolfram, & J. P. Baker. 1977. Effect of diet on cecal pH and feeding behavior of horses. *J. Anim. Sci.* 45:87–93.

2637 Zapata, I., J. A. Serpell, & C. E. Alvarez. 2016. Genetic mapping of canine fear and aggression. *BMC Genomics.* 17: 572.

2638 **Zemo, T., & J. O. Klemmedson. 1970. Behavior of fistulated steers on a desert grassland.** *J. Range Manag.* **23:158–163.**

2639 Brinkmann, L., M. Gerken, & A. Riek. 2013. Seasonal changes of total body water and water intake in Shetland ponies measured by an isotope dilution technique. *J. Animal Sci.* 91(8):3750–3758.

2640 **Hansen, B. D., B. Lascelles, X. Duncan, B. W. Keene, A. K. Adams, & A. E. Thomson. 2013. Evaluation of an accelerometer for at-home monitoring of spontaneous activity in dogs.** *Am. J. Vet. Res.* **68:468–475.**

2641 Zoller, B., L. Rhodes, & R. G. Smith. 2017. Capromorelin increases food consumption, body weight, growth hormone, and sustained insulin-like growth factor 1 concentrations when administered to healthy adult Beagle dogs. *J. Vet. Pharmacol. Ther.* 40(2):140–147.

2642 Akdemir, D., & J. I. Sanchez. 2016. Efficient breeding by genomic mating. *Front. Genet.* 7:210.

2643 Albanese, V., A. S. Munsterman, F. J. DeGraves, & R. K. Hanson. 2013. Evaluation of intra-abdominal pressure in horses hat crib. *Vet. Surg.* 42(6):658–662.

2644 **Albuquerque, N., K. Guo, A. Wilkinson, B. Resende, & D. S. Mills. 2018. Mouth-licking by dogs as a response to emotional stimuli.** *Behav. Proc.* **146:42–45.**

2645 Albuquerque, N., K. Guo, A. Wilkinson, C. Savalli, E. Otta, & D. Mills. 2016. Dogs recognize dog and human emotions. *Biol. Lett.* 12:20150883.

2646 Allen, E., C. Sheaffer, & K. Martinson. 2013. Forage nutritive value and preference of cool-season grasses under horse grazing. *Agron. J.* 105(3):679–684.

2647 Andersen, H., A. G. Kongsted, & M. Jakobsen. 2020. Pig elimination behavior—A review. *Appl. Anim. Behav. Sci.* 222:104888.

2648 Appleby, M. C., J. A. Mench, & B. O. Hughes. 2004. *Poultry behaviour and welfare.* CABI.

2649 Arahori, M., H. Chijiiwa, S. Takagi, B. Bucher, H. Abe, M. Inoue-Murayama, & K. Fujita. 2017. Microsatellite polymorphisms adjacent to the oxytocin receptor gene in domestic cats: Association with personality? *Front. Psychol.* 8:2165.

2650 Arden, R., & M. J. Adams. 2016. A general intelligence factor in dogs. *Intelligence.* 55:79–85.

2651 Arden, R., M. K. Bensky, & M. J. Adams. 2016. A review of cognitive abilities in dogs, 1911 through 2016: More individual differences, please! *Curr. Dir. Psychol. Sci.* 25(5):307–312.

2652 Arteaga, L., H. G. Rödel, M. T. Elizalde, D. González, & R. Hudson. 2013. The pattern of nipple use before weaning among littermates of the domestic dog. *Ethology.* 119(1):12–19.

2653 Asher, L., G. C. W. England, R. Sommerville, & N. D. Harvey. 2020. Teenage dogs? Evidence for adolescent-phase conflict behaviour and an association between attachment to humans and pubertal timing in the domestic dog. *Biol. Lett.* 16(5).

2654 Auer, U., Z. Kelemen, V. Engl, & F. Jenner. 2021. Activity time budgets—A potential tool to monitor equine welfare? *Animals.* 11(3):850.

2655 Balogh, O., N. Borruat, A. Andrea Meier, S. Hartnack, & I. M. Reichler. 2018. The influence of spaying and its timing relative to the onset of puberty on urinary and general behaviour in Labrador Retrievers. *Reprod. Domest. Anim.* 53(5):1184–1190.

2656 **Banerjee, K., C. F. Chabris, V. E. Johnson, J. J. Lee, F. Tsao, & M. D. Hauser. 2009. General intelligence in another primate: Individual differences across cognitive task performance in a new**

world monkey (Saguinus oedipus). *PLoS ONE.* 4(6):e5883.

2657 Baragli, P., L. Banti, V. Vitale, & C. Sighieri. 2014. Effect of aging on behavioural and physiological responses to a stressful stimulus in horses (*Equus caballus*). *Behaviour.* 151(11):1513–1533.

2658 Bartošová, J., M. Komárková, J. Dubcová, L. Bartoš, & J. Pluháček. 2011. Concurrent lactation and pregnancy: Pregnant domestic horse mares do not increase mother-offspring conflict during intensive lactation. *PLoS ONE.* 6(8):e22068.

2659 Bellegarde, L. G. A., M. J. Haskell, C. Duvaux-Ponter, A. Weiss, A. Boissy, & H. W. Erhard. 2017. Face-based perception of emotions in dairy goats. *Appl. Anim. Behav. Sci.* 193:51–59.

2660 Benjamin, A., & K. Slocombe. 2018. "Who's a good boy?!" Dogs prefer naturalistic dog-directed speech. *Anim. Cogn.* 21:353–364.

2661 Bloom, T., & H. L. Friedman. 2013. Classifying dogs' *(Canis familiaris)* facial expressions from photographs. *Behav. Proc.* 96:1–10.

2662 Benson-Amram, S., B. Dantzer, G. Stricker, E. M. Swanson, & K. E. Holekamp. 2016. Brain size predicts problem-solving ability in mammalian carnivores. *Proc. Natl. Acad. Sci.* 113(9):2532–2537.

2663 Birkl, P., A. Bharwani, J. B. Kjaer, W. Kunze, P. McBride, P. Forsythe, & A. Harlander-Matauschek. 2018. Differences in cecal microbiome of selected high and low feather-pecking laying hens. *Poult. Sci.* 97(9):3009–3014.

2664 Blois-Heulin, C., C. Rochais, S. Camus, C. Fureix, A. Lemasson, C. Lunel, E. Bezard, & M. Hausberger 2015. Animal welfare: Could adult play be a false friend? *Anim. Behav. Cogn.* 2(2):156–185.

2665 Bonnell, M. K., & S. M. McDonnell. 2016. Evidence for sire, dam, and family influence on operant learning in horses. *J. Equine Vet. Sci.* 36:69–76.

2666 Boogert, N. J., R. C. Anderson, S. Peters, W. A. Searcy, & S. Nowicki. 2011. Song repertoire size in male song sparrows correlates with detour reaching, but not with other cognitive measures. *Anim. Behav.* 81(6):1209–1216.

2667 Boyland, N. K., D. T. Mlynski, R. James, L. J. N. Brent, & D. P. Croft. 2016. The social network structure of a dynamic group of dairy cows: From individual to group level patterns. *Appl. Anim. Behav. Sci.* 174:1–10.

2668 Brady, K., L. Hewison, H. Wright, H. Zulch, N. Cracknell, & D. Mills. 2018. A spatial discounting test to assess impulsivity in dogs. *Appl. Anim. Behav. Sci.* 202:77–84.

2669 Braem, M., L. Asher, S. Furrer, I. Lechner, H. Würbel, & L. Melotti. 2017. Development of the "Highly Sensitive Dog" questionnaire to evaluate the personality dimension "Sensory Processing Sensitivity" in dogs. *PLoS ONE.* 12(5):e0177616.

2670 Bray, E. E., E. L. MacLean, & B. A. Hare. 2014. Context specificity of inhibitory control in dogs. *Anim. Cogn.* 17(1):15–31.

2671 Bray, E. E., E. L. MacLean, & B. A. Hare. 2015. Increasing arousal enhances inhibitory control in calm but not excitable dogs. *Anim. Cogn.* 18(6):1317–1329.

2672 Bray, E. E., M. D. Sammel, D. L. Cheney, J. A. Serpell, & R. M. Seyfarth. 2017. Effects of maternal investment, temperament, and cognition on guide dog success. *Proc. Natl. Acad. Sci. U. S. A.* 114(34):9128–9133.

2673 Briard, L., J. Deneubourg, & Petit, O. 2021. Group behaviours and individual spatial sorting before departure predict the dynamics of collective movements in horses. *Anim. Behav.* 174:115–125.

2674 Briefer, E. F., C. C. -R. Sypherd, P. Linhart, L. M. C. Leliveld, M. P. de la Torre, E. R. Read, C. Guérin, *et al.* 2022.

Classification of pig calls produced from birth to slaughter according to their emotional valence and context of production. *Sci. Rep.* 12:3409.

2675 Siniscalchi, M., S. d'Ingeo, M. Minunno, & A. Quaranta. 2018. Communication in dogs. *Animals.* 8(8):131.

2676 Siniscalchi, M., S. d'Ingeo, S. Fornelli, & A. Quaranta. 2018. Lateralized behavior and cardiac activity of dogs in response to human emotional vocalizations. *Sci. Rep.* 8(1):77.

2677 Nawroth, C., N. Albuquerque, C. Savalli, M. -S. Single, & A. G. McElligott, 2018. Goats prefer positive human emotional facial expressions. *R. Soc. Open Sci.* 5:180491.

2678 Broom, D. M., & A. F. Fraser. 2015. *Domestic animal behaviour and welfare,* 5th ed. CABI.

2679 Brucks, D., S. Marshall-Pescini, L. J. Wallis, L. Huber, & F. Range. 2017. Measures of dogs' inhibitory control abilities do not correlate across tasks. *Front. Psychol.* 8(MAY):849.

2680 Bulmer, L., S. McBride, K. Williams, & J.-A. Murray. 2015. The effects of a high-starch or high-fibre diet on equine reactivity and handling behaviour. *Appl. Anim. Behav. Sci.* 165:95–102.

2681 Bulmer, L. S., J.-A. Murray, N. M. Burns, A. Garber, F. Wemelsfelder, N. R. McEwan, & P. M. Hastie. 2019. High-starch diets alter equine faecal microbiota and increase behavioural reactivity. *Sci. Rep.* 9(1):18621.

2682 Burattini, B., K. Fenner, A. Anzulewicz, N. Romness, J. McKenzie, B. Wilson, & P. McGreevy. 2020. Age-related changes in the behaviour of domestic horses as reported by owners. *Animals.* 10(12).

2683 **Burnett, E., C. L. Brand, D. G. O'Neill, C. L. Pegram, Z. Belshaw, K. B. Stevens, & R. M. A. Packer. 2022. How much is that doodle in the window? Exploring motivations and behaviours of UK owners acquiring**

designer crossbreed dogs (2019-2020). *Canine Med. Genet.* 9(1):8.

2684 Buzek, A., K. Serwańska-Leja, A. Zaworska-Zakrzewska, & M. Kasprowicz-Potocka. 2022. The shape of the nasal cavity and adaptations to sniffing in the dog (*Canis familiaris*) compared to other domesticated mammals: A review article. *Animals.* 12:517.

2685 Camerlink, I., C. Proßegger, D. Kubala, K. Galunder, & J. L. Rault. 2021. Keeping littermates together instead of social mixing benefits pig social behaviour and growth post-weaning. *Appl. Anim. Behav. Sci.* 235:105230.

2686 Camerlink, I., K. Scheck, T. Cadman, & J. Rault. 2022. Lying in spatial proximity and active social behaviours capture different information when analysed at group level in indoor-housed pigs. *Appl. Anim. Behav. Sci.* 246:105540.

2687 Cannas, S., B. Tonini, B. Belà, R. Di Prinzio, G. Pignataro, D. Di Simone, & A. Gramenzi. 2021. Effect of a novel nutraceutical supplement (Relaxigen Pet dog) on the fecal microbiome and stress-related behaviors in dogs: A pilot study. *J. Vet. Behav.* 42:37–47.

2688 **Carpenter, P. A., M. A. Just, & P. Shell. 1990. What one intelligence test measures: A theoretical account of the processing in the Raven progressive matrices test. *Psychol. Rev.* 97(3):404–431.**

2689 Carreira, L. M. 2016. Using Bronson equation to accurately predict the dog brain weight based on body weight parameter. *Vet. Sci.* 3(4).

2690 Carreiro, C., V. Reicher, A. Kis, & M. Gácsi. 2022. Attachment towards the owner is associated with spontaneous sleep EEG parameters in family dogs. *Animals.* 12(7):895.

2691 Horn, J., N. E. Mateus-Pinilla, R. Warner, & E. J. Heske. 2011. Home range, habitat use, and activity patterns of free-roaming domestic cats. *J. Wildl. Manag.* 75(5):1177–1185.

2692 Chacha, J., P. Szenczi, D. González, S. Martínez-Byer, R. Hudson, & O. Bánszegi. 2020. Revisiting more or less: Influence of numerosity and size on potential prey choice in the domestic cat. *Anim. Cogn.* 23(3):491–501.

2693 Charlton, K., & E. Frasnelli. 2023. Does owner handedness influence paw preference in dogs? *Anim. Cogn.* 26:425–433.

2694 Chen, F. L., M. Zimmermann, J. P. Hekman, K. A. Lord, B. Logan, J. Russenberger, E. A. Leighton, & E. K. Karlsson. 2021. Advancing genetic selection and behavioral genomics of working dogs through collaborative science. *Front. Vet.* Sci. 8.

2695 Christensen, J. W., L. P. Ahrendt, R. Lintrup, C. Gaillard, R. Palme, & J. Malmkvist. 2012. Does learning performance in horses relate to fearfulness, baseline stress hormone, and social rank? *Appl. Anim. Behav. Sci.* 140(1):44–52.

2696 Christensen, J. W., L. P. Ahrendt, J. Malmkvist, & C. Nicol. 2021. Exploratory behaviour towards novel objects is associated with enhanced learning in young horses. *Sci. Rep.* 11(1):1428.

2697 Cieri, R. L., S. E. Churchill, R. G. Franciscus, J. Tan, & B. Hare. 2014. Craniofacial feminization, social tolerance, and the origins of behavioral modernity. *Curr. Anthropol.* 55(4):419–443.

2698 Cole, E. F., J. Morand-Ferron, A. E. Hinks, & J. L. Quinn. 2012. Cognitive ability influences reproductive life history variation in the wild. *Curr. Biol.* 22(19):1808–1812.

2699 Cooper, J. J., N. Cracknell, J. Hardiman, H. Wright, & D. Mills. 2014. The welfare consequences and efficacy of training pet dogs with remote electronic training collars in comparison to reward based training. *PLoS ONE.* 9(9):e102722.

2700 Correia-Caeiro, C., K. Guo, & D. Mills. 2021. Bodily emotional expressions are a primary source of information for dogs, but not for humans. *Anim. Cogn.* 24:267–279.

2701 Craddock, H. A., A. Godneva, D. Rothschild, Y. Motro, D. Grinstein, Y. Lotem-Michaeli, T. Narkiss, E. Segal, & J. Moran-Gilad. 2022. Phenotypic correlates of the working dog microbiome. *npj Biofilms Microbiomes.* 8(1):66.

2702 Croston, R., C. L. Branch, D. Y. Kozlovsky, R. Dukas, & V. V. Pravosudov. 2015. Heritability and the evolution of cognitive traits. *Behav. Ecol.* 26(6):1447–1459.

2703 **Cummins, D. D., & Cummins, R. 1999. Biological preparedness and evolutionary explanation. *Cognition.* 73(3):B37–B53.**

2704 da Cruz, A. B., S. Hirata, M. E. dos Santos, & R. S. Mendonça. 2023. Show me your best side: Lateralization of social and resting behaviors in feral horses. *Behav. Proc.* 206:104839.

2705 Dai, F., A. D. Costa, L. Bonfanti, C. Caucci, G. Di Martino, R. Lucarelli, B. Padalino, & M. Minero. 2019. Positive reinforcement-based training for self-loading of meat horses reduces loading time and stress-related behavior. *Front. Vet. Sci.* 6:350.

2706 **Darwin, C. 1859. *On the origin of species by means of natural selection, or the preservation of favoured races in the struggle for life.* London: John Murray.**

2707 Davies, A. C., C. J. Nicol, & A. N. Radford. 2015. Effect of reward downshift on the behaviour and physiology of chickens. *Anim. Behav.* 105:21–28.

2708 Davis, K. M., M. E. Iwaniuk, R. L. Dennis, P. A. Harris, & A. O. Burk. 2020. Effects of grazing muzzles on behavior and physiological stress of individually housed grazing miniature horses. *Appl. Anim. Behav. Sci.* 231:105067.

2709 de Fombelle, A., V. Julliand, C. Drogoul, & E. Jacotot. 2001. Feeding and microbial disorders in horses: 1-Effects of an abrupt incorporation of two levels of barley in a hay diet on microbial profile and activities. *J. Equine Vet. Sci.* 21(9):439–445.

2710 de Mouzon, C., M. Gonthier, & G. Leboucher. 2023. Discrimination of cat-directed speech from human-directed speech in a population of indoor companion cats (Felis catus). *Anim. Cogn.* 26:611–619.

2711 De Santis, M., S. Seganfreddo, M. Galardi, F. Mutinelli, S. Normando, & L. Contalbrigo. 2021. Donkey behaviour and cognition: A literature review. *Appl. Anim. Behav. Sci.* 244:105485.

2712 Delank, K., S. Reese, M. Erhard, & A. C. Wöhr. 2023. Behavioral and hormonal assessment of stress in foals (Equus caballus) throughout the weaning process. *PLoS ONE.* 18(1):e0280078.

2713 Delgadillo, J. A., L. A. Espinoza-Flores, J. A. Abecia, H. Hernández, M. Keller, & P. Chemineau. 2022. Sexually active male goats stimulate the endocrine and sexual activities of other males in seasonal sexual rest through the "buck-to-buck effect." *Domest. Anim. Endocrinol.* 81:106746.

2714 Delgado, M., & J. Hecht. 2019. A review of the development and functions of cat play, with future research considerations. *Appl. Anim. Behav. Sci.* 214:1–17.

2715 Delgado, M. M., B. S. G. Han, & M. J. Bain. 2022. Domestic cats (*Felis catus*) prefer freely available food over food that requires effort. *Anim. Cogn.* 25(1):95–102.

2716 Deniz, M., K. T. De Sousa, M. F. Moro, M. M. D. Vale, J. R. Dittrich, L. G. Filho, & M. J. Hötzel. 2021. Social hierarchy influences dairy cows' use of shade in a silvopastoral system under intensive rotational grazing. *Appl. Anim. Behav. Sci.* 244:105467.

2717 **Desforges, E., A. Moesta, & M. J. Farnworth. 2016. Effect of a shelf-furnished screen on space**

utilisation and social behaviour of indoor group-housed cats (*Felis silvestris catus*). *Appl. Anim. Behav. Sci.* 178:60–68.

2718 Desforges, J., C. Sonne, M. Levin, U. Siebert, S. De Guise, & R. Dietz. 2016. Immunotoxic effects of environmental pollutants in marine mammals. *Environ. Int.* 86:126–139.

2719 Destrez, A., P. Grimm, & V. Julliand. 2019. Dietary-induced modulation of the hindgut microbiota is related to behavioral responses during stressful events in horses. *Physiol. Behav.* 202:94–100.

2720 Destrez, A., P. Grimm, F. Cézilly, & V. Julliand. 2015. Changes of the hindgut microbiota due to high-starch diet can be associated with behavioral stress response in horses. *Physiol. Behav.* 149:159–164.

2721 Destrez, A., M. Costes-Thiré, A. S. Viart, F. Prost, B. Patris, & B. Schaal. 2021. Male mice and cows perceive human emotional chemosignals: A preliminary study. *Anim. Cogn.* 24:1205–1214.

2722 **Di Giminiani, P., V. L. M. H. Brierley, A. Scollo, F. Gottardo, E. M. Malcolm, S. A. Edwards, & M. C. Leach. 2016. The assessment of facial expressions in piglets undergoing tail docking and castration: Toward the development of the piglet grimace scale. *Front. Vet. Sci.* 3:100.**

2723 Dollion, N., A. Paulus, N. Champagne, N. St-Pierre, É. St-Pierre, M. Trudel, & P. Plusquellec. 2019. Fear/reactivity in working dogs: An analysis of 37 years of behavioural data from the Mira Foundation's future service dogs. *Appl. Anim. Behav. Sci.* 221:104864.

2724 Dror, S., A. Sommese, Á. Miklósi, A. Temesi, & C. Fugazza. 2022. Multisensory mental representation of objects in typical and Gifted Word Learner dogs. *Anim. Cogn.* 25(6):1557–1566.

2725 Dudde, A., L. Schrader, S. Weigend, L. R. Matthews, & E. Krause. 2018. More eggs but less social and more fearful?

Differences in behavioral traits in relation to the phylogenetic background and productivity level in laying hens. *Appl. Anim. Behav. Sci.* 209:65–70.

2726 Duffrene, J., O. Petit, B. Thierry, R. Nowak, & V. Dufour. 2022. Both sheep and goats can solve inferential by exclusion tasks. *Anim. Cogn.* 25(6):1631–1644.

2727 Dutrow, E. V., J. A. Serpell, & E. A. Ostrander. 2022. Domestic dog lineages reveal genetic drivers of behavioral diversification. *Cell.* 185(25):4737–4755.

2728 Edgar, J. L., Paul, E. S., & Nicol, C. J. 2013. Protective mother hens: Cognitive influences on the avian maternal response. *Anim. Behav.* 86(2):223–229.

2729 Elzerman, A. L., T. DePorter, A. Beck, & J. Collin. 2019. Conflict and affiliative behavior frequency between cats in multi-cat households: A survey-based study. *J. Fel. Med. Surg.* 22(8):705–717.

2730 Evangelista, M. C., J. Benito, B. P. Monteiro, R. Watanabe, G. M. Doodnaught, D. S. J. Pang, & P. V. Steagall. 2020. Clinical applicability of the Feline Grimace Scale: Real-time versus image scoring and the influence of sedation and surgery. *PeerJ.* 8:e8967.

2731 Eyre, R., M. Trehiou, E. Marshall, L. Carvell-Miller, A. Goyon, & S. McGrane. 2022. Aging cats prefer warm food. *J. Vet. Behav.* 47:86–92.

2732 **Falconer, D. S., & T. F. C. Mackay. 1996.** *Introduction to quantitative genetics.* **London: Prentice Hall.**

2733 Fan, Z., Z. Bian, H. Huang, T. Liu, R. Ren, X. Chen, X. Zhang, *et al.* 2023. Dietary strategies for relieving stress in pet dogs and cats. *Antioxidants.* 12(3).

2734 Farhoody, P., I. Mallawaarachchi, P. M. Tarwater, J. A. Serpell, D. L. Duffy, & C. Zink. 2018. Aggression toward familiar people, strangers, and conspecifics in gonadectomized and intact dogs. *Front. Vet. Sci.* 5(FEB):18.

2735 **Farmer, K., K. Krüger, R. W. Byrne, & I. Marr. 2018. Sensory laterality in affiliative interactions in domestic horses and ponies (*Equus caballus*). *Anim. Cogn.* 21(5):631–637.**

2736 Favati, A., O. Leimar, & H. Løvlie. 2014. Personality predicts social dominance in male domestic fowl. *PLoS ONE.* 9(7):e103535.

2737 Febrer, K., T. L. Jones, C. A. Donnelly, & M. S. Dawkins. 2006 . Forced to crowd or choosing to cluster? Spatial distribution indicates social attraction in broiler chickens. *Anim. Behav.* 72(6):1291–1300. Behavioral, demographic, and management influences on equine responses to negative reinforcement. *J. Vet. Behav.* 29:11–17.

2738 **Fermo, J. L., M. A. Schnaider, A. H. P. Silva, & C. F. M. Molento. 2019. Only when it feels good: Specific cat vocalizations other than meowing. *Animals.* 9:878.**

2739 Ferrando, E., & C. D. Dahl. 2022. An investigation on the olfactory capabilities of domestic dogs (*Canis lupus familiaris*). *Anim. Cogn.* 25(6):1567–1577.

2740 Ferreira, V. H. B., V. Guesdon, L. Calandreau, & P. Jensen. 2022. White Leghorn and Red Junglefowl female chicks use distal and local cues similarly, but differ in persistency behaviors, during a spatial orientation task. *Behav Processes.* 2022;200:104669.

2741 Feuerbacher, E. N., & C. D. Wynne. 2015. Shut up and pet me! Domestic dogs (*Canis lupus familiaris*) prefer petting to vocal praise in concurrent and single-alternative choice procedures. *Behav. Proc.* 110:47–59.

2742 Finka, L. R., & R. Foreman-Worsley. 2021. Are multi-cat homes more stressful? A critical review of the evidence associated with cat group size and wellbeing. *J. Fel. Med. Surg.* 24(2):65–76.

2743 Finn, J. L., B. Haase, C. E. Willet, D. van Rooy, T. Chew, C. M. Wade, N. A. Hamilton, & B. D. Velie. 2016.

The relationship between coat colour phenotype and equine behaviour: A pilot study. *Appl. Anim. Behav. Sci.* 174:66–69.

2744 Fischer, G.J. 1975. The behaviour of chickens. In E. S. E. Hafez (Ed.), *The behaviour of domestic animals.* Baillière Tindall.

2745 **Fleurance, G., N. Rossignol, & B. Dumont. 2022. Diurnal observations of feeding choices in grazing horses correctly predict their daily diet composition. *Appl. Anim. Behav. Sci.* 252:105652.**

2746 Forbes, J. M. 2006. Food choice and intake in chickens. In *Feeding in domestic vertebrates*, pp. 108–119. CABI.

2747 Foris, B., M. Zebunke, J. Langbein, & N. Melzer. 2019. Comprehensive analysis of affiliative and agonistic social networks in lactating dairy cattle groups. *Appl. Anim. Behav. Sci.* 210:60–67.

2748 Fortin, M., M. Valenchon, F. Lévy, L. Calandreau, C. Arnould, & L. Lansade. 2018. Emotional state and personality influence cognitive flexibility in horses (*Equus caballus*). *J. Comp. Psychol.* 132(2):130–140.

2749 **Foster, J. A., & K.-A. McVey Neufeld. 2013. Gut-brain axis: How the microbiome influences anxiety and depression. *Trends Neurosci.* 36(5):305–312.**

2750 Fox, A. E., & D. L. Belding. 2015. Reducing pawing in horses using positive reinforcement. *J. Appl. Behav. Anal.* 48(4):936–940.

2751 Foyer, P., E. Wilsson, & P. Jensen. 2016. Levels of maternal care in dogs affect adult offspring temperament. *Sci. Rep.* 6(1):1–8.

2752 French, J. M. 1998. Mother–offspring relationships in donkeys. *Appl. Anim. Behav. Sci.* 60:253–258.

2753 Freymond, S. B., D. Bardou, S. Beuret, I. Bachmann, K. Zuberbühler, & E. F. Briefer. 2019. Elevated sensitivity to tactile stimuli in stereotypic horses. *Front. Vet. Sci.* 6:162.

2754 Fritz, W. F., S. E. Becker, & L. S. Katz. 2021. Urine from domesticated male goats (*Capra hircus*) provides attractive olfactory cues to estrous females. *Appl. Anim. Behav. Sci.* 236:105252.

2755 Fugazza, C., Á. Pogány, & Á. Miklósi. 2016. Recall of others' actions after incidental encoding reveals episodic-like memory in dogs. *Curr. Biol.* 26(23):3209–3213.

2756 Fugazza, C., B. Turcsan, A. Sommese, S. Dror, A. Temesi, & A. Miklósi. 2022. A comparison of personality traits of gifted word learner and typical border collies. *Anim. Cogn.* 25(6):1645–1652.

2757 Gabor, V., & M. Gerken. 2018. Study into long-term memory of a complex learning task in Shetland ponies (*Equus caballus*). *Appl. Anim. Behav. Sci.* 198:60–66.

2758 **Garnham, L., & H. Løvlie. 2018. Sophisticated Fowl: The complex behaviour and Cognitive Skills of chickens and red junglefowl. *Behav. Sci.* 8:13-miss.**

2759 Gibson, J. M., S. A. Scavelli, C. J. Udell, & M. A. R. Udell. 2014. Domestic dogs (*Canis lupus* familiaris) are sensitive to the "human" qualities of vocal commands. *Anim. Behav. Cogn.* 1:281–295.

2760 Gmel, A. I., A. Zollinger, C. Wyss, I. Bachmann, & S. B. Freymond. 2022. Social box: Influence of a new housing system on the social interactions of stallions when driven in pairs. *Animals.* 12(9):1077.

2761 Gnanadesikan, G. E., B. Hare, N. Snyder-Mackler, & E. L. MacLean. 2020. Estimating the heritability of cognitive traits across dog breeds reveals highly heritable inhibitory control and communication factors. *Anim. Cogn.* 23(5):953–964.

2762 **Gobbo, E., & M. Zupan. 2020. Dogs' sociability, owners' neuroticism and attachment style to pets as predictors of dog aggression. *Animals.* 10(2):315.**

2763 González-Pech, P. G., J. Ventura-Cordero, R. A. Torres-Fajardo, P. R. Jaimez-Rodríguez, J. F. de J. Torres-Acosta, & C. A. Sandoval-Castro. 2021. Comparing the browsing behavior of inexperienced kids versus adult goats on heterogeneous vegetation. *Appl. Anim. Behav. Sci.* 236:105240.

2764 Górecka-Bruzda, A., E. Jastrzębska, M. Drewka, Z. Nadolna, K. Becker, & L. Lansade. 2022. Female horses are more socially dependent than geldings kept in riding clubs. *Appl. Anim. Behav. Sci.* 254:105714.

2765 Górecka-Bruzda, A., J. Jaworska, M. Siemieniuch, Z. Jaworski, C. R. Stanley, I. Wocławek-Potocka, & L. Lansade. 2022. Human-controlled reproductive experience may contribute to incestuous behavior observed in reintroduced semi-feral stallions (*Equus caballus*). *Theriogenology.* 180:82–86.

2766 Gould, K., P. Iversen, S. Sikkink, R. Rem, & J. Templeton. 2022. Persistence and gazing at humans during an unsolvable task in dogs: The influence of ownership duration, living situation, and prior experience with humans. *Behav. Processes.* 201:104710.

2767 Goursot, C., S. Düpjan, A. Tuchscherer, B. Puppe, & L. M. C. Leliveld. 2019. Visual laterality in pigs: Monocular viewing influences emotional reactions in pigs. *Anim. Behav.* 154:183–192.

2768 Greening, L., & S. D. McBride. 2022. A review of equine sleep: Implications for equine welfare. *Front. Vet. Sci.* 9:916737.

2769 Greening, L., J. Downing, D. Amiouny, L. Lekang, & S. McBride. 2021. The effect of altering routine husbandry factors on sleep duration and memory consolidation in the horse. *Appl. Anim. Behav. Sci.* 236:105229.

2770 Grillaert, K., & E. Hartmann. 2022. Aggression, erection, and masturbation in feral Pottoka ponies and Implications for equine welfare. *Animals.* 12:421.

2771 Guhl, A. M. 1958. The development of social organisation in the domestic chick. *Anim. Behav.* 6(1–2):92–111.

2772 Ha, D., & Ha, J. 2017. A subjective domestic cat (*Felis silvestris catus*) temperament assessment results in six independent dimensions. *Behav. Proc.* 141:351–356.

2773 Hall, N. J., F. Péron, S. Cambou, L. Callejon, & C. D. L. Wynne. 2017. Food and food-odor preferences in dogs: A pilot study. *Chem. Senses.* 42(4):361–370.

2774 Hao, Z., J. Dai, D. Shi, Z. Xu, D. Chen, B. Zhao, H. Teng, & Q. Jiang. 2014. Association of a single nucleotide polymorphism in HOXB9 with developmental dysplasia of the hip: A case-control study. *J. Orthop. Res.* 32(2):179–182.

2775 Hare, B. 2017. Survival of the friendliest: Homo sapiens evolved via selection for prosociality. *Annu. Rev. Psychol.* 68(1):155–186.

2776 Hare, B., M. Brown, C. Williamson, & M. Tomasello. 2002. The domestication of social cognition in dogs. *Science* 298(5598):1634–1636.

2777 Hare, B., A. Rosati, J. Kaminski, J. Bräuer, J. Call, & M. Tomasello. 2010. The domestication hypothesis for dogs' skills with human communication: A response to Udell et al. (2008) and Wynne et al. (2008). *Anim. Behav.* 79(2):e1–e6.

2778 Harman, H. H., & W. H. Jones. 1966. Factor analysis by minimizing residuals (minres). *Psychometrika.* 31(3):351–368.

2779 Hart, B. L., & Hart, L. A. 1985. Selecting pet dogs on the basis of cluster analysis of breed behavior profiles and gender. *J. Am. Vet. Med. Assoc.* 186(11):1181–1185.

2780 Hart, B. L., & L. A. Hart. 2022. The perfect puppy: Breed selection and care by veterinary science for behavior and neutering age, pp. 1–332. Academic Press.

2781 Hart, B. L., & M. F. Miller. 1985. Behavioral profiles of dog breeds. *J. Am. Vet. Med. Assoc.* 186(11):1175–1180.

2782 Hartmann, E., T. Rehn, J. W. Christensen, P. P. Nielsen, & P. McGreevy. 2021. From the horse's perspective: Investigating attachment behaviour and the effect of training method on fear reactions and ease of handling—A pilot study. *Animals.* 11(2).

2783 Haselmann, A., M. D. L. Wenter, W. Knaus, B. Fuerst-Waltl, Q. Zebeli, & C. Winckler. 2022. Forage particle size and forage preservation method modulate lying behaviour in dairy cows. *Appl. Anim. Behav. Sci.* 254:105711.

2784 Hayward, J. J., M. G. Castelhano, K. C. Oliveira, E. Corey, C. Balkman, T. L. Baxter, M. L. Casal, *et al.* 2016. Complex disease and phenotype mapping in the domestic dog. *Nat. Commun.* 7:10460.

2785 **Hecht, E. E., J. B. Smaers, W. D. Dunn, M. Kent, T. M. Preuss, & D. A. Gutman. 2019. Significant neuroanatomical variation among domestic dog breeds. *J. Neurosci.* 39(39):7748–7758.**

2786 Henry, S., S. Briefer, M.-A. Richard-Yris, & M. Hausberger. 2007. Are 6-month-old foals sensitive to dam's influence? *Dev. Psychobiol.* 49(5):514–521.

2787 Hernandez, S. M., K. A. T. Loyd, A. C. Newton, M. Gallagher, B. L. Carswell, & K. Abernathy. 2018. Activity patterns and interspecific interactions of free-roaming, domestic cats in managed Trap-Neuter-Return colonies. *Appl. Anim. Behav. Sci.* 202:63–68.

2788 Herrmann, E., M. V. Hernández-Lloreda, J. Call, B. Hare, & M. Tomasello. 2009. The structure of individual differences in the cognitive abilities of children and chimpanzees. *Psychol. Sci.* 21(1):102–110.

2789 **Hiestand, L. 2011. A comparison of problem-solving and spatial orientation in the wolf (Canis lupus) and dog (Canis familiaris). *Behav. Genet.* 41(6):840–857.**

2790 Hintze, S., S. Smith, A. Patt, I. Bachmann, & H. Würbel. 2016. Are eyes a mirror of the soul? What eye wrinkles reveal about a horse's emotional state. *PLoS ONE.* 11:e0164017.

2791 Hocking, P., C. E. Channing, D. C. Waddington, & R. Jones. 2001. Age-related changes in fear, sociality and pecking behaviours in two strains of laying hen. *Br. Poul. Sci.* 42(4):414–423.

2792 Hodgson, S., P. Bennett-Skinner, B. Lancaster, S. Upton, P. Harris, & A. D. Ellis. 2022. Posture and pull pressure by horses when eating hay or haylage from a hay net hung at various positions. *Animals.* 12(21).

2793 **Holcomb, F. R., K. S. Multhaup, S. R. Erwin, & S. E. Daniels. 2022. Spaced training enhances equine learning performance. *Anim. Cogn.* 25(3):683–690.**

2794 Holcova, K., E. Koru, Z. Havlicek, & P. Rezac 2021. Factors associated with sniffing behaviors between walking dogs in public places. *Appl. Anim. Behav. Sci.* 244:105464.

2795 **Holtby, A. R., T. J. Hall, B. A. McGivney, H. Han, K. J. Murphy, D. E. MacHugh, L. M. Katz, & E. W. Hill. 2023. Integrative genomics analysis highlights functionally relevant genes for equine behaviour. *Animal Genetics.* 00:1–13.**

2796 Hooks, K. B., Konsman, J. P., & O'Malley, M. A. 2018. Microbiota-gut-brain research: A critical analysis. *Behav. Brain Sci.* 42:e60.

2797 **Hopkins, W. D., J. L. Russell, & J. Schaeffer. 2014. Report chimpanzee intelligence is heritable. *Curr. Biol.* 24:1649–1652.**

2798 Horowitz, A., E. West, M. Ball, & B. Bagwell. 2021. Can dogs limbo? Dogs' perception of affordances for negotiating an opening. *Animals.* 11(3).

2799 Horschler, D. J., & MacLean, E. L. 2019. Leveraging brain–body scaling relationships for comparative studies. *Anim. Cogn.* 22(6):1197–1202.

2800 Houpt, K. A., D. M. Zahorik, & J. A. Swartzman-Andert. 1990. Taste aversion learning in horses. *J. Anim. Sci.* 68(8):2340–2344.

2801 Howe, L. M., M. R. Slater, H. W. Boothe, H. P. Hobson, J. L. Holcom, & A. C. Spann. 2001. Long-term outcome of gonadectomy performed at an early age or traditional age in dogs. *J. Am. Vet. Med. Assoc.* 218(2):217–221.

2802 **Hsu, Y., & J. A. Serpell. 2003. Development and validation of a questionnaire for measuring behavior and temperament traits in pet dogs. *J. Am. Vet. Med. Assoc.* 223(9):1293–1300.**

2803 Hubbard, A., M. J. Foster, & C. L. Daigle. 2021. Social dominance in beef cattle—A scoping review. *Appl. Anim. Behav. Sci.* 241:105390.

2804 **Huck, M., & S. Watson. 2019. The use of animal-borne cameras to video-track the behaviour of domestic cats. *Appl. Anim. Behav. Sci.* 217: 63–72.**

2805 Huo, X., M. Wongkwanklom, T. Phonraksa, & P. Na-Lampang. 2020. Effects of playing classical music on behavior of stabled horses. *Vet. Integ. Sci.* 19(2):259–267.

2806 Ilska, J., M. J. Haskell, S. C. Blott, E. Sánchez-Molano, Z. Polgar, S. E. Lofgren, D. N. Clements, & P. Wiener. 2017. Genetic characterization of dog personality traits. *Genetics.* 206(2):1101–1111.

2807 Ison, S. H., S. Jarvis, S. A. Hall, C. J. Ashworth, & K. M. D. Rutherford. 2018. Periparturient behavior and physiology: Further insight into the farrowing process for primiparous and multiparous sows. *Front. Vet. Sci.* 5(JUN):122.

2808 **Jakovcevic, A., A. M. Elgier, A. E. Mustaca, & M. Bentosela. 2010.** Breed differences in dogs' (*Canis familiaris*) gaze to the human face. *Behav. Proc.* 84(2):602–607.

2809 Jardat, P., L. Calandreau, V. Ferreira, C. Gouyet, C. Parias, F. Reigner, & L. Lansade. 2022. Pet-directed speech improves horses' attention toward humans. *Sci. Rep.* 12:4297.

2810 Jardat, P., M. Ringhofer, S. Yamamoto, C. Gouyet, R. Degrande, C. Parias, F. Reigner, *et al.* 2023. Horses form cross-modal representations of adults and children. *Anim. Cogn.* 26:369–377.

2811 **Jardim-Messeder, D., K. Lambert, S. Noctor, F. M. Pestana, M. E. de Castro Leal, M. F. Bertelsen, A. N. Alagaili, *et al.* 2017. Dogs have the most neurons, though not the largest brain: Trade-off between body mass and number of neurons in the cerebral cortex of large carnivoran species. *Front. Neuroanat.* 11.**

2812 Jarvis, J. R., S. M. Abeyesinghe, C. E. McMahon, & C. M. Wathes. 2009. Measuring and modelling the spatial contrast sensitivity of the chicken (*Gallus g. domesticus*). *Vis. Res.* 49:1448–1454.

2813 **Jensen, H. H., H. Meilby, S. Nielsen, & P. Sandøe. 2022. Movement patterns of roaming companion cats in Denmark—A study based on GPS tracking. *Animals.* 12(14):1748.**

2814 **Johnson-Ulrich, L., & K. E. Holekamp. 2020. Group size and social rank predict inhibitory control in spotted hyaenas. *Anim. Behav.* 160:157–168.**

2815 **Johnson, P. J., R. Elders, P. Pey, & R. Dennis. 2016. Clinical and magnetic resonance imaging features of inflammatory versus neoplastic medial retropharyngeal lymph node mass lesions in dogs and cats. *Vet. Radiol. Ultrasound.* 57(1):24–32.**

2816 Johnston, A. M., A. M. Arre, M. J. Bogese, & L. R. Santos. 2021. How do communicative cues shape the way that dogs (Canis familiaris) encode objects? *J. Comp. Psychol.* 135:534–544.

2817 Johnston, A. M., L. W. Chang, K. Wharton, & L. R. Santos. 2021. Dogs (*Canis familiaris*) prioritize independent exploration over looking back. *J. Comp. Psychol.* 135:370–381.

2818 **Joly-Mascheroni, R. M., A. Senju, & A. J. Shepherd. 2008. Dogs catch human yawns. *Biol. Lett.* 4(5):446–448.**

2819 Kang, H. M., N. A. Zaitlen, C. M. Wade, A. Kirby, D. Heckerman, M. J. Daly, & E. Eskin. 2008. Efficient control of population structure in model organism association mapping. *Genetics.* 178(3):1709–1723.

2820 Karenina, K., & A. Giljov, 2018. Chapter 5 – Mother and offspring lateralized social behavior across mammalian species. In *Cerebral lateralization and cognition: Evolutionary and developmental investigations of behavioral biases,* vol. 238, pp. 115–141. Elsevier.

2821 Karenina, K., A. Giljov, J. Ingram, V. J. Rowntree, & Y. Malashichev. 2017. Lateralization of mother–infant interactions in a diverse range of mammal species. *Nat. Ecol. Evol.* 1(2):30.

2822 Karlsson, E. K., I. Baranowska, C. M. Wade, N. H. Salmon Hillbertz, M. C. Zody, N. Anderson, T. M. Biagi, *et al.* 2007. Efficient mapping of mendelian traits in dogs through genome-wide association. *Nat. Genet.* 39(11):1321–1328.

2823 **Kasbaoui, N., C. Bienboire-Frosini, P. Monneret, J. Leclercq, E. Descout, A. Cozzi, & P. Pageat. 2022. Influencing elimination location in the domestic cat: A semiochemical approach. *Animals* 12(7):896.**

2824 Kauter, A., L. Epping, T. Semmler, E.-M. Antao, D. Kannapin, S. D. Stoeckle, H. Gehlen, *et al.* 2019. The gut microbiome of horses: Current research on equine enteral microbiota and future perspectives. *Anim. Microbiome* 1(1):14.

2825 **Keagy, J., J.-F. Savard, & G. Borgia, 2009. Male satin bowerbird problem-solving ability predicts mating success. *Anim. Behav.* 78(4):809–817.**

2826 Kim, H. H., S. C. Yeon, K. A. Houpt, H. C. Lee, H. H. Chang, & H. J. Lee. 2006. Effects of ovariohysterectomy on reactivity in German shepherd dogs. *Vet. J.* 172(1):154–159.

2827 King, S. R. B., K. A. Schoenecker, & M. J. Cole. 2022. Effect of adult male sterilization on the behavior and social associations of a feral polygynous ungulate: The horse. *Appl. Anim. Behav. Sci.* 249:105598.

2828 Kirchoff, N. S., M. A. R. Udell, & T. J. Sharpton. 2019. The gut microbiome correlates with conspecific aggression in a small population of rescued dogs (*Canis familiaris*). *PeerJ.* 2019(1):e6103.

2829 Kis, A., A. Gergely, Á. Galambos, J. Abdai, F. Gombos, R. Bódizs, & J. Topál. 2017. Sleep macrostructure is modulated by positive and negative social experience in adult pet dogs. *Proc. Roy. Soc. B: Biol. Sci.* 284(1865):20171883.

2830 Kockaya, M., N. Ercan, Y. S. Demirbas, & G. Da Graça Pereira. 2018. Serum oxytocin and lipid levels of dogs with maternal cannibalism. *J. Vet. Behav.* 27:23–26.

2831 Kokocińska-Kusiak, A., M. Woszczyło, M. Zybala, J. Maciocha, K. Barłowska, & M. Dzięcioł. 2021. Canine olfaction: Physiology, behavior, and possibilities for practical applications. *Animals.* 11: 2463.

2832 Konno, A., T. Romero, M. Inoue-Murayama, A. Saito, & T. Hasegawa. 2016. Dog breed differences in visual communication with humans. *PloS ONE.* 11(10):e0164760.

2833 **Kotrschal, A., B. Rogell, A. Bundsen, B. Svensson, S. Zajitschek, I. Brännström, S. Immler, *et al.* 2013. Artificial selection on relative brain size in the guppy reveals costs and benefits of evolving a larger brain. *Curr. Biol.* 23(2):168–171.**

2834 Koyasu, H., H. Takahashi, M. Yoneda, S. Naba, N. Sakawa, I. Sasao, M. Nagasawa, & T. Kikusui, 2022. Correlations between behavior and hormone concentrations or gut microbiome imply that domestic cats (Felis silvestris catus) living in a group are not like 'groupmates.' *PLoS ONE.* 17(7):e0269589.

2835 Kozlowski, C. P., E. Baskir, H. L. Clawitter, A. D. Franklin, T. Thier, M. Fischer, D. M. Powell, & C. S. Asa. 2021. Behavioral interactions and glucocorticoid production of Somali wild ass (Equus africanus somaliensis) mothers and foals. *Appl. Anim. Behav. Sci.* 240:105337.

2836 Krichbaum, S., & L. Lazarowski. 2022. Reward type affects dogs' performance in the cylinder task. *Anim. Behav. Cogn.* 9(3):287–297.

2837 Krueger, K., L. Trager, K. Farmer, & R. Byrne. 2022. Tool use in horses. *Animals.* 12(15).

2838 Lamoot, I., Vandenberghe, C., Bauwens, D., & Hoffmann, M. 2005. Grazing behaviour of free-ranging donkeys and Shetland ponies in different reproductive states. *J. Ethol.* 23(1):19–27.

2839 **Lampe, M., J. Bräuer, J. Kaminski, & Z. Virányi. 2017. The effects of domestication and ontogeny on cognition in dogs and wolves. *Sci. Rep.* 7(1):11690.**

2840 Lansade, L., & Simon, F. 2010. Horses' learning performances are under the influence of several temperamental dimensions. *Appl. Anim. Behav. Sci.* 125(1):30–37.

2841 **Lansade, L., C. Bonneau, C. Parias, & S. Biau. 2019. Horse's emotional state and rider safety during grooming practices, a field study. *Appl. Anim. Behav. Sci.* 217:43–47.**

2842 Lansade, L., J. Lemarchand, F. Reigner, C. Arnould, & A. Bertin. 2022. Automatic brushes induce positive emotions and foster positive social interactions in group-housed horses. *Appl. Anim. Behav. Sci.* 246:105538.

2843 Lansade, L., F. Lévy, C. Parias, F. Reigner, & A. Górecka-Bruzda. 2022. Weaned horses, especially females, still prefer their dam after five months of separation. *Animals.* 16(10):100636.

2844 Lansade, L., M. Trösch, C. Parias, A. Blanchard, E. Gorosurreta, & L. Calandreau. 2021. Horses are sensitive to baby talk: Pet-directed speech facilitates communication with humans in a pointing task and during grooming. *Anim. Cogn.* 24:999–1006.

2845 **Lansade, L., R. Nowak, A. L. Lainé, C. Leterrier, C. Bonneau, C. Parias, & A. Bertin. 2018. Facial expression and oxytocin as possible markers of positive emotions in horses. *Sci. Rep.* 8:14680.**

2846 **Anderson, K. H., Y. Yao, P. J. Perry, J. D. Albright, & K. A. Houpt. 2022. Case distribution, sources, and breeds of dogs presenting to a veterinary behavior clinic in the United States from 1997 to 2017. *Animals.* 12:576.**

2847 Lanthony, M., M. Danglot, M. Špinka, & M. Hausberger. 2022. Dominance hierarchy in groups of pregnant sows: Characteristics and identification of related indicators. *Appl. Anim. Behav. Sci.* 254:105683.

2848 Larssen, R., & L. S. V. Roth. 2022. Regular positive reinforcement training increases contact-seeking behaviour in horses. *Appl. Anim. Behav. Sci.* 252:105651.

2849 Leach, H. M. 2003. Human domestication reconsidered. *Curr. Anthropol.* 44(3):349–368.

2850 Lee, H. S., H. Louton, A. Schwarzer, E. Rauch, A. Probst, N. Shamsaei, P. S. Schmidt, *et al.* 2016. Effects of multiple daily litter applications on the dust bathing behaviour of laying hens kept in an enriched cage system. *Appl. Anim. Behav. Sci.* 178:51–59.

2851 Lesch, R., K. Kotrschal, I. Schöberl, A. Beetz, J. Solomon, & W. T. Fitch. 2019. Talking to dogs: Companion animal-directed speech in a stress test. *Animals.* 9:417.

2852 Tate, A. J., H. Fischer, A. E. Leigh, & K. M. Kendrick. 2006. Behavioural and neurophysiological evidence for face identity and face emotion processing in animals. *Philos. Trans. R. Soc. Lond. B Biol. Sci.* 361(1476):2155–2172.

2853 Lesimple, C., C. Sankey, M. A. Richard, & M. Hausberger. 2012. Do horses expect humans to solve their problems? *Front. Psychol.* 3(AUG):306.

2854 **Liehrmann, O., A. Viitanen, V. Riihonen, E. Alander, S. E. Koski, V. Lummaa, & L. Lansade. 2022. Multiple handlers, several owner changes and short relationship lengths affect horses' responses to novel object tests. *Appl. Anim. Behav. Sci.* 254:105709.**

2855 Lonardo, L., C. J. Völter, C. Lamm, & L. Huber. 2021. Dogs follow human misleading suggestions more often when the informant has a false belief. *Proc. Roy. Soc. B Biol. Sci.* 288(1955):20210906.

2856 Loy, J., L. Wills, S. King, K. Jenkins, S. Ellis, & H. Randle. 2021. A preliminary study of the effects of the number of consecutive days of training and days off on foal recall. *J. Vet. Behav.* 46:62–68.

2857 Lundberg, P., E. Hartmann, & L. S. V. Roth. 2020. Does training style affect the human-horse relationship? Asking the horse in a separation–reunion experiment with the owner and a stranger. *Appl. Anim. Behav. Sci.* 233:105144.

2858 Luz, M. P., C. M. Maia, H. C. Gonçalvez, & J. F. Filho. 2021. Influence of workload and weather conditions on rolling behaviour of horses and mules. *Behav. Proc.* 189:104433.

2859 Maarschalkerweerd, R. J., N. Endenburg, J. Kirpensteijn, & B. W. Knol. 1997. Influence of orchiectomy on canine behaviour. *Vet. Rec.* 140:617–619.

2860 **Mach, N., A. Foury, S. Kittelmann, F. Reigner, M. Moroldo, M. Ballester, D. Esquerré, *et al.* 2017. The effects of weaning methods on gut microbiota composition and horse physiology. *Front. Physiol.* 8.**

2861 Mach, N., A. Ruet, A. Clark, D. Bars-Cortina, Y. Ramayo-Caldas, E. Crisci, S. Pennarun, *et al.* 2020. Priming for welfare: Gut microbiota is associated with equitation conditions and behavior in horse athletes. *Sci. Rep.* 10(1):8311.

2862 **Maclean, E. L. 2016. Unraveling the evolution of uniquely human cognition. *Proc. Natl. Acad. Sci.* 113(23):6348–6354.**

2863 **MacLean, E. L., B. Hare, C. L. Nun, E. Addess, F. Amic, R. C. Anderson, F. Aureli, *et al.* 2014. The evolution of self-control. *Proc. Natl. Acad. Sci.* 111(20):E2140–E2148.**

2864 Back, M., & K. Houpt. 2023. Short communication: The patterns and physiology of salt intake by horses. *J. Vet Behav.* 67:17–19.

2865 **MacLean, E. L., E. Herrmann, S. Suchindran, & B. Hare. 2017. Individual differences in cooperative communicative skills are more similar between dogs and humans than chimpanzees. *Anim. Behav.* 126:41–51.**

2866 MacLean, E. L., N. Snyder-Mackler, B. M. vonHoldt, & J. A. Serpell. 2019. Highly heritable and functionally relevant breed differences in dog behaviour. *Proc. Roy. Soc. B Biol. Sci.* 286(1912):20190716.

2867 Malavasi, R., & L. Huber. 2016. Evidence of heterospecific referential communication from domestic horses (Equus caballus) to humans. *Anim. Cogn.* 19(5):899–909.

2868 Manrique, L. P., O. Bánszegi, R. Hudson, & P. Szenczi. 2021. Repeatable individual differences in behaviour and physiology in juvenile horses from an early age. *Appl. Anim. Behav. Sci.* 235:105227.

2869 **Marchei, P., S. Diverio, N. Falocci, J. Fatjó, J. L. Ruiz-de-la-Torre, & X. Manteca. 2009. Breed differences in behavioural development in kittens.** *Physiol. Behav.* **9:522–531.**

2870 Marchei, P., S. Diverio, N. Falocci, J. Fatjó, J. L. Ruiz-de-la-Torre, & X. Manteca. 2011. Breed differences in behavioural response to challenging situations in kittens. *Physiol. Behav.* 102(3):276–284.

2871 **Marino, L. 2017. Thinking chickens: A review of cognition, emotion, and behavior in the domestic chicken.** *Anim. Cogn.* **20(2):127–147.**

2872 Maroudas, A. 1980. *Metabolism of cartilaginous tissue: A quantitative approach*. Tunbridge Wells, England: Pitman.

2873 **Marshall-Pescini, S., C. Frazzi, & P. Valsecchi. 2016. The effect of training and breed group on problem-solving behaviours in dogs.** *Anim. Cogn.* **19(3):571–579.**

2874 Marshall-Pescini, S., Z. Virányi, & F. Range. 2015. The effect of domestication on inhibitory control: Wolves and dogs compared. *PLoS ONE.* 10(2):e0118469.

2875 **Martinson, K. L., M. S. Wells, & C. C. Sheaffer. 2016. Horse preference, forage yield, and species persistence of 12 perennial cool-season grass mixtures under horse grazing.** *J. Equine Vet. Sci.* **36:19–25.**

2876 **Matzel, L. D., Y. R. Han, H. Grossman, M. S. Karnik, D. Patel, N. Scott, S. M. Specht, & C. C. Gandhi. 2003. Individual differences in the expression of a "general" learning ability in mice.** *J. Neurosci.* **23(16):6423–6433.**

2877 Mazzatenta, A., M. C. Veronesi, G. Vignola, P. Ponzio, A. Carluccio, & I. De Amicis. 2019. Behavior of Martina Franca donkey breed jenny-and-foal dyad in the neonatal period. *J. Vet. Behav.* 33:81–89.

2878 **McConnell, I., L. Marker, & N. Rooney. 2022. Preliminary investigation into personality and effectiveness of livestock guarding dogs in Namibia.** *J. Vet. Behav.* **48:11–19.**

2879 McGreevy, P. D., D. Georgevsky, J. Carrasco, M. Valenzuela, D. L. Duffy, & J. A. Serpell. 2013. Dog behavior co-varies with height, bodyweight and skull shape. *PLoS ONE.* 8(12):e80529.

2880 **McGreevy, P. D., J. Righetti, & P. C. Thomson. 2005. The reinforcing value of physical contact and the effect on canine heart rate of grooming in different anatomical areas.** *Anthrozoos.* **18(3):236–244.**

2881 McKinney, C. A., B. C. M. Oliveira, D. Bedenice, M.-R. Paradis, M. Mazan, S. Sage, A. Sanchez, & G. Widmer. 2020. The fecal microbiota of healthy donor horses and geriatric recipients undergoing fecal microbial transplantation for the treatment of diarrhea. *PLoS ONE.* 15(3):e0230148.

2882 **McVey, A., A. Wilkinson, & D. S. Mills. 2018. Social learning in horses: The effect of using a group leader demonstrator on the performance of familiar conspecifics in a detour task.** *Appl. Anim. Behav. Sci.* **209:47–54.**

2883 Mehrkam, L. R., & C. D. L. Wynne. 2014. Behavioral differences among breeds of domestic dogs (Canis lupus familiaris): Current status of the science. *Appl. Anim. Behav. Sci.* 155:12–27.

2884 **Melvin, M. V., E. Costello, & J. D. Colpoys. 2020. Enclosed versus ring feeders: Effects of round-bale feeder type on horse behavior and welfare.** *J. Vet. Behav.* **39:41–46.**

2885 Mendes, J. W. W., B. Resende, & C. Savalli. 2021. Effect of different experiences with humans in dogs' visual communication. *Behav. Proc.* 192:104487.

2886 Mendonça, T., C. Bienboire-Frosini, I. Kowalczyk, J. Leclercq, S. Arroub, & P. Pageat. 2019. Equine activities influence horses' responses to different stimuli: Could this have an impact on equine welfare? *Animals.* 9(6).

2887 Merkies, K., Y. Sudarenko, & A. Hodder. 2022. Can ponies (*Equus caballus*) distinguish human facial expressions? *Animals.* 12(18).

2888 Mikkola, S., M. Salonen, E. Hakanen, S. Sulkama, & H. Lohi. 2021. Reliability and validity of seven feline behavior and personality traits. *Animals.* 11(7).

2889 Miklósi, Á., E. Kubinyi, J. Topál, M. Gácsi, Z. Virányi, & V. Csányi. 2003. A simple reason for a big difference: Wolves do not look back at humans, but dogs do. *Curr. Biol.* 13(9):763–766.

2890 Miyashita, Y., S. Nakajima, & H. Imada. 2000. Differential outcome effect in the horse. *J. Exp. Anal. Behav.* 74(2):245–253.

2891 Moehlman, P. D. 1998. Feral asses (*Equus africanus*): Intraspecific variation in social organization in arid and mesic habitats. *Appl. Anim. Behav. Sci.* 60(2):171–195.

2892 Moll, H., & Tomasello, M. 2007. Cooperation and human cognition: The Vygotskian intelligence hypothesis. *Trans. R. Soc. B Biol. Sci.* 362(1480):639–648.

2893 Mongillo, P., G. Bono, L. Regolin, & L. Marinelli. 2010. Selective attention to humans in companion dogs. *Canis familiaris. Anim. Behav.* 80(6):1057–1063.

2894 Mongillo, P., A. Scandurra, B. D'Aniello, & L. Marinelli. 2017. Effect of sex and gonadectomy on dogs' spatial performance. *Appl. Anim. Behav. Sci.* 191:84–89.

2895 Mueller, C., L. Sroka, M.-L. Hass, S. Aboling, A. These, & I. Vervuert. 2022. Rejection behaviour of horses for hay contaminated with meadow saffron (Colchicum autumnale L.). *J. Anim. Physiol. Anim. Nutr.* 106(2):327–334.

2896 Murata, K., M. Nagasawa, T. Onaka, N. Kanemaki, S. Nakamura, K. Tsubota, K. Mogi, & T. Kikusui. 2022. Increase of tear volume in dogs after reunion with owners is mediated by oxytocin. *Curr. Biol.* 32:R869–R870.

2897 Murphy, B. R., A. Wagner, O. McGlynn, F. Kharazyan, J. C. Browne, & J. Elliott. 2014. Exercise influences circadian gene expression in equine skeletal muscle. *Vet. J.* 201(1):39–45.

2898 Murray, L. W., K. Byrne, & R. B. D'Eath. 2013. Pair-bonding and companion recognition in domestic donkeys, *Equus asinus. Appl. Anim. Behav. Sci.* 143(1):67–74.

2899 Nakamura, K., A. Takimoto-Inose, & T. Hasegawa. 2018. Cross-modal perception of human emotion in domestic horses (*Equus caballus*). *Sci. Rep.* 8:8660.

2900 Fuchs, C., C. Kiefner, S. Reese, M. Erhard, & A.-C. Wöhr. 2016. Narcolepsy: Do adult horses really suffer from a neurological disorder or rather from a recumbent sleep deprivation/rapid eye movement (REM)-sleep deficiency? *Equine Vet. J.* 48:9.

2901 Nasr, M. A. F., W. J. Browne, G. Caplen, B. Hothersall, J. C. Murrell, & C. J. Nicol. 2013. Positive affective state induced by opioid analgesia in laying hens with bone fractures. *Appl. Anim. Behav. Sci.* 147(1):127–131.

2902 Navas González, F. J., J. Jordana Vidal, J. M. León Jurado, A. K. McLean, & J. V. Delgado Bermejo. 2019. Dumb or smart asses? Donkey's (*Equus asinus*) cognitive capabilities share the heritability and variation patterns of human's (*Homo sapiens*) cognitive capabilities. *J. Vet. Behav.* 33:63–74.

2903 Nawroth, C., M. Ebersbach, & E. von Borell. 2013. A note on pigs' knowledge of hidden objects. *Arch. Anim. Breed.* 56(1):861–872.

2904 Nawroth, C., M. Ebersbach, & E. von Borell. 2013. Are juvenile domestic pigs

(Sus scrofa domestica) sensitive to the attentive states of humans?—The impact of impulsivity on choice behaviour. *Behav. Proc.* 96:53–58.

2905 **Nawroth, C., Z. M. Martin, & A. G. McElligott. 2020. Goats follow human pointing gestures in an object choice task. *Front. Psychol.* 11:915.**

2906 Nelini, C., D. Bobbo, & G. G. Mascetti. 2010. Local sleep: A spatial learning task enhances sleep in the right hemisphere of domestic chicks (*Gallus gallus*). *Exp. Brain Res.* 205(2):195–204.

2907 Nicol, C. J. 2015. The behavioural biology of chickens. British Poultry Science, CABI.

2908 Nicol, C. 2007. How animals learn from each other. *Appl. Anim. Behav. Sci.* 100(1–2):58–63.

2909 Nicol, C. J. 2004. Development, direction, and damage limitation: Social learning in domestic fowl. *Anim. Learn. Behav.* 32(1):72–81.

2910 Padalino, B., M. Zappaterra, M. Felici, C. Ricci-Bonot, L. Nanni Costa, K. Houpt, & A. Tateo. 2023. Factors associated with house-soiling in Italian cats. *J. Feline Med. Surg.* 25(11):1098612X231202482.

2911 **Nicol, C. J., G. Caplen, P. Statham, & W. J. Browne. 2011. Decisions about foraging and risk trade-offs in chickens are associated with individual somatic response profiles. *Anim. Behav.* 82:255–262.**

2912 Niittynen, T., V. Riihonen, L. R. Moscovice, & S. E. Koski. 2022. Acute changes in oxytocin predict behavioral responses to foundation training in horses. *Appl. Anim. Behav. Sci.* 254:105707.

2913 **Ntalampiras, S., L. A. Ludovico, G. Presti, E. P. Previde, M. Battini, S. Cannas, C. Palestrini, & S. Mattiello. 2019. Automatic classification of cat vocalizations emitted in different contexts. *Animals.* 9:543.**

2914 O'Hanley, K. A., D. L. Pearl, & L. Niel. 2021. Risk factors for aggression in adult cats that were fostered through a shelter program as kittens. *Appl. Anim. Behav. Sci.* 236:105251.

2915 O'Malley, C. I., S. P. Turner, R. B. D'Eath, J. P. Steibel, R. O. Bates, C. W. Ernst, & J. M. Siegford. 2019. Animal personality in the management and welfare of pigs. *Appl. Anim. Behav. Sci.* 218:104821.

2916 Olczak, K., C. Klocek, & J. W. Christensen, 2021. Hucul horses' learning abilities in different learning tests and ue the association with behaviour, food motivation and fearfulness. *Appl. Anim. Behav. Sci.* 245:105498.

2917 **Olczak, K., J. Winther Christensen, & C. Klocek. 2018. Food motivation in horses appears stable across different test situations. *Appl. Anim. Behav. Sci.* 204:60–65.**

2918 Oldham, L., G. Arnott, I. Camerlink, A. Doeschl-Wilson, M. Farish, F. Wemelsfelder, & S. Turner. 2021. Once bitten, twice shy: aggressive and defeated pigs begin agonistic encounters with more negative emotions. *Appl. Anim. Behav. Sci.* 244:105488.

2919 Houpt, K. A. 2023. Feeding behavior of cats. In E. Stelow (Ed.), *Clinical handbook of feline medicine.* Wiley Blackwell.

2920 **Olsen, M. R. 2018. A case for methodological overhaul and increased study of executive function in the domestic dog (Canis lupus familiaris). *Anim. Cogn.* 21(2):175–195.**

2921 **Orihuela, A., & C. S. Galina. 2021. The effect of maternal behavior around calving on reproduction and Wellbeing of Zebu Type Cows and Calves. *Animals.* 11(11).**

2922 Pal, S. K., S. Roy, & B. Ghosh. 2021. Pup rearing: The role of mothers and allomothers in free-ranging domestic dogs. *Appl. Anim. Behav. Sci.* 234:105181.

2923 Palestrini, C., S. M. Mazzola, B. Caione, D. Groppetti, A. M. Pecile, M. Minero, & S. Cannas. 2021. Influence of gonadectomy on canine behavior. *Animals.* 11(2):553.

2924 Parker, H. G., D. L. Dreger, M. Rimbault, B. W. Davis, A. B. Mullen, G. Carpintero-Ramirez, & E. A. Ostrander. 2017. Genomic analyses reveal the influence of geographic origin, migration, and hybridization on modern dog breed development. *Cell Rep.* 19(4):697–708.

2925 **Parker, H. G., L. V. Kim, N. B. Sutter, S. Carlson, T. D. Lorentzen, T. B. Malek, G. S. Johnson, *et al.* 2004. Genetic structure of the purebred domestic dog. *Science.* 304(5674):1160–1164.**

2926 Parker, M., E. Challet, B. Deputte, B. Ract-Madoux, M. Faustin, & J. Serra. 2022. Seasonal effects on locomotor and feeding rhythms in indoor cats. *J. Vet. Behav.* 48:56–67.

2927 **Parker, M., J. Serra, B. Deputte, B. Ract-Madoux, M. Faustin, & E. Challet. 2022. Comparison of locomotor and feeding rhythms between indoor and outdoor cats living in captivity. *Animals.* 12(18):2440.**

2928 Patt, A., L. Gygax, B. Wechsler, E. Hillmann, R. Palme, & N. M. Keil. 2012. The introduction of individual goats into small established groups has serious negative effects on the introduced goat but not on resident goats. *Appl. Anim. Behav. Sci.* 138(1–2):47–59.

2929 Pearson, C., P. Filippi, L. Lush, & L. A. González. 2021. Automated behavioural monitoring allows assessment of the relationships between cow and calf behaviour and calves' survivability and performance. *Appl. Anim. Behav. Sci.* 245:105493.

2930 Pérez Manrique, L., R. Hudson, O. Bánszegi, & P. Szenczi. 2019. Individual differences in behavior and heart rate variability across the preweaning period in the domestic horse in response to an ecologically relevant stressor. *Physiol. Behav.* 210:112652.

2931 **Persson, M. E., L. S. V. Roth, M. Johnsson, D. Wright, & P. Jensen. 2015. Human-directed social behaviour in dogs shows significant heritability. *Genes Brain Behav.* 14(4):337–344.**

2932 Plaza, J., C. D. M. Palacios, J. Abecia, J. T. Nieto, M. Sánchez-García, & H. Lu. 2022. GPS monitoring reveals circadian rhythmicity in free-grazing sheep. *Appl. Anim. Behav. Sci.* 251:105643.

2933 Pongrácz, P., & S. S. Sztruhala. 2019. Forgotten, but not lost—Alloparental behavior and pup–adult interactions in companion dogs. *Animals.* 9:1011.

2934 Pongrácz, P., C. Molnár, A. Miklósi, & V. Csányi. 2005. Human listeners are able to classify dog (*Canis familiaris*) barks recorded in different situations. *J. Comp. Psychol.* 119:136–44.

2935 Potter, A. A., & D. S. Mills. 2015. Domestic cats (Felis silvestris catus) do not show signs of secure attachment to their owners. *PLoS ONE.* 10(9):e0135109.

2936 Powell, L., B. Lee, C. L. Reinhard, M. Morris, D. Satriale, J. Serpell, & B. Watson. 2022. Returning a shelter dog: The role of owner expectations and dog behavior. *Animals.* 12(9).

2937 **Powell, L., D. Stefanovski, C. Siracusa, & J. Serpell. 2020. Owner personality, owner-dog attachment, and canine demographics influence treatment outcomes in canine behavioral medicine cases. *Front. Vet. Sci.* 7:630931.**

2938 Prescott, N. B., & C. M. Wathes. 1999. Spectral sensitivity of the domestic fowl (*Gallus g. domesticus*). *Br. Poul. Sci.* 40:332–339.

2939 Proops, L., K. Grounds, A. V. Smith, & K. McComb. 2018. Animals remember previous facial expression that specific humans have exhibited. *Curr. Biol.* 28(9):1428–1432.

2940 Puurunen, J., E. Hakanen, M. Salonen, S. Mikkola, S. Sulkama, C. Araujo, & H. Lohi. 2020. Inadequate socialisation, inactivity, and urban living environment are associated with social fearfulness in pet dogs. *Sci. Rep.* 10(1):1-10.3227.

2941 **Quaranta, A., S. d'Ingeo, R. Amoruso, & M. Siniscalchi. 2020. Emotion recognition in cats. *Animals.* 10:1107.**

2942 Racca, A., K. Guo, K. Meints, & D. S. Mills. 2012. Reading faces: Differential lateral gaze bias in processing canine and human facial expressions in dogs and 4-year-old children. *PLoS ONE.* 7(4):e36076.

2943 **Raffan, E., R. J. Dennis, C. J. O'Donovan, J. M. Becker, R. A. Scott, S. P. Smith, D. J. Withers, *et al.* 2016. A deletion in the canine POMC gene is associated with weight and appetite in obesity-prone labrador retriever dogs. *Cell Metab.* 23(5):893–900.**

2944 Range, F., J. Jenikejew, I. Schröder, & Z. Virányi. 2014. Difference in quantity discrimination in dogs and wolves. *Front. Psychol.* 5(NOV):1299.

2945 Rankins, E. M., & C. L. Wickens. 2020. A systematic review of equine personality. *Appl. Anim. Behav. Sci.* 231:105076.

2946 Rehkämper, G., A. Perrey, C. W. Werner, C. Opfermann-Rüngeler, & A. Görlach. 2000. Visual perception and stimulus orientation in cattle. *Vis. Res.* 40:2489–2497.

2947 Reicher, V., A. Kis, P. Simor, R. Bódizs, F. Gombos, & M. Gácsi, 2020. Repeated afternoon sleep recordings indicate first-night-effect-like adaptation process in family dogs. *J. Sleep Res.* 29(6):e12998.

2948 Reimert, I., J. Bolhuis, B. Kemp, & T. Rodenburg. 2014. Emotions on the loose: emotional contagion and the role of oxytocin in pigs. *Anim. Cogn.* 18(2):517–532.

2949 Reimert, I., T. Rodenburg, W. Ursinus, B. Kemp, & J. Bolhuis. 2014. Responses to novel situations of female and castrated male pigs with divergent social breeding values and different backtest classifications in barren and straw-enriched housing. *Appl. Anim. Behav. Sci.* 151:24–35.

2950 **Ren, X., H. Yang, Y. Zhao, S. Su, X. Wang, H. Bao, D. Bai, *et al.* 2017. Association analysis between major temperament traits and diversification of the candidate gene in Mongolian horse (*Equus caballus*). *J. Agric. Biotechnol.* 25(3):405–414.**

2951 Rocha, C. E., E. da C. de Carvalho, F. C. G. S. de Castro, I. L. G. de S., Xavier, R. J. Young, M. S. Palhares, J. M. da Silva Filho, *et al.* 2020. Is mare sexual behavior affected by age and can it predict ovulation? *Appl. Anim. Behav. Sci.* 224:104937.

2952 **Rochais, C., S. Henry, & M. Hausberger. 2018. "Hay-bags" and "Slow feeders": Testing their impact on horse behaviour and welfare. *Appl. Anim. Behav. Sci.* 198:52–59.**

2953 Rørvang, M. V., J. W. Christensen, J. Ladewig, & A. McLean. 2018. Social learning in horses-fact or fiction? *Front. Vet. Sci.* 5:212.

2954 Rørvang, M. V., L. P. Ahrendt, & J. W. Christensen. 2015. Horses fail to use social learning when solving spatial detour tasks. *Anim. Cogn.* 18(4):847–854.

2955 Rørvang, M. V., & J. W. Christensen. 2018. Attenuation of fear through social transmission in groups of same and differently aged horses. *Appl. Anim. Behav. Sci.* 209:41–46.

2956 Rosvold, E. M., R. C. Newberry, T. Framstad, & I. L. Andersen. 2018. Nest-building behaviour and activity budgets of sows provided with different materials. *Appl. Anim. Behav. Sci.* 200:36–44.

2957 Rovee-Collier, C. K., B. A. Clapp, & G. H. Collier. 1982. The economics of food choice in chicks. *Physiol. Behav.* 28(6):1097–1102.

2958 Rudman, R. 1998. The social organisation of feral donkeys (Equus asinus) on a small Caribbean island (St. John, US Virgin Islands). *Appl. Anim. Behav. Sci.* 60(2–3):211–228.

2959 Rumpel, A. S., M. M. Alievi, J. F. Filho, C. E. P. Rozo, L. a. H. Schuster, A. Da Silva, & M. P. Ferreira. 2021. Can the training regimen influence night time physical activity in racehorses? *Vet. Anim. Sci.* 14:100208.

2960 Rutkauskaite, A., & P. Jensen. 2022. Domestication effects on social information transfer in chickens. *Anim. Cogn.* 25(6):1473–1478.

2961 Rutter, S. M., & I. J. H. Duncan. 1991. Shuttle and one-way avoidance as measures of aversion in the domestic fowl. *Appl. Anim. Behav. Sci.* 30(1):117–124.

2962 Sabiniewicz, A., K. Tarnowska, R. Świątek, P. Sorokowski, & M. Laska. 2020. Olfactory-based interspecific recognition of human emotions: Horses (*Equus ferus caballus*) can recognize fear and happiness body odour from humans (*Homo sapiens*). *Appl. Anim. Behav. Sci.* 230:105072.

2963 **Sackman, J. E., & K. A. Houpt. 2019. Equine personality: Association with breed, use, and husbandry factors. *J. Equine Vet. Sci.* 72:47–55.**

2964 Sahu, B. K., A. Parganiha, & A. K. Pati. 2020. Behavior and foraging ecology of cattle: A review. *J. Vet. Behav.* 40:50–74.

2965 Salonen, M., S. Mikkola, J. E. Niskanen, E. Hakanen, S. Sulkama, J. Puurunen, & H. Lohi. 2023. Breed, age, and social environment are associated with personality traits in dogs. *iScience.* 26(5).

2966 **Salonen, M., K. Vapalahti, K. Tiira, A. Mäki-Tanila, & H. Lohi. 2019. Breed differences of heritable behaviour traits in cats. *Sci. Rep.* 9(1):7949.**

2967 Santos, N. R., A. Beck, T. Blondel, C. Maenhoudt, & A. Fontbonne. 2020. Influence of dog-appeasing pheromone on canine maternal behaviour during the peripartum and neonatal periods. *Vet. Rec.* 186(14):449–449.

2968 **Sarrafchi, A., & H. J. Blokhuis. 2013. Equine stereotypic behaviors: Causation, occurrence, and prevention. *J. Vet. Behav.* 8(5):386–394.**

2969 Scandurra, A., A. Alterisio, A. Di Cosmo, A. D'Ambrosio, & B. D'Aniello. 2019. Ovariectomy impairs socio-cognitive functions in dogs. *Animals.* 9(2).

2970 **Schjelderup-Ebbe, T. 1922. Beiträge zur Sozialpsychologie des Haushuhns [Observation on the social psychology of domestic fowls]. Zeitschrift für Psychologie und Physiologie der Sinnesorgane. Abt. 1. *Zeitschrift für Psychologie.* 88:225–252.**

2971 Proctor, H. S., & Gemma Carder, G. 2014. Can ear postures reliably measure the positive emotional state of cows? *Appl. Anim. Behav. Sci.* 161:20–27.

2972 **Schneider, R., G. W. Randolph, G. Dionigi, C.-W. Wu, M. Barczynski, F.-Y. Chiang, Z. Al-Quaryshi, *et al.* 2018. International neural monitoring study group guideline 2018 part I: Staging bilateral thyroid surgery with monitoring loss of signal. *Laryngoscope.* 128(Suppl):S1–S17.**

2973 Schork, I. G., I. A. Manzo, M. R. De Oliveira, F. D. N. Costa, R. Palme, R. H. Young, & C. S. De Azevedo. 2022. How environmental conditions affect sleep? An investigation in domestic dogs (*Canis lupus familiaris*). *Behav. Proc.* 199:104662.

2974 Schuetz, A., K. Farmer, & K. Krueger. 2017. Social learning across species: Horses (Equus caballus) learn from humans by observation. *Anim. Cogn.* 20(3):567–573.

2975 Scott, J. P., & J. L. Fuller. 2012. *Genetics and the social behavior of the dog.* University of Chicago Press.

2976 **Seganfreddo, S., D. Fornasiero, M. De Santis, L. Contalbrigo,**

F. Mutinelli, & S. Normando. 2022. Investigation of donkeys learning capabilities through an operant conditioning. *Appl. Anim. Behav. Sci.* 255:105743.

2977 Seyfang, J., K. J. Plush, R. N. Kirkwood, A. J. Tilbrook, & C. R. Ralph. 2018. The sex ratio of a litter affects the behaviour of its female pigs until at least 16 weeks of age. *Appl. Anim. Behav. Sci.* 200:45–50.

2978 Shen, C., X. Tong, R. Chen, S. Gao, X. Liu, A. P. Schinckel, Y. Li, *et al.* 2020. Identifying blood-based biomarkers associated with aggression in weaned pigs after mixing. *Appl. Anim. Behav. Sci.* 224:104927.

2979 Shouldice, V. L., A. M. Edwards, J. A. Serpell, L. Niel, & J. A. B. Robinson. 2019. Expression of behavioural traits in Goldendoodles and Labradoodles. *Animals.* 9(12).

2980 Simon, T., E. Frasnelli, K. Guo, A. Barber, A. Wilkinson, & D. S. Mills. 2022. Is there an association between paw preference and emotionality in pet dogs? *Animals.* 12(9).

2981 Simon, T., K. Guo, E. Frasnelli, A. Wilkinson, & D. S. Mills. 2022. Testing of behavioural asymmetries as markers for brain lateralization of emotional states in pet dogs: A critical review. *Neurosci. Biobehav. Rev.* 143:104950.

2982 Siniscalchi, M., S. d'Ingeo, & A. Quaranta. 2016. The dog nose "KNOWS" fear: Asymmetric nostril use during sniffing at canine and human emotional stimuli. *Behav. Brain Res.* 304:34–41.

2983 Smit, M., R. A. Corner-Thomas, K. Weidgraaf, & D. Thomas. 2022. Association of age and body condition with physical activity of domestic cats (*Felis catus*). *Appl. Anim. Behav. Sci.* 248:105584.

2984 Smith, A. V., L. Proops, K. Grounds, J. Wathan, S. K Scott, & K. McComb. 2018. Domestic horses (*Equus caballus*) discriminate between negative and positive human nonverbal vocalisations. *Sci. Rep.* 8:13052.

2985 Smith, A. A., L. P. Posner, R. E. Goldstein, J. W. Ludders, H. N. Erb, K. W. Simpson, & R. D. Gleed. 2004. Evaluation of the effects of premedication on gastroduodenoscopy in cats. *J. Am. Vet. Med. Assoc.* 225(4):540–544.

2986 Smith, A. V., L. Proops, K. Grounds, J. Wathan, & K. McComb. 2016. Functionally relevant responses to human facial expressions of emotion in the domestic horse (*Equus caballus*). *Biol. Lett.* 12(2):20150907.

2987 Snigdha, S., L.-A. Christie, C. De Rivera, J. A. Araujo, N. W. Milgram, & C. W. Cotman. 2012. Age and distraction are determinants of performance on a novel visual search task in aged Beagle dogs. *Age (Dordr).* 34(1):67–73.

2988 Sommese, A., Á. Miklósi, Á. Pogány, A. Temesi, S. Dror, & C. Fugazza. 2022. An exploratory analysis of head-tilting in dogs. *Anim. Cogn.* 25(3):701–705.

2989 Somppi, S., H. Törnqvist, J. Topál, A. Koskela, L. Hänninen, C. M. Krause, & O. Vainio. 2017. Nasal oxytocin treatment biases dogs' visual attention and emotional response toward positive human facial expressions. *Front. Psychol.* 8:1854.

2990 Smith, A. V., L. Proops, K. Grounds, J. Walthan, & K. McComb. 2016. Horses discriminate between facial expressions of conspecifics. *Biol. Lett.* 12:20150907.

2991 Souris, A., P. Kaczensky, R. Julliard, & C. Walzer. 2007. Time budget-, behavioral synchrony- and body score development of a newly released Przewalski's horse group Equus ferus przewalskii, in the Great Gobi B strictly protected area in SW Mongolia. *Appl. Anim. Behav. Sci.* 107(3–4):307–321.

2992 Spasskaya, N. N., V. N. Voronkova, A. V. Letarov, Y. A. Ermilina,

E. A. Nikolaeva, E. A. Konorov, Y. A. Stolpovsky, & S. V. Naidenko. 2022. Features of reproduction in an isolated island population of the feral horses of the Lake Manych-Gudilo (Rostov Region, Russia). *Appl. Anim. Behav. Sci.* 254:105712.

2993 Sroka, L., C. Müller, M.-L. Hass, A. These, S. Aboling, & I. Vervuert. 2022. Horses' rejection behaviour towards the presence of *Senecio jacobaea* L. in hay. *BMC Vet. Res.* 18(1):25.

2994 **Stäbler, R., D. Patzkéwitsch, S. Reese, M. Erhard, & S. Hartmannsgruber. 2022. Behavior of domestic pigs under near-natural forest conditions with *ad libitum* supplementary feeding. *J. Vet. Behav.* 48:20–35.**

2995 Stachurska, A., M. Różańska-Boczula, & E. Wnuk-Pawlak. 2021. The difference in the locomotor activity of horses during solitary and paired release. *Pferdeheilkunde.* 37(1):50–55.

2996 Stachurska, A., A. Wiśniewska, W. Kędzierski, M. Różańska-Boczula, & I. Janczarek, 2021. Behavioural and physiological changes in a herd of Arabian mares after the separation of individuals differently ranked within the dominance hierarchy. *Animals.* 11(9):2694.

2997 Staff, T. P. O. N. E. 2014. Correction: The welfare consequences and efficacy of training pet dogs with remote electronic training collars in comparison to reward based training. *PLoS ONE.* 9(10):e110931.

2998 Staiger, E. A., J. D. Albright, & S. A. Brooks. 2016. Genome-wide association mapping of heritable temperament variation in the Tennessee Walking Horse. *Genes Brain Behav.* 15(5):514–526.

2999 Starling, M., A. Fawcett, B. Wilson, J. Serpell, & P. McGreevy. 2019. Behavioural risks in female dogs with minimal lifetime exposure to gonadal hormones. *PLoS ONE.* 14(12):e0223709.

3000 **Stelow, E. A., M. J. Bain, & P. H. Kass. 2016. The relationship between coat color and aggressive behaviors in the domestic cat. *J. Appl. Anim. Welf. Sci.* 19(1):1–15.**

3001 Sundman, A.-S., M. E. Persson, A. Grozelier, L.-L. Halldén, P. Jensen, & L. S. V. Roth. 2018. Understanding of human referential gestures is not correlated to human-directed social behaviour in Labrador retrievers and German shepherd dogs. *Appl. Anim. Behav. Sci.* 201:46–53.

3002 **Takagi, S., M. Arahori, H. Chijiiwa, A. Saito, H. Kuroshima, & K. Fujita. 2019. Cats match voice and face: Cross-modal representation of humans in cats (*Felis catus*). *Anim. Cogn.* 22:901–906.**

3003 Tallet, C., M. Rakotomahandry, C. Guérin, A. Lemasson, & M. Hausberger. 2016. Postnatal auditory preferences in piglets differ according to maternal emotional experience with the same sounds during gestation. *Sci. Rep.* 61 6 (1):1–8.

3004 Tamioso, P. R., C. F. Maiolino Molento, X. Boivin, H. Chandèze, S. Andanson, É. Delval, D. Hazard, *et al.* 2018. Inducing positive emotions: Behavioural and cardiac responses to human and brushing in ewes selected for high vs low social reactivity. *Appl. Anim. Behav. Sci.* 208:56–65.

3005 Tesfai, R. T., F. Parrini, N. Owen-Smith, & P. D. Moehlman. 2021. African wild ass drinking behaviour on the Messir Plateau, Danakil Desert, *Eritrea. J. Arid Environ.* 185:104327.

3006 **Tobey, B. A., G. A. Mario, R. David, & M. Nicolas. 2017. Dog-directed speech: Why do we use it and do dogs pay attention to it? *Proc. Roy. Soc. B.* 284:20162429.**

3007 Topál, J., Á. Miklósi, V. Csányi, & A. Dóka. 1998. Attachment behavior in dogs (*Canis familiaris*): A new application of Ainsworth's (1969) Strange Situation Test. *J. Comp. Psychol.* 112(3):219–229.

3008 Trösch, M., E. Bertin, L. Calandreau, R. Nowak, & L. Lansade. 2020. Unwilling or willing but unable: Can horses interpret human actions as goal directed? *Anim. Cogn.* 23:1035–1040.

3009 **Trösch, M., F. Cuzol, C. Parias, L. Calandreau, R. Nowak, & L. Lansade. 2019. Horses categorize human emotions cross-modally based on facial expression and non-verbal vocalizations. *Animals.* 9:862.**

3010 Trösch, M., M. Ringhofer, S. Yamamoto, J. Lemarchand, C. Parias, F. Lormant, & L. Lansade. 2019. Horses prefer to solicit a person who previously observed a food-hiding process to access this food: A possible indication of attentional state attribution. *Behav. Proc.* 166:103906.

3011 **Turcsán, B., E. Kubinyi, & Á. Miklósi. 2011. Trainability and boldness traits differ between dog breed clusters based on conventional breed categories and genetic relatedness. *Appl. Anim. Behav. Sci.* 132(1):61–70.**

3012 Turner, S. P., M. C. Jack, & A. B. Lawrence. 2013. Precalving temperament and maternal defensiveness are independent traits but precalving fear may impact calf growth. *J. Anim. Sci.* 91(9):4417–4425.

3013 **Udell, M. A. R., N. R. Dorey, & C. D. L. Wynne. 2010. What did domestication do to dogs? A new account of dogs' sensitivity to human actions. *Biol. Rev.* 85(2):327–345.**

3014 **Udell, M. A. R., M. Ewald, N. R. Dorey, & C. D. L. Wynne. 2014. Exploring breed differences in dogs (*Canis familiaris*): Does exaggeration or inhibition of predatory response predict performance on human-guided tasks? *Anim. Behav.* 89:99–105.**

3015 Ungerfeld, R., A. Fernández-Werner, Ö. Gökdal, O. Atay, & A. Freitas-de-Melo. 2021. Lambs identify their mothers' bleats but not a picture of her face. *J. Vet. Behav.* 46:69–73.

3016 **Urrutia, A., O. Bánszegi, P. Szenczi, & R. Hudson. 2022. Emergence of personality in weaning-age kittens of the domestic cat? *Dev. Psychobiol.* 64(5):e22281.**

3017 Valenchon, M., J. Deneubourg, A. P. Nesterova, & O. Petit. 2022. Does a high social status confer greater levels of trust from groupmates? An experimental study of leadership in domestic horses. *Behav. Proc.* 201:104708.

3018 **van den Berg, M., V. Giagos, C. Lee, W. Y. Brown, A. J. Cawdell-Smith, & G. N. Hinch. 2016. The influence of odour, taste and nutrients on feeding behaviour and food preferences in horses. *Appl. Anim. Behav. Sci.* 184:41–50.**

3019 Laan, J. E., C. M. Vinke, J. A. Van Der Borg, & S. S. Arndt. 2021. Restless nights? Nocturnal activity as a useful indicator of adaptability of shelter housed dogs. *Appl. Anim. Behav. Sci.* 241:105377.

3020 **Vékony, K., F. Prónik, & P. Pongrácz. 2022. Personalized dominance—A questionnaire-based analysis of the associations among personality traits and social rank of companion dogs. *Appl. Anim. Behav. Sci.* 247:105544.**

3021 **Vestergaard, K. S., J. A. Hogan, & J. P. Kruijt. 1990. The development of a behavior system: Dustbathing in the Burmese Red Junglefowl I. The influence of the rearing environment on the organization of dustbathing. *Behaviour.* 112(1–2):99–116.**

3022 Völter, C. J., & L. Huber. 2021. Dogs' looking times and pupil dilation response reveal expectations about contact causality. *Biol. Lett.* 17(12):20210465.

3023 Wallis, L. J., F. Range, C. A. Müller, S. Serisier, L. Huber, & Z. Virányi. 2014. Lifespan development of attentiveness in domestic dogs: Drawing parallels with humans. *Front. Psychol.* 5(FEB):71.

3024 Watts, E. T., C. N. Johnson, S. Carver, C. Butler, A. M. Harvey, & E. Z. Cameron. 2020. Maternal protectiveness in feral horses: responses to intraspecific and interspecific sources of risk. *Anim. Behav.* 159:1–11.

3025 Webb, L. E., B. Engel, K. Van Reenen, & E. A. Bokkers. 2017. Barren diets increase wakeful inactivity in calves. *Appl. Anim. Behav. Sci.* 197:9–14.

3026 Weller, J. E., I. Camerlink, S. P. Turner, M. Farish, & G. Arnott. 2019. Playful pigs: Early life play-fighting experience influences later life contest dynamics. *Anim. Behav.* 158:269–279.

3027 **Wells, D. L. 2021. Paw preference as a tool for assessing emotional functioning and welfare in dogs and cats: A review. *Appl. Anim. Behav. Sci.* 236:105148.**

3028 Wells, D. L., & P. G. Hepper. 2006. Prenatal olfactory learning in the domestic dog. *Anim. Behav.* 72(3):681–686.

3029 Wells, D. L., & L. J. McDowell. 2019. Laterality as a tool for assessing breed differences in emotional reactivity in the domestic cat, *Felis silvestris catus*. *Animals.* 9(9):647.

3030 Wells, D. L., P. G. Hepper, A. D. S. Milligan, & S. Barnard. 2019. Lack of association between paw preference and behaviour problems in the domestic dog, *Canis familiaris. Appl. Anim. Behav. Sci.* 210:81–87.

3031 Westgarth, C., & O. H. P. Burman. 2016. Can sleep and resting behaviours be used as Indicators of welfare in shelter dogs (*Canis lupus familiaris*)? *PLoS ONE.* 11(10):e0163620.

3032 Wilhelmy, J., J. Serpell, D. Brown, & C. Siracusa. 2016. Behavioral associations with breed, coat type, and eye color in single-breed cats. *J. Vet. Behav.* 13:80–87.

3033 Williams, M., C. N. Davis, D. L. Jones, E. S. Davies, P. Vasina, D. Cutress, M. T. Rose, *et al.* 2021. Lying behaviour of housed and outdoor-managed pregnant sheep. *Appl. Anim. Behav.* 241.105370.

3034 Wilson, C., N. Hall, E. O. Aviles-Rosa, K. Campbell, G. Arnott, & C. Reeve. 2023. The effect of repeated testing on judgement bias in domestic dogs (Canis familiaris). *Anim. Cogn.* 26(2):477–489.

3035 Wiśniewska, A., I. Janczarek, I. Wilk, E. Tkaczyk, M. Mierzicka, C. Stanley, & A. Górecka-Bruzda. 2021. Heterospecific fear and avoidance behaviour in domestic horses (*Equus* caballus*). Animals.* 11(11):3081.

3036 Wiśniewska, A., I. Janczarek, I. Wilk, E. Tkaczyk, M. Mierzicka, C. Stanley, & A. Górecka-Bruzda. 2022. Correction: Wiśniewska et al. Heterospecific fear and avoidance behaviour in domestic horses (*Equus caballus*). *Animals.* 2021, 11:3081.

3037 Wofford, J. A., B. Zollers, L. Rhodes, M. Bell, & E. Heinen. 2018. Evaluation of the safety of daily administration of capromorelin in cats. *J. Vet. Pharmacol. Ther.* 41(2):324–333.

3038 Wolframm, I. A., & R. G. J. Meulenbroek. 2012. Co-variations between perceived personality traits and quality of the interaction between female riders and horses. *Appl. Anim. Behav. Sci.* 139(1):96–104.

3039 **Woods, H., M. Li, U. A. Patel, B. D. X. Lascelles, D. J. Samson, & M. E. Gruen. 2020. A functional linear modeling approach to sleep–wake cycles in dogs. *Sci. Rep.* 10:1–8.**

3040 Yarnell, K., C. K. Hall, C. Royle, & S. P. Walker. 2015. Domesticated horses differ in their behavioural and physiological responses to isolated and group housing. *Physiol. Behav.* 143:51–57.

3041 **Yildirim, F., A. Küreksiz, F. Yildirim, & A. Küreksiz. 2022. How frequently do and what time Thoroughbred and Haflinger breeding horses perform particular behaviors in paddock areas? *GSC Biol. Pharm. Sci.* 21(1):229–237.**

3042 Yokomori, T., A. Ohnuma, T. Tozaki, T. Segawa, & T. Itou. 2023. Identification of personality-related candidate genes in thoroughbred racehorses using a bioinformatics-based approach involving functionally annotated human genes. *Animals.* 13(4).

3043 Yun, J., & A. Valros, 2015. Benefits of prepartum nest-building behaviour on parturition and lactation in sows—A review. *Asian-Australasian J. Anim. Sci.* 28(11):1519–1524.

3044 Zakošek Pipan, M., L. Kajdič, A. Kalin, T. Plavec, & I. Zdovc. 2020. Do newborn puppies have their own microbiota at birth? Influence of type of birth on newborn puppy microbiota. *Theriogenology.* 152:18–28.

3045 Zapata, I., M. L. Lilly, M. E. Herron, J. A. Serpell, & C. E. Alvarez. 2022. Genetic testing of dogs predicts problem behaviors in clinical and nonclinical samples. *BMC Genomics.* 23(1):102.

3046 **Zimmerman, P. R., S. A. F. Buijs, J. Bolhuis, & L. J. Keeling. 2011. Behaviour of domestic fowl in anticipation of positive and negative stimuli.** *Anim Behav.* **81(3):569–577.**

3047 Zink, M. C., P. Farhoody, S. E. Elser, L. D. Ruffini, T. A. Gibbons, & R. H. Rieger. 2014. Evaluation of the risk and age of onset of cancer and behavioral disorders in gonadectomized Vizslas. *J. Am. Vet. Med. Assoc.* 244(3):309–319.

3048 Ahola, M. K., K. Vapalahti, & H. Lohi. 2017. Early weaning increases aggression and stereotypic behaviour in cats. *Sci. Rep.* 7:10412.

3049 Alegría-Morán, R. A., S. A. Guzmán-Pino, J. I. Egaña, J. I. Valeria Sotomayor, & J. Figueroa. 2019. Food preferences in cats: effect of dietary composition and intrinsic variables on diet selection. *Animals.* 9(6):372.

3050 Andersen, P. H., S. Broomé, M. Rashid, J. Lundblad, K. Ask, Z. Li, E. Hernlund, *et al.* 2021. Towards machine recognition of facial expressions of pain in horses. *Animals.* 11(6):1643.

3051 Behnke, A. C., K. R. Vitale, & M. A. R. Udell. 2021. The effect of owner presence and scent on stress resilience in cats. *Appl. Anim. Behav. Sci.* 243:105444.

3052 Briefer Freymond, S., D. Bardou, S. Beuret, I. Bachmann, K. Zuberbühler, & E. F. Briefer. 2019. Elevated sensitivity to tactile stimuli in stereotypic horses. *Front. Vet. Sci.* 6:162.

3053 Brown, S. M., R. Peters, I. M. Nevison, & A. B. Lawrence. 2018. Playful pigs: Evidence of consistency and change in play depending on litter and developmental stage. *Appl. Anim. Behav. Sci.* 198:36–43.

3054 Caicoya, A. L., A. Schaffer, R. Holland, L. von Fersen, M. Colell, & F. Amici. 2023. Innovation across 13 ungulate species: problem solvers are less integrated in the social group and less neophobic. *Proc. R. Soc. B* 290:20222384.

3055 Calder, C., & J. Albright. 2021. Chicken behavior. In C. B. Greenacre, & T. Y. Morishita (Eds.), *Backyard poultry medicine and surgery*. Hoboken, NJ: Wiley Blackwell.

3056 Cameron, K. E., A. Siddall, & L. A. Bizo. 2021. Comparison of paired- and multiple-stimulus preference assessments using a runway task by dogs. *Int. J. Comp. Psychol.* 34:1–14.

3057 Cannas, S., B. Tonini, B. Bela, R. Di Prinzio, G. Pignataro, D. Di Simone, & A. Gram. 2021. Effect of a novel nutraceutical (Relaxigen Pet dog) on the fecal microbiome and stress-related behaviors in dogs: A pilot study. *J. Vet. Behav.* 42:37–47.

3058 Chapagain, D., F. Range, L. Huber, & Z. Virányi. 2018. Cognitive aging in dogs. *Gerontology.* 64(2):165–171.

3059 da Cordoni, G., M. Gioia, E. Demuru, & I. Norscia. 2021. The dark side of play: Play fighting as a substitute for real fighting in domestic pigs, Sus scrofa. *Anim. Behav.* 175:21–31.

3060 Delgado, M., & J. Julie Hecht. 2019. A review of the development and functions of cat play, with future research considerations. *Appl. Anim. Behav. Sci.* 214:1–17.

3061 Fenner, K., R. Freire, A. McLean, & P. McGreevy. 2019. Behavioral, demographic, and management influences on equine responses to negative reinforcement. *J. Vet. Behav.* 29:11–15.

3062 Fenner, K., G. Caspar, M. Hyde, C. Henshall, N. Dhand, F. Probyn-Rapsey, K. Dashper, *et al.* 2019. It's all about the sex, or is it? Humans, horses and temperament. *PLoS ONE.* 14(5):e0216699.

3063 Feuerbacher, E. N., & Wynne, C. D. L. 2015. Shut up and pet me! Domestic dogs (Canis lupus familiaris) prefer petting to vocal praise in concurrent and single-alternative choice procedures. *Behav. Proc.* 110:47–59.

3064 Fuchs, C., C. Kiefner, S. Reese, M. Erhard, & A. Wöhr. 2016. Narcolepsy: Do adult horses really suffer from a neurological disorder or rather from a recumbent sleep deprivation/rapid eye movement (REM)-sleep deficiency. *Equine Vet. J.* 48(9).

3065 González, F. J. N., J. J. Vidal, A. K. Mclean, & J. V. Delgado Bermejo. 2020. Nonparametric analysis of noncognitive determinants of response type, intensity, mood, and learning in donkeys (*Equus asinus*). *J. Vet. Behav.* 40:21–35.

3066 Gough, W., & B. McGuire. 2015. Urinary posture and motor laterality in dogs (Canis lupus familiaris) at two shelters. *Appl. Anim. Behav. Sci.* 168:61–70.

3067 Hawken, P. A. R., C. Fiol, & D. Blache. 2012. Genetic differences in temperament determine whether lavender oil alleviates or exacerbates anxiety in sheep. *Physiol. Behav.* 105:117–1123.

3068 Heuschele, D. J., D. Catalano, K. Martinson, & J. Wiersma. 2018. Consumer knowledge and horse preference for different colored oats. *J. Equine Vet. Sci.* 71:6–12.

3069 **Horn, J. A., N. Mateus-Pinilla, & R. E. Warner. 2011. Home range, habitat use, and activity patterns of free-roaming domestic cats. *J. Wildlife Manag.* 75 (5):1177–1185.**

3070 Hu, J., T. A. Johnson, H. Zhang, & H. W. Cheng. 2022. The Microbiota-Gut-Brain Axis: Gut microbiota modulates conspecific aggression in diversely selected laying hens. *Microorganisms.* 10(6):10811081.

3071 Humphrey, T., L. Proops, J. Forman, R. Spooner, & K. McComb. 2020. The role of cat eye narrowing movements in cat human communication. *Sci. Rep.* 10:16503.

3072 Dawson, J. S., & P. B. Siegel. 1967. Behavior patterns of chickens to ten weeks of age. *Poul. Sci.* 43:615–622.

3073 Jacobs, L. N., E. A. Staiger, J. D. Albright, & S. A. Brooks. 2016. The MC1R and ASIP coat color loci may impact behavior in the horse. *J. Heredity.* 107(3):214–219.

3074 Jung, Y., H. Jung, Y. Jang, D. Yoon, & M. Yoon. 2021. Classification of behavioral signs of the mares for prediction of the pre-foaling period. *J. Anim. Reprod. Biotech.* 36(2):99–105.

3075 Karl, S., M. Boch, A. Zamansky, D. van der Linden, I. C. Wagner, C. J. Völter, C. Lamm, & L. Huber. 2020. Exploring the dog–human relationship by combining fMRI, eye-tracking and behavioural measures. *Sci. Rep.* 10:22273

3076 King, S., C. Asa, J. Pluhacek, K. Houpt, & J. Ransom. 2016. Behavior of horses zebras and asses. In J. Ransom & J. Pluhacek (Eds.), *Wild equids*, pp. 23–40. Baltimore, MD: Johns Hopkins University Press.

3077 Kour, H., K. P. Patison, N. J. Corbet, & D. L. Swain. 2018. Validation of accelerometer use to measure suckling behaviour in Northern Australian beef calves. *Appl. Anim. Behav. Appl.* 202:1–6.

3078 Krueger, K. S., C. Wohr, C. K. Hemele, I. Marr, & K. Farmer. 2022. Laterality in horse training: Psychological and physical balance and coordination and strength rather than straightness. *Animals.* 12(8):1042.

3079 Lach, G., H. Schellekens, T. G. Dinan, & J. F. Cryan. 2018. Anxiety, depression, and the microbiome: A role for gut peptides. *Neurotherapeutics.* 15:36–59.

3080 Lansade, L., M. F. Bouissou, & X. Boivin. 2007. Temperament in preweanling horses: Development of reactions to humans and novelty, and startle responses. *Dev. Psychobiol.* 49:501–513.

3081 Laurijs, K. A., E. F. Briefer, I. Reimert, & L. E. Webb. 2021. Vocalizations in farm animals: A step towards positive welfare assessment. *Appl. Anim. Behav. Sci.* 236:105264.

3082 Lazarowski, L., B. L. Rogers, P. Waggoner, & J. S. Katz. 2019. When the nose knows: Ontogenetic changes in detection dogs' (*Canis familiaris*) responsiveness to social and olfactory cues. *Anim. Behav.* 153:61–68.

3083 Liu, Z., S. Torrey, R. C. Newberry, & T. Widowski. 2020. Play behaviour reduced by environmental enrichment in fast-growing broiler chickens. *Appl. Anim. Behav. Sci.* 232:105098.

3084 Denenberg, S. 2021. *Small animal veterinary psychiatry.* Boston, MA: CABI.

3085 McGuire, B. 2016. Scent marking in shelter dogs: Effects of sex and age. *Appl. Anim. Behav. Sci.* 182:15–22

3086 Mondo, E., M. Barone, M. Soverini, F. D'Amico, M. Cocchi, C. Petrulli, M. Mattioli, *et al.* 2020. Gut microbiome structure and adrenocortical activity in dogs with aggressive and phobic behavioral disorders. *Heliyon.* 6(1):e03311.

3087 Nicol, C. 2006. How animals learn from each other. *Appl. Anim. Behav. Sci.* 100:58–63.

3088 Owczarczak-Garstecka, S. C., & O. H. P. Burman. 2019. Can sleep and resting behaviours be used as indicators of welfare in shelter dogs (*Canis lupus familiaris*)? *PLoS ONE.* 11(10):e0163620.

3089 Papadaki, K., G. P. Laliotis, & L. Bizelis. 2021. Acoustic variables of high-pitched vocalizations in dairy sheep breeds. *Appl. Anim. Behav. Sci.* 241:105398.

3090 Platzer, J., N. Erica, & E. N. Feuerbacher. 2022. Reinforcer efficacy of grain for horses. *J. Exp. Anal. Behav.* 118:1–14.

3091 Polasik, D., A. Konieczna, A. Terman, & A. Dybus. 2021. The association of C789A polymorphism in the dopamine beta-hydroxylase gene (DBH) and aggressive behaviour in dogs. *Acta Vet. Brno.* 90(3):295–299.

3092 Proctor, H. S., & G. Carder. 2014. Can ear postures reliably measure the positive emotional state of cows? *Appl. Anim. Behav. Sci.* 161:20–27.

3093 Rushen, J. 1982. Development of social behavior in chickens: A factor analysis. *Behav. Proc.* 7:319–333.

3094 Salomons, H., K. C. M. Smith, M. Callahan-Beckel, M. Callahan, K. Levy, B. S. Kennedy, E. E. Bray, *et al.* 2021. Cooperative communication with humans evolved to emerge early in domestic dogs. *Curr. Biol.* 31(14):3137–3144.

3095 Seganfreddo, S., D. Diletta Fornasiero, M. De Santis, L. Contalbrigo, F. Mutinelli, & S. Normando. 2019. Food preferences in cats: Effect of dietary composition and intrinsic variables on diet selection. *Animals.* 9:372.

3096 Seganfreddo, S., D. Diletta Fornasiero, M. De Santis, L. Contalbrigo, F. Mutinelli, & S. Normando. 2022. Investigation of donkeys learning capabilities through an operant conditioning. *Appl. Anim. Behav. Sci.* 255:105734.

3097 Tate, A. J., H. Fischer, A. E. Leigh, & K. M. Kendrick. 2006. Behavioural and neurophysiological evidence for face identity and face emotion processing in animals. *Trans. R. Soc.* 361:2155.

3098 Torcivia, C., & S. McDonnell. 2021. Equine discomfort ethogram. *Animals.* 11(2):580.

3099 Vinassa, M., D. Cavallini, D. Galaverna, P. Baragli, F. Raspa, J. Nery, & E. Valle. 2020. Palatability assessment in horses in relation to lateralization and temperament. *Appl. Anim. Behav. Sci.* 232:105110.

3100 Zanker, A., A. C. Wöhr, S. Reese, & M. Erhard. 2011. Qualitative and quantitative analyses of polysomnographic measurements in foals. *Sci. Rep.* 11:1–2. doi: 10.1038/s41598-021-95770-5

3101 Zhang, L., & J. J. McGlone. 2020. Scratcher preferences of adult in-home cats and effects of olfactory supplements on cat scratching . *Appl. Anim. Behav. Sci.* 227:104997.

3102 D'Aniello, B., G. R. Semin, A. Alterisio, M. Aria, & A. Scandurra. 2018. Interspecies transmission of emotional information via chemosignals: From humans to dogs (*Canis lupus familiaris*). *Anim. Cogn.* 21:67–78.

3103 Saito, A., & K. Shinozuka. 2013. Vocal recognition of owners by domestic cats (*Felis catus*). *Anim. Cogn.* 16:685–690.

3104 Schnaider, M. A., M. S. Heidemann, A. H. P. Silva, C. A. Taconeli, & C. F. M. Molento. 2022. Cat vocalization in aversive and pleasant situations. *J. Vet. Behav.* 55:71–78.

3105 King, S., C. Asa, J. Pluhacek, K. Houpt, & J. Ransom. 2016. Behavior of horses zebras and asses. In J. Ransom, & J. Pluhacek (Eds.), *Wild equids*, pp. 23–40. Johns Hopkins University Press.

3107 Stäbler, R., D. Patzkéwitsch, S. Reese, M. Michael Erhard, & S. Hartmannsgruber. 2022. Behavior of domestic pigs under near-natural forest conditions with ad libitum supplementary feeding. *J. Vet. Behav.* 48:20–35.

3108 Christensen, J. W., C. G. Strøm, K. Nicová, C. Lafaige de Gaillard, C. P. Sandøe, & H. Skovgård. 2022. Insect-repelling behaviour in horses in relation to insect prevalence and access to shelters. *Appl. Anim. Behav. Sci.* 247:105560.

3109 Ungerfeld, R., A. Freitas-de-Melo, R. Nowak, & F. Lévy. 2018. Preference for the mother does not last long after weaning at 3 months of age in sheep. *Appl. Anim. Behav. Sci.* 205:28–33.

3110 Ozella, L., E. Price, J. Langford, K. E. Lewis, C. Cattuto, & D. P. Croft. 2022. Association networks and social temporal dynamics in ewes and lambs. *Appl. Anim. Behav. Sci.* 246:105515.

3111 Bentosela, M., A. Jakovcevic, A. M. Elgier, A. E. Mustaca, & M. R. Papiniu. 1996. Incentive contrast in domestic dogs (*Canis familiaris*). *J. Comp. Psychol.* 123:125–130.

3112 Bray, E., G. E. Gnanadesikian, D. J. Horschler, K. M. Levy, B. S. Kennedy, T. R. Famula, & E. L. MacLean. 2021. Early emerging and highly heritable sensitivity to human communication in dogs. *Curr. Biol.* 31:3132–3136.

3113 Junttila, S., A. Valros, K. Maki, H. Vaataja, E. Reunanen, & K. Tiira. 2022. Breed differences in social cognition, inhibitory control, and spatial problem-solving ability in the domestic dog (*Canis familiaris*). *Sci. Rep.* 12:22529.

3114 Krueger, K., S. Schwarz, I. Marr, & K. Farmer. 2022. Laterality in horse training: Psychological and physical balance and coordination and strength rather than straightness. *Animals.* 12:1042.

3115 Hu, J., T. A. Johnson, H. Zang, & H. W. Chen. 2022. The Microbiota–Gut–Brain axis: Gut microbiota modulates conspecific aggression in diversely selected laying hens. *Microorganisms.* 10(6):1081/

3116 Karl, S., M. Boch, A. Zamansky, D. van der Linden, I. C. Wagner, C. J. Völter, C. Lamm, & L. Huber. 2020. Exploring the dog–human relationship by combining fMRI, eye-tracking and behavioural measures. *Sci Rep.* 10:22273.

3117 Herron, M. E., F. S. Shofer, & I. R. Reisner. 2009. Survey of the use and outcome of confrontational and non-confrontational training methods in client-owned dogs showing undesired behaviors. *Appl. Anim. Behav. Sci.* 117:47–54.

3118 Zhang, L., K. B. Needham, S. Juma, X. Si, & F. Martin. 2021. Feline communication strategies when presented with an unsolvable task: The attentional state of the person matters. *Anim. Cogn.* 24:1109–1119.

3119 Raun, K., P. von Voss, & L. B. Knudsen. 2007. Liraglutide, a once-daily human glucagon-like peptide-1 analog, minimizes food intake in severely obese minipigs. *Obesity.* 15(7):1710–1716.

3120 Arias-Esquivel, A. M., C. J. Kwang, P. Fan, J. Lance, S. DeNotta, & C. Wickens. 2023. Gut microbiome characteristics of horses with history of cribbing behavior: An observational study. *J. of Vet. Behav.* 12:008.

Index

Domestic Animal Behavior for Veterinarians and Animal Scientists, Seventh Edition. Katherine A. Houpt.
© 2024 John Wiley & Sons, Inc. Published 2024 by John Wiley & Sons, Inc.
Companion website: www.wiley.com/go/houpt/7e